A REPRINT *of THE*
LONG-LOST CLASSIC

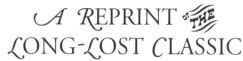
THE
COMPLETE
HERBALIST

BY DR. O. PHELPS BROWN

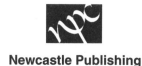

Newcastle Publishing
North Hollywood, California

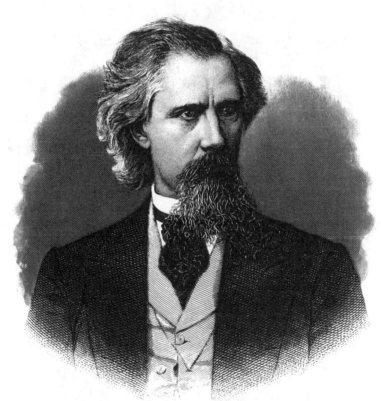

Yours truly,
Dr. O. P. Brown

THE
COMPLETE
HERBALIST

Cover design by Michele Lanci-Altomare

ISBN: 0-87877-184-0
A Newcastle book
First printing 1993.
10 9 8 7 6 5 4 3 2 1
Printed in the United States of America.

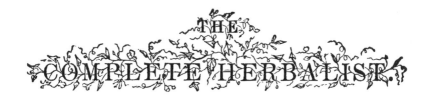

THE COMPLETE HERBALIST.

A BRIEF HISTORY OF MEDICINE.

IN presenting this work on Crude Organic Remedies—the Constituents of Plants, and their Officinal Preparations—I do not propose to "run a tilt" against any of the systems of Medical Practice, however much some of them may be opposed to common sense and reason, and to the Divine ordinances of Nature ; nor shall I treat with contempt the teachings and practices of great and wonderful names, or oppose the pride, interest, expectation, and conscientious convictions of a learned, honorable, and influential profession ; my object is simply to present many new and curious, if not startling facts, not only well worthy of the earnest consideration of the more intelligent portion of the community, who demand reasons the most profound to lead them to conviction of a TRUTH, but of the great mass of humbler people, who desire, amid all the great *Reforms* in human society, above all things to secure a " *sound mind in a sound body*," and to feel something of that exalted state of happiness which alone can arise from the possession of the most robust and rubicund physical and moral HEALTH.

It must be palpable to every thinking mind that Therapeutical and Pharmaceutical science is the very foundation of the "HEALING ART DIVINE." In the language of Holy Writ, " *The Lord has created medicines out of the earth, and he that is wise will not abhor them.*"*

> Yea, happy he that can the knowledge gain,
> To know the Eternal God made naught in vain."

The use of medicine is no doubt coincident with the History of the Human Race ; but writers generally agree that medicine first became a profession among the Egyptians. The priests of the earlier nations

---

Ecclesiastes xxxviii, 4.

were the practitioners of the Healing Art, but it does not seem that women were excluded from the right of administering medicine for the purpose of healing the sick, since mention is made of a certain Queen ISIS, who became greatly celebrated among them, and was worshipped as a "GODDESS OF HEALTH." Although the practitioners among the Egyptians, Assyrians, and Jews were in the habit of employing incantations, which, of course, produced their good and bad impressions through the medium of the imagination, yet their efficiency in curing diseases was mainly due to their knowledge of the medicinal virtues of many of the vegetable products of Nature. They seemed to look up as high as the *stars* to know the reason of the operation of the Herbs in the various affections of the human race.

Among the Greeks, HIPPOCRATES first caused medicine to be regarded as a *science*, while ÆSCULAPIUS was the first who made medicine an exclusive study and practice. His sons, MACHAON and PODALIRIUS, are celebrated in Homer's "Iliad" for their medical skill as surgeons in the Greek armies or during the Trojan war. Two daughters also of Æsculapius, PANAKEIA and HYGEIA, were no less distinguished than their renowned brothers; the latter being the inventor of many valuable herbal preparations, whose success in curing diseases won for her, as in the case of Queen Isis of Egypt, the proud honor and deification of the Greeks as an especial "GODDESS OF HEALTH." We have no knowledge that Æsculapius or his immediate followers, the Asclepiadæ, ever conceived the idea of curing disease by drug or mineral preparations. Ablutions, bandages, fomentations, ointments, etc., were administered externally, and preparations of aromatic herbs, roots, flowers, balms, gums, etc., constituted their whole materia medica for all *internal* ailments. Next the Pythagorean school became famous, and these were the first to visit the sick at their homes.

The next most prominent medical practitioner after these was HIPPOCRATES, the "Coan Sage," who, being one of the most sagacious, observing, and industrious men that ever lived, was entitled the "*Father of Medicine.*" He traveled much in foreign countries, devoting himself with untiring energy to the study and practice of medicine. His writings were numerous, and even to this day his doctrines are extensively recognized. His practice was consistently founded on the phenomena of Nature as exhibited in human beings during health and disease. His materia medica was derived almost wholly from the vegetable kingdom. His internal remedies were purgatives, sudorifics, diuretics, and injections, while his external were ointments, plasters, liniments, etc. The great principle which directed all his operations was the supposed operations of Nature in superintending and regulating all the actions of the system. This mode of practice had the good effect of enabling the practitioner to make himself well acquainted with all the phenomena of disease, and thus to diagnosticate correctly, and to meet the varied indications by the administration of some *herbal* remedy, which would induce the crisis requisite to the removal of disease and restoration to sound or vigorous health.

About three hundred years before the Christian era, the Ptolemies founded a medical school in Alexandria, Egypt. The most famous of the professors were ERASISTRATUS and HEROPHILUS, who dissected the bodies of criminals obtained from government. They opposed bleeding and violent remedies, trusting more to nature than to art. Herophilus paid particular attention to the action of the heart, and was the first to give anything like an accurate description of the various kinds of *pulse*, though Praxagoras of Cos, the last of the Asclepiadæ, had before observed the relation which exists between the pulse and the general condition of the system. From that time to the present the pulse has been, as it were, the guide for determining the character, extent, and probable cause of the disease afflicting the patient, and the description of treatment required to produce a change for the better. I, however, derive great assistance from the temperament, age, sex, etc.

We pass over the days of the Dogmatics and Empirics, the Pneumatics, and other sects of medical practitioners (who, though they employed *herbal* remedies as a general rule, were strangely given to the promulgations of theories and doctrines utterly at variance with the most ordinary ratiocinations of Philosophy and Reason), until we come to the period when GALEN first made his appearance, at the request of the Emperor AURELIUS. Galen was a native of Pergamos, born A.D. 130, having traveled much and written largely on subjects directly or indirectly connected with medicine before settling himself at Rome. He was entirely independent in his opinions, paid very little respect to authority, and so great was his learning and wisdom, and rare skill in medicine, that he came to be regarded by many as an "Oracle." Thoroughly educated in all the schools of philosophy, he selected from them all except the Epicurean, which he totally rejected. His treatment of disease was principally by Herbal remedies. From Galen have sprung the sect that is now generally known as Eclectics, who do not confine remedies exclusively to the herbal practice, but employ many of the mineral substances upon which the Allopathic and Homœopathic systems of medicine of the present day are based.

About the middle of the seventeenth century, on the death of PAULUS, the Greek school of medicine terminated, the Arabians having conquered a large portion of the semi-civilized world, and destroyed an immense Alexandrian library. The Arabian physicians soon adopted the opinions of Galen, but, owing to the invention of chemistry, it was speedily made subservient to medicine. They produced medical works, some of which have enjoyed great celebrity, without having really added anything substantial to medical science as previously understood. With AVERROES terminated the Arabic or Saracenic School of medicine, the great reputation of which is mainly owing to the circumstance, that from the eighth to the twelfth centuries, when all Europe was sunk in deep barbarism, the principal remains of a taste for literature and science existed among the Moors and Arabs. Their physicians added many vegetable products and a few metallic oxides in the catalogue of remedies. From the employment of chemical and mineral remedies by the Arabian physicians may be dated the disastrous consequences of medical science that were subsequently inaugurated by that Prince of Quacks—PARACELSUS.

After the Arabians, from the twelfth to the fifteenth century, the practice of medicine was chiefly confined to the hands of the priests, who, being men of great learning and followers of Æsculapius, Hippocrates, and Galen, became the principal physicians, and a little medicine was taught in the monasteries; for a long time the Benedictine monks of Monte Casino enjoyed in this respect great reputation. The Jews also became celebrated physicians; and though not allowed to administer medicines to Christians, yet obtained access to the courts, and even to the palace of the Roman pontiffs.

The European feudal system was at length greatly shaken by the Crusades. MAHOMET the second, about the middle of the fifteenth century, captured Constantinople, and soon after the ruin of the Byzantine empire the *Reformation* occurred, and about the same time the art of printing was invented. These events gave a powerful impulse to the world of mind, and reawakened investigation into all the departments of science, literature, and the arts; but, although many works were writ ten, very few facts were gleaned concerning the physiological, anatomi cal, and pathological phenomena incident to the Structure, Health, and Disease of the human being.

The alchemic art, however, was at length transferred from Arabia into European countries, and medical chairs were established in various Universities on the continent during the thirteenth century, and finally LINACRE, who had been educated at Oxford, and having traveled in Italy, and spent some time at the court of Florence, returned to England, and succeeded in founding medical professorships at Oxford and Cambridge, from which circumstance was laid the foundation of the London College of Physicians. Thus chemistry, after having been employed in various pharmaceutical processes, was applied to physiology, pathology, and therapeutics. The chemical doctors were very wild and extravagant in advancing unnatural theories; but they had an ever-present champion in the name of Galen, who was well entitled to be called the "Prince of Medical Philosophers." He *was* a philosopher—a *natural* philosopher; for he studied Nature closely, deeply, profoundly, and de-duced his indications of cure from an accurate observation of her laws. His system, however, was destined to be utterly overthrown by an adventurous vagrant, whose quackery never had its equal on earth. This impudent and unprincipled charlatan was none other than Paracelsus, to whom the medical world is more indebted for the *mineral* drugging system than to all other physicians who have ever lived. He introduced the *mercurial* and *antimonial* practice, which still constitutes the great strength of the popular materia medica of the day, and which also continues to exhibit its terribly devastating power on all human constitutions that come under its sway or influence. In the fulness of his pride, pomp, and arrogance, Paracelsus burned, with great solemnity, the works of Galen and Avicenna, declaring that he had found the philosopher's stone, and that mankind had no further use for the medical works of others. He lived a disappointed vagabond, and died prematurely at the age of forty-eight, his famous *elixir vitæ* having failed to save him from a most horrible fate. Still his abominable doctrines prevailed, and his infatuated followers have added several hundred other chemical or mineral preparations to the materia medica of the great Quicksilver Quack. At the present day, among a certain class of physicians, there is hardly a disease in the catalogue of human ailments in which the employment of mercury, antimony, arsenic, and other deadly drugs is not employed.

During the seventeenth century the doctrines of Hippocrates again rose to some consideration in medical philosophy. Anatomy made progress. HARVEY discovered the circulation of the blood; others traced out the absorbent system, and explained the functions and structure of the lungs; while BOYLE disengaged chemistry from the mystery by which it was surrounded, and explained its *true province* to be, "not the manufacture of solid gold, nor liquid nostrums, nor gaseous theories, but an investigation into the change of properties which bodies experience in their action upon each other."

From this time to the beginning of the eighteenth century, notwithstanding many facts had accumulated in chemistry, anatomy, and physiology, physicians, as a body, held no more natural views of the *true nature* of disease than were advanced by Hippocrates, three thousand years before. Indeed, it is positively certain that none of the most eminent *new* schools or sects of the present day had been more successful in curing diseases than were Hippocrates, Galen, and Sydenham. Meantime, however, there have arisen physicians, who, while they readily received all new facts in respect to the structure of the human organism, still adhered to the instinctive inductions of Nature, and treated diseases with most abundant success by means of Herbal preparations alone. We have at this day as bright a galaxy of names—scholars, philosophers, philanthropists, and humanitarians—as ever adorned any age of the world, devoting themselves with a zeal and industry worthy of all praise to the study and practice of medicine, but, failing to perceive the *grand results* anticipated in their laborious researches after truth, do not hesitate to admit that our actual information does not increase in any degree in proportion to our experience. All their array of learning, and their multitudinous writings, have only served to make confusion worse confounded, and all from the very simple fact that they have neglected to follow the requirements of Nature and common sense, in maintaining the Herbal Practice as the only true and philosophical foundation of the Healing Art. Amidst all the jarrings, conflicts, and dogmas of the medical world, is it any wonder that the great masses are rapidly losing all confidence in Medical Science, and crying for a more natural system of medication—even one founded in the principles of irrefragable Nature? With this view I have devoted many years of my life, and having traveled in numerous lands, I feel that I am now qualified, from a long medical experience and deep research into the physiology of Plants, to present to the world of suffering humanity all those curative elements best calculated to ensure perfect health, and the utmost length of life, to all who may feel disposed to be guided by the doctrines and system of medication which it is the object of this volume to make known.

THE HERBAL WORLD.

IN the foregoing pages we have seen, that from the earliest period in the history of the human race to the present time, the administration of the juices and essences of Herbs and Plants, in all forms of disease, has ever been considered by judicious and philosophical minds as the most rational and natural means of relieving the economy of all abnormal obstructions and derangements, and restoring all the functions to their original or primitive vigor and healthful working. Notwithstanding the innovations of the *mineral* practice, I have ever held most rigidly to the *Herbal* System of medication; but having failed to meet with the success reasonably anticipated by pursuing the ordinary routine of Therapeutics, I was finally led to reject the many changes in medical doctrines and practice, and start forth on a path of investigation of my own into the mysteries of the mineral and vegetable Kingdoms, especially as they might bear upon the health and happiness of the human being; accordingly, early in my professional career I attempted, by proper chemical analyses and practical experiment, to determine the best *specific* means for the healing of the maladies of mankind. The results of these researches, since confirmed by many years' successful medical experience based upon them, have but the more strongly strengthened my opposition to the use of all the mineral preparations of the modern schools of medicine, and to establish my faith all the more firmly in the employment of HERBAL elements exclusively—whether in the materia of roots, barks, seeds, or flowers—as the surest and safest means for the thorough eradication of every form of disease.

In saying all this, however, I do not deny the fact that many mineral substances enter into the composition of the human being, and are necessary for his full health and perfection—as chalk or lime is requisite to form bone, iron to enrich or strengthen the blood, and other mineral substances for the formation of the tissues, as phosphorus for the tissues of the brain and nerves, etc.—but I stoutly contend that all such inorganic substances are taken up by plants and distributed to the various tissues and elements of the human being, either in the way of food or medicine, in exactly the precise quantity requisite for man's perfect health, if rightly used, neither in excess or diminution, agreeably to the laws of Nature; and their virtues are thus prepared and eliminated in a way far superior to any chemical manipulation ever conceived or known to man, with all the elements of chemical science at his command. That this is the case is demonstrated by chemical analyses of plants. Coca contains phosphorus; twinleaf, the salts of potassa, lime, iron, magnèsia, silica, etc.; the houseleek, super-malate of lime; Matico, the salts of lime, iron, sulphur, etc. *Spongia usta*, carbon, silica, sodium, lime, magnesium, iron, and phosphorus, either in combination or free; coffee, chlorogenate of potassa; in fact, all the chemical elements composing the organism of man are also found in plants. The reader will find these chemical elements given in the history of plants. I also refer him to page 385, where, in the article " Treatment of Chronic Diseases," will be found a full explanation of the author's specialty in curing chronic disorders by chemically prepared herbal remedies.

The herbal physician has, moreover, decided advantages over the mineral physician, with reference to the administration of mineral substances. He gives them in natural combinations—in such chemical association which, for exactness and propriety, can only occur in the great laboratory of Nature; while the dispenser of mineral drugs gives them wholly as isolated elementary principles, as furnished by the inorganic chemist, who, like all humans, is liable to err. Let us illustrate this advantage by iodine. The algæ, such as the *fuci* and *laminariæ* (deep-sea-water plants, growing at the depth of three hundred fathoms), furnish this principle in abundance. The mineral physician, not content to administer the alterative in the best possible combination, as it exists in the sea-weed, subjects the plants to chemical operations, releases the iodine, and then either exhibits it by itself or in association with sodium,

1*

potassium, mercury, etc. The true herbal physician acts more wisely ·in this respect : he administers the plant in substance, tincture, extract, etc., and has the consciousness that the iodine which Nature furnishes him is pure, and not the inferior adulterated article of commerce. In plants where its chemical nature may be concentred into one compound principle, and the residue but inert matter, it is judicious to separate it from the plant, but radically wrong to release but one simple elementary mineral quality of the plant.

The advocate of mineral medication may retort by·asking the use of administering the whole plant, when the iodine alone constitutes its therapeutical value. Why give the refuse matter with the iodine? To this sophistical argument and foolish inquiry I will reply, Why eat the whole peach, when its flavor only makes it pleasant as an edible? Why not release the flavor and fatten on that delectable principle?

The best argument, however, in favor of herbal medication, and one which establishes it as the correct philosophy, is the comparison of results from both systems; and with these the author became fully acquainted by practical experiment, and which led him, and not prejudice, to adopt exclusively the herbal system of medication. I may justly claim this system of practice, in its most important relations, as solely my own, and for which I have been the recipient of all encouragement of scientific men and societies; but the homage that I value most, and which afforded the motive and stimulated my ambition, is the gratitude of almost numberless invalids whom I have thus been enabled to cure of diseases which were pronounced, and in fact are, incurable by physicians who rely upon minerals for their agents of cure.

The true theory of *disease* and its *cure* is embodied in two chemical forces, which, like the currents of electricity, are *positive* and *negative.* Thus, if the positive force of disease is manifested upon any organ, it disturbs the harmony and functional action of that organ, and the disorganization will continue as long as the negative force of cure is not placed in antagonism with it, to neutralize the activity of the positive force. When this is done the autonomy of the organ is re-established, and its function becomes again natural and healthful.

Again, if upon discovery any organ or tissue becomes deficient in its chemical elements, it must be supplied by such plants as contain them; or if any organ or tissue becomes surcharged with its chemical constituents, negative chemical elements must be exhibited to reduce them to their normal quantities. See article on "Treating Diseases Chemically," page 385.

These forces in various ways control the whole organic world. Increase the centrifugal force, and the earth flies into space; remove the centripetal, and it rushes headlong to the sun. If they are as they exist, coequal, the earth rolls on in its orbit in grand precision and admirable harmony.

Having thus philosophized, and finally realized that the entire universe was composed of *contrary* elements—of *negative* and *positive* principles—yet that the whole worked, or acted, in the most perfect harmony, agreeably to the wisdom of a Great First Cause, when such elements were not disarranged or disturbed by any *violation* of the laws of pristine *Nature*, I was soon led to a *logical deduction* of the general laws which govern the virtues or medicinal properties of all the varieties of plants, with a view to employ them as remedial agents in the cure of disease. In a word, I found in the being, MAN, an epitome of all creation—found in his organism all the elements of universal nature—and necessarily discerned that, as there are summer and winter, night and day, in regular and systematic succession, such alternations of nature could not but have the most important influences in respect to the health and diseases of the human being—Heaven's last, most perfect work. I realized that, in accordance with the various operations of nature, man remained in health, or became afflicted with disease. Hence it became necessary for me to fully understand or comprehend the *cause* of any departure from the normal or natural condition of man, and to provide the cure, or the remedy best adapted for the restoration of the equilibrium of the functions of his entire organism.

I ascertained by experiment what was before a preconceived idea, that plants afforded the best agents to antagonize the force of disease, and to re-establish the integrity of any organ or tissue assailed. The discovery was made apparent, however, that indiscriminate selection of medicinal plants was injudicious, and that the curative property of a plant was developed only in proportion as certain essential conditions were provided. These conditions proved to be those necessary to the full health of man, viz., proper climate, air, and food.

The first great essential of a plant which is to be selected for its medical qualities is its nativity. If indigenous to the locality or country wherein found, it is a proper one to select. Plants that are introduced from other countries are lessened or deprived of their virtues, unless they meet in their new home all the essential conditions possessed in their native place.

The *geographical* distribution of plants is affected by climatic influences, constituents of soil, heat, moisture, altitude of situation, etc. The flowers, shrubs, and trees which adorn the plains of India and South America, are not the same with those which clothe the valleys of England and North America. Nor are their *medicinal* properties the same, however those herbal products may resemble each other. The plants which flourish on the sea-shore of Great Britain are not the same as those on the coast of Africa, nor are these, again, allied to the maritime vegetation of Chili, South America. Nearly all the beautiful plants which adorn our green-houses are natives of a limited space near

the Cape of Good Hope, as are also many of our most beautiful bulbs;
but the *medicinal* properties of all become *weakened and changed* by
transplantation. The curious stafelias, that smell so offensively, are
found wild only in South Africa. They are there used for *medical*
purposes by the Aborigines. The trees that bear balsam grow principally in Arabia and on the banks of the Red Sea. The umbelliferous and
cinciferous plants spread across Europe and Asia. The *Cacti* are found
only in tropical America, while the lobiatæ and cariophyllacea are seldom discovered but in Europe. The peculiar ranges and centres of
vegetation, as they are termed, are all owing to chemical, climatic, and
electrical influences, and yield their *medicinal* properties in exact *ratio of
quality*, in accordance with the latitudes or places in which they are
indigenous.

From the many facts existing, we must believe that there is not a
single disease in man that may not have its remedy or cure, in some
herb or other, if we but knew *which* plant, and *where* to find it, in this,
or that, or any clime or portion of the world—agreeably to the providence of Nature.

This fact or law is proven in the lower animal kingdom. Who has
not often seen not only our familiar domestic animals, but many of the
untamed creatures of the forests, fields, and air, seek out some one or
peculiar herb, when laboring under sickness or derangement of the
functions of its organism?

Truly, Nature has wisely implanted a *definite* instinct in every organic creature, in order to serve for its health, or for its restoration to
health from disease. In man, however, such instinct is not so plainly
marked, but to him has been given reason and judgment, and (in some
few of the race) a disposition to investigate the laws and mysteries of
creation, in order to secure his own highest health and perfection, and
to find the means for the healing of his kind, when they have become
diseased through ignorance, perversion, and violation of the immutable
ordinances of Creation.

As the proverb says, "There are sermons in stones, and books in running brooks;" so do we behold volumes of wisdom in all the herbal kingdom—in every emerald and variegated leaf, in every tinted blossom—in
all, there is a voiceless language, eternally singing significant psalms in
praise of "HIM who doeth all things well."

Thus we find that *adaptation* is the *law* of the universe—and no-
where is it more vividly portrayed than in the growth and development
of the *Herbal* world.

It will thus be seen that it is only by carefully studying the physiology or functions, or nature of plants, we can derive instruction for the
proper regulation or government of our own organisms. The causes
which influence the growth and development of plants, are conditions

necessary to be understood, in order to preserve the health or integrity of our systems.

Dependent upon the causes I have already named, the plants, also, may lose their medicinal virtues; while much will be owing to the season of the year when they are gathered, in order to adapt them to medico-chemical purposes.

For instance, in the Spring of the year the common *Nettle* plant may afford a palatable food for man; but if selected at a later period, instead of serving as a savory vegetable, or purifier of morbid elements from the blood and system of man, might be converted into or *act* as a virulent or dangerous poison upon his organism.

In China the *Ginseng* (so called from the two Chinese words *gen sing*, "first of plants") plant or root is regarded—weight for weight—as silver, for medicinal purposes; whereas the same herb grown in America, or other countries, does not possess a tithe of the value of the Chinese production for healing purposes.

The American chamomile, though in all respects the same as the European, is positively inert in its medicinal qualities.

There must be, therefore, I repeat, a combination of influences to insure the full development of perfection of any plant. There must be not only internal but external stimuli, to develop the virtues of the herb. The external, as we have seen, consist of certain nutritious matters contained in the soil, water, atmospheric gases, electricity, light, and heat, besides the elements of oxygen, both in its combined or simple form, nitrogen, etc.

If we take a stem cut from a pine tree, in the forests of North Carolina, and place it in contact with the trunk of a healthy growing pine, the former would destroy the latter in the course of the season. The worms generated in the severed or decayed stem will pass to the living tree, and rapidly cause its destruction.

Any farmer knows that if the lordly oak be felled in June it will pass into a state of decay in the course of from four to eight weeks; but if it be cut down at a proper season (which is in Fall and early Spring, when the tree is nearly destitute of sap), it affords the best timber for the building of ships. It may be of interest, also, to state that at such times the transplantation of trees should be made. The tree should be removed at night, and set out in the same relative position to the sun as in its former aspect. If these rules are followed, no tree will rarely ever die, unless its most vital parts are too extensively injured.

We all know that a plant stripped of its leaves will soon perish. Among the reasons for this is, that the absorption by the roots is insufficient to supply all the materials for its nourishment. Let us look a little more closely into these phenomena of nature. There must be a certain number of stages for all herbal growths. First, the ascending sap dissolves the nutritive deposits of the root and stem, and conveys them to assist in the development of leaves and flowers. Hence it is evident that if the root, bark, or stem be gathered at this season, it will prove deficient in medicinal virtues, or be altogether inert. The leaves also will be found worthless for remedial purposes. On the other hand, if we wait a little longer, or until the plant is fully developed, we will find that either the bark or root, the leaves or flowers, are full of rare medicinal virtues.

The *precise* moment when all the assimilative processes of the plant have been perfected—whether it be Summer or Winter, Spring or Autumn—*is the time to gather it* for a remedial agent in disease, inasmuch as we know that the laws of chemical decomposition and recombination know no rest; hence, as in the case of the nettle, while it may be a good food in its earlier stages of development, it would prove a poison in a more advanced stage of its growth.

The peculiar properties of herbs as medicines will often depend upon the greenness or ripeness of the plant, and other circumstances attendant upon its cutting, and the length of time it is kept after being gathered.

For instance, the concrete juice of the Manna ash (*Fraxinus Ornus*)— the manna of commerce—increases in purgative qualities by age. The Oak-bark, for tanning hides, improves in value for a period of four or five years after it has been stripped from the trunk; in the same manner, its medicinal properties are either diminished or improved, according to the season when the bark is gathered, or the manner in which it is converted into tannic acid for medical or scientific purposes.

It must be apparent to all, that herbs are liable to suffer from the vicissitudes of soil, climate, season, etc., and, as a matter of course, from these causes will vary the medicinal principles attributed to them.

Repeated analysis demonstrates the fact, that specimens of the same plant, grown in different localities, will vary infinitely in the proportions of the medicinal principles yielded. Take, for example, the Butterfly-weed, or Pleurisy-root (*Asclepias Tuberosa*), which grows in the barren and sandy soil of New Jersey, and it will be found to yield from one to two hundred per cent. of its medicinal virtues more than the same plant grown in the rich alluvial soils of the West. Hence, when given as medicine, the quantity must correspond accordingly—be either increased or diminished, in order to secure its proper curative effects upon the system. Thus it is seen that a medicine, prepared from plants culled at an improper season, will prove entirely inert or useless, while the same herb, gathered at a proper time in a proper climate, especially and properly prepared, would secure the restoration of a patient from disease to health.

There is likewise a wide difference between the virtues of a plant growing in a wild or *natural* condition from that of the same herb when artificially cultivated. The transference of plants from their native locations, to soils prepared by the hands of man, induces many changes in their individual elements. Many plants formerly used for medicines are now cultivated for the table alone. The small acid root of the *Brassica Rupa* has become the large and nutritious article of diet known as the *turnip*. The dandelion, when grown in natural localities, possesses well-defined medical properties, all of which are lost when the plant is artificially cultivated. In the cultivated plant the proportions of starch, grape-sugar, and other non-medical principles are largely increased, while that which is gathered in its wild or native state is known to possess rare virtues in affections of the liver, kidneys, and respiratory organs. In the cultivated rose the stamens are converted into petals. The castor-oil plant in Africa is a woody tree—in our gardens it is an annual. The mignonette, in Europe, is an annual plant, but becomes perennial in the sandy deserts of Egypt.

I repeat, from what has been seen it is evident that all herbs, perhaps, possess some property suitable for medical purposes. These virtues may be found in the root of one plant, in the bark of another, in the leaves of another, in the blossoms of another, in the seeds of another, or in the whole combined. Even the *color* of the flower has much to do with the therapeutic properties of the plant--as, for instance, the *Blue Vervain*, as used in my Fits and Dyspepsia remedy, is the only kind that is used for medical purposes—all the other species being entirely useless, or else more or less dangerous.

In fact, it is evident to the comprehension of the simplest mind that climatic influences have much to do with the full development of plants. This may be illustrated in the *Tobacco* raised in Cuba and that grown in Connecticut—the one being grown in a Southern and the other in a Northern climate. The poison *nicotine* is derived from the tobacco plant; the exhilarating *caffeine* and *theine* are obtained from the coffee berry and tea plant. Thus it is possible that some therapeutic agent or other may be derived from every plant grown on the surface of the globe.

The Red Men of the American forests are never at a loss to know which plant is best, nor the time it should be gathered, to cure them of disease. They know how to treat their complaints in physic, surgery, and midwifery with a skill that far surpasses that of many a learned doctor of the big medical schools, with all their science, and the medical teachings of physicians for upwards of four thousand years. What other guide have the poor Indians—those untutored savages of the woods—but their reason and their instinct, and their practical experience in the use of herbs?

This is the same in the East Indies, South America, South Sea

Islands, Patagonia, Africa, and other lands. The negroes in the interior parts of Africa possess a knowledge of the medicinal properties of plants which is really surprising, and, by consequence, are rarely afflicted with disease. The art of healing in Sumatra consists in the application of plants, in whose medicinal virtues they are surprisingly skilled. In fact, the Sumatrans have a degree of botanical knowledge that surprises the European or American. They become acquainted at an early age not only with the names, but the qualities and properties of every shrub and herb among that exuberant variety with which their country abounds.

In gathering herbs for medical purposes, we should not only know the season when they should be culled, but we should be qualified to comprehend the principles of which the plant is composed—whether they be resins, alkaloids, or neutrals—and be able also to separate the one ingredient or element from the other, as a *distinct* medicinal property, or combine the whole for the purpose of a *compound* medical agent.

Plants by their appearance often invite the invalid to cull them for his restoration, and assume such shapes as to suggest their curative

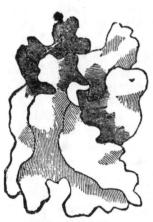

Lungwort.

properties. For instance, herbs that simulate the shape of the *Lungs*, as Lungwort (*see figure adjoining*), Sage, Hounds-tongue, and Comfrey, are all good for pulmonary complaints.

Plants which bear in leaves and roots a *heart*-like form, as Citron Apple, Fuller's Thistle, Spikenard, Balm, Mint, White-beet, Parsley, and Motherwort, will yield medicinal properties congenial to that organ. Vegetable productions like in figure to the *ears*, as the leaves of the Coltfoot or Wild Spikenard, rightly prepared as a conserve and eaten, improve the hearing and memory; while *oil* extracted from the shells of sea-snails, which have the turnings and curvings of the ears, tends wonderfully to the cure of deafness. A decoction of Maiden Hair and the moss of Quinces, which plants resemble the *hairs of the head*, is good for baldness. Plants resembling the human *nose*, as the leaves of the Wild Water Mint, are beneficial in restoring the *sense of smell*. Plants having a semblance of the *Womb*, as Birthwort, Heart Wort, Ladies' Seal or Briony, conduce much to a safe *accouchement*. Shrubs and Herbs resembling the bladder and gall, as Nightshade and Alkekengi, will relieve the gravel and stone. Liver-shaped plants, as *Liverwort* (*see the following figure*), Trinity, Agaric, Fumitory, Figs, etc., all are efficacious in *bilious* diseases. Walnuts, Indian nuts,

Leeks, and the root of Ragwort, because of their form, when duly prepared will further generation and prevent sterility. Herbs and seeds in shape like the teeth, as Toothwort, Pine-kernel, etc., preserve the dental organization. Plants of knobbed form, like knuckles or joints, as Galingale, and the knotty odoriferous rush, *Calamus*, are good for diseases of the spine and reins, foot, gout, knee swellings, and all joint pains whatsoever. Oily vegetable products, as the Filbert, Walnut, Almond, etc., tend to fatness of the body.

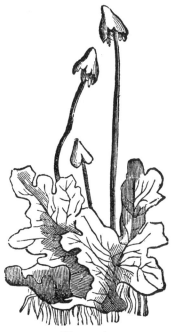

Liverwort.

Plants naturally *lean*, as Sarsaparilla or long-leaved *Rosa Solie* emaciate those who use them.

Fleshy plants, such as Onions, Leeks, and Colewort, make flesh for the eaters. Certain plants, as the Sensitive plant, Nettles, the roots of Mallows, and the herb *Neurus*, when used as *outward* applications, fortify and brace the *nerves*. Milky herbs, as Lettuce and the fruit of the Almond and Fig trees, propagate *milk*. Plants of a *serous* nature, as Spurge and Scammony, purge the noxious humors between the flesh and the skin. Herbs whose acidity turns milk to curd, such as Galium and the seeds of Spurge, will lead to procreation. Rue mixed with Cummin will relieve a sore breast, if a poultice of them be applied, when the milk is knotted therein ; while plants that are *hollow*, as the stalks of Grain, Reeds, Leeks, and Garlic, are good to purge, open, and soothe the hollow parts of the body. Many more instances of such adaptation of herbs and plants to diseases of the body might be cited if deemed necessary.

The *vitality* of plants may be destroyed by giving them deleterious or poisonous substances, such as arsenic, mercury, etc. In fact, *mineral* poisons act on plants and herbs in nearly the same way they do upon human beings or other animals.

The *color* of plants is generally under the influence of *solar* light ; hence, plants grown in darkness become etiolated or blanched. The *green* of leaves is due to *nitrogen*, while in proportion as the *oxygen* of the air predominates, the leaves put on varied tints, as the beautiful red and crimson assumed by some leaves in Autumn.

The *color of flowers*, as a general rule, is influenced by *solar* light, though the *magnetic* condition of the soil has much to do with the color. For instance, the petals of the common butter-cup are of as brilliant a yellow in town gardens enveloped in the smoke of London as on any country hill, while the tints of the rose remain, when languishing for lack of a clear atmosphere. The flowers of the common hydrangea, which are naturally *pink*, may be made *blue* by planting the shrub in soil impregnated with iron. So will certain medical preparations of iron turn *blue* the human flesh. The color of the flower of the tulips can be turned into white, yellow, brown, purple, and a beautiful tint of rose, by transplanting the plants from a poor soil to a rich one, and *vice versâ*.

The *fragrances* of flowers and plants have their physiological or medical uses. The use of the fragrance in leaves, bark, and wood, is apparently to preserve them from the attacks of insects; as the smell of the red and Bermuda cedars (of which pencils are made) and of Camphor, also a *vegetable* product, is to keep moths and other vermin from attacking substances with which they are in contact.

Plants sometimes distil or secrete medicinal or nutritive fluids, which are contained in convenient receptacles. Such plants invariably grow far from the haunts of men, away from the course of streams or vicinity of ponds. Whose ordination is it that such plants have such a habitude? It is that Providence who, in his bountiful beneficence, places them where the traveler may not die of thirst or disease on his way of discovery. This is most beautifully illustrated in the *Nepenthes distillatoria*

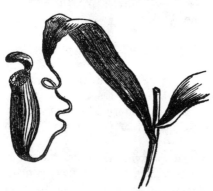

Nepenthes distillatoria.

(see cut), in which the leaves terminate in a most singular manner, forming a sort of urn or vase, surmounted by a cover, which opens and shuts as occasion requires. This vessel is suspended at the extremity of a thread-like appendage to a winged petiole, which would seem to be altogether unfit to support it. An officer of marines writes as follows: "Three days after my arrival at Madagascar I lost myself during a short excursion into the interior, and was overtaken with an excessive lassitude, accompanied with a devouring thirst. After a long walk I was on the point of yielding to despair, when I perceived close to me, suspended to leaves, some small vases, somewhat like those used to preserve fresh water. I began to think I was under one of those hallucinations by which the sick are often visited in fever, when the refreshing draught seems to fly from their parched lips. I approached it, however, with some hesitation, threw a rapid glance at the pitchers : judge of my happiness when I found them filled with a pure and transparent liquid. The draught I partook gave me the best idea I have realized of the nectar served at the table of the gods." Plants of such description become extinct if civilization approaches their domain.

Plants have attributes other than medical which are of interest to the general reader besides the botanist.

In many instances there seems to be a striking affinity between the herbal and animal kingdom, and other instances of the repelling character. For instance, a most remarkable instance of irritability by contact is that exhibited by the "Venus's Fly-Trap," *Dionæa muscipula*, a native of Canada, and nearly allied to the common "Sun-Dew" of the British commons. Its flowers have nothing remarkable about them, ex-

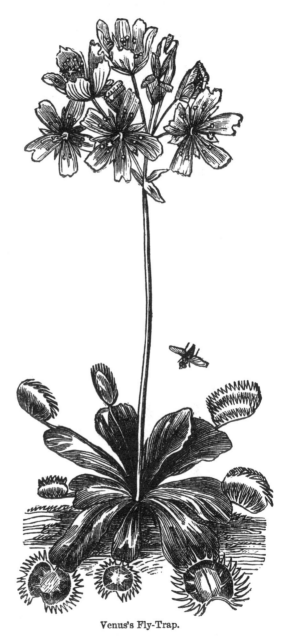

Venus's Fly-Trap.

cept that their petals roll up when they are about to decay; but the leaves are very curiously constructed. They have broad leaf-like petioles, at whose extremity there are two fleshy tubes, which form the real leaf, and which are armed with strong, sharp spines, three on the blade of each lobe, and a fringe of larger spines round the margin.

When an insect touches the base of the central spines the leaf collapses, and the poor insect is caught, been either impaled by the central spines or entrapped by the others. The leaf then remains closed, the fringe of long spines being firmly interlaced and locked together till the body of the insect has wasted away. This apparatus being the nearest approach to a stomach which has yet being observed in plants, an experiment was tried some years ago of feeding a *dionæa* (Venus's Fly-Trap) with very small particles of raw meat, when it was found that the leaves closed in the same way as they would have done over an insect, and did not open again until the meat was consumed. The leaves of this plant possess medicinal properties, which, when properly prepared in tincture or decoction, have been found of exceeding efficacy in many diseases of the digestive organs of the human being.

Sarracenia, or Side-Saddle flower, the leaves of which are pitcher-shaped, resembling an old-fashioned side-saddle, six of which generally belong to each plant. Each of these pitchers will hold nearly a wine-glassful, and are generally filled with water and aquatics, which undergo decomposition, or a sort of *digestion*, and serve as a nutriment to the plant.

This animal characteristic is also illustrated in the *sensitive plant* (Mimosa Sensitiva), which the slightest touch suffices to make it close its folioles. If we cut with scissors the extreme end of one foliole the others immediately approach in succession. This irritation is not local, but communicates from circle to circle, and propagates itself from leaf to leaf. Up to a certain point it gets accustomed to outside interference. Touching it again and again will habituate it to the movement and fail to respond, as if it were owing in the first instance to fright.

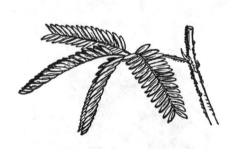

Sensitive Plant.

The sleep of plants vaguely recalls to us the sleep of animals. Their period of sleep is mostly at night, and any interested person may observe this habit in a variety of plants, as many of them when asleep are difficult to recognize in their bearing. The leaves are rolled up, or become reversed, as in the genus *Sida* and the *Lupinus*. The Vetch, the Sweet-pea, the Broad Bean, in their sleep rest their leaves during the night one against the other.

Parental solicitude is displayed in the orach-root (*Atriplex hortensis*). The leaves of this plant fall back upon the young shoots, and enclose them whenever the effects of the atmosphere would injure them. This is also seen in the chickweed at night.

The folding of some flowers in the absence of the sun, and the opening of others as soon as that luminary has withdrawn his beams, are ascribable to various causes. The white marigold closes its flowers on the approach of rain, and the dwarf *Colendrina* folds up its bright crimson corolla about four o'clock every afternoon; while, on the contrary, the plant commonly called *Four o'clock*, whose flower remains closed all day, opens precisely at the hour of four. The evening primrose will not open its large yellow flower till the sun has sunk below the horizon. On the other hand, the Sun-flower is always seen bending its face (*vis-à-vis*) in the direction of the sun, and follows its course during the entire diurnal round, from its rise in the Orient, or East, in the morning, to its decline in the Hesperian region, or west, in the evening. The *Silphium laciniatum*, or compass-weed, always points its leaves towards the north star. The Night-blowing Cereus only expands its flowers about midnight. Indeed, some flowers are so regular in their opening or shutting, that the great botanist, LINNÆUS, formed what he called "*Flora's Timepiece*," in which each hour was represented by the flower which opened or closed at that particular time. An arrangement of this kind may be seen in the following

FLORAL CLOCK:

Between 3 and 4 A.M .... Bind-weed of the hedgerows.
At 5 A.M................Naked stalked Poppy and most of the Chichoraceæ.
Between 5 and 6 A.M......Nipplewort and the Day Lily.
At 6 A.M................Many of the Solanaceæ (Night-shade) family.
Between 6 and 7 A.M......Sow Thistle and Spurrey.
At 7 A.M................Water Lilies, Lettuces.
At 7 to 8 A.M............Venus' Looking-Glass.
At 8 A.M.................Wild Pimpernel.
At 9 A.M.................Wild Marigold.
At 9 to 10 A.M............Ice Plant.
At 11 A.M.................Purslain, Star of Bethlehem.
At 12.....................Most of the Ficoid, or Mesembryanthemum family.
At 2 P.M.................Scilla Pomeridiana.
Between 5 and 6 P.M......Silene Noctiflora.
Between 6 and 7 P.M......Marvel of Peru.
Between 7 and 8 P.M......Cereus Grandiflorus, Tree Primrose.
At 10 P.M................Purple Convolvulus.

In addition to the above, I would remark that certain equinoctial flowers open and close at a fixed time in the same day; on the morrow, and for several following days, they again open and shut at the same regular hours. The Star of Bethlehem opens several days in succession at eleven in the morning, and closes at three. The *Ficoides Noctiflora* blows several days in succession at seven in the evening, and closes about six or seven in the morning.

Besides the cases in which flowers open and shut their corollas by the influence of light, instances are known in which merely the petals roll up by day, and resume their natural shape after sunset. A remarkable circumstance respecting the effect of atmospheric influence is, that the same causes do not affect all plants, and yet no peculiarity of construction has been discovered in those so affected to distinguish them from those that are not.

Every student of nature can witness much more that is of general interest regarding the habits, so to speak, and characteristics of plants. They have been a favorite theme in all ages. Lovers have dwelt on them and given them a language. Nearly every one delights in the flowering plants. Who would refuse a bouquet of choice flowers? This attachment to flowers was pathetically illustrated in the Highland emigrants in Canada, who wept when they found that the heather would not grow in their newly-adopted soil. And well they might, for it is the flower of their native mountains, and associated with all their brightest and tenderest recollections. In the age of chivalry the daisy was renowned; and St. Louis, of France, took it and a lily for a device in his ring, as emblematical of his wife and country. The thistle, like the famous geese of Rome, saved Scotland, and for this reason it is the national emblem of that country. During the Danish invasion, one of their soldiers placed his naked foot on the spiny leaves of a thistle, and instinctively uttered a cry which awoke the slumbering Scots, who turned upon their foes, defeated, and drove them from their land.

The poetry attached to plants, however, is not of immediate concern in this volume. It is their medicinal properties which engages our study and demands our labors. Yet I could not so well establish their superior fitness as curative agents above the mineral drug unless I gave that which is of general interest. One fact will be apparent to the reader, that plants have life, and hence are eminently suitable to give life to the suffering patient. The lifeless inorganic mineral has none, and can give no vital element.

EPITOME OF BOTANY.

THAT the reader may more intelligently understand the description of the medicinal plants in this book, the author has deemed it prudent to preface the part of this work dedicated to Herbal Materia Medica with a brief analysis of the plant, as made by the botanist. This becomes particularly necessary, inasmuch as a plant cannot be accurately described unless scientific language be employed; but, nevertheless, throughout this whole work it has been the aim of the author to use the plainest language, and not to weary the reader by as pedantic employment of technical terms and scientific language.

Nothing more will be given than the anatomy of the plant, as nothing of systematic botany need be known to the reader to recognize the plant, or to acquaint himself with the medicinal properties thereof. If he has not a common acquaintance with a medicinal plant, but desires it for domestic medication, it is important that he should know that he employs the proper herb, and not use one which simulates it. It has therefore been the aim of the author to give accurate descriptions of the herbs, so that the gatherer may not err in his selection of the plant which his case may need.

All parts of the plant are used in medicine—sometimes the seed only; in others the flower, the leaves, root, rhizome; in others two or more of these parts, and, again, in others the whole plant.

ANATOMY OF A PLANT.

THE ROOT.

The root of a plant is that portion which is usually found in the earth, the stem and leaves being in the air. The point of union is called the collar or neck of the plant.

A fibrous root is one composed of many spreading branches, as that of barley.

A conical root is one where it tapers regularly from the crown to the apex, as that of the carrot.

A fusiform root is one when it tapers up as well as down, as that of the radish.

A napiform root is one when much swollen at the base, so as to become broader than long, as that of the turnip.

A fasciculated root is one when some of the fibres or branches are thickened.

A tuberiferous root is one when some of the branches assume the form of rounded knobs, as that of the potato.

A **palmate** root is one when these knobs are branched.

Aerial roots are those emitted from the stem into the open air, as that of Indian corn.

A **rhizoma,** or root stock, is a prostrate stem either subterranean or resting on the surface, as that of calamus, or blood-root.

A **tuber** is an enlargement of the apex of a subterranean branch of the root, as that of the common potato or artichoke.

A **cormus** is a fleshy subterranean stem of a round or oval figure, as in the Indian turnip.

A **bulb** is an extremely abbreviated stem clothed with scales, as that of the lily.

THE STEM.

The stem is that portion of the plant which grows in an opposite direction from the root, seeking the light, and exposing itself to the air. All flowering plants possess stems. In those which are said to be stemless, it is either very short, or concealed beneath the ground.

An **herb** is one in which the stem does not become woody, but dies down to the ground at least after flowering.

A **shrub** is a woody plant, branched near the ground, and less than five times the height of man.

A **tree** attains a greater height, with a stem unbranched near the ground.

The stem of a tree is usually called the **trunk;** in grasses it has been termed the **culm.**

Those stems which are too weak to stand erect are said to be **decumbent, procumbent,** and **prostrate.**

A **stolon** is a form of a branch which curves or falls down to the ground, where they often strike root.

A **sucker** is a branch of subterraneous origin, which, after running horizontally and emitting roots in its course, at length rises out of the ground and forms an erect stem, which soon becomes an independent plant, as illustrated by the rose, raspberry, etc.

A **runner** is a prostrate, slender branch sent off from the base of the parent stem.

An **offset** is a similar but shorter branch, with a tuft of leaves at the end, as in the houseleek.

A **spine** is a short and imperfectly developed branch of a woody plant, as exhibited in the honey-locust.

A **tendril** is commonly a slender leafless branch, capable of coiling spirally, as in the grape vine.

THE LEAF.

The leaf is commonly raised on an unexpanded part or stalk which is called the **petiole,** while the expanded portion is termed the **lamina.**

limb, or blade. When the vessels or fibres of the leaves expand immediately on leaving the stem, the leaf is said to be **sessile.** In such cases the petiole is absent. When the blade consists of a single piece the leaf is **simple;** when composed of two or three more with a branched petiole, the leaf is **compound.**

The distribution of the veins or framework of the leaf in the blade is termed **venation.**

A **lanceolate** leaf has the form of a lance.

An **ovate** leaf has the shape of ellipsis.

A **cuneiform** leaf has the shape of a wedge.

A **cordate** leaf has the shape of a heart.

A **reniform** leaf has the shape of a kidney.

A **sagittate** leaf is arrow-shaped.

A **hastate** leaf has the shape of an ancient halberd.

A **peltate** leaf is shaped like a shield.

A **serrate** leaf is one in which the margin is beset with sharp teeth, which point forward towards the apex.

A **dentate** leaf is one when these teeth are not directed towards the apex.

A **crenate** leaf has rounded teeth.

A **sinuate** leaf has alternate concavities and convexities.

A **pinnate** leaf has the shape of a feather.

A **pectinate** leaf is one having very close and narrow divisions, like the teeth of a comb.

A **lyrate** leaf has the shape of a lyre.

A **runcinate** leaf is a lyrate leaf with sharp lobes pointing towards the base, as in the dandelion.

A **palmate** leaf is one bearing considerable resemblance to the hand.

A **pedate** leaf is one bearing resemblance to a bird's foot.

An **obovate** leaf is one having the veins more developed beyond the middle of the blade.

When a leaf at its outer edge has no dentations it is said to be **entire.** When the leaf terminates in an acute angle it is **acute,** when in an obtuse angle it is **obtuse.** An obtuse leaf with the apex slightly depressed is **retuse,** or if more strongly notched, **emarginate.** An obovate leaf with a wider or more conspicuous notch at the apex become **obcordate,** being a cordate leaf inverted. When the apex is cut off by a straight transverse line the leaf is **truncate;** when abruptly terminated by a small projecting point it is **mucronate;** and when an acute leaf has a narrowed apex it is **acuminate.** In ferns the leaves are called **fronds.**

THE FLOWER.

The flower assumes an endless variety of forms, and we shall assume in the dissection merely the typical form of it.

2

The organs of a flower are of two sorts, viz. : 1st. Its leaves or envelopes ; and 2d, those peculiar organs having no resemblance to the envelopes. The envelopes are of two kinds, or occupy two rows, one above or within the other. The lower or outer row is termed the **Calyx**, and commonly exhibits the green color of the leaves. The inner row, which is usually of more delicate texture and forms the most showy part of the flower, is termed the **Corolla**. The several parts of the leaves of the Corolla are called **Petals**, and the leaves of the Calyx have received the analogous name of **Sepals**. The floral envelopes are collectively called the **Perianth**.

The essential organs enclosed within a floral envelope are also of two kinds and occupy two rows one within the other. The first of these, those next within the petals, are the **Stamens**. A stamen consists of a stalk called the **Filament**, which bears on its summit a rounded body termed the **Anther**, filled with a substance called the **Pollen**.

The seed-bearing organs occupy the centre or summit of a flower, and are called **Pistils**. A pistil is distinguished into three parts, viz. : 1st, the **Ovary**, containing the **Ovales**; 2d, the **Style**, or columnar prolongation of the ovary ; and 3d, the **Stigma**, or termination of the style.

All the organs of the flower are situated on, or grown out of, the apex of the flower-stalk, into which they are inserted, and which is called the **Torus** or **Receptacle**.

A plant is said to be **monœcious**, where the stamens and pistils are in separate flowers on the same individual, **diœcious**, where they occupy separate flowers on different individuals, and **polygamous** where the stamens and pistils are separate in some flowers and united in others, either on the same or two or three different plants.

THE FRUIT.

The principal kinds may be briefly stated as follows :—

A **follicle** is the name given to such fruit as borne by the larkspur or milkweed.

A **legume** or pod is the name extended to such fruit as the pea or bean.

A **drupe** is a stone fruit, as the plum, apricot, etc.

An **achenium** is the name of the fruit as borne by the butter-cup, &c.

A **cremocarp** is the fruit of the Poison Hemlock and similar plants.

A **caryopsis** is such fruit as borne by the wheat tribe.

A **nut** is exemplified by the fruit of the oak, chestnut, &c.

A **samara** is the name applied to the fruit of the maple, birch, and elm.

A **berry** is a fruit fleshy and pulpy throughout, as the grape, gooseberry, &c.

A **pome** is such as the apple, pear, &c.

A **pepo** is the name applied to the fruit of the pumpkin, cucumber, &c.

A **capsule** is a general term for all dry fruits, such as lobelia, &c.

A **silique** is such fruit as exhibited in Shepherd's purse, &c.

A **cone** or **strobile** is a collective fruit of the fir tribe, magnolia, &c.

THE SEED.

The seed, like the ovule of which it is the fertilized and matured state, consists of a **nucleus,** usually enclosed within two **integuments,** The outer integument or proper seed coat is variously termed the **episperm, spermoderm,** or **testa.**

An **annual** plant is one which springs from the seed, flowers and dies the same year.

A **biennial** plant, such as the radish, carrot, beet, &c., does not flower the first season.

A **perennial** plant is one not absolutely depending upon the stock of the previous season, but annually produces new roots and new accumulations.

MEDICINAL PROPERTIES AND PREPARATIONS.

EVERY herb employed in the cure of diseases, whether in its natural state or after having undergone various preparations, belongs to the Herbal Materia Medica, in the extended acceptation of the term. It shall, however, be our purpose only to describe each separate herb in its living state, or the medicinal part thereof, and not dwell much upon the forms usually prepared by the apothecary or physician. In this portion of our work we propose to give an account of all the most important medicinal herbs necessary for the cure of diseases. No herb, however, is to be despised or regarded as worthless because of its not finding mention in .this work; but, as previously stated, that each and every plant has its virtues, though to describe all recognized as medicinal would make the work too voluminous, and in price far exceed the reach of the million. The various properties of medicinal agents ·have been designated as follows :—

ABSORBENTS or ANTACIDS are such medicines that counteract acidity of the stomach and bowels.

ALTERATIVES are medicines which, in certain doses, work a gradual cure by restoring the healthy functions of different organs.

ANODYNES are medicines which relieve pain.

ANTHELMINTICS are medicines which have the power of destroying or expelling worms from the intestinal canal.

ANTISCORBUTICS are medicines which prevent or cure the scurvy.

ANTISPASMODICS are medicines given to relieve spasm, or irregular and painful action of muscles or muscular fibres, as in Epilepsy, St. Vitus' Dance, etc.

AROMATICS are medicines which have a grateful smell and an agreeable pungent taste.

ASTRINGENTS are those remedies which, when applied to the body, render the solids dense and firmer.

CARMINATIVES are those medicines which dispel flatulency of the stomach and bowels.

CATHARTICS are medicines which accelerate the action of the bowels, or increase the discharge by stool.

DEMULCENTS are medicines suited to prevent the action of acrid and stimulating matters upon the mucous membranes of the throat, lungs, etc.

DIAPHORETICS are medicines that promote or cause perspirable discharge by the skin.

DIURETICS are medicines which increase the flow of urine by their action upon the kidneys.

EMETICS are those medicines which produce vomiting.

EMMENAGOGUES are medicines which promote the menstrual discharge.

EMOLLIENTS are those remedies which, when applied to the solids of the body, render them soft and flexible.

ERRHINES are substances which, when applied to the lining membrane of the nostrils, occasion a discharge of mucous fluid.

EPISPASTICS are those which cause blisters when applied to the surface.

ESCHAROTICS are substances used to destroy a portion of the surface of the body, forming sloughs.

EXPECTORANTS are medicines capable of facilitating the excretion of mucus from the chest.

NARCOTICS are those substances having the property of diminishing the action of the nervous and vascular systems, and of inducing sleep.

RUBEFACIENTS are remedies which excite the vessels of the skin and increase its heat and redness.

SEDATIVES are medicines which have the power of allaying the actions of the systems generally, or of lessening the exercise of some particular function.

SIALAGOGUES are medicines which increase the flow of the saliva.

STIMULANTS are medicines capable of exciting the vital energy, whether as exerted in sensation or motion.

TONICS are those medicines which increase the tone or healthy action, or strength of the living system.

PHARMACEUTIC PREPARATIONS.

ACETA or VINEGARS are medicinal preparations where vinegar is used as the dissolving agent.

ÆTHEREA or ETHERS are ethereal tinctures.

AQUÆ or WATERS consist of water impregnated with some medicinal substance, as a volatile oil.

CATAPLASMS are external applications or poultices.

CERATES are agents intended for external application, and are composed of wax, spermaceti, combined with fatty matter, and in which resins and powders, etc., are frequently amalgamated.

CONFECTIONS are medicines in the form of a conserve.

DECOCTIONS are solutions procured from the various parts of herbs by boiling them in water.

DRAGEES are sugar-coated pills.

ENEMAS or INJECTIONS. These consist of medicinal agents in the form of infusion, decoction, or mixture, and designed to be passed into the rectum and other passages.

EXTRACTS. When an infusion, decoction, or tincture is reduced to a soft solid mass, by evaporation, it is termed an extract.

FLUID-EXTRACTS. These are concentrated medicinal principles, not reduced to a solid or nearly semi-fluid consistence, the evaporation not being carried so far as in ordinary extracts. (See page 475)

INFUSIONS are solutions of vegetable principles in water, effected without boiling.

LINIMENTS. These preparations are designed for external application, and should always be of such a consistence as will render them capable of easy application to the skin with the naked hand or flannel.

LOTIONS. These comprise all compounds used as external washes in which vegetable substances are dissolved.

MIXTURES are either liquid or solid compounds, and which are suspended in aqueous fluids by the intervention of some viscid matter, as mucilage, albumen, etc.

OILS are the products of various herbs by distillation with water.

PILLS are medicinal properties formed into a mass and rolled into globular forms. A *bolus* is a large pill.

PLASTERS are designed for external application; the medicinal agent is usually spread on cloth or chamois leather.

POWDERS are medicinal herbs in a pulverized state.

SATURATES are similar to fluid-extracts, being, however, prepared without the employment of heat.

SYRUPS are liquid medicines of a viscid consistence, produced by concentrated solutions of sugar alone or mixed with honey.

TINCTURES. These are preparations obtained by subjecting medicinal herbs to the action of alcohol.

TROCHEES or LOZENGES are medicinal substances in powder, which are formed into solid cakes by the aid of sugar and gum.

UNGUENTA or OINTMENTS are fatty matters, in which are incorporated certain medicines, and are designed for external use.

WINES. These are tinctures of medicinal agents which are insoluble in water, or which do not require as stimulant a solvent as alcohol, but which are capable of yielding their virtues to wine.

WEIGHTS AND MEASURES.

THAT no error may occur, I will here append the weights and measures employed in pharmacy, together with the symbols designating each quantity. It is necessary to understand but two measures, as the author has conformed all the solid or liquid quantities to these measures. These are :—

1ST.—APOTHECARIES' WEIGHT.

20 grains (gr.) ....1 scruple.
3 scruples (Ə) ....1 drachm.
8 drachms (ʒ) ....1 ounce.
12 ounces (℥)...........................1 pound (℔).

The doses of powders, extracts, and all such that are not fluid are intended to correspond with this weight.

2D.—APOTHECARIES' MEASURE.

60 minims (♏) ....1 fluid drachm.
8 fluid drachms (f ʒ) ....1 fluid ounce.
16 fluid ounces (f ℥).....................1 pint.
8 pints (O)..............................1 gallon (cong).

The quantities of all fluids mentioned in this book agree with this measure, though the word fluid or the symbol (f) is omitted in most instances.

It is not to be supposed, however, that in all families measuring graduates are to be found ; hence a comparison of these measures with tea, dessert, and table spoons, etc., becomes necessary to simplify the fluid measure. The weight of any quantity I should always advise to be correctly ascertained by scales :—*

COMPARISON.

A *drop* corresponds with a minim.
A teaspoonful " " " fluid drachm.
A dessertspoonful " " " three fluid drachms.
A tablespoonful " " " one-half fluid ounce.
A wineglassful " " " two fluid ounces.
A teacupful " " " gill (4 f $\mathfrak{Z}$).

In the body of this work the quantity has been stated, with but few exceptions, in which each medicine must ordinarily be given to produce its peculiar effects upon the adult patient. But there are circumstances which modify the dose, and demand attention, the most important of which is the age ; hence the following table, exhibiting the dose proportioned to the age, should receive careful reference in domestic practice :—

TABLE.

The dose for a person of age being 1 or 1 drachm.
That of a person from 14 to 21 years will be $\frac{2}{3}$ or 2 scruples.
   7 to 14 " " " $\frac{1}{2}$ or $\frac{1}{2}$ drachm.
   4 to 7 " " " $\frac{1}{3}$ or 1 scruple.
  of 4 " " " $\frac{1}{4}$ or 15 grains.
   3 " " " $\frac{1}{6}$ or 10 grains.
   2 " " " $\frac{1}{8}$ or 8 grains.
   1 " " " $\frac{1}{12}$ or 5 grains.
   $\frac{1}{2}$ " " " $\frac{1}{16}$ or 4 grains.

The following rule, however, is a little more simple :—
For children under 12 years the dose of most medicines must be diminished in the proportion of the age to the age increased by 12 ; thus, at two years the dose will be $\frac{1}{7}$ of that for adults, viz. :—

$$\frac{2}{2+12} = \frac{2}{14} \text{ or } \frac{1}{7} ; \text{ at 4, it will be } \frac{4}{4+12} = \frac{4}{16} \text{ or } \frac{1}{4}.$$

---

* The weights used in the British Pharmacopœia are the Imperial or avordupois pound, ounce, and grain, and the terms *drachm* and *scruple*, as designating specific weights, are discontinued. The ounce contains 437½ grains, and the pound 7,000 grains. The Imperial Measure contains 8 fluid drachms to the ounce, 20 fluid ounces to the pint, and 8 pints to the gallon.

HERBAL MATERIA MEDICA.

ACACIA VERA.

COMMON NAMES. *Gum Arabic, Egyptian Thorn.*
MEDICINAL PART. *The concrete juice or gum.*
Description.—Acacia Vera is a small tree or shrub, but sometimes attains the height of forty feet. The leaves are bipinnate and smooth, leaflets eight or ten pairs. Spines sharp and in pairs. Flowers in globose heads, and the fruit a legume.

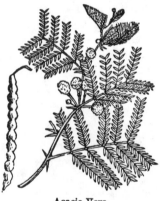

Acacia Vera.

History.—The tree inhabits the southern portion of Asia and the upper portion of Africa. The gum flows naturally from the bark of the trees, in the form of a thick and rather frothy liquid, and speedily concretes into tears ; sometimes the discharge is promoted by wounding the trunk and branches. The more ruptured the tree, the more gum it yields. The best quality of Gum Arabic is colorless, or very pale yellow-white, shining, transparent in small fragments, hard but pulverable, inodorous, and of a sweet and viscous taste. It invariably forms a white powder. Cold or hot water dissolves its own weight, forming a thick mucilaginous solution.

Properties and Uses.—The gum is nutritive and demulcent, and exerts a remarkably soothing influence upon irritated or inflamed mucous surfaces, by shielding them from the influence of deleterious agents, atmospheric air, etc. It is useful, in diarrhœa and dysentery, to remove griping and painful stools, in catarrh, cough, hoarseness, consumption, gonorrhœa, and all inflammatory conditions of the mucous surfaces. For lung diseases it is especially an indispensable vehicle in which to carry the necessary curative and powerful corrective agents, while at the same time its nutritive qualities also exert a good influence, often supplying the place of food where the stomach is too weak to partake of anything else. It may be given almost *ad libitum* in powder, lozenge, or solution, alone or combined with syrups, decoctions, etc. It constitutes the menstruum of my well-known Acacian Balsam, see page 470.

ADDER'S TONGUE (ERYTHRONUM AMERICANUM).

COMMON NAMES. *Dog-Tooth Violet, Serpent's Tongue, etc.*
MEDICINAL PARTS. *The bulb and leaves.*

Description.—This is a perennial plant, springing from a bulb at some distance below the surface. The bulb is white internally and fawn-colored externally. The leaves are two, lanceolate, pale green, with purplish or brownish spots, and one nearly twice as wide as the other. It bears a single drooping yellow flower, which partially closes at night and on cloudy days. Fruit a capsule.

History.—This beautiful little plant is among the earliest of our spring flowers, and is found in rich open grounds, or in thin woods throughout the United States, flowering in April or May. The leaves are more active than the roots; both impart their virtues to water.

Properties and Uses.—It is emetic, emollient, and antiscorbutic when fresh; nutritive when dried. The fresh root simmered in milk, or the fresh leaves bruised and often applied as a poultice to scrofulous tumors or ulcers, together with a free internal use of an infusion of them, is highly useful as a remedy for scrofula. The expressed juice of the plant, infused in cider, is very beneficial in dropsy, and for relieving hiccough, vomiting, and hematemesis, and bleeding from the lower bowels.

AGRIMONY (AGRIMONIA EUPATORIA).

COMMON NAMES. *Cockleburr or Sticklewort.*
MEDICINAL PARTS. *The root and leaves.*

Description.—Agrimony has a reddish, tapering, not creeping root, with brown stems covered with soft silky hairs; two or three feet high; leaves alternate, sessile, interruptedly pinnate. The stipule of the upper leaves large, rounded, dentate, or palmate. The flowers grow at the top of the stem, are yellow, small, and very numerous, one above another in long spikes, after which come rough heads hanging downwards, which will stick to garments or anything that rubs against them.

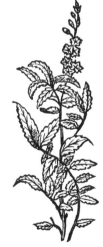

History.—This perennial plant is found in Asia, Europe, Canada, and the United States, along roadsides, and in fields and woods, flowering in July or August. Both the flowers and roots are fragrant, but harsh and astringent to the taste, and yield their properties to water or alcohol.

Properties and Uses.—It is a mild tonic, alterative, and astringent. Useful in bowel complaints, chronic

Agrimony.

mucous diseases, chronic affections of the digestive organs, leucorrhœa,

2*

certain cutaneous diseases, etc. A strong decoction, sweetened with honey, is an invaluable cure for scrofula, if persisted in for a length of time. It is exceedingly useful in gravel, asthma, coughs, and obstructed menstruation. As a gargle for sore throat and mouth, it is very service able.

Dose.—Powder, one teaspoonful; decoction, a wineglassful.

ALDER (Prinos Verticillatus).

Common Name. *Winterberry.*
Medicinal Parts. *The bark and berries.*
Description.—This is an indigenous shrub of irregular growth, with a stem six or eight feet in height; bark grayish and alternate branches. The leaves are ovate, acute at the base, olive green in color, smooth above and downy beneath. Flowers small and white; calyx small and six-cleft; corolla divided into six obtuse segments. Fruit a berry.

History.—Black Alder is common throughout the United States and England, growing in moist woods, swamps, etc., flowering from May to July, and maturing its fruit in the latter part of autumn. It yields its virtues to water by decoction or infusion. The bark has a bitterish, sub astringent taste, and the berries have a sweetish taste.

Properties and Uses.—It is tonic, alterative, and astringent. It is very beneficial in jaundice, diarrhœa, gangrene, dropsy, and all diseases attended with great weakness. Two drachms of the powdered bark and one drachm of powdered golden seal infused in a pint of boiling water, and, when cold, taken in the course of the day, in doses of a wineglass-ful, and repeated daily, has proved very efficacious in dyspepsia. Ex ternally the decoction forms an excellent local application in gangrene, indolent ulcers, and some affections of the skin. The berries are cathar-tic and vermifuge, and form, with cedar apples, a pleasant and effectual worm medicine for children.

Dose.—Powdered bark, half a drachm to a drachm; decoction, a tea-spoonful three or four times a day.

ALE HOOF (Nepeta Glechoma).

Common Names. *Gill-go-by-the-ground, Ground Ivy, Cat's-Foot, Turnhoof, &c.*
Medicinal Part. *The leaves.*
Description.—This plant is a perennial gray, hairy herb, with a pro-cumbent creeping stem, varying in length from a few inches to one or two feet. The leaves have petioles, cordate, and hairy on both sides. The flowers are bluish purple. The corolla is about three times as long as the calyx.

History.—This plant is common to the United States and Europe, where it is found in shady places, waste grounds, dry ditches, &c. It flowers in May or August. The leaves impart their virtues to boiling water by infusion. They have an unpleasant odor, and a harsh, bitterish, slightly aromatic taste.

Properties and Uses.—It is stimulant, tonic, and pectoral, and is useful in diseases of the lungs and kidneys, asthma, jaundice, hypochondria, and monomania. An infusion of the leaves is very beneficial in lead-colic, and painters who make use of it are seldom, if ever, troubled with that affection. The fresh juice snuffed up the nose often cures the most inveterate headache

Dose.—Powder, half a drachm to a drachm; infusion, one or two fluid ounces.

ALL-HEAL (PRUNELLA VULGARIS).

COMMON NAMES. *Hercules Wound Wort, Panay, etc.*
MEDICINAL PART. *The root.*
Description.—This shrub sometimes attains the height of five feet, but is usually much smaller. The stem is strong and round, with many joints, with some leaves thereat. The leaves consist of five or six pair of wings, and when chewed have a bitterish taste. The root is thick and long, the juice of which is hot and biting. The flower is a small and yellow one, and the seeds whitish yellow, short and flat.

History.—This plant is found in England and other parts of Europe. In England it flowers usually until the end of summer, but in other parts of Europe it flowers from May to December.

Properties and Uses.—All-heal is a pungent and bitter tonic and antispasmodic. It has also vermifuge properties, and is slightly diuretic. It is excellent for cramps, fits, falling sickness, convulsions, etc. (inferior, however, to Blue Vervain). In obstructions of the liver it serves a good purpose. It sometimes cures the toothache by inserting cotton saturated with the juice into the decayed places of the teeth.

ALMONDS (AMYGDALUS COMMUNIS).

AMYGDALA AMARA, *Bitter Almonds;* AMYGDALA DULCIS, *Sweet Almonds.*
MEDICINAL PART. *The kernels.*
Description.—The almond tree is from ten to eighteen feet high, with a pale-brown rugged bark, and dividing into many branches. The leaves are of a bright light green, two to four inches long, and about three-fourths of an inch wide. Flowers are moderately large, pink or white, sessile, in pairs, and appearing before the leaves. Calyx reddish, petals variable in size. The fruit is a hoary drupe; stone oblong or

ovate, hard in various degrees, always rugged and pitted with irregular holes.   Both the bitter and sweet almonds come from this tree.

History.—The almond tree is indigenous to most of the southern parts of Asia and Barbary, but is cultivated in Southern Europe.   The best of the sweet kind comes from Malaga.   The sweet kernel is without odor, and of a pleasant flavor; that of the bitter is also inodorous, unless rubbed with water, when it exhales a smell similar to Prussic acid.   Its taste is similar to that of peach-meats.   Both varieties contain oil—the sweet a fixed oil, the bitter both a fixed and an essential oil, impregnated with Prussic acid.   The oil of bitter almonds has a golden color, an agreeable odor, an acid bitter taste, combustible, and is a poison acting in the same manner as Prussic acid.   One drachm of this oil, dissolved in three drachms of alcohol, forms the "essence of almonds" much used by confectioners, perfumers, etc.   The oil is also much used by soap-makers.

Properties and Uses.—Triturated with water, sweet almonds produce a white mixture called *emulsion*, or *milk of almonds*, bearing a remarkable analogy with animal milk.   It is used as a demulcent and vehicle for other medicines.   The oil is demulcent in small quantity, in larger doses laxative.   It is frequently employed in cough, diseases dependent upon intestinal irritation, and for mitigating acrimonious urine in calculous affections.

Dose.—Of the oil, a teaspoonful.

ALNUS RUBRA (Tag Alder).

COMMON NAMES.   *Common Alder*, *Smooth Alder*.
MEDICINAL PART.   *The bark.*

Description.—This is a well-known shrub, growing in clumps, and forming thickets on the borders of ponds and rivers, and in swamps. The stems are numerous, and from six to fifteen feet high.   The leaves are obovate, acuminate, smooth, and green, from two to four inches long.

History.—The Alnus Rubra is indigenous to Europe and America, and blossoms in March and April.   The bark is the part used medicinally.

Properties and Uses.—The bark is universally acknowledged to be alterative and emetic, and is especially recommended for scrofula, secondary syphilis (inferior, however, to Rock Rose or Stillingia), and cutaneous diseases, of which there are many varieties, some of which have and some of which have not been classified.   The active principle of *Alnus Rubra*, as prepared for practitioners, is called *Alnuin*, and is most excellent in cases of dyspepsia produced by inactivity of the gastric glands.

AMARANTH (Amaranthus Hypochondriasis).

COMMON NAMES. *Prince's Feather, Red Cock's Comb, etc.*
MEDICINAL PART. *The leaves.*

Description.—This is an annual herb, with a stout upright stem, from
from three to four feet high. The leaves are ob-
long, lanceolate, mucronate, green, with a red
purplish spot, clustered flowers, five stamens.

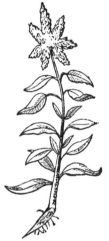

History.—This plant is a native of the Middle
States, where it is cultivated in gardens as an ornamental plant, but contains more medicinal virtues
in its wild state. It flowers in August. The leaves
impart their virtues to water.

Properties and Uses.—Amaranth is astringent.
The decoction drank freely is a valuable domestic
remedy for menorrhagia, diarrhœa, dysentery, and
hemorrhage from the bowels. It is useful as a
local application to ulcers of the mouth and throat,
as an injection for leucorrhœa, and as a wash to
foul, indolent ulcers.

ANEMONE (Anemone Nemorosa).

Amaranth.

COMMON NAME. *Wind Flower.*
MEDICINAL PARTS. *Root, herb, and seed.*

Description.—This is a delicate and pretty plant, with a creeping root,
simple erect stem, six to nine inches high, bearing but a single flower ;
leaves ternate ; sepals, four to six ; stamens and ovaries numerous.

History.—This plant is common to Europe and the United States,
bearing purplish and white flowers in April and May. The *Meadow
Anemone* of Europe is the most active in its medicinal qualities. Its
active principle is called *Anemonine.* This plant affords the *Pulsatilla*
of the *Homœopaths.*

Properties and Uses.—Anemone in solution has been applied externally to scald head, ulcers, syphilitic nodes, paralysis, cataract, and
opacity of the cornea, with benefit. A decoction is sometimes used as
an emmenagogue for secondary syphilis, whooping-cough, etc. The
leaves, fresh and bruised, act as a rubefacient. Care should be taken
in its internal administration, as it is acrid and poisonous.

A plant of the same family, *Anemone Cylindrica,* is used by the Indians for the cure of the rattle-snake bite. They chew some of the tops
of the plant, swallowing but little of the saliva, then apply it to the bite ;
in a few minutes the bite is rendered harmless.

Dose.—Decoction, a tablespoonful ; anemonine, one grain.

ANGELICA (ANGELICA ATROPURPUREA).

COMMON NAME. *Masterwort.*

MEDICINAL PART. *Root, herb, and seed.*

Description.—This plant is five or six feet high. The root has a purple color; leaves ternate, with large petioles; calyx five-toothed, with equal petals, and the fruit a nut.

History.—The plant is perennial, and grows in fields and damp places, developing greenish-white flowers from May to August. The plant has a powerful, peculiar, but not unpleasant odór, a sweet taste, afterwards pungent; but in drying it loses much of these qualities.

Properties and Uses.—It is aromatic, stimulant, carminative, diaphoretic, expectorant, diuretic, and emmenagogue. It is used in flatulent colic and heart-burn. It is serviceable in diseases of the urinary organs. The *A. Archangelica,* or *Archangel,* may be substituted for this.

Dose.—Decoction, two to four ounces; powder, thirty to sixty grains.

ANISE (PIMPINELLA ANISUM).

COMMON NAME. *Aniseed.*

MEDICINAL PART. *The fruit.*

Description. —Anise has a perennial, spindle-shaped, woody root, and a smooth, erect, branched stem, about ten or twelve inches in height. The leaves are petiolated, roundish, cordate, serrate; flowers small and white, disposed on long stalks. *Calyx* wanting, or minute. The fruit is ovate, about an eighth of an inch long, dull brown, and slightly downy.

History.—It is a native of Egypt, but now cultivated in many of the warm countries of Europe. The Spanish Aniseed is commonly used for medicinal purposes. The odor of anise is penetrating and fragrant, the taste aromatic and sweetish. It imparts its virtues wholly to alcohol, only partially to water. That used in cordials is the *Star Anise,* which is procured from the *Illicium Anisatum,* a plant of Eastern Asia. Its volatile oil is often fraudulently substituted for the European oil of anise.

Properties and Uses.—Stimulant and carminative; used in cases of flatulency, colic of infants, and to remove nausea. Sometimes added to other medicines to improve their flavor or to correct disagreeable effects.

Dose.—Of the seed, twenty to forty grains; essence, thirty drops to a teaspoonful.

ALOES (ALOE SPICATA).

MEDICINAL PART. *The inspissated juice of the leaves.*

Description.—The spiked aloe is an inhabitant of the southern parts of Africa, growing in sandy soil. The stem is woody, round, and about four feet high, and from three to five inches in diameter. The leaves are thick and fleshy, with a few white spots. Spike a foot long; flowers scarlet, and filled with purplish honey. This tree furnishes the *Cape Aloes* of commerce. There are other varieties, the *A. Socotrina* and the *A. vulgaris.* The Socotrine aloes is an inhabitant of Socotra, and the Aloe Vulgaris is generally found in the East Indies and Barbary.

History.—Aloes is of a deep brown or olive color; odor unpleasant, taste peculiar and bitter, powder a bright yellow. These properties change somewhat in the different varieties. It is almost completely dissolved in water.

Properties and Uses.—Aloes is tonic, purgative, emmenagogue, and anthelmintic. As a laxative its applications are limitless. It acts chiefly upon the rectum, causing heat and irritation about the anus; it is therefore improper, unless associated with other medicines, to give it to patients suffering with piles. It promotes the menstrual flow, but when used for this purpose it had better be combined with myrrh. Its chief use is as a purgative, and it should never be given in inflammatory affections, in gastritis or enteritis, or to females liable to sudden uterine evacuation, or during pregnancy.

Dose.—Two to ten grains in pill.

ASARABACCA (ASARUM EUROPÆUM).

COMMON NAMES. *Hazlewort, or Wild Nard.*

MEDICINAL PARTS. *Root and leaves.*

Description.—The stem of this plant is very short, simple round and herbaceous, bearing dark-green reniform leaves; also one drooping flower of purple color, without corolla. The fruit is a capsule.

History.—This is a European plant, growing in moist hilly woods, and flowers from May to August. The root, when dried, has a pepper-like odor, spicy taste, and yields an ash-colored powder; the leaves give a green powder, and have the same medicinal properties as of the root. They impart their virtues to water or alcohol.

Properties and Uses.—Emetic, cathartic, and errhine. Used principally as an errhine in certain affections of the brain, eyes, face, and throat, toothache, and paralysis of the mouth and tongue. It is used by drunkards in France to promote vomiting.

Dose.—Powder, 10 or 12 grains; as an emetic, from one-half to one drachm.

AYA-PANA (AYA-PANA EUPATORIUM).

MEDICINAL PARTS. *The whole plant.*

Description.— While traveling in Paraguay, South America, some years ago, I became acquainted with a species of *Eupatorium* or *Lungwort* called *Aya-pana*, possessed of most extraordinary virtues in consumption and other diseases of the chest. In Paraguay, which is a very paradise on earth, numerous medicinal herbs of exceeding great value grow to the greatest perfection. The *Aya-pana* belongs to the class of *Eupatorium Perfoliatum*, though quite unlike the *Lungwort* and *Thorough-wort*, indigenous to North America. The *Aya-pana* is only found on the eastern slope of the Andes, on the mountain sides, along the sunny banks of streams, and beautifully luxuriant on all the tributaries to the Amazon, and La Plata especially. It is a perennial plant, with numerous erect, round, hairy stems, five to ten feet high, the stalk plain below, but branching out in numerous stems near the top. The leaves grow on the opposite sides of the stalk in pairs, each pair being joined at

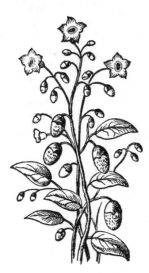

Aya-pana.

the base. The direction of each pair of leaves is at right angles with that of the pair either above or beneath. The leaves are long and narrow, broadest at the base where they coalesce, gradually tapering to a serrated point, wrinkled, palish green on the under surface, and beset with white silken hairs, which add much effect to their greenish-gray color. The flowers are snow-white, slightly tinged with a purplish hue at the end, very numerous, supported on hairy peduncles. The calyx is cylindrical, and composed of imbricated, lanceolate, hairy scales, inclosing from twelve to fifteen tubular florets, having their border divided into five spreading segments. There are five black anthers united in a tube, through which a bifid filiform style projects above the flower, rendering the whole a beautiful and picturesque plant.

History.—It flowers constantly during the dry or sunny season, the blossoms and leaves being only used for medicinal purposes. The flowers are better than the leaves, have an aromatic odor, resembling slightly chamomile, and possess a strong bitter taste, somewhat like horehound or quassia, which virtue is imparted either to water or alcohol. Resin, gum, balsam, and mucilage are among the principal constituents of the flowers. The flowers are gathered in the morning on sunny days, carefully dried in the sun or by artificial heat, when they are put up in bags or cedar boxes, and become ready for medicinal use. Prepared in this way, the flowers and leaves retain their properties for years, improving in their virtues by age, adding to their rich honey-like yellow coloring matter when distilled for medical purposes.

Properties and Uses.—This plant may rightly be regarded as a specific in all forms of pulmonary and bronchial affections. It has also great influence over the valvular action of the heart, in its healthful invigoration of the arterial and venous systems, and its wonderful power in expelling carbonic acid from the air-cells and pulmonary vessels, prior to the elimination of rich vermilion blood through the great aorta of the human economy.

It is one of the ingredients of my "Acacian Balsam" (see page 470), which, with various other remarkable medicinal agents, forms one of the most wonderful remedies for coughs, colds, and consumption ever compounded. The plant is not much known in this country, and only imported by myself, and can consequently not be had in apothecaries'.

BALM (MELISSA OFFICINALIS).

MEDICINAL PART. *The herb.*

Description.—Balm is a perennial herb, with upright, branching, four-sided stems, from ten to twenty inches high. The leaves are broadly ovate, acute, and more or less hairy. The flowers are pale yellow, with ascending stamens.

History.—Balm is a native of France, but naturalized in England and the United States. It grows in fields, along road-sides, and is well known as a garden plant, flowering from May to August. The whole plant is official or medicinal, and should be collected previous to flowering. In a fresh state it has a lemon-like odor, which is nearly lost by drying. Its taste is aromatic, faintly astringent, with a degree of persistent bitterness. Boiling water extracts its virtues. Balm contains a bitter extractive substance, a little tannin, gum, and a peculiar volatile oil. A pound of the plant yields about four grains of the oil, which is of a yellowish or reddish-yellow color, very liquid, and possessing the fragrance of the plant in a high degree. The *Nepeta Citriodora*, a powerful emmenagogue, is sometimes cultivated and employed by mistake for Balm. It has the same odor, but may be distinguished by having both surfaces of the leaves hairy.

Properties and Uses.—It is moderately stimulant, diaphoretic, and antispasmodic. A warm infusion, drank freely, is very serviceable to produce sweating, or as a diaphoretic in fevers. It is also very useful in painful menstruation, and also to assist the courses of females. When given in fevers, it may be rendered more agreeable by the addition of lemon-juice. The infusion may be taken at pleasure.

BALMONY (CHELONE GLABRA).

COMMON NAMES. *Snake head, Turtle bloom. Salt rheum weed.*

MEDICINAL PART. *The leaves.*

Description.—This is a perennial, smooth, herbaceous plant, with

simple erect stem about two or three feet high. The leaves are opposite, sessile, oblong-lanceolate, acuminate, serrate, and of a dark shining
green color. The fruit is a capsule.

History.—This valuable medical plant is found in the United States,
in damp soils, flowering in August and September. The flowers are
ornamental, and vary in color according to the variety of the plant. The
leaves are exceedingly bitter, but inodorous, and impart their virtues to
water and alcohol.

Properties and Uses.—It is tonic, cathartic, and anthelmintic; very
valuable in jaundice, liver diseases, and for the removal of worms. In
small doses it is a good tonic in dyspepsia, debility of the digestive
organs, and during convalescence from febrile and inflammatory diseases. An ointment made from the fresh leaves is valuable for piles,
inflamed breasts, tumors, and painful ulcers.

Dose.—Of the powdered leaves, one drachm; of the tincture, one or
two teaspoonsful; of the active principle, *Chelonin*, one or two grains.

BARBERRY (BERBERIS VULGARIS).

MEDICINAL PART. *Bark and berries.*

Description.—Barberry is an erect, deciduous shrub, from three to
eight feet high, with leaves of an obovate-oval form, terminated by soft
bristles, about two inches long, and one-third as wide. The flowers are
small and yellow, in clusters, and the fruit bright-red oblong berries, in
branches, and very acid.

History.—This shrub is found in the New England States, on the
mountains of Pennsylvania and Virginia, among rocks and hard gravelly
soil. Occasionally it is found in the West on rich grounds. It flowers
in April and May, and ripens its fruit in June. Its active principle is
Berberina.

Properties and Uses.—It is tonic and laxative, indicated in jaundice,
chronic diarrhœa, and dysentery. The berries form an agreeable acidulous draught, useful as a refrigerant in fevers; the bark is bitter and
astringent, and used in the treatment of jaundice. The bark of the root
is the most active; a teaspoonful of the powder will act as a purgative.
A decoction of the bark or berries will be found of service as a wash or
gargle in aphthous sore mouth and chronic ophthalmia.

BAYBERRY (MYRICA CERIFERA).

COMMON NAME. *Wax Myrtle.*

MEDICINAL PART. *The bark of the root.*

Description.—This shrub is branching and partially evergreen, and
varies in height from two to a dozen feet. The flowers appear in May,

before the leaves are fully expanded. The fruits are small and globular, resembling berries, which are at first green, but become nearly white. They consist of a hard stone, inclosing a two-lobed and two-seeded kernel. On the outside of the stone are gunpowder-like grains, and over these is a crust of dry greenish-white wax.

History.—Bayberry is found in woods and fields, from Canada to Florida. The bark of the root is the officinal part, but the wax is also used. Water must be employed to extract the astringent principles of the root-bark, alcohol to extract its stimulating virtues. The period at which the root should be collected is the latter part of fall. Cleanse it thoroughly, and while fresh separate the bark with a hammer or club. Dry the bark thor-

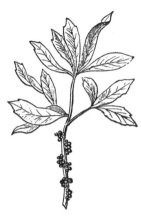

Bayberry.

oughly and keep it in a dry place ; then pulverize, and keep the powder in dark and sealed vessels. In order to obtain the wax, boil the berries in water ; the wax will soon float on the surface, and may be removed when it becomes cold and hardened.

Properties and Uses.—The bark has been successfully used in scrofula, jaundice, diarrhœa, dysentery, and in other cases where astringent stimulants were indicated. Powdered, it has been employed as a snuff, with curative effect, in catarrh of the head and nasal polypus. It is sometimes applied, in poultice form, to old ulcers, sores, tumors, etc. ; but is better for these when combined with Bloodroot. The wax possesses mild astringent with narcotic properties. The real properties of Bayberry bark are found in a preparation called *Myricin*, which is a stimulant and astringent, and can be employed to the best advantage in dysentery with typhoid symptoms, chronic diarrhœa, scrofula, and follicular stomatitis. Its greatest and most salutary influence is exerted over a diseased condition of the mucous surface. Myricin should be administered internally by the advice of a physician acquainted with its virtues. It may be applied externally to sores, ulcers, etc., by anybody ; but its immediate effects must be neutralized by a poultice of slippery elm

ARBERRY (ARCTOSTAPHYLOS UVA-URSI).

COMMON NAME. *The Upland Cranberry.*

MEDICINAL PART. *The Leaves.*

Description.—Bearberry is a small, perennial shrub, having a long fibrous root. The stems are woody and trailing ; bark smooth. The leaves are alternate, evergreen, obovate, acute, and have short petioles. The fruit is a small, scarlet-colored drupaceous berry.

History.—This plant is a perennial evergreen, common in the northern part of Europe and America. It grows on dry, sterile, sandy soils, and gravelly ridges. The berries ripen in winter, although the flowers appear from June to September. The green leaves, picked from the stems in the fall and dried in a moderate heat, are the parts used. These leaves are odorless until reduced to powder, when the odor emitted is like that of dried grass. The powder is of a light brown color, tinged with a yellowish green. The taste is astringent and bitterish. The properties of the leaves are extracted by alcohol or water. A preparation called *Ursin* is made from them.

Properties and Uses.—Uva Ursi is especially astringent and tonic, depending upon these qualities for the most of its good effects. It is particularly useful in chronic diarrhœa, dysentery, profuse menstruation, piles, diabetes, and other similar complaints. It possesses rare curative principles when administered for diseases of the urinary organs, more especially in chronic affections of the kidneys, mucous discharges from the bladder, inflammation of the latter organ, and all derangements of the water-passages. It is also a valuable assistant in the cure of gonorrhœa of long standing, whites, ulceration of the *cervix uteri* (or neck of the womb), pain in the vesical region, etc. Many physicians now rely upon it as the basis of their remedy for gonorrhœa which is accompanied by mucous discharges, and for all kindred afflictions. Its tannic acid gives it great power in rectifying and extirpating the obstinate and disagreeable complaints we have mentioned.

Dose.—The dose of the powder is ten to forty grains; of the decoction, one to two fluid ounces—(to make this, boil a pint and a half of pure water, containing one ounce of uva ursi, down to a pint); of the extract, five to ten grains.

BEARS BED (POLYTRICHIUM JUNIPERUM).

COMMON NAMES. *Hair-cap Moss, Robin's Rye, Ground Moss.*
MEDICINAL PART. *The whole plant.*

Description.—This is an indigenous plant, having a perennial stem, slender, of a reddish color, and from four to seven inches high; leaves lanceolate, and somewhat spreading. The fruit a four-sided oblong capsule.

History.—This evergreen plant is found in high, dry places, along the margins of dry woods, mostly on poor sandy soil. It is of darker green color than the mosses in general. It yields its virtues to boiling water.

Properties and Uses.—This plant is not much known as a remedial agent, but is nevertheless a valuable remedy. It is a powerful diuretic, and very serviceable in dropsy. It is very useful in gravel and urinary obstructions. It causes no nausea or disagreeable sensations in the stomach, and may be used with the hydragogue cathartics with decided advantage in dropsical affections.

BEAD TREE (MELIA AZEDARACH).

COMMON NAME. *Pride of China.*
MEDICINAL PART. *The bark of the root.*

Description.—This is an elegant tree, which attains the height of thirty or forty feet, with a trunk about a foot and a half in diameter. The bark is rough; leaves bipinnate; flowers lilac color; calyx five-parted; corolla has five petals; stamens deep violet; anthers yellow. The fruit is a five-celled bony nut.

History.—It is a native of China, but cultivated in the warm climates of Europe and America. It does not grow to any extent north of Virginia, and flowers early in the spring. Its name of *Bead Tree* is derived from the use to which its hard nuts are put in Roman Catholic countries, viz., for making rosaries. The recent bark of the root is the most active part for medicinal purposes. It has a disagreeably bitter taste and a very unpleasant odor, and imparts its properties to boiling water.

Properties and Uses.—The bark is anthelmintic, and in large doses narcotic and emetic. It is useful in worm fevers and in infantile remittents, in which, although worms are absent, yet the symptoms are similar to those accompanying the presence of worms.

The fruit is somewhat saccharine, and is an excellent remedy to expel worms. Its pulp is used as an ointment for destroying lice and other ectozoa, as well as in treatment of scald head and other diseases of the skin. The oil of the nuts is useful as a local application in rheumatism, cramps, obstinate ulcers, etc.

Dose.—Of the powdered bark, twenty grains; of the decoction (which is the best form for administration—two ounces of the bark to a pint of water, and boiled down to a half a pint), a tablespoonful every one, two, or three hours, till the desired effect is obtained. A purgative should follow its employment.—See "*Renovating Pill*," page 473.

BELLADONNA (ATROPA BELLADONNA).

COMMON NAMES. *Deadly Night-shade, Dwale, Black Cherry, etc.*
MEDICINAL PART. *The leaves.*

Description.—This perennial herb has a thick, fleshy, creeping root, and an annual erect leafy stem about three feet high. Leaves ovate, acute, entire, on short petioles, and of a dull green color. The flowers are dark purple, and fruit a many-seeded berry.

History.—This plant is common to Europe, growing among ruins and waste places, blossoming from May to August, and maturing its fruit in September. The leaves should be gathered while the plant is in flower. They yield their virtues to water and alcohol.

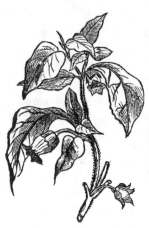

Belladonna.

Properties and Uses. — Belladonna is an energetic narcotic. It is anodyne, antispasmodic, calmative, and relaxant; exceedingly valuable in all convulsive diseases. It is much used as a preventive of scarlatina, and as a cure for whooping-cough. It dilates the pupil of the eyes very measurably, and they should always be watched whenever the plant is administered. In the hands of the educated herbal physician it is a very useful remedy; but I caution my readers not to use it in domestic practice.

BETH-ROOT (Trillium pendulum).

.COMMON NAMES. *Wake Robin, Indian Balm, Ground Lily, etc.*

MEDICINAL PART. *The root.*

Description.—This is an herbaceous, perennial plant, having an oblong tuberous root, from which arises a slender stem from ten to fifteen inches high. The leaves are three in number, acuminate, from three to five inches in diameter, with a very short petiole. The flowers are white, sepals green, petals ovate and acute, styles erect, and stigmas recurved.

History.—This plant is common in the Middle and Western States, growing in rich soils and shady woods, flowering in May and June. There are many varieties, all possessing analogous medicinal properties. These plants may be generally known by their three net-veined leaves, and their solitary terminal flower, which varies in color in the different species, being whitish-yellow and reddish-white. The roots have a faint turpentine odor, and a peculiar aromatic and sweetish taste. When chewed they impart an acid astringent impression to the mouth, causing a flow of saliva and a sensation of heat in the throat and fauces. *Trilline* is its active principle.

Properties and Uses.—It is astringent, tonic, and antiseptic, and is successfully employed in bleeding from the lungs, kidneys, and womb, excessive menstruation, and likewise in leucorrhœa or whites, and cough, asthma, and difficult breathing. Boiled in milk, it is of eminent benefit in diarrhœa and dysentery. The root made into a poultice is very useful in tumors, indolent and offensive ulcers, stings of insects, and to restrain gangrene; and the leaves boiled in lard are a good application to ulcers, tumors, etc. The red Beth-root will check ordinary epistaxis, or bleeding of the nose. The leaves boiled in lard is a good external application in ulcers and tumors. A strong infusion of powdered Beth-root, of from two to four tablespoonfuls, is the most pleasant form of administration of this valuable remedy.

Dose of the powdered root is one drachm, to be given in hot water; of the infusion, two to four ounces.

BIRDS' NEST (MONOTROPA UNIFLORA).

COMMON NAMES. *Ice Plant, Fit Plant, Ova-ova, Indian Pipe.*
MEDICINAL PART. *The root.*
Description.—This plant has a dark-colored, fibrous, perennial root, matted in masses like a chestnut vine, from which arise one or more short ivory-white stems, four to eight inches high, adorned with white, sessile, lanceolate leaves.

History.—This singular plant is found from Maine to Carolina, and westward to Missouri, growing in shady, solitary places, in rich moist soil, or soil composed of decayed wood and leaves. The whole plant is ivory-white, resembling frozen jelly, and when handled melts away like ice. It flowers from June to September. It is evidently a parasite of the roots at the base of trees.

Properties and Uses.—It is tonic, sedative, and antispasmodic. It is useful in fevers, and employed in instances of restlessness, pains, nervous irritability, etc., in place of opium. It cures remittent and intermittent fevers, and may be employed instead of quinine. Prompt success has followed its use in convulsive diseases. The juice of the plant mixed with rose-water forms an excellent application to sore eyes, or as an injection in gonorrhœa. It is very singular that people will use injurious drugs, or permit themselves to take them, when in this queer little herb that grows all around them, and which by its singular character invites attention to it, they can find a sovereign remedy for numberless ills.

Dose.—Of the powdered root, half a drachm to a drachm, two or three times a day.

BITTER ROOT (APOCYNUM ANDROSÆMIFOLIUM).

COMMON NAMES. *Dog's-bane, Milk-weed, etc.*
MEDICINAL PART. *The root.*
Description.—This is a smooth, elegant plant, five or six feet high, with a large perennial root. The leaves are dark-green above, pale beneath, ovate, and about two or three inches long and an inch wide. Corolla white, calyx five-cleft, and stamens five. Fruit a follicle. Every part of the plant is milky.

History.—This plant is indigenous to the United States, growing in dry, sandy soils, and in the borders of woods, from Maine to Florida, flowering from May to August. When any part of the plant is wounded a milky juice exudes. The large, milky root is the part used for medicinal purposes. It possesses an unpleasant amarous taste. It yields its properties to alcohol, but especially to water. Age impairs its medicinal quality.

Properties and Uses.—Emetic, diaphoretic, tonic, and laxative. It is very valuable in all liver or chronic hepatic affections. In conjunction with *Menispermin*, it is excellent in dyspepsia and amenorrhœa. When it is required to promptly empty the stomach, without causing much nausea or a relaxed condition of the muscular system, the powdered root may be given in two or three scruple doses; but much prostration is apt to ensue. As a laxative it is useful in constipation. As a tonic, ten or twenty grains may be given to stimulate the digestive apparatus, and thus effect a corresponding impression on the general system. It is also useful as an alterative in rheumatism, scrofula, and syphilis.

BITTER-SWEET (AMARA DULCIS, SOLANUM DULCAMARA).

COMMON NAMES. *Mortal, Woody Nightshade, Felon Wort, etc.*
MEDICINAL PART. *Bark of root and twigs.*

Description.— Bitter-Sweet is a woody vine, with a shrubby stem several feet in length, having an ashy green bark. Leaves acute, and

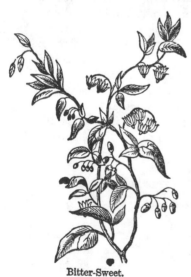

generally smooth, lower one cordate, upper ones hastate. The flowers are purple, and the fruit a scarlet, juicy and bitter berry, which, however, should not be eaten or used.

History.—Bitter-Sweet is common to both Europe and America, growing in moist banks, around dwellings, and in low damp grounds, about hedges and thickets, and flowering in June and July. The berries ripen in autumn, and hang upon the vines for several months. After the foliage has fallen the twigs should be gathered. Boiling water and dilute alcohol extract their virtues.

Properties and Uses.—It is a mild narcotic, diuretic, alterative, diaphoretic, and discutient. It is serviceable

Bitter-Sweet.

in cutaneous diseases, syphilitic diseases, rheumatic and cachectic affections, ill-conditioned ulcers, scrofula, indurations, sores, glandular swellings, etc. In obstructed menstruation it serves a good purpose.

It is of incalculable benefit in leprosy, tetter, and all skin diseases. It excites the venereal functions, and is in fact capable of wide application and use. I regard this plant as important as any in the herbal kingdom, and too little justice is done to it by those under whose care the sick are entrusted. It receives but half the homage that is due to it.

The world knows the virtues of my "Herbal Ointment" (see page 472), and which is in great measure due to Bitter-Sweet, as it is one of the ingredients.

Dose.—Of the decoction, one or two fluid ounces; extract, two to five grains; powdered leaves, ten to thirty grains.

BLUE FLAG (IRIS VERSICOLOR).

MEDICINAL PART. *The rhizome.*

Description.—Blue Flag is an indigenous plant, with a fleshy, fibrous rhizome. The stem is two or three feet in height, round on one side, acute on the other, and frequently branched. The leaves are ensiform, about a foot long, half an inch to an inch wide. The fruit a three-celled capsule.

History.—Blue Flag is common throughout the United States, growing in moist places, and bearing blue or purple flowers from May to July. The root has a peculiar odor, augmented by rubbing or pulverizing, and a disagreeable taste. It imparts its virtues to boiling water, alcohol, or ether. The root should be sliced transversely, dried, and placed in dark vessels, well closed, and placed in a dark place; it will then preserve its virtues for a long time. The *oleo-resin* obtained from it is called Iridin, its active principle.

Properties and Uses.—This is one among our most valuable medicinal plants, capable of extensive use. It is alterative, cathartic, sialogogue, vermifuge, and diuretic. In scrofula and syphilis it acts as a powerful and efficient agent, and I employ it in my special treatment of chronic diseases extensively and successfully. It is useful in chronic hepatic, renal, and splenitic affections, but had best be combined with mandrake, poke, black cohosh, etc. It will sometimes salivate, but it need cause no apprehension; and when this effect is established, it may be distinguished from mercurial salivation by absence of stench, sponginess of the gums, and loosening of the teeth.

Dose.—Powdered root, five to ten grains; Iridin, one grain.

BLUE VERVAIN (VERBENA HASTATA).

COMMON NAMES. *Wild Hyssop, Simpler's Joy.*

MEDICINAL PART. *The root and herb.*

Description.—Vervain is an erect, tall, elegant, and perennial plant,

3

with a four-angled stem three or four feet high, having opposite branches. The leaves are petiolate, serrate, acuminate, and hastate. The flower is a small purplish blue one, sessile, and arranged in long spikes. Seeds, four.

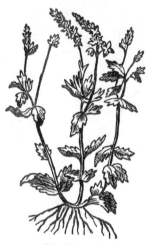

Blue Vervain.

History.— Vervain is indigenous to the United States, and grows along roadsides, and in dry, grassy fields, flowering from June to September. It is also found in England, growing among hedges, by the way-side, and other waste grounds, flowering in July, and the seeds ripening soon after.

Properties and Uses.—Vervain is tonic, expectorant, sudorific, and antispasmodic. It is serviceable in mismenstruation. It is an antidote to poke-poisoning. It expels worms, and is a capital agent for the cure of all diseases of the spleen and liver. If given in intermittent fever, in a warm infusion or powder, it never fails to effect a cure. In all cases of cold and obstinate menstruation it is a most complete and advantageous sudorific. When the circulation of the blood is weak and languid, it will increase it and restore it to its proper operation. The infusion, taken cold, forms a good tonic in cases of constitutional debility, and during convalescence from acute diseases. Its value has been found to be great in scrofula, visceral obstructions, and stone and gravel. It will correct diseases of the stomach, help coughs, wheezing, and shortness of breath, etc., but its virtues are more wonderful still in the effect they produce upon epilepsy, or falling sickness, and fits.

This great—very great—medicinal value of this plant was brought to my attention by an accidental knowledge of the good it had effected in a long-standing case of epilepsy. Its effects in that case were of the most remarkable character, and I was, therefore, led to study most carefully and minutely its medicinal peculiarities. I found, after close investigation and elaborate experiment, that, prepared in a certain way, and compounded with boneset, water-pepper, chamomile blossoms, and the best of whiskey, it has no equal for the cure of fits, or falling sickness, or anything like fits; also for indigestion, dyspepsia, and liver complaints of every grade. A more valuable plant is not found within the whole range of the herbal pharmacopœia. See "*Restorative Assimilant,*" page 469.

The following application is singularly effective in promoting the absorption of the blood, effusion in bruises, and allaying the attendant pain : Take of Vervain, Senna, and White Pepper, of each equal parts; make a cataplasm or plaster by mixing with white of eggs.

It is also most valuable as a cure for diarrhœa, stomachic and enteric pains, bowel complaints, and a superexcellent tonic.

I first brought the notice of physicians to this plant about twelve years ago, previous to which it was unknown as a remedy, but which is now used by very many physicians, whose reports of its virtues in various medical journals, published works, and to me by correspondence, are as flattering as my own.

Dose.—Of the powdered root, from one to two scruples; the dose of the infusion is from two to four wine-glassfuls three or four times a day, if an emetic is desired.

BLACK COHOSH (CIMICIFUGA RACEMOSA).

COMMON NAMES. *Rattleroot, Squaw Root, Black Snake Root.*
MEDICINAL PART. *The root.*

Description.—This plant is a tall, leafy perennial herb, with a large knotty root, having long slender fibres. The stem is simple. smooth, and furrowed, and from three to nine feet high. The flower is a small and fetid one.

History.—It is a native of the United States, inhabiting upland woods and hillsides, and flowering from May to August. The root is the medicinal part. It contains a resin, to which the names of *Cimicifugin* or *Macrotin* have been given; likewise fatty substances, starch, gum, tannic acid, etc. The leaves of *Cimicifuga* are said to drive away bugs; hence its name from *cimex*, a bug, and *fugo*, to drive away.

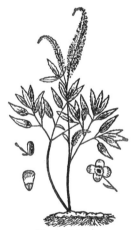

Boiling water takes up the properties of the root but partially, alcohol wholly.

Properties and Uses.—It is a very active and useful remedy in many diseases. It is slightly narcotic, sedative, antispasmodic, and exerts a

Black Cohosh.

marked influence over the nervous system. It is successfully used in cholera, periodical convulsions, fits, epilepsy, nervous excitability, asthma, delirium tremens, and many spasmodic affections, and in consumption, cough, acute rheumatism, neuralgia, and scrofula. Also, very valuable in amenorrhœa, dysmenorrhœa, and other menstrual and uterine affections, leucorrhœa, etc. The saturated tincture of the root is a valuable embrocation in all cases of inflammation of the nerves, tic doulou reux, *crick* in the back or sides, rheumatism, old ulcers, etc. It has an especial affinity for the uterus, and as it reduces very materially the arterial action, it is, hence, very useful in palpitation of the heart, and cardiac affections generally.

It exerts a tonic influence over mucous and serous tissues, and is a superior remedy in a variety of chronic diseases. In my special practice I use it largely, and its use, in conjunction with other indicated remedies, has afforded me flattering success in many chronic affections.

Dose.—Fluid extract, half a drachm to two drachms; solid extract, four to eight grains; of the tincture the dose is from one to three teaspoonsful; of *Cimicifugin* the dose is from one to six grains.

BLAZING STAR (LIATRIS SQUARROSA).

COMMON NAMES. *Gay Feather, Devil's Bit, etc.*
MEDICINAL PART. *The root.*
Description.—There are three varieties of this plant used in medicine. The above is the most common one. It has a tuberous root, and an erect annual stem from two to five feet high, linear leaves, and flowers sessile, and of bright purple color.

Liatris Spicata, or *Button Snake Root*, is very similar to the above.

Liatris Scariosa, or *Gay Feather*, has a perennial tuberous root, with a stout stem from four to five feet high. The leaves are numerous and lanceolate, lower one on long petioles.

History.—The two former are natives of the Middle and Southern States, and the latter is found from New England to Wisconsin. These splendid natives flower from August to September. The roots have a hot bitter taste and an agreeable turpentine odor. The virtues are extracted by alcohol.

Properties and Uses.—These plants are diuretic, tonic, stimulant, and emmenagogue. The decoction is very useful in gonorrhœa, gleet, and kidney diseases. It is also of service in uterine diseases. As a gargle in sore throat it is of great advantage. These plants are used for, and said to have antidotal powers over snake-bites.

BONESET (EUPATORIUM PERFOLIATUM).

COMMON NAME. *Thoroughwort.*
MEDICINAL PARTS. *The tops and leaves.*
Description.—Boneset is an indigenous perennial herb, with a horizontal crooked root; the stems being round, stout, rough and hairy, from one to five feet high, and the leaves veiny, serrate, rough, and tapering to a long point. The flowers are white and very numerous.

History.—Boneset grows in low grounds, on the borders of swamps and streams, throughout the United States, flowering in August and September. Alcohol or boiling water extracts the virtues of the parts used. It has a feeble odor, but a very bitter taste. It contains tannin and the extractive salts of potassa. It is called Boneset on account that it was formerly supposed to cause rapid union of broken bones.

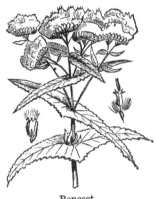

Boneset.

Properties and Uses.—It is a very valuable medicinal agent. The cold infusion or extract is tonic and aperient, the warm infusion diaphoretic and emetic. As a tonic it is very useful in remittent, intermittent, and typhoid fevers, dyspepsia, and general debility. In intermittent fever a stong infusion, as hot as can be comfortably swallowed, is administered for the purpose of vomiting freely. This is also attended with profuse diaphoresis, and, sooner or later, by an evacuation of the bowels. During the intermission the cold infusion or extract is given every hour as a tonic and antiperiodic. In epidemic influenza the warm infusion is valuable as an emetic and diaphoretic, likewise in febrile diseases, catarrh, colds, and wherever such effects are indicated. The warm infusion is also administered to promote the operation of other emetics. *Externally*, used alone or in combination with hops or tansy, etc., a fomentation of the leaves applied to the bowels is very useful in inflammation, spasms, and painful affections.

Boneset is one of the ingredients of my "Restorative Assimilant," and is certainly an excellent adjuvant to the Blue Vervain. (See page 469.)

Dose.—Of the powder, from ten to twenty grains; of the extract, from two to four grains; of the infusion, from two to four wineglassfuls.

BLACK ROOT (LEPTANDRIA VIRGINICA).

COMMON NAMES. *Culver's Physic, Tall Speedwell.*
MEDICINAL PART. *The root.*

Description.—It is perennial, with a simple, straight, smooth, herbaceous stem, and grows from three to four or five feet in height. The leaves are short petioled, whorled in fours to sevens, lanceolate, acuminate, and finely serrated. The flowers are white, nearly sessile, and very numerous. Calyx four-parted, corolla small and nearly white; stamens, two. The fruit is a many-seeded capsule.

History.—This plant is indigenous to the United States, but is to be found in good condition only in limestone countries. It is often discovered in new soil, in moist woods, in swamps, etc., but its medicinal virtues are feeble, excepting when it is found where there is limestone. The root is the part used. It is perennial, irregular, horizontal, woody, and about as thick as the forefinger. It is gathered in the fall of the second year. The fresh root should never be used, as it is very violent and uncertain in its operations. The dried root, after having been properly prepared, is what may be relied upon for beneficial effects. *Leptandrin* is its active principle.

Properties and Uses.—The fresh root is too irritant to be used, although a decoction of it may, with care, be used in intermittent fever. The dried root is laxative, cholagogue, and tonic, and very much used in chronic hepatic diseases. It is an excellent laxative in febrile diseases, and peculiarly applicable in bilious and typhoid fevers. As a laxative and tonic it is very useful in dyspepsia, especially when associated with torpidity of the liver. In diarrhœa and dysentery, as a cathartic it frequently effects a cure in one active dose. This admirable remedy is one of the ingredients of my "Renovating Pill," see page 473.

Dose.—Powdered root, twenty to sixty grains; infusion, half an ounce; leptandrin, one-fourth grain to a grain.

BLOODROOT (Sanguinaria Canadensis).

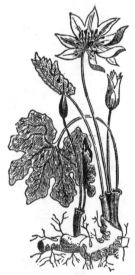

Bloodroot.

Common Name. *Red Puccoon.*
Medicinal Part. *The root.*

Description.—Bloodroot is a smooth, herbaceous, perennial plant, with a fibrous root, which when cut or bruised emits an orange-colored juice. From each bud of the root stalk there springs a single leaf about six inches high, and which is cordate and reniform. The flower is white, stamens short, and anthers yellow. The fruit is a two-valved capsule.

History.—Bloodroot grows throughout the United States, in shaded woods and thickets, and rich soils generally, and flowers from March to June. Although the whole plant is medicinal, the root is the part chiefly used. The fresh root is fleshy, round, and from one to four inches in length, and as thick as the fingers. It presents a beautiful appearance when cut and placed under a microscope, seeming like an aggregation of minute precious stones. The dried root is dark brown outside, bright yellow inside; has a faint virose odor, and a bitter and acrid taste. It may be readily reduced to powder. Its active properties are taken up by boiling water or by alcohol. Age and moisture impair the qualities of the root, and it is of the utmost consequence to get that which has been properly gathered, and not kept too long. It yields several principles, among which are sanguinaria, puccine, chelidonic acid, a yellowish fixed oil, lignin, and gum.

Properties and Uses.—The actions of Bloodroot vary according to administration. In small doses it stimulates the digestive organs, acting as a stimulant and tonic. In large doses it is an arterial sedative. It is useful in bronchitis, laryngitis, whooping-cough, and other affections of the respiratory organs. It excites the energies of a torpid liver, and has proved beneficial in scrofula, amenorrhœa, and dysentery. Applied to fungous growths, ulcers, fleshy excrescences, cancerous affections, the powder acts as an escharotic, and the infusion is often applied with benefit to skin diseases.

Dose.—Of the powder as an emetic, ten to twenty grains; as a stimulant and expectorant, three to five grains; as an alterative, half a grain to two grains. Tincture, twenty to sixty drops.

BOX (BUXUS SEMPERVIRENS).

MEDICINAL PART. *The leaves.*

Description.—Box is a small, dense-leaved, hard-wood evergreen tree. The leaves are ovate, deep shining green, becoming red in autumn; flowers pale yellow; and the fruit a six-seeded globular capsule.

History.—The box tree is a native of the west of Asia, but grows on dry hills and sandy elevations generally in Europe, and but rarely on similar soil in America. A preparation called *Buxina* is obtained from the powdered bark, but the leaves are the parts mainly used in medical practice. They readily impart their virtues to alcohol or water.

Properties and Uses.—It is cathartic, sudorific, and alterative. The preparations of the leaves are excellent for the expulsion of worms, for purging the bowels, and regulating the action of the liver; for breaking fevers, and for purifying the blood and glandular secretions. In syrup it is very valuable as a cure for all diseases of a syphilitic character, and may be used alone to great advantage, where the compound syrup of stillingia cannot be obtained. The stillingia is preferable if it is at all to be had. The dose of a strong decoction, or syrup, of box, is half a fluid ounce, three times a day. In very severe cases the dose may be increased to a fluid ounce; but this should not be undertaken excepting by the advice of a physician. When intestinal worms are to be destroyed or expelled, the powdered leaves are usually administered in, to children, doses of five grains; to adults, in doses of from ten to fifteen grains. It possesses antispasmodic qualities, and has been given with good effect in hysteria, epilepsy, chorea (St. Vitus' Dance), etc. Chips of the wood (decoction) are useful in chronic rheumatism. The chief value of the *Buxus Sempervirens*, however, centres in its antisyphilitic virtues. I combine it with corydalis (Turkey pea) and the compound syrup of stillingia, in such a manner that it will *surely* cure syphilis in the first, second, or third stage; also certain forms of scrofula and scurvy. In other diseases it is no better than many other plants mentioned in this book.

The reader will do well to remember that the common garden box possesses the medical qualities of the *Buxus Sempervirens* to a feeble extent only. The powerful antisyphilitic virtues of which I have spoken can be procured only from the leaves of the tree reared in Asia, the influences of that climate being requisite to perfect them.

BUCHU (BAROSMA CRENATA).

MEDICINAL PART. *The leaves.*

Description.—This plant has a slender, smooth, upright, perennial stem, between two and three feet high. The leaves are opposite, flat, about an inch long, ovate or obovate, acute, serrated, and dotted. The flowers are pink, and fruit an ovate capsule.

History.—The Buchu plant is a native of Southern Africa. It does not grow very prolifically. There are two other varieties from which the leaves are taken, and which are of equal value with the *Barosma Crenata.* The leaves are the parts which are termed officinal. The Hottentots gather these leaves (which emit a sort of minty odor) and powder them. "The powder," says a traveler, "they have named *Booko,* and they use it for *anointing* their bodies." They also distil the leaves, and obtain from them a strong spirituous liquor somewhat resembling pale brandy, which they not only use for convivial purposes, but for the cure of various diseases, particularly those which are located in the stomach, bladder, bowels, and kidneys. A decoction of the leaves is systematically applied by them, with success, we are told, to wounds; but this is an assertion of which we have no direct proof. As we get them, the leaves are nearly, or quite, an inch in length, and from a sixth to half an inch in width, elliptical, lanceolate, slightly acute, or shorter and obtuse; their margin is serrated and glandular, upper surface smooth, and of a clear shining green, the under surface paler, with scattered oil points. They taste and smell like pennyroyal; but are neither heating nor bitter when chewed. They have to be kept very carefully, if their odor and virtues are desired to be thoroughly preserved for any reasonable length of time. The leaves of all the varieties are somewhat similar, and possess about the same qualities. They yield their volatile oil and extractive (upon which their virtues are mainly dependent) to alcohol or water.

Properties and Uses.—Buchu is aromatic and stimulant, diuretic and diaphoretic. It is employed in dyspepsia with a palliative effect, but is chiefly administered in chronic inflammation of the bladder, irritation of the membrane of the urethra, uric acid gravel, diabetes in its first stage, and in incontinence of urine. It is recommended, without good reason, for cutaneous and rheumatic affections. I have no doubt Buchu is of some importance in chronic diseases of the urino-genital organs, for I have tried it; but I am sure that we have many native remedies which are altogether superior, and which are neglected only because the public is so familiar with them that they do not care to give them a fair trial.

Dose.—Of the powder, twenty to thirty grains; infusion, two to four ounces; tincture, one or two drachms; fl. extract, thirty to sixty drops.

BURNING BUSH (Euonymus Atropurpureus).

COMMON NAMES. *Wahoo, Spindle Tree, etc.*
MEDICINAL PART. *The bark of the root.*

Description.—Wahoo is a small shrub or bush, with smooth branches, and from five to ten feet high. The leaves are from two to five inches in length, lanceolate, acute, and finely serrate. Flowers dark purple, and the fruit a crimson, five-celled capsule. There is another variety known as *Euonymus Americanus*, which is equally useful medicinally, and this and the foregoing are both known by the name of *Wahoo* better than by any other title.

History.—These plants grow in many sections of the United States, in woods and thickets, and in river bottoms, flowering in June. The bark of the root has a bitter and unpleasant taste in its natural shape, and yields its qualities to water and alcohol. The active principle is *Euonymin.*

Properties and Uses.—It is tonic, laxative, alterative, diuretic, and expectorant. It is serviceable in dyspepsia, torpid liver, constipation, dropsy, and pulmonary diseases. In intermittents it serves a good purpose.

Dose.—Of the powder, twenty to thirty grains; tincture, one to four drachms; Euonymin, one-eighth to half a grain.

BUTTER WEED (Erigeron Canadense).

COMMON NAMES. *Colt's Tail, Pride Weed, Horse Weed, Canada Flea-Bane.*
MEDICINAL PART. *The whole plant.*

Description.—This is an indigenous, annual herb, with a high bristly, hairy stem, from six inches to nine feet high. The leaves are lanceolate; flowers small, white, and very numerous.

History.—Butterweed is common to the Northern and Middle States,

3*

grows in fields and meadows, by road-sides, and flowers from June to September. It should be gathered when in bloom, and carefully dried. It has a feeble odor, somewhat astringent taste, and yields its virtues to alcohol or water.

Properties and Uses.—It is tonic, diuretic, and astringent. It is useful in gravel, diabetes, dropsy, and in many kidney diseases. It can also be employed in diarrhœa, dysentery, etc. The volatile oil may be used instead of the infusion.

Dose.—Of the powder, half a drachm; infusion, two to four ounces; fl. extract, teaspoonful; oil, from four to six drops on sugar.

CAHINCA (CHIOCOCCA RACEMOSA).

COMMON NAME. *Snow Berry.*

MEDICINAL PART. *The bark of the root.*

Description.—This is a climbing shrub, with a round branched root, and a stem from eight to twelve feet high. The leaves are ovate and smooth; flowers white and odorless, and become yellow and redolent; calyx, five-cleft; corolla, funnel-shaped; stamens, five. The fruit is a small white berry.

History.—This plant is a native of the West Indies, Florida, and South America. The root has a coffee-like taste, of a reddish-brown color, and a disagreeable. odor. It affords the *Cahincic Acid,* its most important medicinal agent.

Properties and Uses.—In medium doses it aids the urinary discharge, increases the action of the heart, and promotes perspiration. It has been found efficient in amenorrhœa, rheumatism, syphilis, etc., and is used in Brazil as an antidote to snake-bites.

Dose.—Of the powder, from twenty to sixty grains.

CALICO BUSH (KALMIA LATIFOLIA).

COMMON NAMES. *Sheep Laurel, Spoonwood, Mountain Laurel, Lamb-kill.*

MEDICINAL PART. *The leaves.*

Description.—This handsome plant is a shrub from four to eight feet high, with crooked stems and a rough bark. The leaves are evergreen, ovate, lanceolate, acute at each end, on long petioles, and from two to three inches long. The flowers are white and numerous. The fruit is a dry capsule.

History. — Sheep Laurel inhabits the rocky hills and elevated grounds of most parts of the United States. Its beautiful flowers appear in June and July. The leaves are reputed to be poisonous to sheep and other animals, and it is said that birds which have eaten them will poison those who eat the birds. The leaves are the officinal part. Attention was called to their medicinal virtues by the use which the Indians make of them, viz., a decoction by which they commit suicide.

Properties and Uses.—The plant, in medicinal doses, is antisyphilitic, sedative to the heart, and somewhat astringent. It is a most efficient agent in syphilis, fevers, jaundice, neuralgia, and inflammation. The preparation should be used with great care and prudence. In cases of poisoning with this plant, either man or beast, whiskey is the best antidote. Externally, stewed with lard, it is serviceable as an ointment for various skin diseases.

Dose.—The saturated tincture of the leaves is the best form of administration. It is given in from ten to twenty drops every two or three hours. Powdered leaves, from ten to twenty grains.

CANCER ROOT (OROBANCHE VIRGINIANA).

COMMON NAME. *Beech Drops.*
MEDICINAL PART. *The plant.*

Description.—This is a parasitic plant, with a smooth, leafless stem from a foot to a foot and a half in height, with slender branches given off the whole length of it. The root is scaly and tuberous.

History.—This plant is native to North America, and generally a parasite upon the roots of beech trees, flowering in August and September. The whole plant is of a dull red color, without any verdure. It has a disagreeable, astringent taste It yields its virtues to water and alcohol.

Properties and Uses.—An eminent astringent. Used with benefit in fluxes and in diarrhœa, but possesses no property of curing cancer. It can be used with advantage in erysipelas. Locally applied to wounds, it prevents or arrests the process of mortification. It is also useful as an application to obstinate ulcers, aphthous ulcerations, etc., etc. It exerts the same influence upon the capillary system as the mineral drug tincture of iron.

CANNABIS INDICA.

COMMON NAME. *Indian Hemp.*
MEDICINAL PART. *The root.*

Description.—This is an herbaceous annual, growing about three feet high, with an erect, branched, angular bright green stem. The leaves are alternate. or opposite, on long lax foot-stalks, roughish, with sharply serrated leaflets tapering into a long, smooth entire point. The male flowers are drooping and long, the females simple and erect. The seeds are small, ash-colored, and inodorous.

History.—Cannabis Indica, or Cannabis Sativa, is a native of the Caucasus, Persia, but grows in the hilly regions of Northern India. It is cultivated in many parts of Europe and Asia; but medicine of value can only be made from the Indian variety, the active principle of the plant being developed only by the heat of the climate of Hindostan. The dried tops and resin are the parts used. The preparations called *Churrus, Gunjah, Bhang, Hashish*, etc., sold in this country, are mostly feeble imitations of the genuine articles, and are comparatively worthless. Even the few specimens of the genuine productions which reach the shops, and are sold at high prices, are crude and inferior, and can in no wise impart the effects which attach to the pure article. It is a matter of great difficulty to procure the genuine article even direct from dealers in India, unless you have had years of experience as a practising herbal physician, and have established business connections in various parts of the world as an importer of rare and pure medicinal herbs, barks, roots, resins, etc.

The *Cannabis Sativa*, or common hemp, possesses similar properties, and can be substituted if the Asiatic hemp is not procurable.

Properties and Uses.—It is narcotic, anodyne, and antispasmodic. It has been successfully employed in gout, neuralgia, rheumatism, lockedjaw, convulsions, chorea, hysteria, and uterine hemorrhage; but it is chiefly valuable as an invigorator of mind and body. Its exhilarating qualities are unequalled, and it is a certain restorative in low mental conditions, as well as in cases of extreme debility and emaciation. In such cases it may be regarded as a real rejuvenator. It should be taken by the advice of one experienced in its uses, in order that its merits may be properly and fairly experienced. The spurious hemp should never be taken, as it produces, what the genuine does not, unpleasant consequences. I have used this article in many a preparation with great success.

CASSIA MARILANDICA.

COMMON NAMES. *American Senna, Wild Senna.*
MEDICINAL PART. *The leaves.*

Description.—This is a perennial herb, growing from four to six feet high, with round, smooth, and slightly hairy stems. The leaves have long petioles, ovate at base; each petiole has eight or ten leaflets, which are oblong, smooth, mucronate, an inch or two long, and quite narrow. The flowers are bright yellow, and the fruit is a legume from two to four inches long.

History.—The American Senna is to be found from New England to Carolina, growing in rich soils here and there. It flowers from June to September, and the leaves are gathered, for their medicinal virtues, while the plant is in bloom. They yield their virtues to alcohol or water.

Properties and Uses.—It is one of the most important herbal cathartics furnished by America, and is mentioned here solely on the ground that it is equally valuable as the foreign Senna, or ordinary Senna of the drug-shops, and costs much less. The analysis of the leaves shows that they contain albumen, mucilage, starch, yellow coloring matter, volatile oil, fatty matter, resin, lignin, and salts of potassa, and lime.

Dose.—Of the powder, from a half-drachm to two and a half drachms; infusion, four or five ounces

CATECHU (ACACIA CATECHU).

COMMON NAMES. *Cutch, Gambir, Terra Japonica.*
MEDICINAL PART. *Extract of the wood.*
Description.—Catechu is a small-sized tree from fifteen to twenty feet high. The bark is thick, and branches spreading. Leaves bipinnate. Flowers numerous, white or pale yellow, and the fruit a legume.
History.—This tree is common to the East Indian continent, thriving in Bengal, and on the Malabar coast. As found in the shops it is in square, round, and irregular pieces, variable in color, friable, odorless, astringent taste. Soluble in hot water, depositing a reddish matter on cooling.
Properties and uses.—This is a strong astringent. In chronic diarrhœa, chronic catarrh, chronic dysentery, it proves beneficial, and it is a valuable agent as a local application in throat diseases, especially such as singers are subject to. The tincture is often useful as a local application to fissured nipples of nursing women.
Dose.—Of the powder, from five to twenty grains; of the tincture, from twenty minims to half an ounce.

CEDRON (SIMABA CEDRON).

MEDICINAL PART. *The seed.*
Description.—*Simaba* is a small tree, with an erect stem about half a foot in diameter, branching luxuriantly at the top. Leaves obovate, large, and serrated; flowers sessile, pale brown, and the fruit a solitary drupe.
History.—This tree grows in New Grenada and Central America. Its value as a medicinal agent has long been known in Costa Rica, Trinidad, etc., and from thence was communicated to scientific gentlemen in France. The seed, which is the part used, is about an inch and a half long, nearly an inch broad, and about half an inch thick. It is hard, but can be easily cut by a common knife. It is inodorous, but tastes like quassia or aloes, and yields its properties to water or alcohol. In South America the properties of these seeds were known as early as the year 1700. At that time they were applied more especially as an antidote to the bites of poisonous serpents, and similar affections.
Properties and Uses.—It is an antispasmodic, and one of the most valuable articles of the kind known to educated herbalists. It is very

useful in all nervous affections, and is administered in one or two grain doses. As it can only be obtained from those who, like myself, import it especially, it is unnecessary to say that it should not be administered without the advice of competent herbal physicians. To give an idea of its value as an antispasmodic, I mention that it is a *cure* for hydrophobia, and an antidote for the majority of acro-narcotic poisons.

CELANDINE (CHELIDONIUM MAJUS).

COMMON NAME. *Tetter Wort.*
MEDICINAL PARTS. *Herb and root.*

Description.—This plant is an evergreen perennial, with a stem from one to two feet in height, branched, swelled at the joints, leafy, round, and smooth; the leaves are smooth, spreading, very deeply pinnatified; leaflets in from two to four pairs, from one and a half to two and a half inches long, and about two-thirds as broad, the terminal one largest, all ovate, cuneately incised or lobed; the lateral ones sometimes dilated at the lower margin, near the base almost as if auricled; color of all, a deep shining green; the flowers are bright yellow, umbellate, on long, often hairy stocks.

History.—Celandine is a pale green, fleshy herb, indigenous to Europe and naturalized in the United States; it grows along fences, by-roads, in waste places, etc., and flowers from May to October. If the plant be wounded, a bright yellow, offensive juice flows out, which has a persistent, nauseous, bitter taste, with a biting sensation in the mouth and fauces. The root is the most intensely bitter part of the plant, and is more commonly preferred. Drying diminishes its activity. It yields its virtues to alcohol or water.

Properties and Uses.—It is stimulant, acrid, alterative, diuretic, diaphoretic, purgative, and vulnerary. It is used internally in decoction or tincture, and externally in poultice or ointment for scrofula, cutaneous diseases, and piles. It is likewise good in hepatic affections, or liver complaints, and exerts a special influence on the spleen. As a drastic hydragogue, or purge, it is fully equal to gamboge. The juice, when applied to the skin, produces inflammations, and even vesications. It has long been known as a caustic for the removal of warts; it is also applied to indolent ulcers, fungous growths, etc., and is useful in removing specks and opacities of the cornea of the eye.

Celandine is from the Greek word *Chelidon*, which signifies a swallow. The ancients assert that if you put out the eyes of young swallows when they are in the nest, the old ones will restore their eyes again with this herb. It is said that we may mar the apple of the bird's eye with a needle, and that the old birds will restore their sight again by means of this herb. Never having made any such cruel experiments, I am not prepared to say whether any such miraculous power of healing loss of sight is a virtue of the plant, or whether it is an instinct or gift inherent of the swallow itself.

Celandine is also used in curing salt-rheum, tetter, or ringworm. It is superior to *arnica* as a vulnerary; an alcoholic tincture of the root (three ounces to a pint) will be found an unrivalled application to prevent or subdue traumatic inflammations.

Dose.—Of the powdered root, from half a drachm to one drachm; of the fresh juice, from twenty to forty drops, in some bland liquid; of the tincture, from one to two fluid drachms; of the aqueous extract, from five to ten grains.

CENTAURY (SABBATIA ANGULARIS).

COMMON NAME. *Rose Pink.*
MEDICINAL PART. *The herb.*

Description.—This plant has a yellow fibrous, biennial root, with an erect, smooth, quadrangular stem, with the angles winged, having many opposite branches, and growing from one to two feet in height. The leaves are opposite, fine-veined, smooth, entire, from one to five inches in length, and from half an inch to one and a half inches wide, clasping the stem. The flowers are numerous, from an inch and a quarter to an inch and a half in diameter, of a rich rose or carnation color, standing, as it were, at the tops of one umbril or tuft, very like those of *St. John's wort*, opening themselves in the day-time and closing at night, after which come seeds in little short husks, in forms like unto wheat corn. There are three varieties of the Centaury in England, one kind bearing white flowers, another yellow, and another red. All have medicinal properties, although the American variety is considered preferable to the European Centaury.

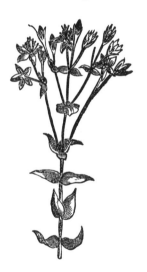

Centaury.

History.—This plant is common to most parts of the United States, growing in moist meadows, among high grass, on the prairies, and in damp, rich soils, flowering from June to September. The whole herb is used. It has a very bitter taste, and yields its virtues to water or alcohol. The best time for gathering it is during the flowering season. In England they use the red Centaury in diseases of the blood, the yellow in choleric diseases, and the white in those of phlegm and water.

Properties and Uses.—It is an excellent tonic. It is used in all fall periodic febrile diseases, both as a preventive and a remedy. It is also serviceable as a bitter tonic in dyspepsia and convalescence from fevers. When administered in warm infusion it is a domestic remedy for worms, and to restore the menstrual secretion.

Dose.—Of the powder, from half a drachm to a drachm ; of the cold infusion, a teacupful every two or three hours ; of the tincture, a wine-glassful ; of the extract, from two to six grains.

CENTURY PLANT (AGAVE AMERICANA).

COMMON NAME.   *South American Agave.*
MEDICINAL PART.   *The inspissated juice.*

Description.—This plant, which is also sometimes called the Century Plant, from an erroneous idea that it blossoms but once in a hundred years, is the largest of all herbaceous plants. It is an evergreen, and does not blossom often.

History.—It flourishes in the warmer latitudes of South America, where its juice is expressed by the natives and allowed to ferment. In this condition it is called *pulque*, and is used as an exhilarating beverage. The natives can drink large quantities of this liquor without getting very much intoxicated ; but it is very severe upon those who are not accustomed to it.

Properties and Uses.—The fresh juice is used by the South Americans to regulate the action of the bowels and kidneys, and is considered very valuable for dyspepsia and diseases of the bladder. The South American women use the juice and the decoction to promote menstruation. I can say of my own knowledge that, in proper combination, it is a superior anti-syphilitic, and that in scorbutic affections it is without many superiors. The dose is from half a fluid ounce to two ounces, three times a day.

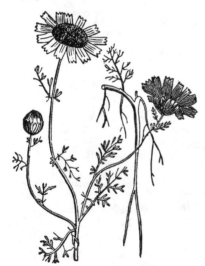

The *Agave Virginica*, or *False Aloe*, is not to be confounded with this, as that plant is a laxative and carminative.

CHAMOMILE (ANTHEMIS NOBILIS).

Chamomile.

MEDICINAL PART.   *The Flowers.*

Description.—This is a perennial herb, with a strong fibrous root. The stems in a wild state are prostrate, but in gardens more upright, about a span long, round, hollow, furrowed, and downy; the leaves pale green, pinnate, sessile, with thread-shaped leaflets. The flower-heads terminal, rather larger than the daisy, and of yellow color, or whitish.

History.—Chamomile is indigenous to Southern Europe; we have also a common or wild Chamomile (*Matricaria Chamomilla*) growing in the United States, but it is not considered as good as the Roman Chamomile for medicinal purposes, which is the kind I use. The white flowers are the best; they have an aromatic, agreeably bitter taste, and peculiar odor. They yield their properties to alcohol and water.

Properties and Uses.—Chamomile is a tonic; one or two teacupfuls of the warm infusion will usually vomit. The cold infusion is highly useful in dyspepsia, and in all cases of weak or irritable stomachs, also in intermittent and typhoid fevers. The oil is carminative and antispasmodic, and is used in flatulency, colic, cramp in the stomach, hysteria, nervous diseases, and painful menstruation.

A poultice of Chamomile will often prevent gangrene, and remove it when present. It is an ingredient in my "Restorative Assimilant," and is a most excellent adjutant and corrigent in that great remedy.

Dose.—Half a drachm to two drachms of the flowers. Of the infusion, half a teacupful to a teacupful; of the oil, five to fifteen drops on sugar.

CHERRY LAUREL (PRUNUS LAUROCERASUS).

MEDICINAL PART. *The leaves.*

Description.—This is a small evergreen shrub or tree with smooth branches. Leaves with short petioles, oval-oblong, serrate, acute, and smooth. Flowers shorter than the leaves, calyx inferior, corolla has five white petals; stamens about twenty; and fruit a round, black, smooth drupe.

History.—Originally a native of Asia Minor, from whence it was introduced into Europe in 1576, and subsequently from Europe to the United States. It is now common in gardens and shrubberies. The leaves have scarcely any odor until bruised, then they have a bitter almond odor; taste very bitter, aromatic, and slightly astringent. They impart their virtues to water and alcohol.

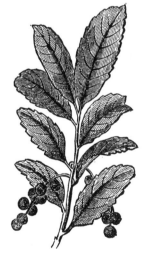

Cherry Laurel.

Properties and Uses.—An excellent sedative. Useful in tic-douloureux, phthisis, spasmodic cough, palpitation of the heart, and in all spasmodic affections.

Dose.—Powdered leaves, four to eight grains; laurel water, ten to thirty drops.

CHICKWEED (STELLARIA MEDIA).

MEDICINAL PART. *The herb.*

Description.—This plant is an annual or biennial weed, from six to fifteen inches in length, with a prostrate, brittle, and leafy stem. The leaves are ovate-cordate; the lower ones on hairy petioles. The flowers are small and white, petals two-parted, stamens three, five, or ten.

History.—It is a common plant in Europe and America, growing in fields and around dwellings, in moist, shady places. It flowers from the beginning of spring till the last of autumn. The seeds are eaten by poultry and birds. The whole herb is used when recent.

Properties and Uses.—It is a cooling demulcent. The fresh leaves bruised and applied as a poultice to indolent, intractable ulcers, even when of many years' standing, will produce most immediate and decided beneficial results, to be changed two or three times a day. The bruised leaves will likewise be found an invaluable application in acute ophthalmia. An ointment made by bruising the recent leaves in fresh lard, may be used as a cooling application to erysipelatous and other forms of ulceration, as well as many forms of cutaneous diseases.

CHOCOLATE ROOT, GEUM RIVALE (*Water Avens*), GEUM VIRGINI-ANUM (*White Avens*).

COMMON NAMES. *Throat Root, Purple Avens.*

MEDICINAL PART. *The root.*

Description.—GEUM RIVALE, or *Purple Avens*, is a perennial, deep green herb; woody root; leaves nearly lyrate, crenate-dentate, and from four to six inches long. The flowers are few and yellowish purple in color.

GEUM VIRGINIANUM, or *Throat Root*, is also a perennial, with a small, crooked root. The stem is two or three feet high. The leaves are pinnate or lyrate; flowers rather small and white; and the fruit an achenium. The former is common to the United States and Europe, flowering in June or July, and the latter only to the United States, flowering from June to August.

History.—These plants, with other varieties, have long been used in domestic practice. The whole herb contains medicinal properties, but the officinal and most efficient part is the root. Boiling water or alcohol extracts their virtues.

Properties and Uses.—Is tonic and astringent. It is used in passive and chronic hemorrhages, chronic diarrhœa and dysentery, leucorrhœa, dyspepsia, pulmonary affections, congestions of the abdominal viscera, etc.

Dose.—Of the powder, from twenty to thirty grains; of the decoction, from two tablespoonfuls to a wineglassful, three or four times a day.

CINCHONA.

COMMON NAMES. *Peruvian Bark, Jesuits' Bark.*
MEDICINAL PART. *The bark.*

Description.—The bark is obtained from the *Cinchona Calisaya, Cinchona Condaminea, Cinchona Succirubra,* and *Cinchona Lancifolia.* These trees are all evergreen trees or shrubs. Their generic character is to have opposite entire leaves; flowers white, or usually roseate or purplish, and very fragrant; calyx a turbinated tube; corolla salver-shaped; stamens, five; anthers, linear; style, simple; stigma, bifid. The fruit a capsule, ovate or oblong, filled with numerous winged seeds. About thirteen varieties of cinchona are known to commerce, but the above are the most important. Of these species the former three yield respectively the pale, yellow, and red cinchona barks, and the fourth is one of the sources of quinine.

History.—Cinchona is a very old discovery, and takes its name from the wife of the Spanish viceroy, Count de Cinchon, who was cured of fever by it, at Lima, about the year 1638. For some time after its introduction into Europe, the Jesuits, who received the bark from their brethren in Peru, alone used it, and kept to themselves the secret of its origin; and their use of it was so successful that it received

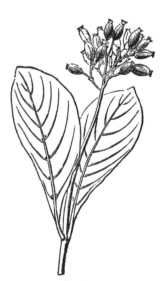

Cinchona.

the name which still clings to it of "Jesuits' Bark." The bark richest in the antiperiodic alkaloids is the Cinchona Calisaya. The geographical range of the cinchonas appears to be exclusively confined to the Andes, within the boundaries of Peru, Bolivia, Equador, and New Granada. Thirteen species furnish the barks of commerce, and all of them are found growing from one to ten thousand feet above the level of the sea. The four species we have named at the head of this article are, however, the only ones recognized by the United States Pharmacopœia, and are the favorites everywhere. Since the seventeenth century these barks have been the study of men versed in medical and chemical science, and they and the preparations made from them rank among the most important articles of the Materia Medica. It contains numerous active principles, but the most important, and one chiefly used, is quinine.

Properties and Uses.—Cinchona bark is tonic, antiperiodic, astringent to a moderate extent, and eminently febrifuge. It is topically (or externally) antiseptic, and is of much value when applied to gangrenous ulcerations, or used for gargles and washes in erysipelas, ulcerated sore throat, mouth, etc. I do not recommend the use of the bark in cases where the stomach is *very much* weakened (although it is employed in every disease in which there is deficient tone), because the woody fibre in the powder will most generally disagree. When taken internally it imparts a sensation of warmth to the stomach, which gradually spreads over the whole body; the pulse becomes stronger and is accelerated, and the various organs are gently stimulated. It may be used with benefit in ordinary cases of dyspepsia, general debility, and all febrile, eruptive, and inflammatory diseases, in whatever stage they may be. In all cases of night-sweating, or great feebleness, it is valuable. As an antiperiodic it is not surpassed by anything else used. When it excites nausea, add an aromatic; if purging, opium; if costiveness, rhubarb.

Quinine is a white flocculent powder, inodorous, and has a very bitter taste. It is very sparingly soluble in warm water, still less so in cold water. It is readily soluble in hot alcohol, and tolerably so in ether. It is always best to administer quinine instead of the bark, unless some of the effects of the other principles are desired.

Dose.—Of the powder, half a drachm to a drachm; fluid extract, ten to sixty drops; of quinine, from one to fifteen grains, according to purpose.

CINQUE-FOIL (POTENTILLA CANADENSIS).

COMMON NAME. *Five-Finger.*
MEDICINAL PART. *The root.*

Description.—This perennial plant has a procumbent stem from two to eighteen inches in length. The leaves are palmate, leaflets obovate, and flowers yellow, on solitary pedicels.

There are two varieties of this plant, the *P. Pamilla*, which is very small and delicate, flowering in April and May, and growing in dry, sandy soils, and the *P. Simplex*, a larger plant, growing in richer soils, and flowering from June to August.

History.—Five-finger is common to the United States, growing by road-sides, on meadow banks and waste grounds, and flowering from April to October. The root is the part used. It has a bitterish, styptic taste, and yields its virtues to water.

Properties and Uses.—It is tonic and astringent. A decoction is useful in fevers, bowel complaints, night sweats, menorrhagia, and other hemorrhages. It makes an excellent gargle for spongy, bleeding gums, and ulcerated mouth and throat.

The POTENTILLA TORMENTILLA, or *Sept-Foil* of Europe, possesses similar qualities, and may be used by my readers in that country if the American root is not to be obtained.

CLEAVERS (GALIUM APARINE).

COMMON NAMES. *Goose Grass, Catchweed, Bed-Straw.*
MEDICINAL PART. *The herb.*

Description.—It is an annual succulent plant, with a weak, procumbent, quadrangular, retrosely-prickled stem, which grows from two to six feet high, and is hairy at the joints. The leaves are one or two inches in length, and two or three lines in breadth; rough on the margin and tapering to the base. The flowers are white, small, and scattered.

History.—This plant is common to Europe and the United States, growing in cultivated grounds, moist thickets, and along banks of rivers, and flowering from June to September. In the green state the plant has an unpleasant odor; but it is inodorous when dried, with an acidulous, astringent, and bitter taste. Cold or warm water extracts the virtues of the plant; boiling water destroys them. The roots dye a permanent red.

Properties and Uses.—It is a most valuable refrigerant and diuretic, and will be found very beneficial in many diseases of the urinary organs, as suppression of urine, calculous affections, inflammation of the kidneys and bladder, and in the scalding of urine in gonorrhœa. It is contra-indicated in diseases of a passive character, on account of its refrigerant and sedative effects on the system, but may be used freely in fevers and all acute diseases. An infusion may be made by macerating an ounce and a half of the herb in a pint of warm water for two hours, of which from two to four fluid ounces may be given three or four times a day when cold. It may be sweetened with sugar or honey. It has also been found useful in many cutaneous diseases, as psoriasis, eczema, lichen, cancer, and scrofula, and is more particularly useful in these diseases when they are combined with strumous diathesis. The best form for administration is that of the inspissated juice, which may be in one or two drachm doses, three times a day.

The plant called GALIUM TINCTORIUM, or *Small Cleavers*, is nervine, anti-spasmodic, expectorant, and diaphoretic. It is used successfully in asthma, cough, and chronic bronchitis, exerting its influence principally upon the respiratory organs. The plant has a pungent, aromatic, pleasant, persistent taste. A strong decoction of the herb may be given in doses of from one to four fluid ounces, and repeated two or three times a day, according to circumstances. The root of this plant will also dye a permanent red.

COCA (ERYTHROXYLON COCA).

MEDICINAL PART. *The herb.*

Description.—I first became acquainted with this most remarkable plant many years ago, while traveling in Bolivia, South America, in the beautiful valleys of the Cordilleras. The Coca is a bush which rarely attains six feet in height, and does not often exceed three. Its foliage is of a bright green, its flowers white, and its fruit small and red. When the plants are just about eighteen inches high they are transplanted from the seed-beds into fields called *cocales*. The ripe leaves are gathered with the fingers. They are dried by spreading them in the sun, sometimes on woollen cloths. The operation requires great care, for the plant must be protected from all dampness, which changes its color, and thus diminishes its value. It is then packed in bags, weighing from fifty to one hundred and fifty pounds, which are often transported to great distances. In the Vice-royalty of Lima, in the latter part of the last century, CASTELNAU represents the consumption of the leaf at three and a half millions of pounds, and worth one million and a quarter of Spanish dollars, while at the same time the total consumption in Peru was two and a half millions of dollars. The importance of the Coca trade, however, is diminishing as the Red Man disappears. The Indians mix the Coca with a small quantity of lime, and constantly carry a small bag of it on all their excursions. They take it from three to six times a day. Dr. GSCHUDI [*Travels in Peru*, page 453] mentions an Indian of sixty-two years of age, who was employed by him, and though at very hard work for five days, took no other nourishment, and rested but two hours of the night. Immediately, or soon after this, he accomplished a journey of one hundred miles in two days, and said that he was ready to do the same thing again if they would give him a new supply of Coca. CASTELNAU says he himself knew of instances as extraordinary. In the time of the Incas the Coca was regarded as sacred.

Properties and Uses.—Its physiological actions are as follows:—

1. It stimulates the stomach and promotes digestion.

2. In large doses it augments animal heat and accelerates the pulse and respiration.

3. It induces slight constipation.

4. In moderate doses, from one to four drachms, it stimulates the nervous system, so as to render it more tolerant of muscular fatigue.

5. In larger doses it gives rise to hallucinations and true delirium.

6. Its most precious property is that of inducing the most pleasant visions ("*phantasmagoria*") without any subsequent depression of the nervous energies.

7. Probably it diminishes some of the secretions.

The Coca has doubtless many other medical properties of a high order, and deserves further investigation.

It stimulates powerfully the digestive functions, while at the same time it exercises a calmative influence over the mucous membranes of the stomach and bowels. In this double action upon the stomach—stimulant and calmative—it resembles Columbo.

It is anti-spasmodic, and is of great service in many nervous disorders, and particularly in *spermatorrhœa* and all debilities of the generative organs.

An infusion of the leaves, or a tincture of the flowers, leaves, and berries may be used in all cases of spermatorrhœa and nervous debility. Combined with other remedies it may be used with great advantage in fevers, pneumonia, pleuritis, neuralgia, hysteria, dysmenorrhœa, amenorrhœa, blenorrhœas (including gonorrhœa and leucorrhœa), chorea, epilepsy, paralysis, after-pains, convulsions, dyspepsia, delirium tremens, etc. My course of concentrated herbal remedies, in which Coca is a principal ingredient, will surely cure spermatorrhœa, seminal weakness, impotence, sterility, and barrenness, and I now use it extensively for all disorders arising from sexual debility. It never yet failed to meet my expectations—hundreds of such cases having been radically cured by its truly miraculous medicinal properties.

COLOCYNTH (CUCUMIS COLOCYNTHIS.)

COMMON NAME. *Bitter Cucumber.*

MEDICINAL PART. *The fruit divested of its rind.*

Description.—Colocynth is an annual plant, with a whitish root, and prostrate, angular, and hispid stems. The leaves are alternate, cordate, ovate, many-lobed, white with hairs beneath. Flowers yellow and solitary; petals small; and fruit globose, smooth, size of an orange, yellow when ripe, with a thin solid rind, and a very bitterish flesh.

History.—This plant is a native of the south of Europe, Asia, and Africa. The fruit assumes a yellow or orange color externally during the autumn, at which

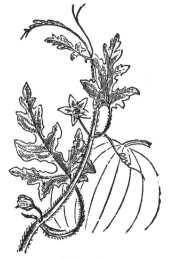

Colocynth.

time it is pulled and dried quickly, either in the stove or sun. That which is deprived of its rind, very white, light spongy, and without seeds, is the best article; all others are more or less inferior in quality.   It contains, besides oils, resins, and gums, bassorin and the sulphates of lime and magnesia.   *Colocynthin* is its active principle.

Properties and Uses.—It is a powerful hydragogue cathartic, producing copious watery evacuations.   It should never be used alone, but be combined with other cathartics.   It may be used advantageously in passive dropsy and cerebral derangements.   In combination with hyoscyamus it loses its irritant properties, and may be so employed whenever its peculiar cathartic effects are desired.   Hippocrates used colocynth as a pessary to promote menstruation.

Dose.—Five to ten grains.

COLT'S FOOT (Tussilago Farfara).

Common Names.   *Cough Wort, Foal's Foot, Horse Hoof, and Bull's Foot.*

Medicinal Part.   *The leaves.*

Description.—Colt's foot has a long, perennial, creeping, fibrous rhizome.   The leaves are erect, cordate, sharply dentate, smooth green above, and pure white and cottony beneath.   They do not appear until the flowers are withered, and are from five to eight inches long, and about an inch broad.   The flowers are large and bright yellow.

History.—This plant grows in Europe, the Crimea, Persia, Siberia, and the East Indies, from the sea-shore to elevations of nearly eight thousand feet.   It also grows in the United States, in wet places, on the sides of brooks, flowering in March and April.   Its presence is a certain indication of a clayey soil.   The leaves are rather fragrant, and continue so after having been carefully dried.   The leaves are the parts used, though all parts of the plant are active, and should always be employed, especially the leaves, flowers, and root.   The leaves should be collected at about the period they have nearly reached their full size, the flowers as soon as they commence opening, and the root immediately after the maturity of the leaves.   When dried, all parts have a bitter, mucilaginous taste, and yield their properties to water or diluted alcohol.

Properties and Uses.—It is emollient, demulcent, and slightly tonic. The decoction is usually administered in doses of from one to three or four fluid ounces, and is highly serviceable in coughs, asthma, whooping-cough, and other pulmonary complaints ; also useful in scrofula.   The powdered leaves form a good errhine for giddiness, headache, nasal obstructions, etc.   It is also used externally in form of poultice in scrofulous tumors.

COLUMBO (Cocculus palmatus).

Medicinal Part.   *The root.*

Description.—Columbo, so important in the present practice of medicine, is a climbing plant, with a perennial sort which is quite thick and branching. The root is covered with a thin brown skin, marked with transverse warts. ✎The stems, of which one or two proceed from the same root, are twining, simple in the male plant, branched in the female, round, hairy, and about an inch or an inch and a half in circumference. The leaves stand on rounded glandular-hairy footstalks, and are alternate, distant, cordate, and have three, seven, or nine lobes and nerves. The flowers are small and inconspicuous.

History.—This plant inhabits the forests near the southeastern coast of Africa, in the neighborhood of Mozambique, where the natives call it *Kalumb*. The root is dug up in the dry season in the month of March, and is cut in slices, strung on cords, and hung up to dry. The odor of Columbo is slightly aromatic; the taste bitter, and also mucilaginous. The root is easily pulverized, but spoils by keeping after having been reduced to a powder. It is best to powder it only as it is required for use. The active principle of Columbo is called *Columbin*. The root also yields *Berberin*, an excellent stomachic, which is produced from the Barberry.

Properties and Uses.—It is one of the purest bitter tonics in the world, and in dyspepsia, chronic diarrhœa, and dysentery, as well as in convalescence from febrile and inflammatory diseases, it can hardly be surpassed as a remedial agent. It is most useful in the remittent and intermittent fevers of hot climates. It is used in many combinations, according to indications.

Dose.—Of the powder, ten to thirty grains; of the infusion, one or two ounces; of the tincture, from one to two drachms.

COMFREY (SYMPHYTUM OFFICINALE).

MEDICINAL PART. *The root.*

Description.—Comfrey has an oblong, fleshy, perennial root, black on the outside and whitish within, containing a glutinous or clammy, tasteless juice, with divers very large, hairy, green leaves lying on the ground, so hairy, or so prickly, that if they touch any tender parts of the hands, face, or body, it will cause it to itch. The stalks are hollowed and cornered, very hairy, having leaves that grow below, but less and less up to the top; at the joints of the stalk it is divided into many branches, at the ends of which stand many flowers, in order one above another, which are somewhat long and hollow like the finger of a glove, of a pale, whitish color; after them come small black seeds. There is another sort which bears flowers of a pale purple color, having similar medicinal properties.

History.—Comfrey is a native of Europe, but naturalized in the United States, growing on low grounds and moist places, and flowering all summer. The root is official and contains a large amount of mucilage, which is readily extracted by water.

4

Properties and Uses.—The plant is demulcent and slightly astringent. All mucilaginous agents exert an influence on mucous tissues, hence the cure of many pulmonary and other affections in which these tissues have been chiefly implicated, by their internal use. Physicians must not expect a *serous* disease to yield to remedies which act on mucous membranes only; to determine the true value of a medicinal agent, they must first ascertain the true character of the affection, as well as of the tissues involved. Again, mucilaginous agents are always beneficial in scrofulous and anæmic habits. Comfrey root is very useful in diarrhœa, dysentery, coughs, hemoptysis or bleeding of the lungs, and other pulmonary affections; also in leucorrhœa and female debility: all these being principally affections of mucous membranes.

It may be boiled in water, wine, or made into a syrup, and taken in doses of from a wineglassful to a teacupful of the preparation, two or three times a day.

Externally the fresh root, bruised, forms an excellent application to bruises, ruptures, fresh wounds, sore breasts, ulcers, white swellings, etc.

CUNDURANGO (EQUATORIA GARCIANA).

MEDICINAL PART. *The bark of the vine.*

Description.—Cundurango, or Condor Vine, a name derived from two words, *cundur* and *angu*, whose marvellous medicinal properties have lately been made known to the world, and which is now so greatly interesting the medical profession, is a climbing vine, resembling much in its habits the grape vine of our forests. The vines are from three to five inches diameter. They are quite flexible when fresh, but when dry very brittle. The bark is externally of a greenish-gray color, and has numerous small warty excrescences. The leaves are large, sometimes reaching six inches in length by five in breadth, opposite, simple, entire, dentate, cordate, and of a dark green color. The flowers are small, arranged in complete umbels; stamens five; petals five; sepals five; and filaments small. The fruit is a pair of pods, and seeds numerous and dark brown. It should be more properly called *Cundurangu*, as there is no *o* in the language of the Incas.

History.—This plant is a native of the Andes Mountains in South America, especially the southern portion of Equador, and found most plentifully in the mountains surrounding the city of Loja. It is generally found on the western exposure of the Andes, at an altitude of 4,000 or 5,000 feet. Its virtues were known to the Indians of the locality for a long time. The tradition is that it was regarded by them as poisonous, and that an Indian woman unintentionally cured her husband, who suffered from a very painful cancer, giving him to drink bowlfuls of decoction of Cundurango, believing and hoping it would prove fatal. It was introduced into medical practice by Dr. Eguiguren, brother of the Governor of the province of Loja, both of whom cured many cases of syphilis and cancerous ulcers in the trial of it. The subject was brought to the notice of our government by our minister at Quito. The Department of State, at once realizing the value of the discovery and the intense interest with which our people would seek after information concerning it, published a circular, setting forth its great value as a remedy. This action of the government at once inspired that confidence to which the plant is entitled. It was tested in a case of cancer afflicting the mother of Vice-President Colfax, and at once asserted its value. It has since been used by progressive physicians, and the success it has given in cancerous and syphilitic affections renders it worthy of the name of a specific, equally as much so as cinchona. It is a singular coincidence that these two specific products of the herbal world should grow in the same regions. The natives insist that there are two varieties of the bark, the *amarillo*, or yellow, and *blanco*, or white; but upon inspection I find they are the same, the difference in color depending upon the strong rays of the sun. When freshly cut the vines give an abundance of milky, viscous juice or sap, the odor of which is balsamic, and flavor decidedly bitter and aromatic. It is not abundant, and hence necessarily of high price.

Properties and Uses.—An unequalled remedy for cancer, syphilis, ulcers, etc. In a short period, when taken, the typical symptoms subside, the pain is diminished, the discharge thickens and becomes less offensive, the tumor becomes softer, the deposits lessen, the expression improves, and a cure is speedily effected. It has also diuretic and tonic powers, and cures many nervous diseases. I have given this remedy competent trials in cases of cancer and syphilis, and the results were so satisfactory as to surprise me, and I am ready to assert that in Cundurango we have a remedy that will rob cancer of its terror, and one that will soon banish it from existence as a disease. Its price is exceedingly high, almost costing its weight in gold; but still that has not deterred me from using it in such cases as I deemed the requirement necessary.

Dose.—Of the powder, one to two drachms; fluid extract, one drachm. (Much that is spurious is sold in market.)

COPAIBA (Copaifera Officinalis).

COMMON NAME. *Balsam of Copaiba.*

MEDICINAL PART. *The oleo-resinous juice.*

Description.—Copaiba is a tall and handsome tree, with many small, crooked branches, and a grayish-brown bark. The leaves are large and equally pinnated, leaflets in pairs of from two to five, petioles short. The flowers are white; calyx four-parted; stamens, ten; fruit obovate, two-valved, and one-seeded.

History.—There are several species which furnish oil of copaiba, all natives of South America and West Indies. The juice is ob· tained by deep incisions being made in the trunk during or following the wet season; the balsam (which, however, is not a balsam, as it contains no benzoic acid) flows freely, being clear, transparent, and fluid, but becoming pale yellowish in time. The oil is unpleasant in smell and taste.

Properties and Uses.—In large doses Copaiba is an irritant, but in proper doses it is stimulant, cathartic, and diuretic. It exerts a favorable influence on the mucous tissues of the system, diminishing excessive secretions, and for this purpose it is chiefly employed. Taken internally it gives warmth to the gastric region, and sometimes provokes nausea and emesis. It is especially useful in chronic mucous affections, as gonorrhœa, bronchitis, diseases of the bladder, gleet, chronic catarrh, diarrhœa, and dysentery, etc., etc. It was formerly regarded as a specific for gonorrhœa, but has lost some of its prestige. Locally it is an excellent application to fistulas, chilblains, old ulcers, etc.

Dose. — From twenty to sixty drops in emulsion with yolk of egg and mint or cinnamon water.

CRANBERRY (High).—(VIBURNUM OPULUS.)

MEDICINAL PART. *The bark.*

Description.—It is a nearly smooth and upright shrub, or small tree, usually from five to twelve feet in height, with several stems from the same root branched above; the leaves are three-lobed, three-veined, broadly-wedged shape, and crenately toothed on the side. The flowers are white, or reddish-white; the fruit ovoid, red, very acid, ripens late, and remains upon the bush after the leaves have fallen. It resembles the common cranberry, and is sometimes substituted for it.

History.—It is indigenous to the northern part of the United States and Canadas, being a handsome shrub, growing in low rich lands, woods, and borders of fields, flowering in June, and presenting at this time a very showy appearance. The flowers are succeeded by red and very acid berries, resembling low cranberries, and which remain through the winter. The bark is the officinal part, as met with in drug-stores. It is frequently put up by Shakers, when it is somewhat flattened from pressure. It has no smell, but has a peculiar, not unpleasant, bitterish, und astringent taste. It yields its properties to water or diluted alcohol. *Viburnine* is its active principle.

Properties and Uses.—It is a powerful antispasmodic, and hence generally known among American practitioners as *Cramp Bark.* It is very effective in cramps and spasms of all kinds, as asthma, hysteria, cramps of females during pregnancy, preventing the attacks entirely if used daily for the last two or three months of gestation.

The following forms an excellent preparation for the relief of spasmodic attacks, viz. : take of Cramp bark, two ounces; scull-cap, skunk cabbage, of each one ounce; cloves, half an ounce; capsicum, two drachms. Have all in powder, coarsely bruised, and add to them two quarts of sherry or native wine. *Dose* of this, half a wineglassful two or three times a day.

It may here be remarked that a poultice of the fruit of the *Low* Cranberry is very efficacious in indolent and malignant ulcers, malignant scarlet fever, applied to the throat; in erysipelas, and other similar diseases. Probably the *High* Cranberry will effect the same result.

Dose.—Of the decoction, or vinous tincture, one glassful two or three times a day.

CRANESBILL (GERANIUM MACULATUM).

COMMON NAMES. *Dove's Foot, Crow Foot, Alum Root, Spotted Geranium, etc.*

MEDICINAL PART. *The root.*

Description.—This plant has a perennial, horizontal, thick, rough, and knotty root, with many small fibres. The stems are grayish-green, erect, round, and a foot or two high. The leaves are spreading and hairy, and the blossoms large, and generally purple, mostly in pairs. The Dove's Foot, or Cranebill, which grows in England, is a different plant, bearing many small bright-red flowers of five leaves apiece, though it possesses medicinal properties similar to the American varieties.

History.—Geranium is a native of the United States, growing in nearly all parts of it, in low grounds, open woods, etc., blossoming from April to June. The root is the officinal part. Its virtues are yielded to water or alcohol. *Geranin* is its active principle.

Properties and Uses.—It is a powerful astringent, used in the second stage of dysentery, diarrhœa, and cholera infantum; in infusion, with milk. Both internally and externally it may be used wherever astringents are indicated, in hemorrhages, indolent ulcers, aphthous sore mouth, ophthalmia, leucorrhœa, gleet, hematuria, menorrhagia, diabetes, and excessive chronic mucous discharges; also to cure mercurial salivation. Relaxation of the uvula may be benefited by gargling with a decoction of the root, as well as aphthous ulceration of the mouth and throat. From its freedom from any nauseous or unpleasant qualities, it is well adapted to infants and persons with fastidious stomachs. In cases of bleeding piles, a strong decoction of the root should be injected into the rectum, and retained as long as possible. Troublesome epistaxis, or bleeding from the nose, wounds, or small vessels, and from the extraction of teeth, may be checked effectually by applying the powder to the bleeding orifice, and, if possible, covering with a compress of cotton. With Aletri's Farinosa (*Unicorn root*) in decoction, and

taken internally, it has proved of superior efficacy in diabetes and in
Bright's disease of the kidneys. A mixture or solution of two parts of
hydrastin and one of geranin will be found of unrivalled efficacy in all
chronic mucous diseases, as in gleet, leucorrhœa, ophthalmia, gastric
affections, catarrh, and ulceration of the bladder, etc. A decoction of
two parts of geranium and one of sanguinaria (*Bloodroot*) forms an 'excellent injection for gleet and leucorrhœa.

Dose of geranium powder, from twenty to thirty grains; of the decoction, a tablespoonful to a wineglassful.

CRAWLEY (CORALLORHIZA ODONTORHIZA).

COMMON NAMES. *Dragon's Claw, Coral root, etc.*

MEDICINAL PART. *The root.*

Description.—This is a singular, leafless plant, with coral-like root-
stocks. The root is a collection of small fleshy tubers; the flowers,
from ten to twenty in number, are of a brownish-green color, and the
fruit a large oblong capsule.

History.—The plant is a native of the United States, growing about
the roots of trees, in rich woods, from Maine to Florida, flowering from
July to October. The entire plant is destitute of verdure. The root
only is used for medical purposes. It is small, dark brown, resembling
cloves, or a hen's claws; has a strong, nitrous smell, and a mucilaginous, slightly bitter, astringent taste.

Properties and Uses.—It is probably the most powerful, prompt, and
certain diaphoretic in the materia medica; but its scarcity and high
price prevents it from coming in general use. It is also sedative, and
promotes perspiration without producing any excitement in the system.
Its chief value is as a diaphoretic in fevers, especially in typhus, and
inflammatory diseases. It has proved effectual in acute erysipelas,
cramps, flatulency, pleurisy, and night-sweats; it relieves hectic fever
without debilitating the patient. Its virtues are especially marked in
the low stages of fevers.

Combined with caulophyllin it forms an excellent agent in amenorrhœa and dysmenorrhœa, or scanty or painful menstruation, and is unsurpassed in after-pains, suppression of lochia, and the febrile symptoms
which sometimes occur at the parturient period.

In fevers Crawley may be advantageously combined with leptandrin
or podophyllin, when it is found necessary to act upon the bowels cr
liver; and mixed with dioscorein it will be found almost a specific in
flatulent and bilious colic.

Dose.—From twenty to thirty grains of the powdered root, given in
water as warm as the patient can drink, and repeated every hour or two,

according to circumstances. The powder should always be kept in well-closed vials. It constitutes the *fever powders* of some practitioners.

CROWFOOT (RANUNCULUS BULBOSUS).

MEDICINAL PARTS. *The cormus and herb.*

Description.—This plant is not to be confounded with the *Geranium maculatum*, which is also called Crowfoot. The cormus or root of this herb is a perennial, solid, fleshy, roundish, and depressed, sending out radicles from its under sides. The root sends up annually erect hairy stems, six to eighteen inches in height. The leaves are on long petioles, dentate and hairy. Each stem supports several solitary golden-yellow flowers; sepals, oblong and hairy; petals, five, cordate; stamens numerous and hairy.

History.—This plant is common in Europe and the United States, growing in fields and pastures, and flowering in May, June, and July. There a great many varieties, but all possess similar qualities, and designated by the general name of *Butter-cup.* When any part of these plants is chewed, it occasions much pain, inflammation, excoriation of the mouth, and much heat and pains in the stomach, if it be taken internally.

Properties and Uses.—This plant is too acrid to be used internally, especially when fresh. When applied externally it is powerfully rubefacient and epispastic. It is employed in its recent state in rheumatic neuralgia and other diseases where vesication and counter-irritation are indicated. Its action, however, is generally so violent that it is seldom used. The beggars use it to produce and keep open sores to excite sympathy. It has been used with success in obstinate cases of nursing sore-mouth—an infusion being made by adding two drachms of the recent root, cut into small pieces, to one pint of hot water, when cold a tablespoonful being given two or three times a day, and the mouth frequently washed with a much stronger infusion.

CUBEBS (PIPER CUBEBA).

MEDICINAL PART. *The berries.*

Description.—This is a perennial plant, with a climbing stem, round branches, about as thick as a goose-quill, ash-colored, and rooting at the joints. The leaves are from four to six and a half inches long by one and a half to two inches broad, ovate-oblong, acuminate, and very smooth. Flowers arranged in spikes at the end of the branches; fruit, a berry rather longer than that of black pepper.

History.—Cubebs is a native of Java and other islands of the Indian Ocean, growing in the forests without cultivation. The fruit is gathered before fully ripe, and then dried. It affords a volatile oil, which is much used. Cubebs has a pleasant, aromatic odor, and a hot, bitter taste. *Cubebin* is the active principle.

Properties and Uses.—It is mildly stimulant, expectorant, stomachic, and carminative. It acts particularly on mucous tissues, and arrests excessive discharges, especially from the urethra. It exercises an influence over the urinary apparatus, rendering the urine of deeper color. It is successfully employed in gonorrhœa, gleet, leucorrhœa, chronic bladder diseases, bronchial affections, and atony of the stomach and bowels.

Dose.—Of the powder, half a drachm to a drachm; tincture, two fluid drachms; oil, ten to thirty drops.

DAISY (LEUCANTHEMUM VULGARE).

COMMON NAMES.   *Ox-eye Daisy, White Weed.*
MEDICINAL PARTS.   *The leaves and flowers.*

Description.—This is a perennial herb, having an erect, branching, and furrowed stem, from one to two feet high. The leaves are few, alternate, lanceolate-serrate, the lower ones petiolate; the upper ones small, subulate, and sessile.

History.—The plant was introduced into the United States from Europe, and is a very troublesome weed to farmers in nearly every section. It bears white flowers in June and July. The leaves are odorous and somewhat acid; the flowers are bitterish; they impart their virtues to water.

Properties and Uses.—It is tonic, diuretic, and anti-spasmodic, and, in large doses, emetic. It is used as a tonic instead of Chamomile flowers, and is serviceable in whooping-cough, asthma, and nervous excitability. Very beneficial externally and internally in leucorrhœa. Its internal use is highly recommended in colliquative perspiration. Externally it is a good application to wounds, ulcers, scald-head, and some other cutaneous diseases. Dose of the decoction, from a wineglassful to a teacupful, two or three times a day. The fresh leaves or flowers will destroy or drive away fleas.

DANDELION (LEONTODON TARAXACUM).

MEDICINAL PART.   *The root.*

Description.—Dandelion is a perennial, top-shaped herb, having a very milky root. The leaves are all radical, shining green in color, sessile, and pinnate. The scape or flower stem is onger than the leaves, five or six inches in height, and bearing a single yellow flower. The fruit is an achenium.

History.—This plant is a native of Greece, but is now found growing abundantly in Europe and the United States, in fields, gardens, and along road-sides, flowering from April to November. The root. only is the officinal part, and should be collected when the plant is in flower. Alcohol or boiling water extracts its properties. The young plant is frequently used as a salad or green, and possesses some slight narcotic properties.

Properties and Uses.—The dried root possesses but little medicinal virtue; but when fresh, is a stomachic and tonic, with slightly diuretic and aperient actions. It has long been supposed to exert an influence upon the biliary organs, removing torpor and engorgement of the liver as well as of the spleen; it is also reputed beneficial in dropsies owing to want of action of the abdominal organs, in uterine obstructions, chronic diseases of the skin, etc. Its virtues, however, are much over-rated.

DEVIL'S BIT (HELONIAS DIOCIA).

COMMON NAMES. *False Unicorn Root, Drooping Star Wort,* etc.
MEDICINAL PART. *The root.*

Description.—This is an herbaceous perennial plant, with a large bulbous root, from which arises a very smooth angular stem one or two feet in height. The cauline leaves are lanceolate, acute, and small; the radical leaves (or those springing from the root) are broader and from four to eight inches in length. The flowers are small, very numerous, greenish-white, disposed in long, terminal, nodding racemes, resembling plumes. The fruit is a capsule.

History.—This plant is indigenous to the United States, and is abundant in some of the Western States, growing in woodlands, meadows, and moist situations, and flowering in June and July.

Properties and Uses.—In large doses it is emetic, and when fresh, sialagogue. In doses of ten or fifteen grains of the powdered root, repeated three or four times a day, it has been found very beneficial in dyspepsia, loss of appetite, and for the removal of worms. It is beneficial in colic, and in atony of the generative organs. It is invaluable in uterine diseases, acting as a uterine tonic, and gradually removing abnormal conditions, while at the same time it imparts tone and vigor to the reproductive organs. Hence, it is much used in leucorrhœa, amenorrhœa, dysmenorrhœa, and to remove the tendency to repeated and successive miscarriage. The plant will kill cattle feeding on it, and the decoction, insects, bugs, and lice.

Dose.—Of the powder, from twenty to forty grains; of the decoction, from a wineglassful to a teacupful.

The *Helonias Bullata,* with purple flowers, and probably some other species possess similar medicinal virtues.

DOCK (RUMEX CRISPUS).

MEDICINAL PART. *The root.*

Description.—There are four varieties of Dock which may be used in medicine : the *Rumex Aquaticus* (Great Water Dock) ; *Rumex Britannica* (Water Dock) ; *Rumex Abtusifolius* (Blunt-leaved Dock) ; and the *R. Crispus*, or Yellow Dock.   They all possess similar medicinal qualities, but the Yellow Dock is the only one entitled to extensive consideration.   It has a deep, spindle-shaped yellow root, with a stem two or three feet high.   The leaves are lanceolate, acute, and of a light green color.   The flowers are numerous, pale green, drooping, and interspersed with leaves below.   The fruit is a nut contracted at each end.

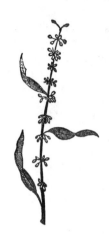

History.—The Docks are natives of Europe, excepting the blunt-leaved, which is indigenous, but they have all been introduced into the United States. Yellow Dock grows in cultivated grounds, waste grounds, about rubbish, etc., flowering in June and July.   The root has scarcely any odor, but an astringent bitter taste, and yields its virtues to water and alcohol.

Dock.

Properties and Uses.—Yellow Dock is an alterative, tonic and detergent, and eminently useful in scorbutic, cutaneous, scrofulous, cancerous and syphilitic affections, leprosy, elephantiasis, etc.   For all impurities of the blood it has no equal, especially if properly compounded with appropriate adjutants and corrigents.   The fresh root bruised in cream, lard, or butter, forms a good ointment for various affections.   This admirable alterative is one of the ingredients of my Blood Purifier (see page 471), in which it is associated with other eminent alteratives, making the compound worthy of the reputation it has achieved.

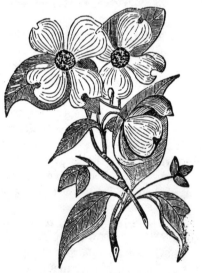

Dogwood.

DOGWOOD (Cornus Florida).

Common Names.   *Boxwood, Flowering Cornel, Green Ozier.*

Medicinal Part.   *The bark.*

Description.—Dogwood is a small indigenous tree from twelve to thirty feet high, with a very hard and compact wood, and covered with a rough and brownish bark.   The tree is of slow growth.   The leaves are opposite, smooth, ovate, acute, dark green above, paler beneath. The flowers are very small, of a greenish yellow color, and constitute the chief beauty of the tree when in bloom. The fruit is an oval drupe of a glossy scarlet color, containing a nut with two cells and two seeds.

History.—This tree grows in various parts of the United States; it flowers in April and May. The fruit matures in autumn. The wood is used for many purposes. The bark yields its virtues to water and alcohol. The chemical qualities are tannic and gallic acids, resin, gum, oil, wax, lignin, lime, potassa, and iron.

Properties and Uses.—It is tonic, astringent, and slightly stimulant. It is an excellent substitute for Peruvian bark, and may be used when the foreign remedy is not to be obtained, or when it fails, or where it cannot be administered. The bark should only be used in its dried state. *Cornine*, its active principle, is much used as a substitute for quinine.

Dogwood, or green ozier, exerts its best virtues in the shape of an ointment. It is detergent in all inflammatory conditions, destructive to morbid growths, and at variance with diseased nutrition. It stimulates granulations, increases the reparative process, induces circulation of healthy blood to the parts, removes effete matter, vitalizes the tissues, and speedily removes pain from the diseased parts. It fulfils these conditions in my great healing remedy, the "Herbal Ointment," see page 472.

Dose.—Of the powder, twenty to sixty grains; extract, five to ten grains; cornine, from one to ten grains.

DRAGON ROOT (ARUM TRIPHYLLUM).

COMMON NAMES. *Wake Robin, Indian Turnip, Jack in the Pulpit, etc.*
MEDICINAL PART. *The cormus or root.*

Description.—This plant has a round, flattened, perennial rhizome; the upper part is tunicated like an onion. The leaves are generally one or two, standing on long, sheathing footstalks; leaflets oval, mostly entire, acuminate, smooth, and paler on the under side.

History.—It inhabits North and South America, is found in wet locations, and flowers from May to June. The whole plant is acrid, but the root is the only part employed. It is of various sizes, turnip-shaped, dark and corrugated externally, and milk-white within, seldom exceeding two and a half inches in diameter. When first dug it is too fiercely acrid for internal employment, as it will leave an impression upon the tongue, lips, and fauces, like that of a severe scald, followed by inflammation and tenderness, which, however, may be somewhat mollified by milk. It exerts no such influence upon the external skin, except upon long and continued application. The root loses its acrimony by age, and should always be used when partially dried. In addition to its acrid principle, it contains a large proportion of starch, with a portion of gum, albumen, and saccharine matter. When the acrid matter is driven off by heat, the root yields a pure, delicate, amylaceous matter, resembling arrow-root, very white and nutritive.

Properties and Uses.—It is acrid, expectorant, and diaphoretic, used in asthma, hooping-cough, chronic bronchitis, chronic rheumatism, pains in the chest, colic, low stages of typhus, and general debility; externally in scrofulous tumors, scald-head, and various skin diseases.

Dose.—Of the grated root, in syrup or mucilage, ten grains, three or four times a day.

ELDER (Sambucus Canadensis).

MEDICINAL PARTS. *The flowers and berries.*

Description.—This is a common, well-known native American plant, from five to twelve feet high, with a shrubby stem, filled with a light and porous pith, especially when young. The bark is rather scabrous and cinereous. The leaves are nearly bipinnate, antiposed. The flowers are numerous, white, in very large level-topped, five-parted cymes, and have a heavy odor. The European Elder, though larger than the American kind, is similar in its general characteristics and properties.

History.—It is an indigenous shrub, growing in all parts of the United States, in low, damp grounds, thickets, and waste places, flowering in June and July, and maturing its berries in September and October. The officinal parts are the flowers, the berries, and the inner bark.

Properties and Uses.—In warm infusion the flowers are diaphoretic and gently stimulant. In cold infusion they are diuretic, alterative, and cooling, and may be used in all diseases requiring such action, as in hepatic derangements of children, erysipelas, erysipelatous diseases, etc. In infusion with Maiden-hair and Beech-drops, they will be found very valuable in all erysipelatous diseases. *The expressed juice of the berries*, evaporated to the consistence of a syrup, is a valuable aperient and alterative; one ounce of it will purge. An infusion of the young leaf-buds is likewise purgative, and sometimes acts with violence. The flowers and expressed juice of the berries have been beneficially employed in scrofula, cutaneous diseases, syphilis, rheumatism, etc. The inner green bark is cathartic; an infusion of it in wine, or the expressed juice, will purge moderately in doses from half a fluid ounce to a fluid ounce. Large doses produce emesis or vomiting. In small doses it produces an efficacious deobstruent, promoting all the fluid secretions, and is much used in dropsy, especially that following scarlatina and other febrile and exanthematous complaints, as well as in many chronic diseases. Beaten up with lard or cream, it forms an excellent discutient ointment, of much value in burns, scalds, and some cutaneous diseases. The juice of the root in half-ounce doses, taken daily, acts as a hydragogue cathartic, and stimulating diuretic, and will be found valuable in all dropsical affections. The inner bark of Elder is hydragogue and emetico-cathartic. Has been successfully used in epilepsy, by taking it from branches one or two years old, scraping off the gray outer bark, and steeping two ounces of it in five ounces of cold or hot water for forty-eight hours. Strain and give a wineglassful every fifteen minutes when the fit is threatening : the patient fasting. Resume it every six or eight days.

ELECAMPANE (INULA HELENIUM).

MEDICINAL PART. *The root.*

Description.—This plant has a thick, top-shaped, aromatic, and pe-rennial root, with a thick, leafy, round, solid stem, from four to six feet high. The leaves are large, ovate, dark green above, downy and hoary beneath, with a fleshy mid-rib. The flowers are of a bright yellow color, and the fruit an achenium.

History.—Elecampane is common in Europe, and cultivated in the United States. It grows in pastures and along road-sides, blossoming from July to September. The root is the part used, and should be gathered in the second year of its development, and during the fall months. It yields its properties to water and alcohol, more especially to the former.

Properties and Uses.—It is aromatic, stimulant, tonic, emmenagogue, diuretic, and diaphoretic. It is much used in chronic pulmonary affec-tions, weakness of the digestive organs, hepatic torpor, dyspepsia, etc.

Dose.—Of the powder, from one scruple to one drachm ; of the infu-sion, one to two fluid ounces.

ERGOT (SECALE CORNUTUM).

COMMON NAMES. *Spurred or Smut Rye.*

MEDICINAL PART. *The degenerated seeds.*

Description.—Ergot is the name given to the fungoid, degenerated seeds of the common rye, which is the result of a parasitic plant called *Oidium Abortifaciens.*

History.—Ergot consists of grains, varying in length, of a violet-black color ; odor fishy, peculiar, and nauseous. Their taste is not very marked, but is disagreeable and slightly acrid. They should be gathered previous to harvest.

Properties and Uses.—Ergot has a remarkable effect upon the human system, and when persisted in for a length of time as an article of food manifests certain symptoms termed *ergotism.* Its chief use as a medicine is to promote uterine contractions in slow, natural labors. It is also useful in checking menorrhagia, uterine hemorrhages, and to expel polypi. It is also employed in gonorrhœa, amenorrhœa, paraplegia, paralysis of the bladder, fever and ague.

This is a valuable remedy to the obstetrician and midwife, but its use should not be persisted in too long, as it often produces dangerous symptoms.

Dose.—Of the powder, five, ten, or fifteen grains; fluid extract, thirty drops.

ERYNGO (ERYNGIUM AQUATICUM).

COMMON NAMES.   *Buttonsnake Root, Rattlesnake's Master, etc.*
MEDICINAL PART.   *The root.*

Description.—This indigenous, perennial herb has a simple stem from one to five feet high. The root is a tuber; the leaves are one or two feet long, half an inch to an inch wide, and taper-pointed. The flowers are white or pale, and inconspicuous.

History.—This plant is indigenous, growing in swamps and low, wet lands from Virginia to Texas, especially on prairie lands, blossoming in August. The root is the officinal part. Water or alcohol extracts its properties.

Properties and Uses.—It is aphrodisiac, exciting venereal desires and strengthening the procreative organs. It is also diuretic, stimulant, diaphoretic, expectorant, and, in large doses, emetic. Very useful in dropsy, nephritic and calculous affections, also in scrofula and syphilis. It is valuable as a diaphoretic and expectorant in pulmonary affections. It is a good substitute for *Senega.* The pulverized root, in doses of two or three grains, is very effectual in hemorrhoids and prolapsus ani. Two ounces of the pulverized root, added to one pint of good Holland gin, is effectual in obstinate cases of gonorrhœa and gleet, to be administered in doses of one or two fluid drachms, three or four times a day. By some practitioners the root is employed as a *specific* in gonorrhœa, gleet, and leucorrhœa; used internally in syrup, decoction, or tincture—and the decoction applied locally by injection. Used externally and internally, it cures the bites of snakes and insects.

Dose.—Of the powder, from twenty to forty grains; of the decoction, which is principally used, from two to four fluid ounces, several times a day.

EYE-BRIGHT (EUPHRASIA OFFICINALIS).

MEDICINAL PART.   *The leaves.*

Description.—This is an elegant little annual plant, with a square, downy, leafy stem, from one to five inches in height. The leaves are entirely opposite, ovate or cordate, and downy; the flowers very abundant, inodorous, with a brilliant variety of colors. The fruit is an oblong pod, filled with numerous seeds.

History.—This plant is indigenous to Europe and America, bearing red or white flowers in July. The leaves are commonly employed; they are inodorous, but of a bitter, astringent taste. Water extracts their virtues.

Properties and Virtues.—Slightly tonic and astringent. Useful in form of infusion or poultice, in catarrhal ophthalmia; also of service in all mucous diseases attended with increased discharges; also, in cough, hoarseness, ear-ache, and head-ache, which have supervened upon catarrhal affections. Four fluid ounces of the infusion taken every morning upon an empty stomach, and also every night at bed-time, has been found successful in helping epilepsy.

FERNS (FILICES).

ROYAL FLOWERING FERN. *Osmunda Regalis.*
COMMON NAME. *Buckhorn Brake.*
MEDICINAL PART. *The root.*

Description.—This Fern has a hard, scaly, tuberous root, quite fibrous, and a whitish core in the centre. The fronds are three or four feet high, bright green, and doubly pinnate. The numerous leaflets are sessile and oblong, some of the upper ones cut.

History.—This beautiful Fern is found in meadows, and low, moist grounds, throughout the United States, blossoming in June. The main root or caudex is the officinal part; it is about two inches long, and has the shape of a buck's horn. It contains an abundance of mucilage, which is extracted by boiling water. The roots should be collected in August, or about the latter part of May, and dried with great care, as they are apt to become mouldy.

The *Osmunda Cinnamomea,* or cinnamon-colored Fern, is inferior to the preceding, but is frequently used for the same medical purposes.

Properties and Uses.—Mucilaginous, tonic, and styptic. Used in coughs, diarrhœa, and dysentery; also used as a tonic during convalescence from exhausting diseases. One root, infused in a pint of hot water for half an hour, will convert the whole into a thick jelly, very valuable in leucorrhœa and other female weaknesses. The mucilage mixed with brandy is a popular remedy as an external application for subluxations and debility of the muscles of the back. For internal use the roots may be infused in hot water, sweetened, and ginger, cinnamon, brandy, etc., added, if not contra-indicated.

FEMALE FERN (POLYPODIUM VULGARE).

COMMON NAMES. *Rock Polypod, Brake Root, Common Polypody.*
MEDICINAL PARTS. *The root and tops.*

Description.—This perennial has a creeping, irregular, brown root. The fronds are from six to twelve inches high, green, smooth, and deeply pinnatified. The fruit on the lower surface of the fronds is in large golden dots or capsules.

History.—This fern is common on shady rocks in woods and mountains throughout the United States. The root has a peculiar and rather unpleasant odor, and somewhat sickening taste. Water extracts its properties.

Properties and Uses.—This plant is pectoral, demulcent, purgative, and anthelmintic. A decoction of syrup has been found very valuable in pulmonary and hepatic diseases. A strong decoction is a good purgative, and will expel tenia and other worms. Dose of the powdered plant, from one to four drachms. Of the decoction or syrup, from one to four fluid ounces, three or four times a day.

MALE FERN (Aspidium Filix Mas).

MEDICINAL PART. *The rhizome.*

Description.—Male Fern has a large, perennial, tufted, scaly rhizome, sending forth yearly several leaves, three or four feet high, erect, oval, lanceolate, acute, pinnate, bright green, and leafy nearly to the bottom; their stalks and midribs having tough, brown, and transparent scales throughout. Leaflets numerous, crowded, oblong, obtuse, and crenate throughout.

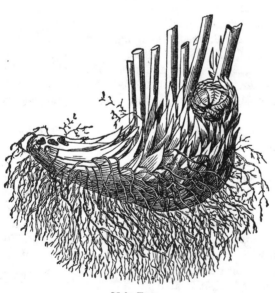

Male Fern.

History.—Male Fern grows in all parts of the United States and Europe. The root has a dark brown epiderm, is almost inodorous, and a nauseous sweet taste. It contains a green fat oil, gum, resin, lignin, tannic acid, pectin, albumen, etc. It should be gathered from June to September. After gathering, it should be carefully prepared, as on the preparation its virtues depend. It loses its virtues in two years if not properly preserved.

Properties and Uses.—It is used for the expulsion of worms, especially tape-worms. It was used as such by Pliny, Dioscorides, Theophrastus, and Galen. It was the celebrated secret remedy of Madame Nouffer, the widow of a Swiss surgeon, who sold her secret to Louis XVI. for 18,000 francs. It is, in fact, a royal anthelmintic, and worthy of all the high commendations it has received from ages past up to the present time. It is one of the ingredients of my " Male Fern Vermifuge." See page 471.

FEVERFEW (PYRETHRUM PARTHENIUM).

MEDICINAL PART. *The herb.*

Description.—Feverfew is a perennial herbaceous plant, with a tapering root, and an erect, round, and leafy stem about two feet high. The leaves are alternate, petiolate, hoary green, with leaflets inclining to ovate and dentate. The flowers are white and compound, and the fruit a wingless, angular, and uniform achenium.

History.—The plant is a native of Europe, but common in the United States ; found occasionally in a wild state, but generally cultivated in gardens, and blossoms in June and July. It imparts its virtues to water, but much better to alcohol.

Properties and Uses.—It is tonic, carminative, emmenagogue, vermifuge, and stimulant. The warm infusion is an excellent remedy in recent colds, flatulency, worms, irregular menstruation, hysteria, suppression of urine, and in some febrile diseases. In hysteria or flatulency, one teaspoonful of the compound spirits of lavender forms a valuable addition to the dose of the infusion, which is from two to four fluid ounces. The cold infusion or extract makes a valuable tonic. The leaves, in poultice, are an excellent local application in severe pain or swelling of the bowels, etc. Bees are said to dislike this plant very much, and a handful of the flower-heads carried where they are will cause them to keep at a distance.

FIGWORT (SCROPHULARIA NODOSA).

MEDICINAL PARTS. *The leaves and root.*

Description.—Figwort has a perennial, whitish, and fibrous root, with a leafy, erect, smooth stem from two to four feet high. The leaves are opposite, ovate ; the upper lanceolate, acute, of deep green color, and from three to seven inches in length. The flowers are small, and dark purple in color. The fruit is an ovate-oblong capsule.

History.—This plant is a native of Europe, but is found growing in different parts of the United States, in woods, hedges, damp copses, and banks, blossoming from July to October. The plants known by the names of *Carpenter's Square, Heal All, Square Stalk,* etc. (*S. Mari-*

landica and *S. Lanceolata*), are all mere varieties of *Figwort*, possessing similar medicinal properties. The leaves and root are the officinal parts, and yield their virtues to water or alcohol. The leaves have an offensive odor, and a bitter, unpleasant taste; the root is slightly acrid.

Properties and Uses.—It is alterative, diuretic, and anodyne; highly beneficial in hepatic or liver diseases, dropsy, and as a general deobstruent to the glandular system when used in infusion or syrup. Externally, in the form of fomentation or ointment, it is valuable in bruises, inflammation of the mammæ, ringworm, piles, painful swellings, itch, and cutaneous eruptions of a vesicular character. The root, in decoction and drunk freely, will restore the lochial discharge when suppressed, and relieve the pains attending difficult menstruation. This plant possesses many valuable and active medicinal properties.

Dose.—Of the infusion or syrup, from a wineglassful to a teacupful.

FIREWEED (Erecthites Hieractifolius).

Medicinal Parts. *The root and herb.*

Description.—This plant has an annual, herbaceous, thick, fleshy, branching, and roughish stem, from one to five feet high. The leaves are simple, alternate, large, lanceolate or oblong, acute, deeply dentate, sessile, and light green. The flowers are whitish, and the fruit an achenium, oblong and hairy.

History.—This indigenous rank weed grows in fields throughout the United States, in moist woods, in recent clearings, and is especially abundant in such as have been burned over. It flowers from July to October, and somewhat resembles the Sowthistle. The whole plant yields its virtues to water or alcohol. It has a peculiar, aromatic, and somewhat fetid odor, and a slightly pungent, bitter, and disagreeable taste.

Properties and Uses.—It is emetic, cathartic, tonic, astringent, and alterative. The latter three qualities are the most valuable. It is an unrivalled medicine in diseases of the mucous tissues. The spirituous extract which I use in my practice is most excellent in cholera and dysentery, promptly arresting the discharges, relieving the pain, and effecting a speedy cure. It is invariably successful in summer complaints of children, even in cases where other means have failed.

FROST-WEED (Helianthemum Canadense).

Common Names. *Rock Rose, Frost Plant, etc.*
Medicinal Part. *The herb.*
Description.—Rock Rose is a perennial herb, with a simple, ascending

downy stem, about a foot high. The leaves are alternate, from eight to twelve inches long, about one-fourth as wide; oblong, acute, lanceolate, erect, and entire. The flowers are large and bright yellow, some with petals, and some without petals. The flowers open in sunshine and cast their petals next day.

History.—It is indigenous to all parts of the United States, growing in dry, sandy soils, and blossoming from May to July. The leaves and stems are cov red with a white down, hence its name. The whole plant is officinal, having a bitterish, astringent, slightly aromatic taste, and yields its properties to hot water. Prof. Eaton, in his work on botany, records this curious fact of the plant : "In November and December of 1816 I saw hundreds of these plants sending out broad, thin, curved ice crystals, about an inch in breadth from near the roots. These were melted away by day, and renewed every morning for more than twenty-five days in succession."

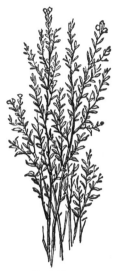

Rock Rose.

Properties and Uses.—This plant has long been used as a valuable remedy for scrofula, in which disease it performs some astonishing cures. It is used in form of decoction, syrup, or fluid extract, but had better be used in combination with other remedies. In combination with *Corydalis Formosa* and *Stillingia* it forms a most valuable remedy. It is tonic and astringent, as well as antiscrofulous. It can be used with advantage in diarrhœa, as a gargle in scarlatina and aphthous ulcerations, and as a wash in scrofulous ophthalmia. Externally, a poultice of the leaves is applied to scrofulous tumors and ulcers. An *oil* has been procured from the plant which is said to be highly valuable in cancerous affections.

The *Helianthemum Corymbosum*, or Frost-weed, growing in the pine barrens and sterile lands of the Southern and Middle States, possesses similar qualities, and may be employed if the former frost-weed is not to be had. This excellent alterative is a constituent of that happy combination of alteratives composing my "Blood Purifier," see page 471.

FUMITORY (FUMARIA OFFICINALIS).

MEDICINAL PART. *The leaves.*

Description.—Fumitory is an annual, glaucous plant, with a sub-erect, much branched, spreading, leafy and angular stem, growing from ten to fifteen inches high. The leaves are mostly alternate. Culpepper, who knew the plant which is now used, better than anybody else, said that "at the top of the branches stand many small flowers, as it were in a long spike one above another, made like little birds, of a reddish purple color, with whitish bellies, after which come small round husks, containing small black seeds.   The root is small, yellow, and not very long, and full of juice when it is young." The fruit, or nut, is ovoid or globose, one-seeded or valveless.   The seeds are crestless.

History.—Fumitory is found growing in cultivated soils in Europe and America, and flowers in May, June, and July.   The leaves are the parts used.   Culpepper recommended the whole plant, but the modern decision is to use the leaves, gathered at the proper times, alone.   They have no odor, but taste bitter under all circumstances.   They are to be used when fresh, and possess the same qualities as Culpepper affixes to the fresh root, viz. : malate of lime and bitter extractive principles.

Properties and Uses.—Its virtues are chiefly tonic, and those who suffer from diseases of the stomach know too well that a tonic, if properly defined, is, simple as it may be, one of the most important remedies for human ailments nature has provided.   Its chief value is found in its action upon the liver.   It is used, in combination, with excellent effect in cutaneous diseases, liver complaints, such as jaundice, costiveness, scurvy, and in debility of the stomach.   An infusion of the leaves is usually given in a wineglass (full) every four hours.   The flowers and tops have been applied, macerated in wine, to dyspepsia, with partial good effect.

GAMBIR PLANT (UNCARIA GAMBIR).

MEDICINAL PART.   *Extract of the leaves and young shoots.*

Description.—Gambir is a stout climbing shrub with round branches. Leaves ovate, lanceolate, acute, smooth, and have short petioles.   Flowers in loose heads, green and pink; calyx short, corolla funnel-shaped; stamens five, and the fruit a two-celled capsule.

History.—It is an inhabitant of the East Indian Archipelago, where it is extensively cultivated.   On the island of Bingtang alone there are 60,000 Gambir plantations.   It affords what is known as *pale catechu.* It is chiefly imported from Singapore.   It is found in cubes which float on water, externally brown, internally pale brick red, breaking easily. Taste bitter, very astringent, and mucilaginous.   Boiling water almost completely dissolves it.   It is used in the arts for tanning.

Properties and Uses.—It is employed as an astringent.   In various affections of the mouth it is an efficacious astringent.   It is also excellent as a stomachic in dyspeptic complaints, especially when accompanied with pyrosis.   It should be used just before taking food.   It is an excellent astringent in chronic diarrhœa and dysentery.

Dose.—From ten to forty grains.

GELSEMIN (GELSEMINUM SEMPERVIRENS).

COMMON NAMES. *Yellow Jessamine, Woodbine, Wild Jessamine.*

MEDICINAL PART. *The root.*

Description.—This plant has a twining, smooth, glabrous stem, with opposite, perennial, lanceolate, entire leaves, which are dark green above and pale beneath. The flowers are yellow, and have an agreeable odor. Calyx is very small, with five sepals, corolla funnel-shaped, stamens five, pistils two, and the fruit a two-celled capsule.

History.—Yellow jessamine abounds throughout the Southern States, growing luxuriantly, and climbing from tree to tree, forming an agreeable shade. It is cultivated as an ornamental vine, and flowers from March to May. The root yields its virtues to water and alcohol. *Gelsemin* is its active principle. It also contains a fixed oil, acrid resin, yellow coloring matter, a heavy volatile oil, a crystalline substance, and salts of potassa, lime, magnesia, iron, and silica.

Properties and Uses.—It is an unrivalled febrifuge, possessing relaxing and antispasmodic properties. It is efficacious in nervous and bilious headache, colds, pneumonia, hemorrhages, leucorrhœa, ague-cake, but especially in all kinds of fevers, quieting all nervous irritability and excitement, equalizing the circulation, promoting perspiration, and rectifying the various secretions, without causing nausea, vomiting, and purging, and is adapted to any stage of the disease. It may follow any preceding treatment with safety. Its effects are clouded vision, double-sightedness, or even complete prostration, and inability to open the eyes. These, however, pass completely off in a few hours, leaving the patient refreshed, and completely restored. When the effects are induced no more of the remedy is required. It is also of great service in various cardiac diseases, spermatorrhœa, and other genital diseases; but its use should be confined entirely to the advice of the physician.

Dose.—The tincture is the form in which it is employed. The dose is from ten to fifty drops in a wineglass half full of water; to be repeated every two hours, as long as required.

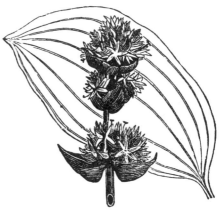

Gentian.

GENTIAN (GENTIANA LUTEA).

MEDICINAL PART. *The root.*

Description.—This plant has a long, thick, cylindrical, wrinkled, ringed, forked, perennial root, brown externally, and yellow within, with a stem three or four feet high, hollow, stout, and erect; leaves ovate-oblong, five-veined, pale, bright green; the blossoms are large, of a bright yellow, in many-flowered whorls; and the fruit is a capsule, stalked, oblong, and two-valved.

History.—This plant is common in Central and Southern Europe, especially on the Pyrenees and Alps, being found from 3,000 to 5,000 feet above the level of the sea. The root affords the medicinal portion, and is brought to America chiefly from Havre and Marseilles. It has a feeble aromatic odor, and a taste at first faintly sweetish, and then purely, intensely, and permanently bitter. It imparts its virtues readily to cold or hot water, alcohol, wine, spirits, or sulphuric ether.

Properties and Uses.—Is a powerful tonic, improves the appetite, strengthens digestion, gives force to the circulation, and slightly elevates the heat of the body. Very useful in debility, exhaustion, dyspepsia, gout, amenorrhœa, hysteria, scrofula, intermittents, worms, and diarrhœa.

Dose.—Of the powder, ten to thirty grains; of the extract, one to ten grains; of the infusion, a tablespoonful to a wineglassful; of the tincture, one or two teaspoonfuls.

Uncrystallized gentianin is a most valuable substitute for quinia, acting as readily and efficaciously on the spleen, in doses of from fifteen to thirty grains, twice a day.

GENTIANA CATESBEI, or the *Blue,* or *American Gentian,* has a perennial, branching, somewhat fleshy root, with a simple, erect, rough stem, eight or ten inches in height, and bears large blue flowers. It grows in the grassy swamps and meadows of North and South Carolina, blossoming from September to December. The root is little inferior to the foreign gentian, and may be used as a substitute for it in all cases, in the same doses and preparations.

GENTIANA QUINQUEFLORA, or *Five-flowered Gentian,* sometimes called Gall-weed, on account of its intense bitterness, is very useful in headache, liver complaint, jaundice, etc. The plant is found from Vermont to Pennsylvania, and a variety of it is common throughout the Western States. It grows in woods and pastures, and flowers in September and October. It may be regarded as a valuable tonic and cholagogue, and deserves further investigation of its therapeutic properties.

There is another kind of gentian (*Gentiana Ochroleuca*), known by the names of Marsh Gentian, Yellowish-white Gentian, Straw-colored Gentian, and Sampson Snake-weed. It has a stout, smoothish, ascending stem, one or two inches in height, its leaves two to four inches long, and three-fourths to an inch and a half in width, with straw-colored flowers two inches long by three-quarters thick, disposed in a dense, terminal cyme, and often in axillary cymes. It is found in Canada and the Southern and Western States, though rarely in the latter, blossoming in September and October; the root is the officinal part, although the tops are often employed. They are bitter, tonic, anthelmintic, and astringent. Used in dyspepsia, intermittents, dysentery, and all diseases of periodicity.

To two ounces of the tops and roots pour on a pint and a half of boiling water, and when nearly cold add a half-pint of brandy. Dose, from one to three tablespoonfuls every half-hour, gradually increasing as the stomach can bear it, lengthening the intervals between the doses. It is also used for bites of snakes, etc.

GILLENIA (GILLENIA TRIFOLIATA).

COMMON NAME. *Indian Physic.*
MEDICINAL PART. *The bark of the root.*
Description.—Gillenia is an indigenous, perennial herb, with an irregular, brownish, somewhat tuberous root, having many long, knotted, stringy fibres. The several stems are from the same root, about two or three feet high, erect, slender, smooth, and of a reddish or brownish color. The leaves are alternate, subsessile; leaflets lanceolate, acuminate, sharply dentated; flowers are white, with a reddish tinge; and the fruit a two-valved, one-celled capsule. Seeds are oblong, brown, and bitter.

History.—This species is found scattered over the United States from Canada to Florida, on the eastern side of the Alleghanies, occurring in open hilly woods, in light gravelly soil. The period of flowering is in May, and the fruit is matured in August. The root yields its virtues to boiling water and alcohol.

Properties and Uses.—It is emetic, cathartic, diaphoretic, expectorant, and tonic. It resembles ipecac in action. It is useful in amenorrhoea, rheumatism, dropsy, costiveness, dyspepsia, worms, and intermittent fever. It may be used in all fevers where emetics are required.

Dose.—As an emetic, twenty to thirty-five grains of the powder, as often as required; as a tonic, two to four grains; as a diaphoretic, six grains in cold water, and repeated at intervals of two or three hours.

GOSSYPIUM HERBACEUM.

COMMON NAME. *Cotton.*
MEDICINAL PART. *The inner bark of the root.*
Description.—Cotton is a biennial or triennial herb, with a fusiform root, with a round pubescent branching stem about five feet high. The leaves are hoary, palmate, with five sub-lanceolate, rather acute lobes; flowers are yellow; calyx cup-shaped, petals five, deciduous, with a purple spot near the base; stigmas, three or five; and the fruit a three or five-celled capsule, with three or five seeds involved in cotton.

History.—It is a native of Asia ; but is cultivated extensively in many parts of the world, and in the Southern portions of America more successfully than anywhere else. The inner bark of the recent root is the part chiefly used in medicine. Its active principle, which is that administered by all educated herbal physicians, is called *Gossypiin.*

Properties and Uses.—The preparation *Gossypiin* is most excellent for diseases of the utero-genital organs. In these diseases it evinces its sole and only virtues, and it ought, on every occasion where it can be procured in its purity, to be used in the stead of *ergot*, or smut rye, in cases of difficult labor. The latter will produce uterine inflammation, and puerperal fever, while gossypiin will achieve the beneficial effects for which ergot is usually administered, and leave the system perfectly free from any prejudicial after-results. The active principle of fresh cotton root forms a most wonderful uterine tonic, and, if correctly prepared, will be found invaluable in sterility, vaginitis, whites, menstrual irregularities, green sickness, etc. I do not recommend the use of the decoction of the root by inexperienced persons. The seeds are said to possess superior anti-periodic properties.

GLOBE FLOWER (CEPHALANTHUS OCCIDENTALIS).

COMMON NAMES. *Button Bush, Pond Dogwood, etc.*
MEDICINAL PART.—*The bark.*
Description.—This is a handsome shrub, growing from six to twelve or more feet high, with a rough bark on the stem, but smooth on the branches. The leaves are opposite, oval, acuminate, in whorls of three, from three to five inches long by two to three wide. The flowers are white, and resemble those of the sycamore, and the fruit a hard and dry capsule.

History.—This plant is indigenous, and found in damp places, along the margins of rivers, ponds, etc., flowering from June to September. The bark is very bitter, and yields its virtues to water and alcohol.

Properties and Uses.—Tonic, febrifuge, aperient, and diuretic. It is used with much success in intermittent and remittent fevers. The inner bark of the root forms an agreeable bitter, and is employed in coughs and gravel. It deserves more notice than it receives, for my experience with it teaches me that it is a valuable medicinal plant.

GOLDEN SEAL (HYDRASTIS CANADENSIS).

COMMON NAMES. *Yellow Puccoon, Ground Raspberry, Turmeric Root, etc.*
MEDICINAL PART. *The root.*
Description.—This indigenous plant has a perennial root or rhizome, which is tortuous, knotty, creeping, internally of a bright yellow color, with long fibres. The stem is erect, simple, herbaceous, rounded, from

six to twelve inches high, bearing two unequal terminal leaves. The two leaves are alternate, palmate, having from three to five lobes, hairy, dark-green, cordate at base, from four to nine inches wide when full grown. The flower is a solitary one, small, white or rose-colored, and the fruit resembles a raspberry, is red, and consists of many two-seeded drupes.

History.—Golden seal is found growing in shady woods, in rich soils, and damp meadows in different parts of the United States and Canada, but is more abundant west of the Alleghanies. It flowers in May and June. The root is the officinal part. Its virtues are imparted to water or alcohol. The root is of a beautiful yellow color, and when fresh is juicy, and used by the Indians to color their clothing, etc.

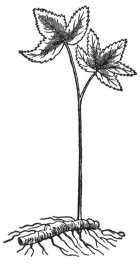

Properties and Uses.—The root is a powerful tonic, at the same time exerting an especial influence upon the mucous surfaces and tissues, with which it comes in contact. Internally, it is successfully administered in dyspepsia, chronic affections of the mucous coats of the stomach, erysipelas; remittent, intermittent, and typhoid fevers; torpor of the liver, and wherever tonics are required. In some instances it proves laxative, but without any astringency, and seems to rank in therapeutical action between rhubarb and blood-root.

A strong decoction of two parts of Golden Seal and one part of Geranium or Cranebill, is very valuable in gleet, chronic gonorrhœa,

Golden Seal.

and leucorrhœa, used in *injection.* It is likewise of much benefit in *incipient stricture, spermatorrhœa,* and *inflammation* and *ulceration of the internal coat of the bladder.* Ulceration of the internal coat of the bladder may be cured by the decoction of Golden Seal alone. It must be injected into the bladder, and held there as long as the patient can conveniently retain it. To be repeated three or four times a day, immediately after emptying the bladder.

Dose.—Of the powder, from ten to thirty grains; of the tincture, from one to two fluid drachms.

GOLD THREAD (COPTIS TRIFOLIA).

COMMON NAME. *Mouth-root.*

MEDICINAL PART. *The root.*

Description.—This plant has a small, creeping, perennial root, of a bright yellow color; the stems are round, slender, and at the base are

5

invested with ovate, acuminate, yellowish scales. The leaves are ever-green, on long, slender petioles; leaflets roundish, acute at base, small and smooth, and veiny and sessile. The flower is a small starry white one, and the fruit an oblong capsule, containing many small black seeds.

History.—Goldthread is found growing in dark swamps and sphagnous woods in the northern parts of the United States, and in Canada, Greenland, Iceland, and Siberia. It flowers early in the spring to July. The root is the medicinal part, and autumn is the season for collect-ing it.

Properties and Uses.—It is a pure and powerful bitter tonic, some-what like quassia, gentian, and columbo, without any astringency. It may be beneficially used in all cases where a *bitter* tonic is required, and is decidedly efficacious as a wash or gargle, when a decoction, in various ulcerations of the mouth. In dyspepsia, and in chronic inflammation of the stomach, equal parts of goldthread and golden seal, made into a decoction, with elixir vitriol added in proper quantity, will not only prove effectual, but in many instances will permanently destroy the appetite for alcoholic beverages.

Dose.—Of the powder or tincture, from half a drachm to a drachm; of the decoction, the dose is from one wineglassful to a teacupful. The tincture, made by adding an ounce of the powdered root to a pint of diluted alcohol, is preferable to the powder. The dose is from twenty drops to a teaspoonful, three times a day.

GUAIAC (GUAIACUM OFFICINALE).

COMMON NAME. *Lignum Vitæ.*
MEDICINAL PARTS. *The wood and resin.*

Description.—This is a tree of slow growth, attaining a height of from thirty to forty feet; stem commonly crooked; bark furrowed; wood very hard, heavy, the fibres crossing each other diagonally. Leaves bijugate; leaflets obovate or oval, obtuse, and evergreen. Flowers light blue, and the fruit an obcordate capsule.

History.—This tree is an inhabitant of the West Indian Islands, and on the neighboring part of the continent. The wood is used by turners for making block-sheaves, pestles, etc., and is very hard and durable. Both the wood and resin are used in medicine. Alcohol is the best solvent.

Properties and Uses.—The wood or resin, taken internally, commonly excites a warmth in the stomach, a dryness of mouth, or thirst. It is an acrid stimulant, and increases the heat of the body and accelerates the circulation. If the body be kept warm while using the decoction, it is diaphoretic; if cool, it is diuretic.

It is used in chronic rheumatism, cutaneous diseases, scrofula, and syphilitic diseases.

Dose.—Decoction of the wood, two to four ounces; of powdered resin, five to twenty grains; tincture, one to four fluid drachms.

HAZEL (WITCH) (HAMAMELIS VIRGINICA).

COMMON NAMES. *Winterbloom, Snapping-hazelnut, Spotted Alder.*
MEDICINAL PARTS. *The bark and leaves.*

Description.—This indigenous shrub consists of several crooked, branching stems, from the same root, from four to six inches in diameter and ten to twelve feet high, covered with a smooth gray bark. The leaves are on short petioles, alternate, oval or obovate; flowers yellow; calyx small, petals four, and the fruit a nut-like capsule or pod.

History.—It grows in damp woods, in nearly all parts of the United States, flowering from September to November, when the leaves are falling, and maturing its seeds the next summer. The barks and leaves are the parts used in medicine. They possess a degree of fragrance, and when chewed are at first somewhat bitter, very sensibly astringent, and then leave a pungent sweetish taste, which remains for a considerable time. Water extracts their virtues. The shoots are used as *divining rods* to discover water and metals under ground by certain adepts in the occult arts.

Properties and Uses.—It is tonic, astringent, and sedative. A decoction of the bark is very useful in hemoptysis, hematemesis, and other hemorrhages or bleedings, as well as in diarrhœa, dysentery, and excessive mucous discharges. It is employed with great advantage in incipient phthisis or consumption, in which it is supposed to unite anodyne influences with its others.

The Indians use it in the form of poultice, in external inflammations, swellings, and all tumors of a painful character.

The decoction may be advantageously used as a wash or injection for sore mouth, painful tumors, external inflammations, bowel complaints, prolapsus ani and uteri, leucorrhœa, gleet, and ophthalmia.

An *Ointment* made with lard, and a decoction of white-oak bark, apple-tree bark, and witch-hazel, is a very valuable remedy for hemorrhoids or piles.

The following forms a useful preparation : Take equal parts of witch-hazel bark, golden seal, and lobelia leaves, the two first made into a strong decoction, after which add the lobelia to the hot liquid, and cover; when cold, strain. This decoction, as a collyrium, will frequently and speedily cure the most obstinate and long-standing cases of ophthalmia.

Dose of the witch-hazel decoction alone, from a wineglassful to a teacupful, three or four times a day.

HELLEBORE (AMERICAN) (VERATRUM VIRIDE).

COMMON NAMES. *Swamp Hellebore, Indian Poke, Itch-weed.*
MEDICINAL PART. *The rhizome.*

Description.—This plant has a perennial, thick, and fleshy rhizome, tunicated at the upper part, sending off a multitude of large whitish roots. The stem is from three to five feet high; lower leaves from six inches to a foot long, oval, acuminate; upper leaves gradually narrower, linear, lanceolate, and all alternate. The flowers are numerous and green, part of them barren.

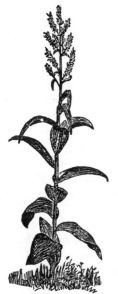

Hellebore.

History.—American Hellebore is native to the United States, growing in swamps, low grounds, and moist meadows, blossoming in June and July. The roots should be gathered in autumn, and as it rapidly loses its virtues, it should be gathered annually and kept in well-closed vessels. When fresh, it has a very strong, unpleasant odor, but when dried is inodorous. It has a sweetish-bitter taste, succeeded by a persistent acridity.

Properties and Uses.—It has many very valuable properties. It is slightly acrid, confining this action to the mouth and fauces. It is unsurpassed by any article as an expectorant. As a diaphoretic, it is one of the most certain of the whole materia medica, often exciting great coolness and coldness of the surface. In suitable doses it can be relied upon to bring the pulse down from a hundred and fifty beats in a minute to forty, or even to thirty. Sometimes it renders the skin merely soft and moist, and at others produces free and abundant perspiration. In fevers, in some diseases of the heart, acute rheumatism, and in many other conditions which involve an excited state of the circulation, it is of exceeding great value. As a deobstruent or alterative, it far surpasses iodine, and therefore used with great advantage in the treatment of cancer, scrofula, and consumption. It is nervine, and never narcotic, which property renders it of great value in all painful diseases, or such as are accompanied with spasmodic action, convulsions, morbid irritability and irritative mobility, as in chorea, epilepsy or fits, pneumonia, puerperal fever, neuralgia, etc., producing these effects without stupefying and torpifying the system, as opium is known to do. As an emetic, it is slow, but certain and efficient, rousing the liver to action, and vomits without occasioning prostration or exhaustion like other emetics, being the more valuable in not being cathartic. It is peculiarly adapted as an emetic in whooping-cough, croup, asthma, scarlet fever, and in all cases where there is much febrile or inflammatory action. As an arterial sedative it stands unparalleled and unequalled, while in small doses it creates and promotes appetite beyond any agent known to medical men. It has recently come into use, and may be justly regarded as one of the most valuable contributions to the list of medicines in a hundred years.

Dose.—Veratrum is usually given in the form of a tincture, the formula being of the dried root, eight ounces to sixteen ounces diluted .835 alcohol, macerating for two weeks, then to be expressed and filtered. To an adult eight drops are given, which should be repeated every three hours, increasing the dose one or two drops every time until nausea or vomiting, or reduction of the pulse to sixty-five or seventy, ensue, then reduce to one-half in all cases. Females and persons from fourteen to eighteen should commence with six drops and increase as above. For children, from two to five years, begin with two drops, and increase one drop only. Below two years of age, one drop is suf-

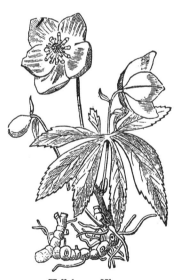

ficient. If taken in so large a dose as to produce vomiting or too much depression, a full dose of morphine or opium, in a little brandy or ginger, is a complete antidote. In pneumonia, typhoid fever, and many other diseases, it must be continued from three to seven days after the symptoms have subsided. In typhoid fever, while using the veratrum, quinia is absolutely inadmissible. It is administered in a little sweetened water, and its employment in moderate doses, or short of nausea, may be continued indefinitely without the least inconvenience.

The HELLEBORUS NIGER, *Black Hellebore*, inhabiting the subalpine and southern parts of Europe, was formerly much used in palsy, insanity, apoplexy, dropsy, epilepsy, etc., but is now more

Helleborus Niger.

or less discarded. It has diuretic and emmenagogue properties, but as it is very toxical in effects, its use is not to be advised in domestic practice.

HENBANE (HYOSCYAMUS NIGER).

MEDICINAL PARTS. *The leaves and seeds.*

Description.—Henbane is a biennial plant. It has a long, thick, spindle-shaped, corrugated root, which is of a brown color externally, but whitish internally. The stem sometimes reaches the height of two feet, but often stops at an altitude of six inches: The leaves are large, oblong, acute, alternate, and of a pale, dull green color. They have long, glandular hairs upon the midrib. The flowers are funnel-shaped, of a dull yellow color, with purple veins and orifice. The seeds are many, small, obovate, and brownish.

History.—Henbane is original with Europe, but has been naturalized in America. It grows in waste grounds, and flowers from July to September. The leaves and seeds are the parts medicinally used. The leaves are collected in the second year, when the plant is in flower ; the seeds are gathered when perfectly ripe. It grows more plentifully than elsewhere in America, in the waste grounds of old settlements, in grave-yards, and around the foundations of ruined houses. Bruise the recent leaves, and they emit a strong narcotic odor, like tobacco. Dry them, and they have little smell or taste. Their virtues are completely extracted by diluted alcohol. The active principle of Henbane is called *Hyosciamia*, but all the recognized preparations are now known by the general name of *Hyoscyamus*.

Properties and Uses.—Henbane is a powerful narcotic, but, unless improperly and injudiciously used, it is not "dangerously" poisonous, as we learn from King. All narcotics are "dangerously" poisonous if dangerously administered. Nature grows wild her most potent medicinal herbs, and those which, if used by persons who understand them, are curative of the very worst afflictions of the human race, are also destructive to a small extent if applied and administered by parties who have not thoroughly studied their properties. Medicinally used, Henbane is calmative, hypnotic, anodyne, and antispasmodic. It is much better than opium, as it does not produce constipation. It is always given, where opium does not agree, with the very best effects. I use it principally to cause sleep, and remove irregular nervous action. Combined with other preparations mentioned in many parts of this volume, it is most excellent for gout, rheumatism, asthma, chronic cough, neuralgia, irritations of the urinary organs, etc. The leaves make fine external preparations for glandular swellings or ulcers, etc. I instruct my patients never to use it, under any circumstances, without the advice of a good herbal physician.

HOARHOUND (Marrubium Vulgare).

MEDICINAL PART. *The herb.*

Description.—This well-known herb has a fibrous, perennial root and numerous annual, bushy stems, leafy, and branching from the bottom to one or two feet in height. The leaves are roundish-ovate, rough and veiny above, woolly on the under surface, one or two inches in diameter; the flowers small and white.

History.—Hoarhound is a native of Europe, but has been naturalized in the United States, where it is very common. It grows on dry, sandy fields, waste grounds, and road-sides, flowering from June to September. The entire plant has a white or hoary appearance; the whole herb is medicinal, and should be gathered before its efflorescence. It has a peculiar, rather agreeable, vinous, balsamic odor, and a very bitter, aromatic, somewhat acrid and persistent taste. Its virtues are imparted to alcohol or water.

Properties and Uses.—A stimulant, tonic, expectorant, and diuretic. It is used in the form of *syrup*, in coughs, colds, chronic catarrh, asthma, and all pulmonary affections. The *warm* infusion will produce perspiration and flow of urine, and is used with great benefit in jaundice, asthma, hoarseness, amenorrhœa, and hysteria. The cold infusion is an excellent tonic in some forms of dyspepsia. It will expel worms and act as a purgative in large doses. It enters into the composition of several syrups and candies.

Dose.—Of the powder, one drachm; of the infusion or syrup, from half to a teacupful.

HOUND'S TONGUE (CYNOGLOSSUM OFFICINALE).

MEDICINAL PARTS. *The leaves and root.*

Description.—This biennial plant has an erect stem one or two feet high. The leaves are hoary, with soft down on both sides, acute, lanceolate, radical ones petiolate, cauline ones sessile, with cordate bases. The flowers are in clusters, calyx downy, corolla reddish purple, and fruit a depressed achenium.

History.—Cynoglossum Officinale grows on the road-sides and waste places of both Europe and America. The leaves and the root are the parts used in medicine; but the preference I give to the root. This, upon being gathered, emits an unpleasant and somewhat heavy odor, which vanishes when it is dried. Its taste is bitter and mawkish. The fresh root is spoken of by several herbalists as being better than the desiccated or dried, but this probably arises from the fact that the roots they used had not been gathered at the proper time, dried in the correct way, or kept in a skilful manner. The dried root is quite as active as the fresh, if prepared by a person who knows its qualities.

Properties and Uses.—It is chiefly valuable for coughs, catarrhs, bleeding from the lungs, and other disorganizations of the respiratory apparatus. The leaves and root are both applied, with great benefit, as a poultice to old ulcers, scrofulous tumors, burns, goitre, and recent bruises and abrasions. In my several remedies the values of many of the plants described at length in these pages are most thoroughly embraced. The object in giving such plants a descriptive space each is to enable the reader, in extraordinary emergencies, to be *his own physician* until he can get a better one, and to show him that what he treads on may, without his knowledge, contain the germs of his rejuvenation.

CYNOGLOSSUM MORRISONI, or *Virginia Mouse-ear, Beggars' Lice, Dysentery Weed*, etc., is an annual weed with an erect hairy, leafy stem, two to four feet high. Leaves three to four inches long, oblong, lanceolate; flowers very small, white, or pale blue. It grows in rocky grounds and among rubbish. The whole plant has an unpleasant odor. The root is the medicinal part. It is very efficacious in diarrhœa and dysentery. The root may be chewed or given in powder or infusion *ad libitum*.

HOPS (HUMULUS LUPULUS).

MEDICINAL PART. *The strobiles or cones.*

Description.—This well-known twining plant has a perennial root, with many annual angular stems. The leaves are opposite, deep green, serrated, venated, and very rough. The flowers are numerous and of a greenish color. Fruit a strobile.

History.—This plant is found in China, the Canary Islands, all parts of Europe, and in many places in the United States. It is largely cultivated in England and the United States for its cones or strobiles, which are used medicinally, and in the manufacture of beer, ale, and porter. The odor of hops is peculiar and somewhat agreeable, their taste slightly astringent and exceedingly bitter. They yield their virtues to boiling water, but a better solvent than water is diluted alcohol. Lupulin is the yellow powder procured by beating or rubbing the strobiles, and then sifting out the grains, which form about one-seventh part of the Hops. Lupulin is in globose kidney-shaped grains, golden yellow and somewhat transparent, and preferable to the Hops itself. *Lupulite* is the bitter principle of Hops, and is obtained by making an aqueous solution of *Lupulin.*

Properties and Uses.—Hops are tonic, hypnotic, febrifuge, antilithic, and anthelmintic. They are principally used for their sedative or hypnotic action—producing sleep, removing restlessness, and abating pain, but sometimes failing to do so. A pillow stuffed with Hops is a favorite way for obtaining sleep. The *lupulin* or its tincture is used in delirium tremens, nervous irritation, anxiety, exhaustion, and does not disorder the stomach, nor cause constipation, as with opium. It is also useful in after-pains, to prevent chordee, suppress venereal desires, etc. Externally, in the form of a fomentation alone, or combined with Boneset or other bitter herbs, it has proved beneficial in pneumonia, pleurisy, gastritis, enteritis, and as an application to painful swellings and tumors. An *ointment*, made by boiling two parts of Stramonium leaves and one of Hops in lard, is an excellent application in salt rheum, ulcers, and painful tumors. It is a powerful antaphrodisiac, composing the genital organs, quieting painful erections in gonorrhœa, etc.

Dose.—Fluid extract, half a drachm to a drachm ; solid extract, five to twenty grains ; tincture (two and a half ounces of hops to one pint of alcohol), three to six drachms ; *infusion* (four drachms to one pint of hot water), a wineglass to a cupful of *Lupulin,* the dose six to ten grains ; *tinct.* of Lupulin (two ounces of Lupulin to one pint of alcohol), one to two teaspoonfuls in sweetened water. Fifteen to twenty grains well rubbed up with white sugar in a mortar is very efficacious in priapism, chordee, and spermatorrhœa.

HOUSE-LEEK (SEMPERVIVUM TECTORUM).

MEDICINAL PART. *The leaves.*

Description.—House-leek has a fibrous root, with several tufts of oblong, acute, extremely succulent leaves. The stem from the centre of these tufts is about a foot high, erect, round, and downy ; flowers large, pale rose-colored, and scentless. Offsets spreading.

History.—This perennial plant is a native of Europe, and is so succulent that it will grow on dry walls, roofs of houses, etc. It flowers in August. It is much cultivated in some places. The leaves contain super-malate of lime.

Properties and Uses.—The fresh leaves are useful as a refrigerant when bruised, and applied as a poultice in erysipelatous affections, burns, stings of insects, and other inflammatory conditions of the skin. The leaves, sliced in two, and the inner surface applied to warts is a positive cure for them. It can be used for many skin diseases. The leaves also possess an astringent property, serviceable in many cases.

HYSSOP (HYSSOPUS OFFICINALIS).

MEDICINAL PARTS. *The tops and leaves.*

Description.—Hyssop is a perennial herb, with square stems. woody at the base, and a foot or two in height, with rod-like branches. The leaves are opposite, sessile, linear, and lanceolate. green on each side ; flowers, bluish-purple, seldom white ; stamens four.

History.—It is an inhabitant of Europe and this country, being raised principally in gardens, and flowers in July. The taste of the leaves is hot, spicy, and somewhat bitter, and yield their virtues to water and alcohol. They contain yellow oil and sulphur.

Properties and Uses.—Stimulant, aromatic, carminative, and tonic. Generally used in quinsy and other sore-throats, as a gargle with sage. As an expectorant it is beneficial in asthma, coughs, etc. The leaves applied to bruises speedily relieve the pain and remove the discoloration.

5*

IBERIS AMARA.

COMMON NAME. *Bitter Candy Tuft.*
MEDICINAL PART. *The seeds.*

Description.—This plant has a herbaceous stem, about a foot in height, with acute, toothed leaves, and bright white flowers.

History.—The leaves, stem, root, and seeds are used; the seeds especially. The plant is an annual, carefully cultivated in Europe, but grows wild also. It flowers in June and July.

Properties and Uses.—The ancients employed it in gout, rheumatism, and diseases of a kindred nature. We use it, compounded with other herbal preparations, for such diseases in their worst forms, and we also use it by itself, in certain proportions, to allay excited action of the heart, particularly where the heart is enlarged. In asthma, bronchitis, and dropsy it is now considered one of the most excellent ingredients of certain cures for those afflictions. The dose is from one to five grains of the powdered seeds.

ICELAND MOSS (CETRARIA ISLANDICA).

MEDICINAL PART. *The plant.*

Description and History.—Iceland Moss is a perennial, foliaceous plant from two to four inches high; a native of Britain and the northern countries of Europe, particularly Iceland. It is diversified in its color, being brownish or grayish-white in some parts, and of a reddish hue in others. It is without odor, with a mucilaginous, bitter, somewhat astringent taste, and when dry the lichen is crisp, cartilaginous, and coriaceous, and is convertible into a grayish-white powder. It swells up in water, absorbing more than its own weight of that fluid, and communicating a portion of its bitterness to it, as well as a little mucilage; when long chewed it is converted into a mucilaginous pulp, and when boiled in water the decoction becomes a firm jelly on cooling.

Properties and Uses.—It is demulcent, tonic, and nutritious. Used as a demulcent in chronic catarrh, chronic dysentery, and diarrhœa, and as a tonic in dyspepsia, convalescence, and exhausting diseases. Boiled with milk it forms an exeellent nutritive and tonic in phthisis and general debility. Its tonic virtues depend upon its *cetrarin*, which, if removed, renders the lichen merely nutritious.

IRON WEED (VERNONIA FASCICULATA).

MEDICINAL PART. *The root.*

Description.—This is an indigenous, perennial, coarse, purplish-green weed, with a stem from three to ten feet high. The leaves are from four to eight inches long, one or two broad, lanceolate, tapering to each end. Corolla showy, and dark purple.

History.—This is a very common plant to the Western States, growing in woods and prairies, and along rivers and streams, flowering from July to September. The root is bitter, and imparts its virtues to water and alcohol.

Properties and Uses.—It is a bitter tonic, deobstruent, and alterative. In powder or decoction the root is beneficial in amenorrhœa, dysmenorrhœa, leucorrhœa, and menorrhagia. It is useful in scrofula and some cutaneous diseases.

Dose.—Of the decoction, one or two fluid ounces; of the tincture, one or two fluid drachms. The leaves or powdered root make an excellent discutient application to tumors.

IVY (AMERICAN) (AMPELOPSIS QUINQUEFOLIA).

COMMON NAMES. *Woodbine, Virginia Creeper, Five Leaves, False Grape, Wild wood-vine.*

MEDICINAL PARTS. *The bark and twigs.*

Description.—This is a woody vine, with a creeping stem, digitate leaves; leaflets acuminate, petiolate, dentate, and smooth; flowers inconspicuous, greenish, or white; and the fruit a berry, acid, dark blue, and small.

History.—The American Ivy is a common, familiar, shrubby vine, climbing extensively, and, by means of its radiating tendrils, supporting itself firmly on trees, stone walls, churches, etc., and ascending to the height of from fifty to a hundred feet. The bark and the twigs are the parts usually used. Its taste is acrid and persistent, though not unpleasant, and its decoction is mucilaginous. The bark should be collected after the berries have ripened. It is like the ivy of England and other countries.

Properties and Uses.—Alterative, tonic, astringent, and expectorant. It is used principally in form of syrup in scrofula, dropsy, bronchitis, and other pulmonary complaints. An old author affirms that there is a very great antipathy between wine and ivy, and therefore it is a remedy to preserve against drunkenness, and to relieve or cure intoxication by drinking a draught of wine in which a handful of bruised ivy leaves have been boiled.

Dose.—Of the decoction of syrup, from one to four tablespoonfuls, three times a day.

JALAP (IPOMŒA JALAPA).

MEDICINAL PART. *The root.*

Description.—Jalap has a fleshy, tuberous root, with numerous roundish tubercles. It has several stems, which are smooth, brownish, slightly rough, with a tendency to twine. The leaves are on long petioles, the

first hastate, succeeding ones cordate, acuminate, and mucronate.   The
calyx has no bracts; corolla funnel-shaped,
purple, and long.   Fruit a capsule.

Jalap.

History.—This plant grows in Mexico,
at an elevation of nearly six thousand feet
above the level of the sea, near Chicanquiaco
and Xalapa, from which it is exported, and
from which last-named place it also receives
its name.   It is generally imported in bags,
containing one or two hundred pounds.   The
worm-eaten root is the most energetic, as
the active part is untouched by them.   It is
soluble in water and alcohol.

Properties and Uses.—Jalap is irritant
and cathartic, operating energetically, and
produces liquid stools.   It is chiefly employed when it is desired to produce an
energetic influence on the bowels, or to
obtain large evacuations.   In intestinal inflammations it should not be used.

Dose.—Powder, ten grains.

JAMESTOWN WEED (DATURA STRAMONIUM).

COMMON NAMES.   *Thorn-Apple, Stinkweed, Apple-peru, etc.*
MEDICINAL PARTS.   *The leaves and seeds.*

Description.—This plant is a bushy, smooth, fetid, annual plant, two
or three feet in height, and in rich soil even more.   The root is rather
large, of a whitish color, giving off many fibres.   The stem is much
branched, forked, spreading, leafy, of a yellowish-green color.   The
leaves are large and smooth, from the forks of the stem, and are uneven
at the base.   The flowers are about three inches long, erect, large, and
white.   The fruit is a large, dry, prickly capsule, with four valves and
numerous black reniform seeds.   There is the *Datura Tatula*, or purple
Stramonium, which differs from the above in having a deep purple stem,
etc.

History.—Stramonium is a well-known poisonous weed, growing upon
waste grounds and road-sides, in all parts of the United States.   It is
found in very many parts of the world.   The whole plant has a fetid,
narcotic odor, which diminishes as it dries.   Almost every part of the
plant is possessed of medicinal properties, but the officinal parts are the
leaves and seeds.   The leaves should be gathered when the flowers are
full-blown, and carefully dried in the shade.   They impart their properties to water, alcohol, and the fixed oils.   The seeds are small, reniform,
compressed, roughish, dark brown or black when ripe, grayish-brown

when unripe. They yield what is called *Daturia*, which may be obtained by exhausting the bruised seeds with boiling rectified alcohol, and then proceeding as for the active principle of other seeds of a similar character.

Properties and Uses.—In large doses it is an energetic narcotic poison. The victims of this poison suffer the most intense agonies, and die in maniacal delirium. In medicinal doses it is an anodyne, antispasmodic, and is often used as a substitute for opium. It is used with fair effect in cases of mania, epilepsy, gastritis, delirium tremens, and enteritis; also in neuralgia, rheumatism, and all periodic pains. The dried and smoked leaves are useful in spasmodic asthma, but as there are other means much more certain to cure, and less dangerous, I, and other herbalists, seldom or never recommend them. Daturia is seldom employed in medicine, being a very active and powerful poison. I should advise my readers never to employ it, unless they be physicians; but I deemed proper to give it a place in this work, as its medicinal qualities are quite important, if its use is intrusted to proper and educated persons.

JUNIPER (JUNIPERUS COMMUNIS).

MEDICINAL PART. *The berries.*

Description.—This is a small evergreen shrub, never attaining the height of a tree, with many very close branches. The leaves are attached to the stem in threes. The fruit is fleshy, of dark-purplish color, ripening the second year from the flower.

History.—Juniper grows in dry woods and hills, and flowers in May. The American berries contain less virtue than those imported from Europe. The oil is contained in the spirituous liquor called Holland gin. The berries yield their properties to hot water and alcohol.

Properties and Uses.—The berries and oil are stimulating, carminative, and diuretic. It is especially useful in averting mucous discharges, especially from the urethra.

Dose.—Of the berries, from one to two drachms; of the oil, from four to twenty minims.

KINO (PTEROCARPUS MARSUPIUM).

MEDICINAL PART. *Concrete juice.*

Description.—Kino is a leafy tree, with the outer coat of the bark brown, and the inner red, fibrous, and astringent. Branches smooth, leaves alternate; leaflets, from five to seven, alternate, elliptical, and rather emarginate; flowers very numerous, white, with a tinge of yellow; fruit a legume on a long petiole.

History.—Kino is the juice of the tree, obtained by making longitudinal incisions in the bark. It flows freely, is of a red color, and by drying it in the sun it cracks into irregular angular masses. The frag·

ments are reddish, black, translucent, and ruby-red on the edges, inodorous, and very astringent. When chewed it tinges the saliva bloodred. Alcohol dissolves about two-thirds of it. It is chiefly imported from Malabar. It inhabits the Circur mountains and forests of the Malabar coast.

Properties and Uses.—Employed in medicine as an energetic astringent only, principally in obstinate chronic diarrhœa. It is also administered as an astringent in leucorrhœa and sanguineous exudations. As a topical remedy, it is applied to flabby ulcers, and used as a gargle, injection, and wash.

Dose.—Of the powder, from ten to thirty grains.

KIDNEY LIVER-LEAF (HEPATICA AMERICANA).

MEDICINAL PART. *The plant.*

Description.—This is a perennial plant, the root of which consists of numerous strong fibres. The leaves are all radical, on long, hairy petioles, smooth, evergreen, cordate at base, the new ones appearing later than the flowers. The flowers appear almost as soon as the snow leaves the ground in the spring. Fruit an ovate achenium.

HEPATICA ACUTALOBA, or *Heart Liver-leaf,* which possesses the same medicinal qualities, differs from the above in having the leaves with three ovate, pointed lobes, or sometimes five-lobed. They both bear white, blue, or purplish flowers, which appear late in March or early in April.

History.—These plants are common to the United States, growing in woods and upon elevated situations—the former, which is the most common, being found on sides of hills, exposed to the north, and the latter on the southern aspect. The plants yield their virtues to water.

Properties and Uses.—It is a mild, mucilaginous astringent, and is freely used in infusion, in fevers, diseases of the liver; and for bleeding from the lungs, coughs, etc., it is a most valuable curative.

Dose.—Infusion taken *ad libitum.*

KOUSSO (BRAYERA ANTHELMINTICA).

MEDICINAL PART. *The leaves.*

Description.—This is a tree, growing about twenty feet high, with round rusty branches. The leaves are crowded, alternate; leaflets oblong, acute, and serrate; flowers small, greenish, and becoming purple; the fruit so far unknown.

History.—This tree grows upon the table-lands of Northeastern Abyssinia, at an elevation of several thousand feet. The flowers are the parts used. They are gathered when in full bloom, and are used in their fresh state, but are equally valuable when properly dried. After drying they are powdered, and in this form they are mixed with warm water and administered. The value of this medicine has been known for a long time, having been introduced in the French practice over forty years ago. It is quite difficult to procure even the adulterated or spurious article in America or England; the genuine is not to be obtained at any price in the drug-stores. In the stores, however, can be obtained, at great cost, an active resinous principle, extracted from the flowers, and sometimes the unripe fruit, to which the names of *Tæniin* and *Koussin* have been given. The dose of this is set down at twenty grains.

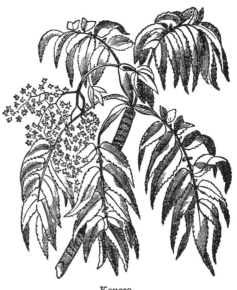

Kousso.

Properties and Uses.—In large doses it will produce heat of the stomach, nausea, and sometimes vomiting, and occasionally will act powerfully on the bowels; but this is only when injudiciously taken. Its chief property is developed in the destruction and expulsion of worms, *especially the tape-worm.* It is the surest of all remedies for that distressing affliction, when compounded with other ingredients which I have mentioned elsewhere. Taken in the proper dose, it seems to have no general effect, but operates wholly and solely upon the worms. The dose of the powdered flowers in infusion is half an ounce to half a pint of warm water. It must be reduced for children. If the medicine does not operate in four hours, use castor-oil. It is one of the ingredients of my Male Fern Vermifuge. (See page 471.)

LADIES' SLIPPER (CYPRIPEDIUM PUBESCENS).

COMMON NAMES. *American Valerian, Umbel, Nerve-root, Yellow-Moccasin flower, Noah's Ark.*

MEDICINAL PART. *The root.*

Description.—This indigenous plant has a perennial, fibrous, fleshy root, from which arise several round leafy stems, from twelve to eighteen inches high. The leaves are from three to six inches long, by two or three broad, oblong, lanceolate, acuminate, pubescent, alternate, generally the same number on each side. Flowers large and very showy, and pale yellow.

History.—This plant grows here in rich woods and meadows, and flowers in May and June. There are several varieties of it, but as they all possess the same medicinal properties, a description of each is not requisite or desirable.

Properties and Uses.—The fibrous roots are the parts used in medicine, and they should be gathered and carefully cleansed in August or September. The properties and uses are various. The preparations made from these roots are tonic and stimulant, diaphoretic, and antispasmodic, and are considered to be unequalled in remedying hysteria, chorea, nervous headache, and all cases of nervous irritability. Combined with a certain foreign plant of a mucilaginous character, and growing near the sea-shore, it is an unfailing cure of fever and ague. The preparation has, however, to be skilfully compounded. . Any one afflicted by fever and ague may write to me for particulars and I will gladly and promptly furnish them. They are also used for delirium, neuralgia, and hypochondria. The form of preparation is an alcoholic extract.

Dose.—From ten to twenty grains; tincture, from one to three fluid drachms; infusion, from one to four fluid ounces. When made into powder, one drachm in warm water is a dose, and may be repeated, in season, as often as may be required.

LARCH (ABIES LARIX).

MEDICINAL PART. *Resinous exudation.*

Description.—Larch is a very lofty and graceful tree, with wide-spreading branches. The buds are alternate, perennial, cup-shaped, scaly, producing annually a pencil-like tuft. Male flowers drooping, about half an inch long, yellow; female flowers erect, larger than the male flowers, and variegated with green and pink; cones erect, ovate, about an inch long, purple when young, reddish-brown when ripe.

History.—The Larch grows in the mountainous regions of Europe, and yields the article of use and commerce known as *Venice turpentine.* The bark contains a large amount of tannic acid.

Properties and Uses.—The medicinal properties are those known to be confined to turpentine.

LARGE FLOWERING SPURGE (EUPHORBIA COROLLATA).

COMMON NAMES. *Blooming Spurge, Milk-weed, Bowman's Root, etc.*

MEDICINAL PART. *The bark of the root.*

Description.—This is a perennial plant with a round, slender, erect stem, one or two feet high, with a yellowish, large, and branching root. The leaves are scattered, sessile, oblong-obovate, smooth in some plants, very hairy in others, and from one to two inches in length. Flowers white and showy, and fruit a three-celled capsule.

History.—This plant grows plentifully in Canada and the United States, in dry fields and woods, and flowers from June to September. The bark of the root is the part used. The plant is readily detected by a milky fluid which exudes from the stem, when that is broken. This fluid, if applied to warts or wens, is of great benefit, in most cases banishing the offensive excrescences.

Properties and Uses.—It is emetic, diaphoretic, expectorant, and epispastic. As an emetic the powdered bark of the root (say from fifteen to twenty grains) is mild, pleasant, and efficacious.

Dose.—As an expectorant it is administered three grains at a time, mixed with honey, molasses, or sugar; as a cathartic, from four to ten grains are required. It is regarded, in doses of fifteen or twenty grains, as one of the very best remedies ever discovered for the dropsy. It has cured hydrothorax and ascites when all other means have failed.

LARKSPUR (DELPHINUM CONSOLIDA).

MEDICINAL PARTS. *The root and seeds.*

Description.—Larkspur is an annual herb, with a simple slender root, a leafy stem, from a foot and a half to two feet high, with alternate spreading branches. The leaves are sessile; flowers bright blue and purple.

DELPHINUM STAPHISAGRIA, or *Stavesacre*, which possesses the same properties as Larkspur, but to a greater degree, is an elegant upright herb, about the same height as Larkspur. Leaves broad, palmate, and petioled. Flowers bluish-gray. Fruit a capsule.

History.—Larkspur is a native of Europe, but has become naturalized in the United States, growing in woods and fields. Stavesacre is native to Europe, growing in waste places.

Properties and Uses.—In medicinal doses emetic, cathartic, and narcotic. It has also vermifuge properties. The whole plant contains an acid principle which is sure death to all kinds of domestic vermin. The flowers and leaves were extensively used in the United States army during the rebellion, to kill lice, and it is pretty well authenticated that the same substance forms the basis of the many preparations offered for the destruction of all noxious insects whose room is better than their company. The flowers are emmenagogue, diuretic, and vermifuge. A tincture of the seeds, it is said, will cure asthma and dropsy. Also a specific for cholera morbus.

Dose.—Two ounces of the seed added to one quart of diluted alcohol makes the tincture, of which ten drops may be given three times a day. This, however, should be used only in extreme cases.

LAVENDER (LAVANDULA VERA AND LAVANDULA SPICA).

MEDICINAL PART. *The flowers.*

Description.—Lavandula Vera is a small shrub from one to two feet high, but sometimes attaining six feet. The leaves are oblong-linear or lanceolate, entire, opposite, and sessile. The flowers are of lilac color, small and in whorls.

Lavandula Spica is more dwarfish and more hoary than the last. Leaves oblong-lanceolate. This plant is not used in medicine, but furnishes the *oil of spike*, much used in the preparation of artistical varnishes and by porcelain painters.

History.—Lavandula Vera grows in the dry soils of Southern Europe, and flowers in July and August. It is largely cultivated in this country. The whole plant is aromatic, but the flowers are the parts used, and should be gathered shortly after their appearance, and carefully dried. The disease to which this plant is subject can only be prevented by not allowing them to grow too closely together.

Properties and Uses.—It is a tonic, stimulant, and carminative, useful mostly in diseases of the nervous system.

LEVER-WOOD (ASTRYA VIRGINICA).

COMMON NAMES. *Iron-wood, Hop-hornbeam.*

MEDICINAL PART. *The inner wood.*

Description.—This small tree of from twenty-five to thirty feet in height is remarkable for its fine, narrow, brownish bark. The wood is white, hard, and strong; leaves oblong-ovate, acuminate, serrate, and somewhat downy. Flowers, fertile and sterile, green, and appear with the leaves.

History.—The inner wood and bark are the parts in which reside the curative virtues, and the latter, which are immense, readily yield to water. The tree flowers in April and May, and is common to the United States. The bark and wood should be gathered in August or September.

Properties and Uses.—Lever-wood is anti-periodic, tonic, and alterative. It is very good in cases of intermittent fever, neuralgia, nervous debility, scrofula, and dyspepsia. It is sometimes administered, with fair success, as a remedy for fever and ague.

Dose.—Decoction, one or two fluid ounces, three or four times a day.

LIFE-ROOT (SENECIO AUREUS).

COMMON NAMES. *Squaw-weed, Ragwort, False Valerian, Golden Senecio,* and *Female Regulator.*

MEDICINAL PARTS. *The root and herb.*

Description.—Life-root has an erect, smoothish stem, one or two feet high. Radical leaves are simple and rounded, mostly cordate and long petioled, lower cauline leaves lyrate, upper ones few, dentate and sessile. Flowers golden-yellow.

History.—The plant is perennial and indigenous, growing on low marshy grounds, and on the banks of creeks. The northern and western parts of Europe are where it is mostly found, and the flowers culminate in May and June. The root and herb are the parts employed for medical purposes. There are several varieties of this plant, but as all possess the same medicinal properties, it is unnecessary to specify them. The whole herb is used of all the varieties.

Properties and Uses.—It is diuretic, pectoral, diaphoretic, and tonic, and exerts a very powerful and peculiar influence upon the reproductive organs of females. This has given it the name of *Female Regulator.* Combined with the Lily, and other native and foreign plants, it is one of the most certain cures in the world for aggravated cases of leucorrhœa ; also in cases of menstrual suppression. It will operate excellently in gravel, and other urinary affections.

Dose.—Ordinary decoction, four ounces.

LILY (MEADOW) (LILIUM CANDIDUM).

MEDICINAL PART. *The root.*

Description.—The thick stem of this plant is from three to four feet high, and arises from a perennial bulb or root. Leaves scattered, lanceolate, and narrowed at the base. Flowers are large, snow-white, and smooth inside.

History.—The Meadow Lily is an exotic. It is a native of Syria and Asia Minor. The flowers are regarded as being very beautiful, but are not used for medical purposes. The plant is principally cultivated for the flowers. The bulb is the part used for its curative properties. Water extracts its virtues.

Properties and Uses.—It is mucilaginous, demulcent, tonic, and astringent. It is chosen by some of our best botanical practitioners as a certain remedy for leucorrhœa and falling of the womb, and for those affections, when combined with Life-Root and other herbal preparations, is without an equal. Sometimes the recent root is used to advantage in dropsy. Boiled in milk, it is also useful for ulcers, inflammations, fever-sores, etc. I use it in combination with other indicated plants as an injection in leucorrhœa, with very gratifying success.

LION'S FOOT (NABULUS ALBUS).

COMMON NAMES. *White Lettuce, Rattle-snake Root.*
MEDICINAL PART. *The plant.*

Description.—This indigenous perennial herb has a smooth stem, stout and purplish, from two to four feet high. Radical leaves angular-hastate, cauline ones lanceolate, and all irregularly dentate.

History.—This plant grows plentifully in moist woods and in rich soils, from New England to Iowa, and from Canada to Carolina. The root, leaves, and juice of the plant are employed.

Properties and Uses.—A decoction of the root taken internally will operate most favorably in cases of dysentery. The milky juice of the plant is taken internally, while the leaves, steeped in water, are applied as a poultice (and frequently changed) for the bite of a serpent.

LOBELIA (LOBELIA INFLATA).

COMMON NAMES. *Indian Tobacco, Wild Tobacco.*
MEDICINAL PARTS. *The leaves and seeds.*

Description.—Lobelia is an annual or biennial indigenous plant, with a fibrous root, and an erect, angular, very hairy stem, from six inches to three feet in height. The leaves are alternate, ovate-lanceolate, serrate, veiny, and hairy ; flowers small, numerous, pale-blue ; fruit a two-celled ovoid capsule, containing numerous small brown seeds.

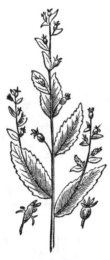
Lobelia.

History.—Lobelia flowers from July to November, and grows in nearly all parts of the United States, in fields, woods, and meadows. The whole plant is active, and the stalks are used indiscriminately with the leaves by those who are best acquainted with its properties. The root is supposed to be more energetic, medicinally, than any other part of the plant. The proper time for gathering is from the last of July to the middle of October. The plant should be dried in the shade, and then be preserved in packages or covered vessels, more especially if it be reduced to powder. It was used in domestic practice by the people of New England long before the time of Samuel Thompson, its assumed discoverer.

Properties and Uses.—Administered internally it is emetic, nauseant, expectorant, relaxant, sedative, anti-spasmodic, and secondarily cathartic, diaphoretic, and astringent. It is extensively used to subdue spasms, and will give relief in epilepsy, tetanus, cramps, hysteria, chorea, and convulsions ; but it is merely a temporary relief when administered internally, and if not used with great skill and caution in that way, may do as much harm as good. Applied externally, in the form of an ointment, combined with healing and soothing barks and roots, it is decidedly the best counter-irritant known to mankind. In this shape its equal has never been discovered, and probably never will be. This is one of the ingredients of the "Herbal Ointment," a full description of which will be found on page 472 of this work. There are any number of officinal preparations of Lobelia, but it is the opinion of the author that its chief value consists in being made into an ointment, with other rare and potent ingredients. There is nothing in nature that can favorably compare with it in this form. In other shapes it may be useful ; but it is also dangerous unless given with care.

LOUSEWORT (Gerardia Pedicularia).

Common Names. *Fever-weed, American Foxglove, etc.*
Medicinal Part. *The herb.*
Description.—The stem of this plant is bushy, tall, two or three feet in height. The leaves are numerous, opposite, ovate-lanceolate ; flowers large, yellow, and trumpet-shaped ; calyx five-cleft, corolla yellow, and fruit a two-celled capsule.
History.—This most elegant plant grows in dry copses, pine ridges, and barren woods and mountains, from Canada to Georgia, flowering in August and September. Water or alcohol extracts its virtues.
Properties aud Uses.—It is diaphoretic, antiseptic, and sedative. Used principally in febrile and inflammatory diseases ; a warm infusion produces a free and copious perspiration in a short time. Very valuable in ephemeral fever.
Dose.—Of the infusion, from one to three fluid ounces.

LUNGWORT (Pulmonaria Officinalis).

Medicinal Part. *The leaves.*
Description.—This rough plant has a stem about one foot high. The radical leaves ovate, cordate ; cauline one, ovate and sessile. Flowers, blue ; calyx, five-angled ; corolla, funnel-shaped ; stigma, emarginate ; and the fruit a roundish, obtuse achenium. (See Illustration, page 16.)
History.—Lungwort is a herbaceous perennial, growing in Europe and this country in northern latitudes. In Europe it is a rough-leaved plant, but in this country the entire plant is smooth, which exhibits the peculiar climatic influence. It is showy, and freely cultivated. It flowers in May. The leaves are used for medical purposes. They are without any particular odor. Water extracts their properties.
Properties and Uses.—It is demulcent and mucilaginous, and in decoction very useful in bleeding from the lungs, and bronchial and catarrhal affections, and other disorders of the respiratory organs. Its virtues seem to be entirely expended upon the lungs, and it is certainly an efficacious remedial agent for all morbid conditions of those organs. It is an ingredient in the "Acacian Balsam," see page 470.

MADDER (RUBIA TINCTORUM).

MEDICINAL PART. *The root.*

Description.—This plant has a perennial, long, cylindrical root, about the thickness of a quill, and deep reddish-brown. It has several herbaceous, brittle stems. The leaves are from four to six in a whorl, lanceolate, mucronate, two or three inches long, and about one-third as wide. Flowers small and yellow.

History.—Madder is a native of the Mediterranean and Southern European countries. The drug is chiefly imported from Holland and France. The root is collected in the third year of the plant, when it is freed from its outer covering and dried. It is valued as a dye-stuff for its red and purple.

Properties and Uses.—It is sometimes used to promote the menstrual and urinary discharges, but is not in very great favor. Combined in a preparation with other ingredients, it is of some considerable remedial value.

Dose.—Thirty grains, three or four times a day. If used frequently, it will color the bones red.

MAD-DOG WEED (ALISMA PLANTAGO).

COMMON NAME. *Water Plantain.*

MEDICINAL PART. *The leaves.*

Description.—This perennial herb has all radical, oval, oblong, or lanceolate leaves, from four to six inches in length, on long radical petioles. The flowers are small and white, and the fruit a three-cornered achenium.

History.—It inhabits the North American continent as well as Europe, grows in watery places, and flowers in July.

Properties and Uses.—It was once considered a capital remedy for hydrophobia, hence its name; but experience has demonstrated that as a cure for this horrible infliction it is impotent. In urinary diseases and affections, an infusion of the leaves, which must be dried and powdered, is very efficacious.

Dose.—Of the infusion above mentioned, from four to six fluid ounces, three or four times a day. The fresh leaves, when bruised, form a very good but mild counter-irritant.

MAIDENHAIR (ADIANTUM PEDATUM).

MEDICINAL PART. *The herb.*

Description.—This is a most delicate and graceful fern, growing from twelve to fifteen inches high, with a slender, polished stalk. Frond pedate, with pinnate branches.

History.—Maidenhair is perennial, and grows throughout the United

States in deep woods, on moist, rich soil. The leaves are bitterish and somewhat aromatic, and part with their virtues upon being immersed in boiling water.

Properties and Uses.—It is refrigerant, expectorant, tonic, and sub-astringent. A decoction of the plant is most gratefully cooling in febrile diseases, and it is a great benefit in coughs, catarrh, hoarseness, influenza, asthma, pleurisy, etc. The decoction, or syrup, can be used freely.

MAGNOLIA (MAGNOLIA GLAUCA).

COMMON NAMES. *White Bay, Beaver-tree, Sweet Magnolia, Swamp Sassafras, etc.*

MEDICINAL PART. *The bark.*

Description.—This tree varies in height from six to thirty feet, being taller in the South than in the North. The leaves are alternate, petioled, entire, and of elliptical shape. The flowers are large and solitary, and of grateful odor. The fruit is a cone.

History.—The therapeutical virtues of these trees are found in the bark and fruit. ·The bark of both the trunk and the root is employed. The odor is aromatic, and the taste bitterish, warm, and pungent. It is gathered during the spring and summer. It has smooth and ash-colored bark, elegant, odoriferous, cream-colored flowers, and can be found in morasses from Massachusetts to the Gulf of Mexico. It flowers from May to August. There are other varieties which do not require especial mention or description.

Properties and Uses.—The bark is an aromatic, tonic bitter, and is also anti-periodic. It is used much in the stead of cinchona, and will remedy the intermittent fevers when cinchona has failed. It is used frequently as a substitute for Peruvian Bark, as it can be continued for a longer time and with more safety. Properly prepared it may be used as a substitute for tobacco, and will break the habit of tobacco-chewing.

Dose.—In powder, half-drachm or drachm doses, five or six times a day. The infusion is taken in wineglassful doses, five or six times a day. The tincture, made by adding two ounces of the cones to a pint of brandy, will be found beneficial in dyspepsia and chronic rheumatism.

MALLOW (COMMON) (MALVA SYLVESTRIS).

COMMON NAME. *High-mallow.*

MEDICINAL PART. *The Herb.*

Description.—This plant is a perennial, and has a round stem two or three feet high, and a tapering, branching, whitish root. The leaves are alternate, deep green, soft, and downy. The flowers are large, numerous, and of purple color ; calyx five-cleft ; petals five ; stamens indefinite ; pollen large, whitish.

History.—The mallow is a native of Europe, but is naturalized in this country. It grows abundantly in fields, waysides, and waste places, and flowers from May to October. The whole plant, especially the root, abounds in mucilage.

Properties and Uses.—It possesses the properties common to mucilaginous herbs, and an infusion thereof forms an excellent demulcent in coughs, irritations of the air-passages, flux, affections of the kidney and bladder, etc. In inflammatory conditions of the external parts, the bruised herb forms an excellent application, making, as it does, a natural emollient cataplasm.

MALVA ROTUNDIFOLIA, or *Low-mallow*, called by children, who are fond of eating the fruit, *cheeses*. possesses similar qualities.

MANDRAKE (PODOPHYLLUM PELTATUM).

COMMON NAMES.　*May-Apple, Wild Lemon, Raccoon-berry, Wild Mandrake.*

MEDICINAL PART.　*The root.*

Description.—This plant, which is illustrated by a cut, is an indigenous perennial herb, with a jointed, dark-brown root, about half the size of

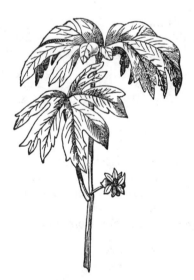

the finger, very fibrous, and internally yellow. The stem is simple, round, smooth, erect, about a foot high, dividing at the top into two petioles, from three to six inches long, each supporting a leaf. The leaves are large, palmate, oftener cordate, smooth, yellowish-green on top, paler beneath. The flower is solitary in the fork of the stem, large, white, and somewhat fragrant. The fruit is fleshy, of a lemon color, and in flavor resembles the strawberry.

There is another plant called *mandrake*, but which is the *Atropa Mandragora*, a plant belonging to the night-shade family. The cut I give of this plant is quite truthful. It is not used in medicine. It inhabits the shores of the Mediterranean, and found

Mandrake.

lurking in dark woods, in the gloomy thickets on the banks of sluggish rivers. It is fetid, poisonous, and repulsive. Even its golden fruit has this nauseous odor. How, then, came it ever to usurp its dominion over men? Its strong narcotic powers may have had some influence; but the peculiar form of its root, in which the resemblance of the human shape, as will be observed, is quite apparent, probably led to its use in magic.

In popular belief, it became invested with half-human attributes; and cries and groans attested its pain when torn from the ground. Gathered with peculiar rites under the shadow of a gallows, it caused money to multiply, but death overtook the daring searcher for mandrake who committed an error in the ritual. There is nothing new under the sun, and as no small number of the old-time magical effects are renewed under new names, our book may reach some spot where the mandrake has been brought forward by some new schemer, and play its part in deluding the silly.

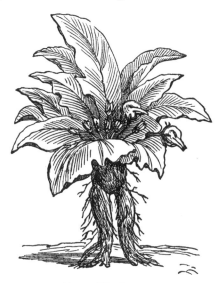

Atropa Mandragora.

History. — The Mandrake is found throughout the United States, in low, shady situations, rich woods, and fields, and flowers in May and June. The fruit matures in September and October. It is scarcer in New England than elsewhere. The Indians were well acquainted with the virtues of this plant. The proper time for collecting the root is in the latter part of October or early part of November, soon after the fruit has ripened. Its active principle is *Podophyllin*, which acts upon the liver in the same manner, but far superior to mercury, and with intelligent physicians it has dethroned that noxious mineral as a cholagogue.

Properties and Uses.—Mandrake is cathartic, emetic, alterative, anthelmintic, hydragogue, and sialagogue. It is an active and certain cathartic. As a deobstruent it has no superior, acting through and upon all the tissues of the system, and its action continues for a long time. In bilious and typhoid febrile diseases it is very valuable as an emeto-cathartic, breaking up the disease quickly. In chronic liver diseases it has no equal in the whole range of medicine. It can also be used as an alterative. In constipation it acts upon the bowels without disposing them to subsequent costiveness. It is also very beneficial in uterine diseases, and its office as a great remedy is extensive. It is one of the ingredients of my "Renovating Pill." See page 473.

Dose.—Of the powdered root, as a cathartic, from ten to thirty grains; of the tincture, from ten to forty drops.

6

MATICO (PIPER ANGUSTIFOLIUM).

MEDICINAL PART.   *The leaves.*

Description.—This is a tall shrub, presenting a singular appearance from its pointed stem and branches.   The leaves are harsh, short-stalked, oblong-lanceolate, and acuminate.   Flowers her-maphrodite.

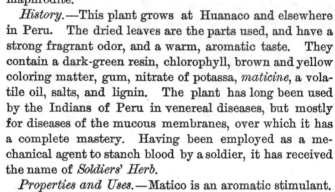

History.—This plant grows at Huanaco and elsewhere in Peru.   The dried leaves are the parts used, and have a strong fragrant odor, and a warm, aromatic taste.   They contain a dark-green resin, chlorophyll, brown and yellow coloring matter, gum, nitrate of potassa, *maticine*, a vola-tile oil, salts, and lignin.   The plant has long been used by the Indians of Peru in venereal diseases, but mostly for diseases of the mucous membranes, over which it has a complete mastery.   Having been employed as a me-chanical agent to stanch blood by a soldier, it has received the name of *Soldiers' Herb.*

Properties and Uses.—Matico is an aromatic stimulant. It is extremely useful to arrest discharges from mucous surfaces, leucorrhœa, gonorrhœa, and catarrh of the blad-der.   As a topical agent for stanching blood it is excel-lent, and is used by surgeons to arrest venous hemorrhage.

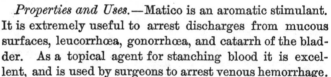

Matico Leaf.

For the above affections Matico serves its office well, but its greatest use and efficacy is exhibited in nasal catarrh.   It is an absolute specific for this disease.   I have long employed it—even before it was admitted in the various pharmacopœias—in my special treatment for catarrh, and I have yet to find a case in which it failed.   I use it both internally and topically, and combine it with such other remedial agents as are sug-gested by the character of each individual case.   Catarrh (see page 262) has long been regarded by the profession as incurable, but in this remedy the incontrovertible aphorism that "every disease has its speci-fic" is still further exemplified, and human progress will ere long com-plete the analogy, if they but investigate the majestic tree, the lowly shrub, or creeping herb.

MECHAMECK (CONVOLVULUS PANDURATUS).

COMMON NAMES.   *Wild Jalap, Man-in-the-Earth, Man-in-the-Ground, Wild Potato.*

MEDICINAL PART.   *The root.*

Description.—This has a perennial, very large tapering root, from which arise several long, round, slender, purplish stems, from four to eight feet high.   The leaves are cordate at base, alternate, and acuminate, and about two or three inches long. Flowers large and white, opening in the forenoon; fruit an oblong, two-celled capsule.

History.—Mechameck belongs to the United States, and grows in light, sandy soils. It flowers from June to August, but is rarely found in northern latitudes. The root is the officinal part. Its best solvent is alcohol or spirits. Water will extract its active properties.

Properties and Uses.—It is a cathartic if powdered and taken in doses of from forty to sixty grains. The infusion, taken in wineglassful doses every hour, is useful in dropsy, strangury, and calculous affections. It seems to exert an influence over the lungs, liver, and kidneys, without excessive diuresis or catharsis. The milky juice of the root is said to be a protection against the bite of the rattlesnake.

MEADOW SAFFRON (COLCHICUM AUTUMNALE).

MEDICINAL PARTS. *The cormus and seeds.*

Description.—The cormus of this plant is large, ovate, and fleshy. The leaves are dark-green, very smooth, obtuse, above a foot long, an inch and a half broad, keeled, produced in the spring along with the capsules. Flowers several, bright-purple, with a white tube appearing in the autumn without the leaves. Fruit a capsule, seeds whitish and polished.

History.—It grows in meadows and low, rich soils in many parts of Europe, and is common in England. The plant is annual or perennial, according to the manner in which it is propagated. The root resembles that of the tulip, and contains a white acrid juice. The bulb should be gathered about the beginning of July, and the seeds early in August. *Colchicia* is the active principle.

Properties and Uses.—It is sedative, cathartic, diuretic, and emetic. Used in gout and gouty rheumatism, dropsy, palpitation of the heart; care should be used in its employment. The tincture is the best form of administration, of which the dose is from twenty to sixty drops.

MONKSHOOD (ACONITUM NAPELLUS).

COMMON NAME. *Wolf's-bane.*

MEDICINAL PARTS. *Leaves and root.*

Description.—This plant has a small napiform root, and simple, straight, erect stems, about five feet high. The leaves are alternate, petioled, dark-green above, paler beneath. The flowers are large, deep bluish-purple, sometimes white, and hairy; fruit a capsule.

History.—This perennial herb is a native of most parts of Europe, growing in wooded hills and plains, and is much cultivated in gardens. It flowers in May and June. All parts of the plant contain powerfully poisonous properties; but the root is the part most generally employed for medical purposes. It yields *Aconitina.*

Properties and Uses.—Although Aconite in the hands of the intelligent physician is of great service, it should not be used in domestic practice. In improper doses all preparations of aconite act as an energetic acro-narcotic poison. As a sedative and anodyne, it is useful in all febrile and inflammatory diseases, and, indeed, in all affections in which there is an increase of nervous, vascular, or muscular action. In acute rheumatism, pneumonia, peritonitis, gastritis, and many other acute disorders, it has been used with the most decided advantage. Its action is more especially displayed in the highest grades of fever and inflammation.

Dose.—The best preparation is the alcoholic extract, formed by evaporating a tincture made of a pound of aconite and a quart of alcohol. The dose of this is one-eighth of a grain.

MOSS (CORSICAN), (FUCUS HELMINTHICORTON).

MEDICINAL PART. *The whole plant.*

Description.—This marine plant has a cartilaginous, tufted, entangled frond, with branches marked indistinctly with transverse streaks. The lower part is dirty-yellow, the branches more or less purple.

History.—It is found growing on the Mediterranean coast, and especially on the Island of Corsica. It is cartilaginous in consistence, is of a dull and reddish-brown color, has a bitter, salt, and nauseous taste, but its odor is rather pleasant. Water dissolves its active principles.

Properties and Uses.—It is an excellent anthelmintic. The influence it exercises upon the economy is entirely inappreciable, but it acts very powerfully on intestinal worms. Dr. Johnson says: "It destroys any worms domiciliating in the bowels as effectually as choke-damps would destroy the life of a miner." This excellent vermifuge plant is one of the ingredients of my Male Fern Vermifuge, see page 471.

Dose.—From ten to sixty grains, mixed with molasses or syrup, or in infusion.

The FUCUS VESICULOSIS, *Sea-wrack,* or *Bladder Fucus,* possesses analogous properties.

MOTHERWORT (LEONURUS CARDIACA).

MEDICINAL PARTS. *The tops and leaves.*

Description.—This perennial plant has stems from two to five feet in height. The leaves are opposite, dark-green, rough, and downy. The flowers are purplish or whitish-red; calyx, rigid and bristly; corolla, purplish; anthers in pairs, and fruit an oblong achenium.

History.—Motherwort is an exotic plant, but extensively introduced into the United States, growing in fields and pastures, and flowering from May to September. It has a peculiar, aromatic, not disagreeable odor, and a slightly aromatic bitter taste. It yields its properties to water and alcohol.

Properties and Uses.—It is antispasmodic, emmenagogue, nervine, and laxative. In amenorrhœa from colds it is excellent, if given in warm infusion. It is very useful in hysteria, nervous complaints, pains peculiar to females, delirium tremens, wakefulness, liver affections, etc., etc. It is a very valuable remedy for many purposes, and deserves greater attention than it receives.

Dose.—Decoction, two to four ounces; extract, three to six grains.

MULLEIN (VERBASCUM THAPSUS).

MEDICINAL PARTS. *The leaves and flowers.*

Description.—This biennial plant has a straight, tall, stout, woolly, simple stem. The leaves are alternate, oblong, acute, and rough on both sides. The flowers are of a golden-yellow color; calyx, five-parted; corolla, five-lobed; stamens, five; and fruit, a capsule or pod.

History.—Mullein is common in the United States, but was undoubtedly introduced from Europe. It grows in recent clearings, slovenly fields, and along the side of roads, flowering from June to August. The leaves and the flowers are the parts used. They have a faint, rather pleasant odor, and a somewhat bitterish, albuminous taste, and yield their virtues to boiling water.

Properties and Uses.—It is demulcent, diuretic, anodyne, and antispasmodic, the infusion being useful in coughs, catarrh, bleeding from the mouth or lungs, diarrhœa, dysentery, and piles. It may be boiled in milk, sweetened, and rendered more palatable by aromatics, for internal use, especially bowel complaints. A fomentation of the leaves in hot vinegar and water forms an excellent local application for inflamed piles, ulcers, and tumors, mumps, acute inflammation of the tonsils, malignant sore throat, etc. A handful of them may be also placed in an old teapot, with hot water, and the steam be inhaled through the spout, in the same complaints.

MYRRH (BALSAMODENDRON MYRRHA).

MEDICINAL PART. *The resinous exudation.*

Description.—This plant has a shrubby, arborescent stem, spinescent branches, a very pale gray bark, and yellowish-white wood. The leaves are ternate, on short petioles; leaflets, obovate; flowers, unknown.

History.—The Myrrh-tree grows in Arabia, and in the regions between Abyssinia and the Red Sea. The juice flows naturally, like cherry-tree gum, upon the bark. At first it is soft and pale yellow, but by drying becomes hard, darker and redder, and forms the medicinal *Gum Myrrh.* It is readily powdered, and has a peculiar, agreeable, balsamic odor, and a bitter, aromatic, not unpleasant taste.

Properties and Uses.—It is a stimulant of the mucous tissues, and used to promote expectoration, as well as menstruation; and is highly useful in enfeebled conditions of the body, excessive mucous secretion, chronic catarrh, leucorrhœa, etc. Also in laryngitis, bronchitis, humoral asthma, and other diseases of the air-tubes, accompanied with profuse secretion, but expelled with difficulty. It is valuable in suppressed menses and cases of anæmia; also as a local application to indolent sores, gangrenous ulcers, aphthous or sloughy sore throat, spongy and ulcerated condition of the gum, caries of the teeth, etc.

Dose.—In powder and pill, ten to thirty grains; of the tincture, from half to two teaspoonfuls.

NARROW LEAF VIRGINIA THYME (PYCANTHEMUM VIRGINICUM).

COMMON NAME. *Prairie Hyssop.*
MEDICINAL PART. *The plant.*
Description.—This pubescent plant has a simple stem, growing from one to two feet high. The leaves are sessile, entire, and linear; flowers are white, and fruit an achenium.
History.—It is found in low grounds, dry hills, and plains, from Ohio and Illinois extending southward, and flowering in July and August. The whole plant is used, and has the taste and odor peculiar to the mint family.
Properties and Uses.—It is diaphoretic, stimulant, antispasmodic, carminative, and tonic. A warm infusion is very useful in puerperal, remittent, and other forms of fever, coughs, colds, catarrhs, etc., and is also of much benefit in spasmodic diseases, especially colic, cramp of the stomach, and spasms of infants. The cold infusion is a good tonic and stimulant during convalescence from exhausting diseases. It forms a most certain remedy for catarrh when combined with other native and foreign herbs and roots.
Dose.—From one to four fluid ounces of the warm or cold infusion, several times a day.
The *P. Pilosum*, *P. Aristatum* or *Wild Basil*, and *P. Incanum*, have similar properties.

NETTLE (URTICA DIOCA).

COMMON NAME. *Great Stinging Nettle.*
MEDICINAL PARTS. *The root and leaves.*
Description.—This is a perennial, herbaceous, dull-green plant, armed with small prickles, which emit an acrid fluid when pressed. The stem is from two to four feet high; root creeping and branching. The leaves are opposite, cordate, lance-ovate, and conspicuously acuminate. Flowers are small and green.
History.—The Common Nettle is well known both in America and in

Europe, and grows in waste places, beside hedges and in gardens, flowering from June to September. The leaves and root are the parts used. The prickles of the Common Nettle contain Formic Acid. The young shoots have been boiled and eaten as a remedy for scurvy.

Properties and Uses.—It is astringent, tonic, and diuretic. In decoction they are valuable in diarrhœa, dysentery, and piles ; also in hemorrhages, scorbutic and febrile affections, gravel, and other nephritic complaints. The leaves of the fresh Common Nettle stimulate, inflame, and raise blisters upon those portions of the skin to which they may be applied, and they have, as a natural consequence, often been used as a powerful rubefacient. They are also an excellent styptic, checking the flow of blood from surfaces almost immediately upon their application. The seeds and flowers are given in wine for agues.

Dose.—Of the powdered root or leaves, from twenty to forty grains ; of the decoction, from two to four fluid ounces.

URTICA URENS, or *Dwarf Nettle*, possesses similar qualities, and is very efficacious in uterine hemorrhage.

URTICA PAMILA, *Cool-weed, Rich-weed,* or *Stingless Nettle,* has also active properties. It gives relief in inflammations, painful swellings, erysipelas, and the topical poison of-rhus.

NET LEAF PLANTAIN (GOODYERA PUBESCENS).

COMMON NAMES. *Scrofula-weed, Adder's Violet, Rattle-snake Leaf,* etc.

MEDICINAL PART. *The leaves.*

Description.—The scape or stem of this plant is from eight to twelve inches high, springing from a perennial root. The leaves are radical, ovate, and dark green. The flowers are white, numerous, and pubescent.

History.—This herb grows in various parts of the United States, in rich woods and under evergreens, and is commoner southward than northward, although there is a variety (*Goodyera Repens*) which is plentiful in colder regions of America. It bears yellowish-white flowers in July and August. The leaves are the parts employed, and yield their virtues to boiling water.

Properties and Uses.—It is anti-scrofulous, and is known to have cured severe cases of scrofula. The fresh leaves are steeped in milk and applied to scrofulous ulcers as a poultice, or the bruised leaves may be laid on them, and in either case they must be removed every three hours ; at the same time an infusion must be taken as freely as the stomach will allow. It is also good as a wash in scrofulous ophthalmia. In my opinion scrofula is one of the most obstinate and many-shaped afflictions to which the human race is subjected, but in the production of this and

other native and foreign plants, nature has shown her great charity
and kindness towards us.

NIGHTSHADE (GARDEN) (SOLANUM NIGRUM).

MEDICINAL PART. *The leaves.*

Description.—This is a fetid, narcotic, bushy herb, with a fibrous
root, and an erect, branching, thornless stem, one or two feet high.
Leaves are ovate, dentated, smooth, and the margins have the appearance as if gnawed by insects. Flowers white or pale-violet ; fruit, a
berry.

History.—This plant is also called Deadly Nightshade, but is not to
be confounded with Belladonna. It is found growing along old walls,
fences, and in gardens, in various parts of the United States, flowering
in July and August. The leaves yield their virtues to water and alcohol.

Properties and Uses.—It is a narcotic and sedative, producing, when
given in large doses, sickness and vertigo. One to three grains of the
leaves, infused in water, will produce a copious perspiration and purge
on the day following. They have been freely used in cancer, scurvy,
and scrofulous affections, in the form of an ointment. Very small
doses are taken internally. These should always be prescribed, and
their effects watched by a physician. It is better to use the plant only
in the form of an ointment. The berries are poisonous, and will produce torpor, insensibility, and death.

NORWAY PINE (ABIES EXCELSA).

MEDICINAL PART. *The concrete juice.*

Description.—This is a large tree, often having a diameter exceeding
four feet, and attaining an altitude of one hundred and forty feet.
Leaves are short, scattered, mucronate, dark-green, and glossy above.

History.—It is an inhabitant of Germany, Russia, and Norway, and
other northern parts of Europe, as well as of Asia. It affords the *Frankincense* of commerce, which, when boiled in water and strained, forms
the officinal *Burgundy Pitch.*

Properties and Uses.—Burgundy Pitch is generally used externally
to produce a redness of the surface, with a slight serous exhalation. It
is employed as a counter-irritant in chronic diseases of the lungs,
stomach, intestines, etc , and is regarded with favor as a local application in rheumatic affections.

NUX VOMICA (STRYCHNOS NUX VOMICA).

MEDICINAL PART. *The seeds.*

Description.—This is a moderate-sized tree, with a short and pretty

thick trunk. The wood is white, hard, and bitter. The leaves are opposite, oval, and smooth on both sides.
Flowers small, greenish-white, funnel-
shaped, and have a disagreeable odor.
The fruit is a berry, round, and about
the size of a large apple, enclosing five
whitish seeds.

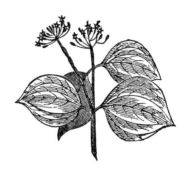

History.—It is an inhabitant of Cor-
omandel, Ceylon, and other parts of
the East Indies. The active principles of the seeds are *strychnine* and
brucia.

Properties and Uses.—It is an energetic poison, exerting its influence

Nux Vomica.

chiefly upon the cerebro-spinal system. It is supposed to affect the
spinal cord principally. It is a favorite medicine for paralysis and nervous debility generally. If a poisonous dose is given it will produce
spasms like tetanus or lock-jaw. It is tonic, and increases the action
of various excretory organs. Where want of nervous energy exists it is
an admirable remedy. Its range of service is quite extensive, and valuable for many indications; but as great caution is required in its administration, it should only be employed by the educated physician.

OAK—WHITE, RED, AND BLACK (QUERCUS ALBA, RUBRA, AND
TINCTORIA).

MEDICINAL PART. *The bark.*

Description.—These forest-trees vary in size, according to the climate
and soil. In diameter they are from three to six feet; in height, from
sixty to a hundred feet. They are too well known to require any botanical description.

History.—Quercus is a very extensive and valuable genus, consisting
of many species, a large proportion of which grow in the United States.
Their usual character is that of astringent, and the three above described
are those which have been more particularly employed in medicine. The
bark of the tree is the portion used. White oak bark is the one chiefly
used in medicine. It is of a pale brownish color, faintly odorous, very
astringent, with a slight bitterness, tough, breaking with a stringy or
fibrous fracture, and not readily powdered. It contains a very large
proportion of tannic acid. Black oak bark is also used as an astringent
externally, but is rarely employed internally, as it is liable to derange
the bowels. It is also used in tanning and for dyeing. Red oak bark
also contains considerable tannin, and is chiefly applied externally in the
treatment of cancers, indolent ulcers, etc.

Properties and Uses.—The bark is slightly tonic, powerfully astrin-
6*

gent, and antiseptic. It is useful internally in chronic diarrhœa, chronic mucous discharges, passive hemorrhages, and wherever an internal astringent is required. In colliquative sweats the decoction is usually combined with lime-water. The gargle and injection are extensively used for sore throat, whites, piles, etc. A bath of the decoction is often advantageous in cutaneous diseases, but should only be used when ordered by a physician.

Dose.—Of the decoction, one or two fluid ounces ; of the extract, from five to twenty grains.

QUERCUS INFECTORIA, or *Dyers' Oak*, is a small shrub, which furnishes the morbid excrescences, *Galls*, which, or the gallic acid obtained from them, may be used wherever an astringent is called for.

OLD MAN'S BEARD (CHIONANTHUS VIRGINICA).

COMMON NAMES. *Fringe Tree, Poison Ash.*
MEDICINAL PART. *Bark of the root.*
Description.—This is a shrub or small tree, growing from eight to twenty-five feet high. The leaves are opposite, oval, oblong, veiny, and smooth ; flowers are in dense panicles ; calyx very small ; corolla snow-white, consisting of four petals ; and fruit a fleshy, oval, purple drupe.

History.—This plant is very ornamental, and is much cultivated in gardens, from Pennsylvania to Tennessee. It grows on river-banks and on elevated places, presenting clusters of snow-white flowers in May and June. The bark of the root, which imparts its properties to water or alcohol, is the part used.

Properties and Uses.—The bark is aperient, alterative, and diuretic, with some narcotic properties. An infusion is recommended for bilious, typhoid, and intermittent fevers. To convalescents who are suffering from the effects of exhaustive diseases it is an excellent tonic and restorative. It can be used to advantage as a poultice for ulcers, wounds, and external inflammations.

Dose.—Of the infusion, from the half a fluid ounce to two fluid ounces, repeated several times through the day, according to the influence it exerts upon the system.

OLD FIELD BALSAM (GNAPHALIUM POLYCEPHALUM).

COMMON NAMES. *Indian Posy, Sweet-scented Life Everlasting, White Balsam, etc.*
MEDICINAL PART. *The herb.*
Description.—This indigenous herbaceous annual has an erect, whitish, woolly, and much branched stem, one or two feet high. The leaves are alternate, sessile, lanceolate, acute, and entire ; flowers tubular and yellow.

History.—Old Field Balsam is found in Canada and various parts of the United States, growing in old fields and on dry barren lands, flowering in July and August. The leaves have a pleasant, aromatic smell, and are the parts used. They readily yield their properties to water.

Properties and Uses.—It is an astringent. Ulcerations of the mouth and throat are relieved by chewing the leaves and blossoms. In fevers a warm infusion is found to be very serviceable; also in quinsy, and pulmonary and bronchial complaints. It is also valuable, in infusion, for diseases of the bowels and hemorrhages; and the leaves, applied to bruises, indolent tumors, and other local affections, are very efficacious.

ANTEMARIA MARGARITACEA, or *Pearl-flowered Life Everlasting*, a perennial, possesses similar medicinal qualities.

OPIUM (PAPAVER SOMNIFERUM).

COMMON NAME. *Poppy.*

MEDICINAL PART. *Concrete juice of unripe capsule.*

Description.—An annual herb, with an erect, round, green, smooth stem, from two to four feet high. Leaves large, oblong, green; margins wavy, incised, and toothed; teeth sometimes tipped with a rigid hair. Flowers large, calyx smooth, and the fruit a large, smooth, globose capsule. There are two varieties, the *black* and *white*.

History.—A native of Asia and Egypt. It grows apparently wild in some parts of Europe and in England, but has escaped the gardens. Cultivated in Asia Minor, Egypt, Persia, and India, for the opium obtained from it. The white variety is cultivated on the plains of India, and the black in the Himalayas. Its virtues have been known to the ancients; for Homer speaks of the poppy growing in gardens. Poppy capsules contain a small quantity of the principles found in opium, and the effect is similar, but much weaker than it possesses. They are used medicinally; but opium is almost universally used.

Properties and Uses.—Opium is a narcotic and stimulant, acting under various circumstances as a sedative, antispasmodic, febrifuge, and diaphoretic. It is anodyne, and extensively used for that purpose. It contains many active principles, morphia and codeia being, however, the most important. There is no herbal medicine more extensively used, as well as abused, than Opium, and though a valuable remedy, its indiscriminate use is pernicious, as it is capable of doing great harm. Laudanum and paregoric are the forms mostly used in domestic practice, but the "soothing syrups" and "carminatives" found in every nursery and household all contain Opium in some form, and work a great deal of mischief.

Dose.—Opium, one grain; laudanum, twenty drops; paregoric, a teaspoonful.

PAPOOSE ROOT (CAULOPHYLLUM THALICTROIDES).

COMMON NAMES. *Blue Cohosh, Squaw Root, etc.*
MEDICINAL PART. *The root.*

Description.—This is a smooth, glaucous plant, purple when young, with a high, round stem, one to three feet high. Leaves biternate or triternate, leaflets oval, petiolate, pale beneath, and from two to three inches long. The flowers appear in May or June.

History.—It is a handsome perennial plant, growing in all parts of the United States, near running streams, and in low, moist, rich grounds; also in swamps and on islands. The seeds, which ripen in August, make a decoction which closely resembles coffee. The berries are dry and rather mawkish. Its active principle is *Caulophyllin.*

Properties and Uses.—It is principally used as an emmenagogue, parturient, and antispasmodic. It also possesses diuretic, diaphoretic, and anthelmintic properties. It is employed in rheumatism, colic, cramps, hiccough, epilepsy, hysteria, uterine inflammation, etc. It is a valuable remedy in all chronic uterine diseases, but should be given in combination with such other remedies as the case requires.

Dose.—Of the decoction, from two to four fluid ounces, three or four times a day.

PAREIRA BRAVA (CISSAMPELOS PAREIRA).

COMMON NAMES. *Velvet Leaf, Ice Vine.*
MEDICINAL PART. *The root.*

Description.—This plant is a shrub, with a round woody root and smooth stems. Leaves roundish, peltate, subcordate, and smooth above when full grown. Flowers small, and the fruit a scarlet, round, reniform, shrivelled berry.

History.—This is a native of the West India Islands and the Spanish Main. It is sometimes imported under the name of *abuta* or *butua* root. It comes in cylindrical pieces, sometimes flattened, and some as thick as a child's arm, and a foot or more in length. The alkaloid obtained from it has been called *Cissampelin*, or *Pelosin.*

Properties and Uses.—Tonic, diuretic, and aperient. Used in chronic inflammation of the bladder, and various disorders of the urinary organs. It is also serviceable in leucorrhoea and gonorrhoea. It is highly beneficial in calculous affections, rheumatism, and jaundice.

Dose.—Of the infusion, one to four ounces; extract, ten to twenty grains.

PARSLEY (PETROSELINUM SATIVUM).

MEDICINAL PART. *The root.*

Description.—This biennial plant has a fleshy, spindle-shaped root, and an erect, smooth, branching stem. The radical leaves are biter-nate, bright green, and on long petioles; leaflets wedge-shaped. Flow-ers white or greenish, and petals rounded and barely emarginate.

History.—Although Parsley is reared in all parts of the civilized world as a culinary vegetable, it is a native of Europe. The root is the officinal part. From the seeds French chemists have succeeded in ob-taining an essential oil, named *Apiol,* which has proved to be a good substitute for quinia in intermittent fevers, and for ergot as a partu-rient.

Properties and Uses.—It is diuretic, and very excellent in dropsy, especially that following scarlatina and other exanthematous diseases. It is also frequently used to remedy retention of urine, strangury, and gonorrhœa. The seeds are sometimes used as carminatives. They kill vermin in the head. The leaves, bruised, are a good application for contusions, swelled breasts, and enlarged glands. The bruised leaves applied to the breasts are used by wet-nurses to "dry up" the milk.

Dose.—Of the oil, for diuretic purposes, three or four drops a day; of the infusion, two to four fluid ounces, three or four times a day.

PARTRIDGE BERRY (MITCHELLA REPENS).

COMMON NAMES. *One Berry, Checkerberry, Winter Clover, Deer-berry, Squaw-vine, etc.*

MEDICINAL PART. *The vine.*

Description.—This indigenous evergreen herb has a perennial root, from which arises a smooth and creeping stem. The leaves are ovate, slightly cordate, opposite, flat and dark-green; flowers are white, often tinged with red, in pairs, very fragrant, and have united ovaries. Calyx four-parted; corolla funnel-shaped; stamens four, inserted on the co-rolla. The fruit is a dry berry-like double drupe.

History.—Partridge Berry is indigenous to the United States. It grows both in dry woods and swampy places, and flowers in June and July. The berry is bright scarlet and edible, but nearly tasteless. The leaves, which look something like clover, remain green throughout the winter. The whole plant is used, readily imparting its virtues to alcohol or boiling water.

Properties and Uses.—Partridge Berry is parturient (producing or promoting child-birth, or labor), diuretic, and astringent. In all uterine diseases it is highly beneficial. The Indian women use it for weeks before confinement, in order to render parturition safe and easy. Ladies who wish to use it for that purpose, however, should consult an herbal physician of experience for a proper, safe, and effectual preparation. The remedy is exclusively American, not being used, or even noticed, by European practitioners.

Dose.—Of a strong decoction, from two to four fluid ounces, three or four times a day. The berries are good for dysentery. They are also highly spoken of as a cure for sore nipples. The application for the nipples is made by boiling a strong decoction of the leaves down to a thick liquid, and then adding cream to it. It is not, however, equal to the Herbal Ointment, for an account of which see page 472.

PENNYROYAL (HEDEOMA PULEGIOIDES).

COMMON NAMES. *Tickweed, Squawmint, etc.*
MEDICINAL PART. *The herb.*
Description.—This is an indigenous annual plant, with a fibrous, yellowish root, and an erect, branching stem, from six to twelve inches high. The leaves are half an inch or more long, opposite, oblong, and on short petioles ; floral leaves similar. The flowers are quite small and light-blue in color.

History.—This plant should not be confounded with the *Mentha pulegioides,* or *European Pennyroyal.* It grows in barren woods and dry fields, and particularly in limestone countries, flowering from June to September and October, rendering the air fragrant to some distance around it. It is common to nearly all parts of the United States. It is said to be very obnoxious to fleas.

Properties and Uses.—It is stimulant, diaphoretic, emmenagogue, and carminative. The warm infusion, used freely, will promote perspiration, restore suppressed lochia or after-flow, and excite the menstrual discharge when recently checked. It is very much used by females for this last purpose—a large draught being taken at bedtime, the feet being previously bathed in hot water.

PEONY (PÆONIA OFFICINALIS).

MEDICINAL PART. *The root.*
Description.—Peony has many thick, long-spreading, perennial roots, running deep into the ground, with an erect, herbaceous, large, green, and branching stem, about two or three feet high. The leaves are large ; leaflets ovate-lanceolate and smooth. The flowers are large, red, and solitary ; and fruit a many-seeded, fleshy follicle.

History.—This plant is indigenous to Southern Europe, and is cultivated in gardens in the United States and elsewhere, on account of the elegance of its large flowers, which appear from May to August. The root is the officinal part. This, with the seeds and flowers, yields its virtues to diluted spirits.

Properties and Uses.—It is antispasmodic and tonic, and can be advantageously employed in chorea, epilepsy, spasms, and various nervous affections. An infusion of value is made by adding an ounce of the root, in coarse powder, to a pint of a boiling liquid, composed of one part of *good* gin and two parts of water.

Dose.—Two or three fluid ounces (sweetened), three or four times a day.

PERUVIAN BALSAM (MYROSPERMUM PERUIFERUM).

MEDICINAL PART. *The balsamic exudation.*

Description.—The tree from which this is procured is large, with a thick, straight, smooth trunk, and a coarse, gray, compact, heavy, granulated bark. The bark is of a pale straw color, filled with resin, which, according to its quantity, changes the color to citron, yellow, red, or dark chestnut; smell and taste grateful, balsamic, and aromatic. The leaves are pinnate; leaflets alternate, oblong or ovate, acuminate, and emarginate. The flowers are in axillary racemes, and the fruit is a pendulous, straw-colored samara.

History.—The tree is common to the forests of Peru, and flowers from July to October. The natives call it *Quinquino.* It contains a large amount of balsamic juice, which yields copiously when the bark is incised. Balsam of Peru, in thin layers, has a dark, reddish-brown color; in bulk it is black, or of the color of molasses. The natives steep the fruit in rum, call the liquid *balsamito,* and use it largely for medical purposes.

Properties and Uses.—It is expectorant and stimulant, acting especially on mucous tissues. Its reparative action on the lungs in consumption is decided, removing the secretions, healing the ulcers, and expelling the tuberculous matter. In all chronic diseases of the lungs and bronchial tubes it is without a superior. Externally it can be applied to old ulcers, wounds, ringworm, etc.

This valuable remedy is one of the ingredients of my "Acacian Balsam," wherein it is properly combined with many other valuable associates.

PINKROOT (SPIGELIA MARILANDICA).

COMMON NAMES. *Carolina Pink* or *Worm Grass.*
MEDICINAL PART. *The root.*

Description.—This herbaceous, indigenous plant has a perennial, very fibrous, yellow root, which sends up several erect, smooth stems of purplish color, from six to twenty inches high. The leaves are opposite, sessile, ovate-lanceolate, acute, or acuminate, entire, and smooth. Flowers few in number and club-shaped. Fruit a double capsule.

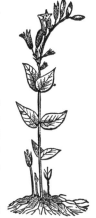

Pinkroot.

History.—It inhabits the Southern States, and is seldom found north of the Potomac. It was used by the Indians as an anthelmintic before the discovery of America, and was formerly collected for the market by the Creeks and

Cherokees in the northern part of Georgia, but since their removal the supply comes from the far Southwest.

Properties and Uses.—It is an active and certain vermifuge, especially among children.   Given alone it is very apt to produce various unpleasant symptoms, increased action of the heart, dizziness, etc.   I extract from the root a resinous principle, to which I have given the name of *Spigeliin*, which has all of the virtues of the root, but does not produce any derangement.   I employ the Spigeliin in my "Male Fern Vermifuge."   See page 471.

PIPSISSEWA (CHIMAPHILA UMBELLATA).

COMMON NAMES.   *Wintergreen, Prince's Pine, Ground Holly, etc.*
MEDICINAL PART.   *The whole plant.*

Description.—This is a small evergreen, nearly herbaceous, perennial herb, with a creeping rhizome, from which spring several erect stems, woody at their base, and from four to eight inches high.   The leaves are from two to three inches long, on short petioles, and of dark green-color, paler below. The flowers are of light-purple color, and exhale a fragrant odor.   The pollen is white, and the fruit is an erect five-celled capsule.

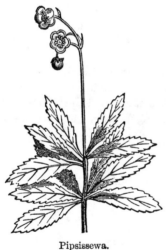
Pipsissewa.

History.—This plant is indigenous to the north temperate regions of both hemispheres, and is met with in dry, shady woods, flowering from May to August.   The leaves have no odor when dried, but when fresh and rubbed they are rather fragrant.   Boiling water or alcohol extracts their virtues.   They contain resin, gum, lignin, and saline substances.

Properties and Uses.—It is diuretic, tonic, alterative, and astringent. It is especially useful in scrofula and chronic rheumatism.   In diseases of the kidneys and dropsy it exerts a decided curative power.   In urinary diseases it is preferable to uva ursi, on account of being less obnoxious to the stomach.   In dropsy it cannot be so well depended upon without the use of some more active measures in combination with it.

PLEURISY ROOT (ASCLEPIAS TUBEROSA).

COMMON NAMES.   *Butterfly-weed, Wind-root, Tuber-root.*
MEDICINAL PART.   *The root.*

Description.—This plant has a perennial, large, fleshy, white, fusiform root, from which numerous stems arise, growing from one to three feet high, which are more or less erect, round, hairy, green or red, and growing in bunches from the root. The leaves are alternate, lanceolate, hairy, dark green above, and paler beneath.

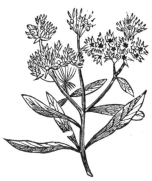

The flowers are numerous, erect, and of a beautifully bright orange color. The fruit is a long, narrow, green follicle. Seeds are ovate, and terminate in long silken hairs.

History.—It is a native of the United States, more particularly of the Southern States, inhabiting gravelly and sandy soils, and flowering in July and August. The root is the medicinal part. When fresh it has a disagreeable, slightly acrimonious taste, but when dried the taste is slightly bitter. Boiling water extracts its virtues. *Asclepin* is the active principle.

Pleurisy Root.

Properties and Uses.—Pleurisy Root is much used in decoction or infusion, for the purpose of promoting perspiration and expectoration in diseases of the respiratory organs, especially pleurisy, inflammation of the lungs, catarrhal affections, consumption, etc. It is likewise carminative, tonic, diuretic, and antispasmodic, but does not stimulate. Acute rheumatism, fever, dysentery, etc., are benefited by a free use of the warm infusion. It is also highly efficacious in some cases of dyspepsia. In uterine difficulties it has also been found of great value. Its chief use, however, is in bronchial and pulmonary complaints, and it serves its indications in these complaints most admirably. It is one of the ingredients of my Acacian Balsam. See page 470.

Dose.—Of the powder, twenty to sixty grains, three or four times a day. Of a *strong* tincture, one or two wineglasses full four or five times a day, until perspiration is produced.

POKE (PHYTOLACCA DECANDRA).

COMMON NAMES. *Pigeon-berry, Garget, Scoke, Coakum, etc.*

MEDICINAL PARTS. *The root, leaves, and berries.*

Description.—This indigenous plant has a perennial root of large size, frequently exceeding a man's leg in diameter, fleshy, fibrous, easily cut or broken, and covered with a thin brownish bark. The stems are annual, about an inch in diameter, round, smooth, when young green, and grow from five to nine feet in height. The leaves are scattered, petiolate, smooth on both sides, and about five inches long and three broad. The flowers are numerous, small, and greenish-white in color; and the berries are round, dark-purple, and in long clusters.

History.—This plant is common in many parts of the country, growing in dry fields, hillsides, and roadsides, and flowering in July and August. It is also found in Europe and northern parts of Africa. The leaves should be gathered just previous to the ripening of the berries. The berries are collected when fully matured. *Phytolaccin* is its active principle.

Properties and Uses.—Poke is emetic, cathartic, alterative, and slightly narcotic. The root excites the whole glandular system, and is very useful in syphilitic, scrofulous, rheumatic, and cutaneous diseases. It is an excellent remedy for the removal of mercurio-syphilitic affections. Very few, if any, of the alteratives have superior power to Poke, if it is properly gathered and prepared for medicinal use. It is an ingredient in my "Blood Purifier," which will be found fully described on page 471.

POMEGRANATE (PUNICA GRANATUM).

MEDICINAL PARTS. *The rind of the fruit, and bark of the root.*

Description.—This is a small tree or shrub. The leaves are opposite, entire, smooth, and two or three inches long. The flowers are large, red, two or three, and nearly sessile. Calyx five-cleft, corolla consists of five much crumpled petals. The fruit is a large pericarp, quite pleasant in flavor, and quite watery.

History.—The Pomegranate is Asiatic, but has been naturalized in the West Indies and the Southern States.

Properties and Uses.—The flowers and rind of the fruit are astringent, and are used for the arrest of mucous discharges, hemorrhages, night-sweats, and diarrhœa accompanying consumption. They are also very good for intermittent fever and tape-worm. The bark of the root is used as a specific for tape-worm, but its chief virtues are healing and balsamic, if taken for ulcerations of the lungs.

Dose.—The dose of the rind or flowers in powder is from one to two scruples, and in decoction from one to three fluid ounces.

PRICKLY ASH (XANTHOXYLUM FRAXINEUM).

COMMON NAMES. *Yellow-wood, Toothache-bush, etc.*

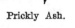

Prickly Ash.

MEDICINAL PARTS. *The bark and berries.*

Description.—This indigenous shrub has a stem ten or twelve feet high, with alternate branches, which are armed with strong conical prickles. The leaves are alternate and pinnate, leaflets ovate and acute. The flowers are small, greenish, and appear before the leaves. The fruit is an oval capsule, varying from green to red in color.

History.—It is a native of North America, growing from Canada to Virginia, and west to the Mississippi, in woods, thickets, and on river banks, and flowering in April and May. The medicinal parts render their virtues to water and alcohol. *Xanthoxyline* is its active principle.

Properties and Uses.—Prickly Ash is stimulant, tonic, alterative, and sialagogue. It is used as a stimulant in languid states of the system, and as a sialagogue in paralysis of the tongue and mouth. It is highly beneficial in chronic rheumatism, colic, syphilis, hepatic derangements, and wherever a stimulating alterative is required. Dose of the powder, from ten to thirty grains, three times a day. The berries are stimulant, carminative, and antispasmodic, acting especially on the mucous tissues.

The *Aralia Spinosa*, or Southern Prickly Ash, differs from Xanthoxylum, both in botanical character and medicinal virtues.

PRIVET (LIGUSTRUM VULGARE).

COMMON NAMES. *Privy, Prim, etc.*
MEDICINAL PART. *The leaves.*

Description.—This is a smooth shrub, growing five or six feet high. The leaves are dark-green, one or two inches in length, about half as wide, entire, smooth, lanceolate, and on short petioles. The flowers are small, white, and numerous, and fruit a spherical black berry. In England the Privet is carried up with many slender branches to a reasonable height and breadth, to cover arbors, bowers, and banqueting houses, and brought or wrought into many fantastic forms, as birds, men, horses.

History.—It is supposed to have been introduced into America from England, but it is indigenous to Missouri, and found growing in wild woods and thickets from New England to Virginia and Ohio. It is also cultivated in American gardens. The leaves are used for medicinal purposes. They have but little odor, and an agreeable bitterish and astringent taste. They yield their virtues to water or alcohol. The berries are reputed cathartic, and the bark is said to be as effectual as the leaves, as it contains sugar, mannite, starch, bitter resin, bitter extractive, albumen, salts, and a peculiar substance called *Ligustrin.*

Properties and Uses.—The leaves are astringent. A decoction of them is valuable in chronic bowel complaints, ulcerations of stomach and bowels, or as a gargle for ulcers of mouth and throat. It is also good as an injection for ulcerated ears with offensive discharges, leucorrhœa, etc. This ingredient I use in a wash for leucorrhœa, which never fails to cure.

333

Dose.—Of the powdered leaves thirty to sixty grains, three times a day; of the decoction two to four teacupfuls.

QUASSIA (PICRÆNIA EXCELSA).

COMMON NAMES. *Bitter-wood, Bitter-ash.*
MEDICINAL PART. *The wood.*

Description.—This is a tree growing from fifty to one hundred feet high, with an erect stem, three or more feet in diameter at the stem. The bark is grayish and smooth. The leaves are alternate, unequally pinnate; leaflets opposite, oblong, acuminate, and unequal at the base. Flowers are small, pale or yellowish-green. Fruit three drupes, about the size of a pea. The *Quassia Amara*, or bitter quassia, is a shrub, or moderately-sized branching tree, having a grayish bark.

History.—*Quassia Amara* inhabits Surinam, Guiana, Colombia, Panama, and the West India Islands. It flowers in November and December. The bark, wood, and root, which are intensely bitter, are used to the greatest advantage in malignant fevers. For the medicinal parts of this tree, as they seldom reach England or America, we get as a substitute the *Picræna Excelsa* of Jamaica and other neighboring islands, which flowers in October and November, and in the two succeeding months matures its fruit.

Properties and Uses.—Quassia is tonic, febrifuge, and anthelmintic. Cups made of the wood have been used for many years by persons requiring a powerful tonic. Any liquid standing in one of these vessels a few moments will become thoroughly impregnated by its peculiar medicinal qualities. Wherever a bitter tonic is required, Quassia is an excellent remedy.

Dose.—Of the powder, thirty grains; of the infusion, from one to three fluid ounces; of the tincture, one or two fluid drachms, and of the extract, from two to ten grains.

QUEEN OF THE MEADOW (EUPATORIUM PURPUREUM).

COMMON NAMES. *Gravel-root, Joe-pie, Trumpet-weed.*
MEDICINAL PART. *The root.*

Description.—This is a herbaceous plant, with a perennial, woody root, with many long dark-brown fibres, sending up one or more solid green, sometimes purplish, stems, five or six feet in height. The leaves are oblong-ovate or lanceolate, coarsely serrate, and from three to six in a whorl. The flowers are tubular, purple, often varying to whitish.

History.—Queen of the Meadow grows in low places, dry woods or meadows, in the Northern, Western, and Middle States of the American Union, and flowers in August and September. The root is the officinal part. It has a smell resembling old hay, and a slightly bitter, aromatic taste, which is faintly astringent but not unpleasant. It yields its properties to water by decoction or spirits.

Properties and Uses.—It is diuretic, stimulant, astringent, and tonic. It is used in all chronic urinary disorders, as well as in hematuria, gout, and rheumatism, with moderate good effect.

Dose.—Of the decoction, from two to four fluid ounces, three or four times a day.

RAGGED CUP (SILPHIUM PERFOLIATUM).

COMMON NAME. *Indian Cup-plant.*

MEDICINAL PART. *The root.*

Description.—This plant has a perennial, horizontal, pitted rhizome, and a large smooth herbaceous stem, from four to seven feet high. The leaves are opposite, ovate, from eight to fourteen inches long by four to seven wide. The flowers are yellowish, and the fruit a broadly ovate winged achenium.

History.—This plant is common to the Western States, and is found growing in rich bottoms, bearing numerous yellow flowers, which are perfected in August. It has a large, long, and crooked root, which is the part used medicinally, and which readily imparts its properties to alcohol or water. It will yield a bitterish gum, somewhat similar to frankincense, which is frequently used to sweeten the breath.

Properties and Uses.—It is tonic, diaphoretic, and alterative. A strong infusion of the root, made by long steeping, or an extract, is said to be one of the best remedies for the removal of ague-cake, or enlarged spleen. It is also useful in intermittent and remittent fevers, internal bruises, debility, ulcers, liver affections, and as a general alterative restorative. The gum is said to be stimulant and antispasmodic. The spleen is an organ whose functions the very best of the old-school physicians cannot define ; but that it is the seat of very many most distressing diseases is a fact which not one of them will pretend to deny. It is, as nearly as can be ascertained by the most laborious research, a dependent of the liver and stomach, and what deranges it deranges both the stomach and the liver.

SILPHIUM GUMMIFERUM, or *Rosin-weed,* and SILPHIUM LACINIATUM, or *Compass-weed,* are used in intermittent fever, and are beneficial in dry, obstinate coughs. They often cure the heaves in horses.

RATTLE BUSH (BAPTISIA TINCTORIA).

COMMON NAMES. *Wild Indigo, Horsefly Weed.*

MEDICINAL PART. *The bark of the root and leaves.*

Description.—The blackish and wood root of this perennial plant sends up a stem which is very much branched, round, smooth, and from two to three feet high. The leaves are small and alternate, leaflets rounded at their extremity; calyx four-cleft, and fruit a short, bluish-black legume.

History.—This small shrub grows in dry places in many parts of the United States, and bears bright yellow flowers in July and August. The fruit is of a bluish-black color in the form of an oblong pod, and contains indigo, tannin, an acid, and *baptisin.* Any portion of the plant, when dried, yields a blue dye, which is, however, not equal in value to indigo. If the shoots are used after they acquire a green color they will cause drastic purgation. Alcohol or water will take up the active properties of this plant. Medicinally, both the root and the leaves are valuable, and deserve to be better known than they are at present as remedial agents. The virtues of the root reside chiefly in the bark.

Properties and Uses.—It is purgative, emetic, astringent, and antiseptic. For its antiseptic qualities or properties it is more highly esteemed than for any other. A decoction of the bark of the root is efficacious in the cure of all kinds of external sores and ulcerations. It is used in decoction or syrup, for scarlatina, typhus, and all cases where there is a tendency to putrescency. As a fomentation it is very useful in ulcers, tumors, sore nipples, etc., and may be so used if you cannot get a superior remedy, as the Herbal Ointment.

Dose.—Of the decoction, one tablespoonful every two or four hours, as required. The decoction is made by boiling one ounce of the powdered bark in two pints of water until they are reduced to one pint.

RED RASPBERRY (Rubus Strigosus.)

Medicinal Parts. *The bark of the root, and leaves.*

Description.—This is a shrubby, strongly hispid plant, about four feet high. Leaves, pinnate; leaflets, oblong-ovate. Flowers, white; corolla, cup-shaped; and fruit, a red berry, of a rich delicious flavor.

History.—The Red Raspberry grows wild, and is common to Canada and the Northern and Middle United States. It grows in hedges and thickets, and upon neglected fields. It flowers in May, and its fruit ripens from June to August. The leaves and bark of the root are the parts used medicinally. They impart their properties to water, giving to the infusion an odor and flavor somewhat similar to black tea.

Properties and Uses.—It is very useful as an astringent. An infusion or decoction of the leaves has been found an excellent remedy in diarrhœa, dysentery, and cholera infantum, and all diseases of a kindred nature. It is somewhat freely used as a wash and injection for leucorrhœa, gleet, gonorrhœa, and prolapsus uteri and ani. The decoction of the leaves combined with cream will suppress nausea and vomiting. It is sometimes used as an aid in labor, and has been efficacious in promoting uterine contractions when *ergot* has failed. This plant is one of the ingredients of my prepared remedy for the above diseases.

Dose.—Of the decoction, from one to four fluid ounces, several times a day. Of the pulverized root bark, which is sometimes used, from twenty to thirty grains.

The *Rubus Trivialis*, or *Dewberry*, and *Rubus Villosus*, or *Blackberry*, contain similar medical qualities, and may be used instead.

RED ROOT (CEANOTHUS AMERICANUS).

COMMON NAMES. *New Jersey Tea, Wild Snow-ball.*

MEDICINAL PART. *The bark of the root.*

Description.—This plant has a large root with a red or brownish bark, tolerably thick, and body of dark-red color. The stems are from two to four feet high, slender, with many reddish, round, smooth branches. The leaves are ovate or oblong-ovate, serrate, acuminate, rather smooth above, and cordate at the base. The flowers are minute and white, and fruit a dry capsule.

History.—This plant is very abundant in the United States, especially in the western portions thereof. It grows in dry woodlands, bowers, etc., and flowers from June to August. The leaves are sometimes used as a substitute for Chinese tea, which, when dried, they much resemble. The root, which is officinal, contains a large amount of Prussic acid. *Ceanothine* is the name that has been given to its active principle.

Properties and Uses.—Red Root is astringent, expectorant, sedative, anti-spasmodic, and anti-syphilitic. It is used with great good effect in dysentery, asthma, chronic bronchitis, whooping-cough, and consumption. It is also successfully used as a gargle in aphthæ of children, sore mouth subsequent to fevers, and sore throats.

Dose.—Of decoction, one tablespoonful three times a day.

RHATANY (KRAMERIA TRIANDRIA).

MEDICINAL PART. *The root.*

Description.—The root of this plant is horizontal, very long, with a thick bark. The stem is round and procumbent, branches two or three feet long ; when young, white and silky ; when old, dark and naked. The leaves are alternate, sessile, oblong and obovate, hoary and entire. The flowers are red on short stalks. Calyx has four sepals, and corolla four petals. The fruit is a dry, hairy drupe.

History.—Rhatany flowers all the year round, and grows upon the sandy, dry, and gravelly hills of Peru. The root is the officinal part, and is dug up in large quantities after the rains. It was made officinal in 1780 by Ruiz, but long before that the natives had used it as a strong astringent for various diseases, afflictions, maladies, and complaints In Portugal, to which the Peruvians send the bulk of the roots gathered, it is used to adulterate red wines. The best method of extracting the medicinal qualities of the root, is to put it powdered in a displacer and pass water through. This will bring a brick-red aqueous solution, which will embrace all the medicinal virtues. There is a false Rhatany, the source of which is unknown.

Properties and Uses.—It is a powerful astringent, and slightly tonic. It is beneficial wherever powerful astringents are required, and may be used to advantage, if properly prepared, for all diseases which call for the application of a decided astringent.

RHEUMATISM ROOT (JEFFERSONIA DIPHYLLA).

COMMON NAMES. *Twin-leaf, Ground-Squirrel Pea.*
MEDICINAL PART. *The root.*

Description.—This plant is perennial, and has a horizontal *rhizoma* or fleshy root, with matted fibrous radicles. The stem is simple, naked, one-flowered, and from eight to fourteen inches in height. The leaves are in pairs, broader than long, ending in an obtuse point, smooth and petioled; flowers, large and white; and fruit an obovate capsule.

History.—This plant is found from New York to Maryland and Virginia, and in many parts of the Western States. It grows chiefly in limestone soil, but also is found in woods and near rivers, irrespective of limestone, and flowers in April and May. The root is the part used, and its virtues are extracted by water or alcohol. A chemical analysis of this plant showed it to contain tannic acid, gum, starch, pectin, fatty resin, bitter matter, similar to polygalic acid, carbonate and sulphate of potassa, lime, iron, magnesia, silica, etc.

Properties and Uses.—It is diuretic, alterative, antispasmodic, and a stimulating diaphoretic. It is successfully used in chronic rheumatism, secondary or mercurio-syphilis, dropsy, in many nervous affections, spasms, cramps, nervous excitability, etc. As a gargle it is useful in diseases of the throat.

Dose.—Of the decoction, from two to four fluid ounces, three or four times a day. Of the saturated tincture, from one to three fluid drachms, three times a day.

RHUBARB (RHEUM PALMATUM).

MEDICINAL PART. *The root.*

Description.—The scientific world happens to be in much argument as to the exact plant or plants from which Rhubarb is produced. It is,

however, well known to all instructed herbalists that Rhubarb is the
root of a Rheum, and that the plant
from which the drug of the shops is
obtained chiefly inhabits Chinese Tartary, and grows wild on the mountains
and highlands of that section of the
globe. That the truth of its botanical
identity is not elicited is owing to a
severe prohibition of the Chinese government. Every sacrifice to obtain the
true plant or the seed has been in vain.

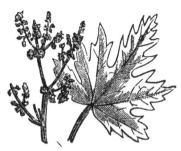

Rheum Palmatum.

History.—There are several varieties
met with in commerce termed the Rus-
sian, Chinese, English, and French Rhubarb, among which the Russian
is considered the best. The names are given, not that they are produced in indicated countries, but of the channels by which they are
thrown upon the market. Rhubarb has a peculiar aromatic odor, bitter, faintly astringent taste, and when chewed tinges the saliva yellow.
It contains oxalate of lime in abundance.

Properties and Uses.—Rhubarb is cathartic, astringent, and tonic; as
a cathartic it acts by increasing the muscular action of the bowels
rather than augmenting their secretions. It is much used as a laxative
for infants, its mildness and tonic qualities making it peculiarly applicable. It is a valuable medicine.

Dose.—Of the powder, as a purgative, from ten to thirty grains. As
a laxative, from five to ten grains. As a tonic, from one to five grains.
Of the tincture or syrup, one to two fluid drachms.

ROSEMARY (ROSMARINUS OFFICINALIS).

MEDICINAL PART. *The tops.*

Description.—Rosemary is an erect, perennial, evergreen shrub, two
to four feet high, with numerous branches of an ash color, and densely
leafy. The leaves are sessile, opposite, and linear, over an inch in
length, dark-green and shining above, and downy. The flowers are
few, bright blue or white. Calyx purplish.

History.—Rosemary is a native of the countries surrounding the
Mediterranean, and is cultivated in nearly every garden for its fragrance and beauty. It flowers in April and May. The parts used in
medicine are the flowering tops.

Properties and Uses.—It is stimulant, antispasmodic, and emmenagogue. The oil is principally employed as a perfume for ointments, liniments, and embrocations.

Dose.—Of the oil, internally, from three to six drops.

7

PYROLA (ROUND-LEAVED) (PYROLA ROTUNDIFOLIA).

COMMON NAMES. *False Wintergreen, Shin-leaf, Canker-Lettuce, Pear-leaf Wintergreen, etc.*

MEDICINAL PART. *The herb.*

Description.—This is a low, perennial, evergreen herb. The leaves are radical, ovate, nearly two inches in diameter, smooth, shining, and thick. The petioles are much longer than the leaf. The flowers are many; large, fragrant, white, and drooping. The fruit is a five-celled, many-seeded capsule.

History.—This plant is common in damp and shady woods in various parts of the United States, flowering in June and July. The whole plant is used, and imparts its medicinal properties to water.

Properties and Uses.—It is astringent, diuretic, tonic, and antispas-modic. The decoction is much used in all skin diseases, and is good to eradicate a scrofulous taint from the system. It is used in injection for whites and various diseases of the womb. The herb is applied with profit as a poultice to ulcers, swellings, boils, felons, and inflammations. The decoction will be found beneficial as a gargle for sore throat and mouth, and as a wash for sore or ophthalmic eyes. Administer it inter-nally for gravel, ulceration of the bladder, bloody urine, and other urinary diseases; also, for epilepsy and other nervous affections.

Dose.—Of the decoction, one fluid ounce, three times a day; of the extract, two to four grains.

SAFFRON (DYERS') (CARTHAMUS TINCTORIUS).

COMMON NAMES. *Safflower, Bastard Saffron.*

MEDICINAL PART. *The flowers.*

Description.—This annual plant has a smooth, striate stem, from one to two feet high, and branching at the top. The leaves are alternate, ovate-lanceolate, sessile, smooth, and shining. The flowers are numer-ous, long, slender, and orange-colored. Corolla five-cleft.

History.—This plant is cultivated in England and America, although it is a native of Egypt and the countries surrounding the Mediterranean. The orange-red florets are the officinal parts. The cultivated Safflower is usually sold in the shops, and contains two coloring matters: the first of which is yellow and soluble in water; the second a beautiful red, and readily soluble in alkaline solutions only.

Properties and Uses.—It will restore the menstrual discharge when the latter has been recently suppressed by cold, if used in warm infu-sion. It will also, when taken in the same form, produce an action of the bowels. In measles, scarlet fever, and other eruptive maladies, it is also considered an excellent diaphoretic. The seeds are sometimes used as purgative and emmenagogue, but, in my opinion, are of no great value. The infusion is made by boiling a drachm or two of the flowers in water, and may be taken tolerably freely.

SAGE (SALVIA OFFICINALIS).

COMMON NAME. *Garden Sage.*
MEDICINAL PART. *The leaves.*
Description.—Sage is a plant with a pubescent stem, erect branches, hoary with down, leafy at the base, about a foot or foot and a half long. The leaves are opposite, entire, petioled, ovate-lanceolate, the lowermost white, with wool beneath. The flowers are blue and in whorls.

History.—Sage is a native of Southern Europe, and has been naturalized for very many years in this country as a garden plant. The leaves and tops should be carefully gathered and dried during its flowering season, which is in June and July. They have a peculiar, strong, aromatic, camphorous odor, and a sharp, warm, slightly bitter taste, which properties are owing to its volatile oil, which may be obtained by distilling the plant with water. It imparts its virtues to boiling water in infusion, but more especially to alcohol.

Properties and Uses.—It is feebly tonic, and astringent, expectorant, diaphoretic, and having properties common to aromatics. The infusion is much valued in cases of gastric debility, checking flatulency with speed and certainty.

The warm infusion will cause active diuresis by checking its diaphoretic tendency. It is called by some a most capital remedy for spermatorrhœa, and for excessive venereal desire, and I am one of those who know from experience in my practice that it is grand for what is termed sexual debility when its use is indicated. The infusion is much used as a gargle for inflammation and ulceration of the throat and relaxed uvula, either alone or combined with vinegar, honey, or sumach.

ST. IGNATIUS' BEAN (IGNATIUS AMARA).

Description.—The Ignatius Amara is a branching tree with long, taper, smooth, scrambling branches. The leaves are veiny, smooth, and a span long. The flowers are long, nodding, and white, and smell like jasmine. The fruit is small and pear-shaped, and the seeds number about twenty, are angular, and are imbedded in a soft pulp.

History.—The tree is indigenous to the Philippine Islands, and the seeds thereof are the St. Ignatius' Bean of the drug-shops. The bean yields its properties best to alcohol, but will also yield them to water. It contains about one-third more strychnia than nux-vomica, but is seldom used for the production of strychnia on account of its extreme scarcity.

Properties and Uses.—Very similar to nux-vomica seeds, but more energetic. It is used in nervous debility, amenorrhœa, chlorosis, epilepsy, worms, etc., with partial good effect, but is a dangerous article however well prepared, and should be used only by the advice of a professional gentleman, upon whose truth and ability you may place the utmost confidence. It should not be employed in domestic practice.

Dose.—Of the powdered seed, one grain ; of the alcoholic extract, one-eighth of a grain.

ST. JOHN'S WORT (HYPERICUM PERFORATUM).

MEDICINAL PARTS. *The tops and flowers.*

Description.—This is a beautiful shrub, and is a great ornament to our meadows. It has a hard and woody root, which abides in the ground many years, shooting anew every year. The stalks run up about two feet high, spreading many branches, having deep-green, ovate, obtuse, and opposite leaves, which are full of small holes, which are plainly seen when the leaf is held up to the light. At the tops of the stalks and branches stand yellow flowers of five leaves apiece, with many yellow threads in the middle, which, being bruised, yield a reddish juice, like blood, after which come small, round heads, wherein is contained small blackish seed, smelling like resin. The fruit is a three-celled capsule.

History.—This plant grows abundantly in this country and Europe, and proves exceedingly annoying to farmers. It flowers from June to August. It has a peculiar terebinthine odor, and a balsamic, bitterish taste. It yields its properties to water, alcohol, and ether.

Properties and Uses.—It is astringent, sedative, and diuretic. It suppresses the urine, and is very applicable in chronic urinary affections, diarrhœa, dysentery, jaundice, menorrhagia, hysteria, nervous affections, hemoptysis, and other hemorrhages. Externally, in fomentation, or used as an ointment, it is serviceable in dispelling hard tumors, caked breasts, bruises, etc.

Dose.—Of the powder, from half a drachm to two drachms ; infusion, one to two ounces.

SANICLE (SANICULA MARILANDICA).

COMMON NAME. *Black-snake Root.*

MEDICINAL PART. *The root.*

Description.—Sanicle is an indigenous, perennial herb, with a smooth, furrowed stem, from one to three feet high. The leaves are digitate, mostly radical, and on petioles from six to twelve inches long. Cauline leaves few, and nearly sessile. The flowers are mostly barren, white, sometimes yellowish, fertile ones sessile.

History.—It is common to the United States and Canada, and is found in low woods and thickets, flowering in June. The fibrous root is aromatic in taste and odor. It imparts its virtues to water and alcohol.

Properties and Uses.—In its action upon the system it resembles valerian very much, possessing nervine and anodyne properties. Domestically, it is used with advantage in intermittent fevers, sore-throat, erysipelas, and cutaneous affections. It is very efficacious in chorea, and is very beneficially employed in various nervous affections.

Dose.—Powder, one drachm ; decoction, from one to four ounces.

SARSAPARILLA (SMILAX OFFICINALIS).

MEDICINAL PART. *The root.*

Description.—The stem of this plant is twining, angular, and prickly, the young shoots being unarmed. The leaves are ovate-oblong, acute, cordate, smooth, and about a foot long. The petioles are an inch long, bearing tendrils above the base. Botanically, nothing is known of the flowers. This plant grows in New Granada, on the banks of the Magdaline, near Bajorque. Great quantities are sent to Mompox and Carthagena, and from thence to Jamaica and Cadiz.

The *Smilax Syphilitica, S. Papyracea, S. Medica, S. China,* and *S. Sarsaparilla* are all members of the same family of plants ; their medicinal qualities are similar, and they form the Sarsaparilla of commerce, with the exception of the S. Sarsaparilla, which is native to the United States, flowering from May to August. The American plant is regarded by some as inert, but why so I do not know. The plant extensively known in the South as *Bamboo Brier*, which is but a species of Sarsaparilla, certainly possesses medicinal qualities equal, if not superior, to commercial Sarsaparilla. Professionally, I employ the Honduras Sarsaparilla, which I regard as the best.

History.—The Sarsaparilla of commerce consists of very long roots, having a thick bark of a grayish or brownish color. They have scarcely any odor, but possess a mucilaginous taste. Those roots that have a deep orange tint are the best, and the stronger the acrid and nauseous qualities, the better are the properties of the root. Water and alcohol extract its medicinal qualities. By chemical analysis it contains *salseparin*, a coloring matter, starch, chloride of potassium, an essential oil, bassorin, albumen, pectic and acetic acid, and the several salts of lime, potassa, magnesia, and oxide of iron.

Properties and Uses.—An alterative. When properly prepared it exerts a favorable change over the system. It has great repute in syphilitic diseases. In several chronic diseases, as of the skin, rheumatic affections, passive dropsy, etc., it is of service. Its chief use, however, is an adjuvant to other alteratives ; its individual properties being too feeble to answer all the conditions required of an alterative.

Dose.—Of the powder, thirty grains ; of the infusion or syrup, four fluid ounces.

SASSAFRAS (Laurus Sassafras).

MEDICINAL PART. *The bark of the root.*

Description.—This is a small tree, varying in height from ten to forty feet. The bark is rough and grayish, that of the twigs smooth and green. The leaves are alternate, petiolate, bright green, very variable in form, smooth above and downy beneath. The flowers appear before the leaves, are small, greenish-yellow ; fruit an oval succulent drupe.

History.—Indigenous to North America, and common to the woods from Canada to Florida, and flowering in the latter part of April or early in May. The bark has an aromatic, agreeable taste, and similar odor. It yields its properties to hot water by infusion, and to alcohol.

Properties and Uses.—It is a warm, aromatic stimulant, alterative, diaphoretic, and diuretic. It is much used in alterative compounds as a flavoring adjuvant. In domestic practice it enjoys a wide field of application and use, especially as a so-called spring-renovator of the blood.

SAVORY (Summer) (Satureja Hortensis).

MEDICINAL PART. *The leaves.*

Description.—This annual plant has a branching, bushy stem, about eighteen inches in height, woody at the base, frequently changing to purple. The leaves are numerous, small, entire, and acute at the end. The flowers are pink-colored. Calyx tubular, corolla bilabiate, stamens diverging.

History.—It is a native of the south of France. It is extensively cultivated for culinary purposes in Europe and America, and flowers in July and August. The leaves are the part employed. They have an aromatic odor and taste analogous to those of thyme.

Properties and Uses.—It is a stimulant, carminative, and emmenagogue. A warm infusion is beneficial in colds, menstrual suppression, and wind colic, for which it is a specific. The oil inserted into the carious teeth will often relieve the tooth-ache.

SATUREJA MONTANA, or *Winter Savory*, possesses similar qualities.

Dose.—From two to four ounces of the infusion, several times a day.

SCULL-CAP (Scutellaria Lateriflora).

COMMON NAMES. *Blue Scull-Cap, Side-Flowering Scull-Cap, Mad-Dogweed,* and *Hood-wort.*

MEDICINAL PART. *The whole plant.*

Description.—Scull-cap has a small, fibrous, yellow, perennial root, with an erect and very branching stem, from one to three feet in height. The leaves are on petioles about an inch long, opposite, thin, subcordate on the stem, ovate on branches, acuminate, acute, and coarsely serrate. The flowers are small, and of a pale-blue color.

History.—It is an indigenous herb, growing in damp places, meadows, ditches, and by the side of ponds, flowering in July and August. The whole plant is medicinal, and should be gathered while in flower, dried in the shade, and kept in well-closed tin vessels. Chemically it contains an essential oil, a yellowish-green fixed oil, chlorophyll, a volatile matter, albumen, an astringent principle, lignin, chloride of soda, salts of iron, silica, etc.

Properties and Uses.—It is a valuable nervine, tonic, and antispasmodic, used in chorea, convulsions, fits, delirium tremens, and all nervous affections, supporting the nerves, quieting and strengthening the system. In delirium tremens an infusion drunk freely will soon produce a calm sleep. In all cases of nervous excitability, restlessness, or wakefulness, etc., it exerts beneficial results.

Dose.—Of the fluid extract, from half to a teaspoonful; of the tincture (four ounces scull-cap to a pint of diluted alcohol), one to two teaspoonfuls; of the infusion, a wineglassful, three times a day.

SENEKA (POLYGALA SENEGA).

COMMON NAME. *Seneca Snake-Root.*

MEDICINAL PART. *The root.*

Description.—This indigenous plant has a perennial, firm, hard, branching root, with a thick bark, and sends up several annual stems, which are erect, smooth, from eight to fourteen inches high, occasionally tinged with red. The leaves are alternate, nearly sessile, lanceolate, with a sharpish point, smooth; flowers white; calyx consists of five sepals, corolla of three petals; and capsules are small, two-celled and two-valved.

History.—It is found in various parts of the United States, in rocky woods and on hill-sides, flowering in July. It is more abundant in the West and South than in the East. The officinal root varies in size from two to four or five lines in diameter, crooked, and a carinate line extends the whole length of it. Its chemical constituents are polygalic, virgineic, pectic, and tannic acids, coloring matter, an oil, cerin, gum, albumen, salts of alumina, silica, magnesia, and iron.

Properties and Uses.—In large doses emetic and cathartic; in ordinary doses it stimulates the secretions, acting particularly as a sialagogue, expectorant, diuretic, diaphoretic, and emmenagogue. In active inflammatory diseases it should not be employed. In protracted pneumonia, commencing stages of croup. humoral asthma, etc., it is a good expectorant.

Dose.—Powder, five to twenty grains; infusion or syrup, half an ounce to two ounces; polygalic acid, one-fourth to one-half grain.

SKUNK CABBAGE (SYMPLOCARPUS FŒTIDUS).

COMMON NAMES. *Skunk-weed, Pole-cat weed, Meadow Cabbage.*
MEDICINAL PARTS. *The roots and seeds.*

Description.—This plant has been a troublesome one for botanists to

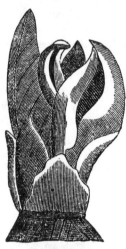

classify; but the term *Symplocarpus* is now generally preferred. It is perennial, having a large, abrupt root, or tuber, with numerous crowded, fleshy fibres, which extend some distance into the ground. The *spathe* appears before the leaves, is ovate, spotted, and striped, purple and yellowish-green, the edges folded inward, and at length coalescing. The flowers are numerous, of a dull purple within the spathe, on a short, oval spadix. Calyx consists of four fleshy, wedge-shaped sepals; corolla, none; stamens, four; seeds round and fleshy, and about as large as a pea.

History.—Skunk Cabbage is a native of the United States, growing in moist grounds, flowering in March and April, and maturing its fruit in August and September, forming a roughened, globular mass, two or three inches in

Skunk Cabbage.

diameter, and shedding its bullet-like fruit, one-third to half an inch in diameter, which are filled with a singular solid, fleshy embryo. The parts used are the seeds and roots, which have an extremely disagreeable odor. Water or alcohol extracts their virtues. Chemically it contains a fixed oil, wax, starch, volatile oil and fat, salts of lime, silica, iron, and manganese.

Properties and Uses.—Internally it is a stimulant, exerting expectorant, antispasmodic, with slightly narcotic influences. It is successfully used in asthma, whooping-cough, nervous irritability, hysteria, fits, epilepsy, convulsions, chronic catarrh, pulmonary and bronchial affections.

Externally, in the form of an ointment, it aids reparative processes, discusses tumors, stimulates granulations, eases pain, etc. It is an ingredient in my world-renowned "Herbal Ointment." (See page 472.)

Dose.—Fluid extract, twenty to eighty drops; tincture (three ounces of root or seed to a pint of alcohol), half a teaspoonful; syrup (two ounces of fluid extract to eight ounces of simple syrup), two or three teaspoonfuls.

SOAP-WORT (SAPONARIA OFFICINALIS).

COMMON NAME. *Bouncing Bet.*
MEDICINAL PARTS. *The root and leaves.*
Description.—This is a stout perennial, herbaceous plant, with a stem

from one to two feet in height. The leaves are lanceolate, smooth; flowers are many, large, flesh-colored, or pale-pink, and often double; fruit an oblong one-celled capsule.

History.—This plant grows in roadsides and waste places in Europe and the United States. It flowers in the early part of July in Europe, but in America in the early part of August. The leaves and root are the parts used medicinally. They have a sweet and bitter taste combined, "with a subsequent persistent pungency and a benumbing sensation." When the root and leaves are subjected to the extractive powers of water they yield a residue something like soap-suds. Their active properties are brought out by either water or alcohol—by the latter particularly. The root gives a principle called *Saponin*, which is very valuable.

Properties and Uses.—It is largely and valuably employed in the treatment of diseases of the liver, scrofulous, syphilitic, and cutaneous afflictions of a severe character; also catarrh, rheumatism, gonorrhœa, whites, and green sickness. Saponin can be prepared only by a competent herbal chemist. In its absence use decoctions of the leaves and roots. Dose of the decoction, from one to two fluid ounces, three times a day. I employ the saponaceous qualities of this plant, which I extract from the root by chemical processes in my laboratory, as a constituent of my "Renovating Pill." (See page 473.)

SOLOMON'S SEAL (CONVALLARIA MULTIFLORA).

MEDICINAL PART. *The root.*

Description.—The stem of this plant is smooth, from one to four feet high, and growing from a perennial root. The leaves are alternate, lanceolate, smooth, and glossy above, paler and pubescent beneath; flowers greenish-white, and fruit a dark-blue or blackish berry. There is another variety, the *Convallaria Racemosa*, the root of which possesses similar qualities to that of Solomon's Seal.

History.—Both plants are to be found throughout the United States and Canada. They flower from May to August. The root, which is the part used, is inodorous, but has a sweetish mucilaginous taste, which is followed by a slight sense of bitterness.

Properties and Uses.—The root is tonic, mucilaginous, and astringent. The decoction is successfully used in whites, pectoral affections, menorrhagia, female debility, inflammation of the stomach and intestines, erysipelas, neuralgia, itch, local inflammations, etc. Dose of the decoction, one to three ounces, three times a day.

SORREL (WOOD) (OXALIS ACETOSELLA).

MEDICINAL PART. *The whole herb.*

Description.—This is a small perennial herb, with a creeping and scaly-toothed root-stock. The leaves are numerous, radical, and on long, weak, hairy stalks; leaflets broadly obcordate, and of yellowish-green color. Flowers white, yellowish at the base, and scentless. Fruit a five-lobed, oblong capsule.

History.—It is indigenous to Europe and this country, growing in woody and shady places, and flowering from April to June. It is inodorous, and has a pleasantly acid taste. The acidity is due to oxalic acid, which, in combination with potassa, forms the binoxolate of that alkali. The "*Salts of Sorrel,*" formerly so much used to remove ink-spots and iron-marks from linen, is merely this salt separated from the plant.

Properties and Uses.—Cooling and diuretic; useful in febrile diseases, hemorrhages, gonorrhœa, chronic catarrh, urinary affections, scurvy, etc. Care is to be observed in its use.

RUMEX ACETOSA, or *Garden Sorrel*, RUMEX ACETOSELLA, or *Sheep Sorrel*, and RUMEX VESICARIUS possess similar qualities.

SQUIRTING CUCUMBER (MOMORDICA ELATERIUM).

MEDICINAL PART. *The feculence of the juice of the fruit.*

Description.—This hispid and glaucous plant has several stems growing from the same root. The leaves are cordate, somewhat lobed, and on long stalks. Flowers monœcious and yellow. Fruit oblong, obtuse at each end, separating from its stalk with violence, and expelling its seeds and mucus with considerable force, in consequence of the sudden contraction of the sides.

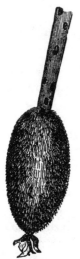

History.—This plant is indigenous to the south of Europe, growing in poor soils, in waste places, and flowering in July. The juice around the seeds is the officinal part, and which, when properly prepared, forms the *Elaterium* of commerce. It must be collected a little before the period of ripening.

Properties and Uses.—It is an energetic hydragogue cathartic, operating with great violence in doses of a few grains, and very apt to cause diffuse inflammation of the stomach and bowels, characterized by vomiting, griping pain, and profuse diarrhœa. It is used chiefly in obstinate dropsy, and as a revulsive in cerebral affections, or wherever a revellent effect is desired. Owing to its active cathartic properties, it is always best to commence with very small doses, from the uncertainty of the preparation.

Squirting Cucumber.

Dose.—From one-eighth to one-half a grain.

STAR-GRASS (ALETRIS FARINOSA).

COMMON NAMES. *Colic-root, Ague-root, Crow-corn, Unicorn root, etc.*
MEDICINAL PART. *The root.*

Description.—This plant has a perennial root, with radical leaves, sessile, lying flat on the ground, ribbed, broad, lanceolate, smooth, the large ones being about four inches long. The flower-stem is from one to three feet high, erect and simple, bearing a bell-shaped flower, which, as it grows old, has a wrinkled, mealy appearance. The fruit is a triangular capsule.

History.—It is indigenous to North America, growing in low grounds, sandy soils, and at the edges of woods. Its flowers are white, and appear from May to August. The root is the part used. Alcohol is the best solvent.

Properties and Uses.—Its root, when thoroughly dried, is an intensely bitter tonic, and in decoction or tincture is of great utility in dyspepsia, general or local debility, flatulent colic, hysteria, etc. It greatly strengthens the female generative organs, affording protection against miscarriage ; and in chlorosis, amenorrhœa, dysmenorrhœa, engorged condition of the uterus, prolapsus of that organ, is a very superior vegetable agent.

Dose.—Of the powdered root, from five to ten grains, three times a day; of the saturated tincture, five to fifteen drops.

STILLINGIA (STILLINGIA SYLVATICA).

COMMON NAMES. *Queen's Root, Queen's Delight, Yawroot, and Silver-leaf.*
MEDICINAL PART. *The root.*

Description.—This perennial herb has a glabrous, somewhat angled stem, from two to four feet high, which, when broken, gives out a milky sap. The leaves are sessile, somewhat leathery, and tapering at the base. The flowers are yellow, and arranged on a terminal spike. Fruit a three-grained capsule.

History. Queen's Root grows in sandy soils, and is a native of the southern part of the United States. The root is the part used. It should be used as soon after being gathered as possible, as age impairs its properties. The latter yield to water, but are better extracted by diluted alcohol. Its properties appear to be owing to a very acrid oil, known as the *Oil of Stillingia.*

Properties and Uses.—In large doses stillingia vomits and purges, accompanied with more or less prostration of the system. In less doses it is an alterative, exerting an influence over the secretory functions unsurpassed by any other known alterative. It is very extensively used in all the various forms of primary and secondary syphilitic affections ; also in scrofulous, hepatic, and cutaneous affections ; also, with combinations of anise or caraway, for laryngitis and bronchitis. The oil, unless well incorporated with some mucilaginous or saccharine substance, should never be used internally. This great alterative is one of the principal constituents in my "Blood Purifier." See page 471.

Dose.—Tincture, half a drachm to a drachm ; decoction, one or two ounces.

STONEROOT (COLLINSONIA CANADENSIS).

COMMON NAMES. *Hardhack, Horseweed, Heal-all, Richweed, Ox-balm, etc.*

MEDICINAL PART. *The plant.*

Description.—This plant has a knobby root, and a four-sided stem, from one to four feet in height. The leaves are thin, broadly ovate, acuminate, coarsely serrate, from six to eight inches long, and from two to four broad. Flowers large, corolla greenish-yellow ; stamens two, and very long ; seeds four, of which two or three are sterile.

History.—This plant grows in moist woods from Canada to Carolina, and flowers from July to September. The whole plant has a strong odor and a pungent and spicy taste. The odor of the fresh root is slightly disagreeable. The whole plant is generally used, and has its value. The chief virtues of the plant are, however, concentrated in the root, which should always be used when fresh. Its active principle is *Collinsonin*, which name is derived from its discoverer, Peter Collinson.

Properties and Uses.—It is used with good effect in chronic catarrh of the bladder (as are other plants mentioned elsewhere), whites, and weak stomach. It exerts a strong influence over all the mucous tissues. It is a very fair stimulant, and a gentle tonic and diuretic. The preparation called *Collinsonin* is *very* valuable as a remedy for hemorrhoids, and all other diseases of the rectum, and for such afflictions I recommend it highly. It is chiefly used in inveterate and chronic cases. The largest dose is five grains ; the average dose two grains. The infusion or decoction of the plant may be moderately used without additional remedies, and in some instances so may the *Collinsonin ;* but in about every case a skilful combination of the latter with other standard preparations is necessary to insure easy and speedy restoration to good health. Stoneroot is used externally—the leaves particularly—in fomentation and poultice, and bruises, wounds, blows, sprains, contusions, cuts, ulcers, sores, etc. I cannot call the attention of the reader too strongly to the effect the preparation called *Collinsonin* has upon all affections of the urinary organs. It should be combined with other indicated remedies.

SUMACH (RHUS GLABRUM).

MEDICINAL PARTS. *The bark and fruit.*

Description.—Sumach is a shrub, from six to fifteen feet high, consisting of many straggling branches, covered with a pale-gray bark, having occasionally a reddish tint. The leaves are alternate, consist of from six to fifteen leaflets, which are lanceolate, acuminate, acutely serrate, shining and green above, whitish beneath, becoming red in the fall. The flowers are greenish red, and fruit a small red drupe, hanging in clusters, with a crimson down, extremely sour to the taste, which is due to malate of lime.

History.—Sumach grows in the thickets and waste grounds of Canada and the United States. It flowers in June and July, but matures its fruit in September and October. The bark and berries are officinal. The berries should be gathered before rains have washed away the acid properties which reside in their external, downy efflorescence. Both the bark and berries yield their active influence to water. Great care is to be taken in the selection of several species of Rhus, as many of them are highly poisonous.

Properties and Uses.—The berries are refrigerant and diuretic; the bark is tonic, astringent, and antiseptic. The bark of the root has sometimes been used with success in decoction or syrup as a palliative of gonorrhœa, leucorrhœa, diarrhœa, hectic fever, dysentery, and scrofula. Combined with the barks of white pine and slippery elm, in certain particular doses of decoction, it will, with other very simple treatment, cure syphilis.

Dose.—From one to three fluid ounces of the decoction of bark. Of the infusion of berries, from one to four fluid ounces.

SWAMP BEGGARS' TICK (BIDENS CONNATA).

MEDICINAL PARTS. *The root and seeds.*

Description.—This herb has a smooth stem, from one to three feet high. The leaves are lanceolate, opposite, serrate, acuminate, and decurrent on the petiole. Flowers, terminal; florets, yellow; and fruit, a wedge-formed achenium.

History.—This is a common weed, found in wet grounds, rich fields, swamps, and ditches, from New England to Missouri. It flowers in August. The root and seeds are employed medicinally, and may be used in decoction, infusion, or tincture.

Properties and Uses.—The root and seeds are emmenagogue and expectorant; the seeds, in powder or tincture, have been used in amenorrhœa, dysmenorrhœa, and some other uterine derangements, and an infusion of the root has proved beneficial in severe cough. It has been used with great success for palpitation of the heart, and for croup. For this latter affliction a strong infusion of the leaves, sweetened with honey, and administered in tablespoonful doses every fifteen minutes until vomiting is produced, is regarded a cure. The leaves heated to the form of a poultice and laid upon the throat and chest in cases of bronchial and laryngeal attacks from exposure to cold, etc., are very beneficial.

BIDENS BIPINNATA, or *Spanish Needles*, and BIDENS FRONDOSA, or *Beggar Tick*, can be employed, medically, the same.

SWEET GUM (LIQUIDAMBAR STYRACIFLUA).

MEDICINAL PART. *The concrete juice.*

Description.—The Sweet Gum tree grows to the height of from fifty to sixty feet. Its bark is gray and deeply furrowed, and there are corky ridges on the branches; the leaves are palmate, rounded, smooth, and shining, fragrant when bruised, and turn a deep red in the fall. Fruit, a kind of strobile.

History.—This tree is very abundant in the Southern and Middle States, and can be found in the moist woods of nearly all parts of the Union. From incisions made in the tree a gum exudes which is resinous and adhesive, and somewhat like white turpentine in appearance.

Properties and Uses.—As a remedy for catarrhs, coughs, and pulmonary affections generally, it is without an equal, although physicians generally do not use it in their practice. It is also very valuable for fever-sores, fistula, scrofula, etc., when made into an ointment.

Dose.—The dose internally is from ten to twenty grains, according to circumstances.

TACAMAHAC (POPULUS BALSAMIFERA).

COMMON NAME. *Balsam Poplar.*

MEDICINAL PART. *The buds.*

Description.—This tree, also called *Tacamahac Poplar*, attains the height of from fifty to seventy feet, with a trunk about eighteen inches in diameter. The branches are smooth, round, and deep brown. The leaves are ovate, gradually tapering, and pointed, deep-green above, and smooth on both sides.

History.—This tree is found in Siberia, and in the northern parts of the United States and Canada. In America it is in blossom in April. The leaf-buds are the officinal part. They should be collected in the spring, in order that the fragrant resinous matter with which they are covered may be properly separated in boiling water, for upon this their virtues depend. They have an agreeable, incense-like odor, and an unpleasant, bitterish taste. The balsamic juice is collected in Canada in shells, and sent to Europe under the name of *Tacamahaca*. Alcohol, or spirits, is the proper solvent. The *Populus Balsamifera* is generally confounded with the *Populus Candicans*, from whose buds we get the virtues known as the *Balm of Gilead ;* but it is much the superior tree for medical purposes.

Properties and Uses.—The buds are stimulant, tonic, diuretic, and anti-scorbutic. In tincture they have been beneficially employed in affections of the stomach and kidneys, and in scurvy and rheumatism. Sometimes they are applied in that form as a remedy for affections of the chest. The bark is known to be tonic and cathartic, and will prove of service in gout and rheumatism.

Dose.—Of a tincture of the buds, from one to four fluid drachms; of an extract of the bark, five to fifteen grains, three times a day.

POPULUS TREMULOIDES, *White Poplar*, or *Aspen*, the well-known tree, furnishes us with *Populin* and *Salacin ;* and is tonic and febrifuge, useful in intermittents. It has also good diuretic properties, and is beneficial in urinary affections, gonorrhœa, gleet, etc.

TANSY (TANACETUM VULGARE).

MEDICINAL PART. *The herb.*

Description.—Tansy has a perennial creeping root, and an erect herbaceous stem, one to three feet high. The leaves are smoothish, dark-green ; flowers, golden-yellow ; fruit, an achenium.

History.—Indigenous to Europe, but has been introduced into this country and cultivated by many; but grows also spontaneously in old grounds, along roads, flowering in the latter part of summer. Drying impairs much of the activity of the plant. It contains volatile oil, wax, stearine, chlorophyll, bitter resin, yellow coloring matter, tannin with gallic acid, bitter extractive gum, and tanacetic acid, which is crystallizable and precipitates lime, baryta, and oxide of lead.

Properties and Uses.—It is tonic, emmenagogue, and diaphoretic. In small doses, the cold infusion will be found useful in convalescence from exhausting diseases, dyspepsia, hysteria, and jaundice. The warm infusion is diaphoretic and emmenagogue. It bears a good reputation in suppressed menstruation, but should be used only when the suppression is due to morbid causes.

THYME (THYMUS VULGARIS).

MEDICNAL PART. *The herb.*

Description.—Thyme is a small undershrub, with numerous erect stems, procumbent at base, and from six to ten inches in height. The leaves are oblong-ovate, lanceolate, and numerous. The flowers are bluish-purple, small, and arranged on leafy whorled spikes.

History.—A native of Europe, but introduced into this country, and extensively cultivated in gardens for culinary purposes. It blossoms in the summer, when it should be collected and carefully dried. It has a strong, pungent, spicy taste and odor, both of which are retained by careful drying. The herb yields its properties to boiling water and alcohol.

Properties and Uses.—Tonic, carminative, emmenagogue, and anti-spasmodic. The cold infusion is beneficial in dyspepsia with weak and irritable stomach. The warm infusion is useful as a parturient, also in hysteria, dysmenorrhœa, flatulence, colic, and to promote perspiration. The leaves are used externally in fomentation.

The THYMUS SERPYLLUS, *Wild Thyme* or *Mother of Thyme*, has similar virtues to the above.

TOLU (MYROSPERMUM TOLUIFERUM).

MEDICINAL PART. *The balsamic exudation.*

Description.—A full botanical description of this tree has not yet been given, but it is supposed that it is similar to the Balsam of Peru tree, differing only in the leaflets, which in this tree are thin, membranous, obovate, taper-pointed; the terminal ones larger than the others.

History.—It is a tree which grows throughout the forests of South America, especially on the elevated parts near Carthagena, Tolu, and in the Magdalena provinces of Columbia. The balsam is obtained by making incisions into the tree, and which flows into wax vessels. It is exported from Carthagena in tin, earthen, and other vessels. It has a pale, yellowish-red or brown color, solid and brittle, an agreeable vanilla-like odor, and a sweetish aromatic taste. It is soluble in alcohol, ether, and essential oils.

Properties and Uses.—It is, like Balsam of Peru, a stimulant, tonic, and expectorant, and cannot be equalled for its curative effects in cases of consumption, catarrh, bronchitis, asthma, and all inflammatory, ulcerated, spasmodic, or other morbid conditions of the respiratory organs and their adjuncts. The balsam dissolved in ether, and the vapor therefrom inhaled, is reported beneficial in coughs and bronchial affections of long standing, and I have no doubt it is so, as its virtues in such complaints are very wonderful.

TURKEY CORN (CORYDALIS FORMOSA).

COMMON NAMES. *Wild Turkey-pea, Stagger-weed, Choice Dielytra.*
MEDICINAL PART. *The root.*

Description.—This indigenous perennial plant has a tuberous root, and a stem from six to ten inches in height. The leaves are radical, rising from ten to fifteen inches high, and somewhat triternate. The scape is naked, eight to twelve inches high, and bearing from six to ten reddish-purple nodding flowers. The fruit is a pod-shaped, many-seeded capsule.

History.—This beautiful little plant flowers very early in the spring, and the root should only be gathered while the plant is in flower. It grows in rich soil, on hills, among rocks, and old decayed timber, and is found westward and south of New York to North Carolina. The alkaloid, *Corydalia*, is the active principle.

Properties and Uses.—Tonic, diuretic, and alterative. In all syphilitic, scrofulous, and cachectic conditions it is one of the best remedies. Its tonic properties render it valuable as an alterative in all enfeebled conditions. Its tonic properties are similar to Gentian, Columbo, and other pure bitters. Its magical properties as an alterative renders it one of the most valuable remedies in the whole range of medicine. Corydalia may be substituted for the herb. It is one of the ingredients in my "Blood Purifier." (See page 471.)

Dose.—Of the infusion, one to four ounces ; saturated tincture, half to two drachms ; corydalia, one-half to a grain.

VALERIAN (VALERIANA OFFICINALIS).

COMMON NAME. *Great Wild Valerian.*
MEDICINAL PART. *The root.*

Description.—This is a large herb, with a perennial, tuberous, fetid root, most aromatic when growing in dry pastures, and a smooth, hollow, furrowed stem, about four feet in height. The leaves are pinnate, opposite ; leaflets, from seven to ten pairs, lanceolate, coarsely serrated, and on long foot-stalks. The flowers are flesh-colored, small, and fragrant.

History.—Valerian is a European plant, growing in wet places, or even in dry pastures, flowering in June and July. Several varieties grow in America, and are used, but the English Valerian is by all odds the best. The officinal part is the root. The taste of the root is warm, camphoraceous, slightly bitter, somewhat acrid, and nauseous. The odor is not considerable ; it is fetid, characteristic, and highly attractive to cats, and, it is said, to rats also. Besides *valerianic acid* the root contains starch, albumen, valerianin, yellow extractive matter, balsamic resin, mucilage, valerianate of potassa, malates of potassa and lime, and phosphate of lime and silica.

Properties and Uses.—Valerian excites the cerebro-spinal system. In large doses it causes headaches, mental excitement; visual illusions, giddiness, restlessness, agitation, and even spasmodic movements. In medicinal doses it acts as a stimulating tonic, anti-spasmodic, and calmative. It is temporarily beneficial in all cases where a nervous stimulant is required. The extract is worthless. The infusion and fluid extract contain all the virtues of the plant.

Dose.—Of the infusion, one or two fluid ounces, as often as may be prescribed by a physician.

VANILLA (VANILLA AROMATICA).

MEDICINAL PART. *The fruit or pods.*

Description.—*Vanilla Aromatica* is a shrubby, climbing, aërial parasite, growing in the clefts of rocks, or attaching itself to the trunks of trees. It suspends itself to contiguous objects, and is truly an aërial plant. The stem is round, about as thick as the finger, from twenty to thirty feet in length, and oftener thicker at the summit than at the base. The leaves are alternate, oblong, entire, on short petioles, green, fleshy, and pointed by a species of abortive tendril. The flowers are yellowish white. The fruit is a species of bean, yellow or buff color, of an agreeable aromatic odor; the beans must be dried with care or they will lose their properties.

History.—Vanilla grows in Mexico and other parts of tropical South America. There are several species which are supposed to furnish the Vanilla of commerce. It yields its virtues to water or alcohol.

Properties and Uses.—It is an aromatic stimulant, and is used, in infusion, in hysteria, rheumatism, and low forms of fever. It is also called an aphrodisiac, powerfully exciting the generative system. Vanilla is said to exhilarate the brain, prevent sleep, increase muscular energy, and stimulate the sexual propensities.

WAFER-ASH (PTELEA TRIFOLIATA).

COMMON NAMES. *Wing-seed, Shrubby Trefoil, Swamp Dogwood, etc.*
MEDICINAL PART. *The bark of the root.*
Description.—This is a shrub from six to eight feet in height, with the leaves trifoliate, and marked with pellucid dots; the leaflets are sessile, ovate, shortly acuminate, downy beneath when young. The flowers are polygamous, greenish-white, nearly half an inch in diameter, and of disagreeable odor. Stamens, mostly four; style short, and fruit a two-celled samara.

History.—Wafer-Ash, or *Ptelea*, is a shrub common to America, growing most abundantly west of the Alleghanies, in shady, moist places and edges of woods, and also in rocky places. It flowers in June. The bark of the root is officinal, and yields its virtues to boiling water. Alcohol, however, is its best solvent. *Ptelein* is its active principle.

Properties and Uses.—It is especially tonic and unirritating. It is said to be very useful as a promoter of the appetite, and as a remedy for general debility. It will be tolerated by the stomach when other tonics are rejected. Some think it equal, in cases of fever (intermittent), to quinia. In convalescence from fever it serves an admirable purpose.

Dose.—Of the powder, ten to thirty grains; of the tincture, one or two drachms; of the extract, five to ten grains; ptelein, one or two grains.

WALNUT (WHITE), (JUGLANS CINEREA).

COMMON NAMES. *Butternut, Oil Nut, etc.*
MEDICINAL PARTS. *Inner bark of the root, and leaves.*
Description.—This indigenous tree attains a height of from thirty to fifty feet, with a trunk about four feet in diameter; the branches are wide-spreading, and covered with a smooth gray bark. The leaves are alternate, twelve to twenty inches long, and consist of seven or eight

pairs of leaflets, which are oblong-lanceolate, and finely serrate. Male and female flowers distinct upon the same tree. Fruit a dark-colored hard nut, kernel oily, pleasant-flavored, and edible.

JUGLANS NIGRA, or *Black Walnut*, a well-known tree, is also medicinal.

History.—Butternut is found throughout the New England, Middle, and Western States, on cold, uneven, rocky soils, flowering in April and May, and maturing its fruit at or about the middle of autumn. Its officinal parts are its leaves and the inner bark of the root. The latter should be gathered from April to July. It contains resin, fixed oil, saccharine matter, lime, potassa, a peculiar principle, and tannic acid. The *Black Walnut* flowers and ripens its fruit at the same time with the *Butternut*. *Juglandin* is the active principle.

Properties and Uses.—Butternut is a gentle and agreeable cathartic, and does not induce constipation after its action. In cases of habitual constipation or other intestinal diseases, it has considerable value. It is used in decoction in cases of fever, and in the murrain of cattle. The juice of the rind of the Black Walnut will cure herpes, eczema, porrigo, etc., and a decoction of it has been used to remove worms. The European walnut has been found to be efficacious in cases of scrofula.

WATER PEPPER (POLYGONUM PUNCTATUM).

COMMON NAME. *Smartweed.*

MEDICINAL PART. *The whole herb.*

Description.—This is an annual plant, with a smooth stem, branched, often decumbent at the base, of reddish or greenish-brown color, and growing from one to two feet high. The leaves are alternate, lanceolate, petiolate, with pellucid dots, wavy, and scabrous on the margin. The flowers are small, greenish-white or purple, and are disposed in loose, slender, drooping, but finally erect spikes.

History.—It is a well-known plant, growing in England and America, in ditches, low grounds, among rubbish, and about brooks and water-courses. It flowers in August and September. The whole plant is officinal. It has a biting, pungent, acrid taste, and imparts its virtues to alcohol or water. It should be collected and made into a tincture while fresh. When it is old it is almost worthless. The English variety of this plant possesses the same properties.

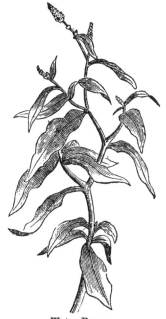

Water Pepper.

Properties and Uses.—It is stimulant, diuretic, emmenagogue, antiseptic, diaphoretic, etc. The infusion in cold water has been found serviceable in gravel, colds and coughs, and in milk sickness. In cholera, the patients wrapped in a sheet moistened with a hot decoction have recovered.

It is used as a wash in chronic erysipelatous inflammations. The fresh leaves bruised with the leaves of May-weed, and moistened with the oil of turpentine, and applied to the skin, will speedily vesicate. The infusion in cold water forms an excellent local application in the sore mouth of nursing women, and in mercurial ptyalism or salivation. The decoction or infusion in hot water is not so active as when prepared in cold or warm water. It has very many virtues; and its office in my "Restorative Assimilant" (see page 469) it performs well.

Dose.—Of the infusion, from a wineglassful to a teacupful, three or four times a day.

WORMSEED (Chenopodium Anthelminticum).

Common Name. *Jerusalem Oak.*
Medicinal Part. *The seeds.*
Description.—This plant has a perennial branched root, with an erect, herbaceous stem, from one to three feet high. The leaves are alternate, oblong-lanceolate, of yellowish-green color, and marked beneath with small resinous particles. The numerous flowers are of the same color as the leaves. Seeds solitary and lenticular.

History.—This plant grows in waste places in almost all parts of the United States, flowering from July to September, and ripening its seeds throughout the fall, at which time they should be collected. The whole plant has a disagreeable odor, and the seeds partake of the same odor.

Properties and Uses.—Anthelmintic and antispasmodic. Excellent to expel the lumbrici from children. The oil is the best form of administration, which may be given in doses of four to eight drops on sugar. The infusion with milk is also given often in wineglassful doses.

WORMWOOD (Artemisia Absinthium).

Medicinal Parts. *The tops and leaves.*
Description.—This is a perennial plant, with a woody root, branched at the crown, and having numerous fibres below. The whole herb is covered with close, silky hoariness; the stems are numerous, bushy, and from one to two feet in height. Their lower part exists for some years, from which young shoots spring forth every year, decaying in cold weather. The leaves are alternate, broadish, and blunted, the lower ones on long peticles, upper ones on shorter, broader, and somewhat winged ones.

History.—Wormwood grows nearly all over the world, from the United States to Siberia. It flowers from June to September. The tops and leaves are the parts used. The dried herb, with the flowers, has a whitish gray appearance, a strong, aromatic odor, and is extremely bitter to the taste. Alcohol or water takes up its active principles. It yields what is known to druggists as *Absinthine.*

Properties and Uses.—It is anthelmintic, tonic, and narcotic. It is used for many diseases, among which may be enumerated intermittent fever, jaundice, worms, want of appetite, amenorrhœa, chronic leucorrhœa, obstinate diarrhœa, etc. It is also used externally in country places as a fomentation for sprains, bruises, and local inflammations. Taken too often, or in large quantities, it will irritate the stomach, and dangerously increase the action of the heart and arteries.

Dose.—Of the powder, ten to twenty grains; infusion, one or two ounces.

Santonin, a well-known anthelmintic, is the peculiar principle obtained from the *Artemisia Santonica.*

Dose.—Three or four grains, twice a day.

YAM (WILD), (DIOSCOREA VILLOSA).

COMMON NAME. *Colic root.*
MEDICINAL PART. *The root.*

Description.—This is a delicate twining vine, with a perennial root. From this root proceeds a smooth, woolly, reddish-brown stem, the sixth of an inch in diameter, and from five to fifteen or eighteen feet long. The leaves average two to four inches in length, and about three-quarters of their length in width. They are glabrous on the upper surface, with soft hairs on the lower. The flowers are of a pale greenish yellow color, and are very small. The seeds are one or two in each cell, and flat.

History.—There are several species of yam-root which grow in the West Indies, and which the natives eat as we do potatoes, but these are not medicinally like the Dioscorea Villosa, which I have described above, and which is a slender vine growing wild in the United States and Canada, and found running over bushes and fences, and twining about the growths in thickets and hedges. The farther south we go the more prolific it is. It flowers in June and July. The root, which is the part used, is long, branched, crooked, and woody. From this is made a preparation called *Dioscorein,* or *Dioscorin,* which contains all its active qualities.

Properties and Uses.—Antispasmodic. Half a pint of the decoction has been used, in almost innumerable cases of bilious colic, with great good effect; the same is also employed for spasm of the bowels, and to allay violent nausea; *especially,* however, the unaccountable nausea of pregnant women. Dioscorein possesses the properties of the crude root in a marvellous degree. I use it mainly for bilious colic; it is the very best relief and promptest cure now known. I also give it in some forms of uterine disease (always, however, combined with other material of a similarly excellent character), but my use of it is chiefly for bilious colic, and for this I commend it to the public.

Dose.—Of the decoction, two to four ounces; tincture, twenty to sixty drops; Dioscorein, one to four grains.

YARROW (ACHILLEA MILLEFOLIUM).

COMMON NAMES. *Milfoil, Thousand Seal, Nose-bleed.*
MEDICINAL PART. *The herb.*

Description.—Yarrow, also called *Thousand Seal,* is from ten to twenty inches high, with a simple stem, branching at the top, and many long, crowded, alternate and dentate leaves spread upon the ground, finely cut, and divided into many parts. The flowers are white or rose-colored, and arrayed in knots upon divers green stalks, which arise from among the leaves. Fruit an oblong, flattened achenium.

History.—Yarrow inhabits Europe and North America; it is found in pastures, meadows, and along road-sides, flowering from May to October. The plant possesses a faint, pleasant, peculiar fragrance, and a rather sharp, rough, astringent taste, which properties are due to tannic and achilleic acid, essential oil, and bitter extractive, alcohol or water being its proper menstruum.

Properties and Uses.—It is astringent, alterative, and diuretic, in decoction. It is efficacious in bleeding from the lungs and other hemorrhages, incontinence of urine, piles, and dysentery. It is valuable in amenorrhœa, or suppressed or restrained menses, flatulency, and spasmodic diseases. It forms a useful injection in leucorrhœa or whites, also in menorrhagia, or profuse or too long continued menstruation. An ointment cures wounds, ulcers, fistulas, and the head bathed in a decoction prevents the falling out of the hair; while the leaves chewed in the mouth will frequently ease the tooth-ache. ACHILLES is supposed to be the first that left the virtues of this herb to posterity, hence the active principle of this plant is called *Achilleine,* which is much used as a substitute for quinia in intermittent fevers in the South of Europe.

Dose.—The infusion of Yarrow is given in doses of from a wineglassful to a teacupful, three or four times a day; the essential oil from five to twenty drops. In menorrhagia or profuse menstruation, a tablespoonful of the saturated tincture may be given three or four times a day.

Achillea Ptarmica, or Sneeze-wort, has leaves entirely different from the Yarrow, and should not be mistaken one for the other. The whole of this plant is pungent, exciting an increased flow of saliva; and the powder of the dried leaves, when snuffed into the nostrils, produces sneezing, which is supposed to be owing to their small, sharp, and marginal teeth.

YELLOW PARILLA (MENISPERMUM CANADENSE).

COMMON NAMES. *Vine-maple, Moonseed.*
MEDICINAL PART. *The root.*

Description.—This plant has a perennial, horizontal, very long woody root, of a beautiful yellow color. The stem is round and climbing, and about a foot in length. The leaves are roundish, cordate, peltate, smooth, glaucous green above, paler below, entire, and four or five inches in diameter. The flowers are in clusters, and are small and yellow. The fruit, a drupe, is about the third of an inch in diameter, and one-seeded.

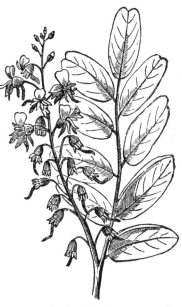
Yellow Parilla.

History.—Yellow Parilla grows in moist woods and hedges, and near streams, from Canada to Carolina, and west to the Mississippi. It flowers in July. The root, which is the part used, has a bitter, lasting, but not unpleasant acrid taste, and yields its virtues to water and alcohol. It is called, not without justice, American Sarsaparilla, and its active principle, known as *menispermin*, shows that it might have received a name less expressive of its merits.

Properties and Uses.—The authors of herbalist dispensatories have set down Yellow Parilla as "tonic, laxative, alterative, and diuretic," and it seems to possess all these qualities. Every plant of medicinal value, however, possesses one virtue which is paramount to all others. Yellow Parilla is essentially and particularly anti-syphilitic, anti-scrofulous, anti-scorbutic, and anti-mercurial. As a purifier of the blood, it is equal to the imported sarsaparilla as we get the latter, and its active principle, *menispermin*, may be used with great good effect in all diseases arising from either hereditary or acquired impurities of the system. It exerts its influence principally on the gastric and salivary glands, and is found expressly beneficial in cases of adhesive inflammation, and where it is found necessary to break up organized deposits, and hasten disintegration of tissue. I use it principally for those diseases arising from a vitiated condition of the blood, but sometimes apply it to dyspepsia. A decoction of the plant may be used to advantage as an embrocation in gouty, rheumatic, and cutaneous affections. The dose of the *menispermin* is from one to four grains. When it produces vomiting reduce the dose.

YELLOW ROOT (XANTHORRHIZA APIIFOLIA).

MEDICINAL PART. *The root.*

Description.—This small, deciduous, indigenous shrub, one to three feet high, has a thick, deep-yellow root, throwing up numerous suckers. The stem is short, woody, and leafy above, with a bright yellow bark and wood. The leaves are pinnate. Flowers small, and of dark-purplish color, and the follicles or capsules, the fruit, are inflated, compressed, and about an inch and a half long.

History.—This plant is found along river-banks in the mountains of Pennsylvania to Florida, being chiefly confined to the mountains. It flowers in March and April. The root is exceedingly bitter, and from four to twelve inches long. Water extracts its virtues. The Indians were well acquainted with it as a dye.

Properties and Uses.—It is a pure bitter tonic, considered by some equal to Columbo. It may be used for all purposes for which bitter tonics are applicable.

Dose.—Of the powder, one or two scruples; decoction, one or two tablespoonfuls.

NOTICE.—The author is at all times willing to furnish correspondents with information as regards medical plants, when incident to correspondence about other matters. But he cannot be expected to devote much time in consideration of the medicinal virtues a certain plant may contain, or to supply its common or botanical name, when it should be gathered, how prepared, and how administered, gratuitously, as his time is too valuable to be thus uncompensated for. Persons sending plants usually have it in such a shape that botanical recognition is rendered extremely difficult, often sending the part having the least distinctive botanical significance, and in many cases send grasses and weeds totally unrecognized in an officinal capacity. To supply the information desired in such cases is therefore tedious, and often unprofitable when secured. To all persons who may send plants, desiring full information with regard to their botanical or medicinal character, my fee will be FIVE DOLLARS. This barely covers absolute expense of chemical analysis, leaving me a mere trifle for my labor. I therefore trust that no one will send without some real medical object in view.

PLANTS.

THEIR COLLECTION AND PRESERVATION.

A Physician who would cure disease, or seek to assist Nature to throw off all morbid accumulations from the body, should have a single eye to the perfection, purity, or quality of the remedial agents he may feel called upon to employ. Plants should be gathered at a proper period, and under correct climatic influences, and always chosen from those in a wild or uncultivated state.

The roots of an annual plant will yield their most active medical properties just before the flowering season, whereas this class of roots are erroneously gathered after the flowering season; in consequence, they are less active, and do not retain their qualities for any reliable time. The roots of the biennial plants are most energetic if gathered when the leaves have fallen from the plant, in the autumn of the FIRST year; while the roots of perennial plants are most active when gathered between the decay of the flowers and leaves and the renewal of verdure of the following Spring. Bulbs are to be collected as soon as matured, or soon after the loss of foliage, in order to secure their most active principles.

Herbaceous stems should be collected after the foliage, but before the blossoms have developed themselves, while ligneous or woody stems should be collected after the decay of the leaves and previous to the vegetation of the succeeding Spring.

Barks are to be gathered in the Spring previous to flowering, or in Autumn after the foliage has disappeared. Spring is the best time to gather resinous barks, and Autumn for the others.

8

Leaves are best when gathered between the period of flowering and maturation of the fruit or seeds. Biennial plants, however, do not perfect themselves the first year, consequently their leaves should be gathered only during the second year of the growth of the plant.

Flowers are to be collected when about to open, or immediately after they have expanded, although I prefer the buds. Flowers, buds, and leaves, are to be gathered in dry weather, after the dew is off from them, or in the evening before it falls, and freed from all impurities. Aromatics should be collected after the flower-buds are formed, while stalks and twigs are best if gathered soon after the decay of the flowers. Berries, succulent fruits, and seeds are to be collected only when ripe, except in some few cases where the medicinal virtue is contained in the unripe article. Roots are to be well washed, rejecting all worm-eaten or decayed portions. Bulbs are cleaned and dried as roots. Barks, stems, twigs, and woods are best dried in a moderate sun-heat, and should be taken every night into a well-ventilated room, where the dew or rain will not touch them, and laid upon sticks, slats, or boards which are some few inches apart, so that the air may be well circulated through. The best method of drying leaves is to strip them from the stem, lay them loosely upon a flooring where the sun shines moderately and the air circulates sufficiently to avoid mould—keep them well stirred. The custom of steaming or moistening leaves in order to pack them more solidly after having been dried, is exceedingly improper, as the articles become thereby much deteriorated in quality and soon get musty.

Seeds are dried in the same manner as stems and leaves. Aromatic herbs and annual plants are dried as advised for leaves similarly prepared.

ESSAYS ON HYGIENE, ETC.

FOOD AND DRINKS.

MAN is an omnivorous creature, partaking of the nature both of the carnivorous and herbiverous animal. Hence, it is reasonable to suppose that man should subsist on a mixed diet, consisting both of animal and vegetable substances. To settle this matter, we must appeal to man's organization. His structure will tell us something we need not mistake. All the works of the Creator show design. Everything he has made has a use, and is so contrived as to be adapted to that use. Lions, tigers, and other animals, for example, which feed on flesh alone, have a short alimentary canal—it being only about three times the length of an animal's body. Animals which eat no flesh—a sheep for example—have very long second stomachs; while the *duodenum*, or second stomach of the human being, is of a medium capacity; which fact, in connection with the peculiar formation of his teeth and his erect or upright position, prove con clusively that man was destined to adapt himself to any clime, and to partake of any kind of food, animal or vegetable, as may be naturally supplied for his subsistence by the hand of Providence. For instance, the inhabitants of the Polar regions subsist principally on animal substances, and that, too, of the most oleaginous or fatty sorts.

Those tribes of men, laborers, hunters, etc., living in cold climates, who subsist almost wholly on flesh, fish, or fowl, devour on an average about seven pounds per diem. In fact, the quantity of animal food consumed by some human beings, who are flesh-eaters in practice, seems almost incredible. Captain Parry relates the case of an Esquimaux lad, who at a meal, which lasted twenty hours, consumed four pounds of raw as well as four pounds of broiled sea-horse flesh, one and a half pints of gravy, besides one and three-quarter pounds of bread, three glasses of raw spirits, one tumbler of strong grog, and nine pints of water. Captain Cochrane states, in a "*Narrative of Travels through Siberian Tartary*," that he has repeatedly seen a Yakut or Largouse eat forty pounds of meat in a day; and it is stated that the men in the Hudson's Bay Company are allowed a ration of seven or eight pounds of ordinary flesh meat per diem.

Charles Francis Hall, in his work called "*Arctic Researches and Life among the Esquimaux*," relates his strange experiences among the tribes of the country, with whom he became, as it were, naturalized. Speaking of the kinds of food they used, and the enormous quantity con sumed, Captain Hall remarks :—" The skin of the Mysticetus (Greenland whale) is a great treat to the Esquimaux, who eat it raw. The ' black skin' is three-fourths of an inch thick, and looks like india-rubber. It is good eating in a raw state, even for a white man, as I know from experience ; but when boiled and soused in vinegar it is most excellent." The Captain afterwards saw the natives cutting up the *krang* (meat) of the whale into such huge slices as their wives could carry ; and as they worked they kept on eating, until boat-load after boat-load was sent over the ice to be deposited in the villages of the vicinity. All day long were they eating, which led the Captain to exclaim : " What enormous stomachs these Esquimaux have ! " He came to the conclusion, however, that the Esquimaux practice of eating their food raw is a good one —at least, for the better preservation of their health. To one educated otherwise, as we civilized whites are, the Esquimaux custom of feeding on uncooked meats is highly repulsive ; but eating meats raw or cooked is entirely a matter of education. " God has made of one blood all nations of men to dwell on the whole face of the earth, and has determined the times before appointed, and the bounds of their habitations." Take the Esquimaux away from the Arctic regions, and they would soon disappear from the face of the earth.

The Esquimaux are a hardy and happy people ; are comparatively free from diseases, and are never known to die of scrofula or consumption, as one of the consequences of eating so enormously of oleaginous or greasy animal substances.

On other hand, in contrast to the gormandizing propensities of the Esquimaux, there are many examples of people living in cold climates subsisting on coarse bread, not exceeding the average amount of one pound of wheat, rye, or corn, daily ; but such persons, unless exceedingly active in their habits, seldom escape from the penalties of scrofula and consumption, for the simple reason that they soon fail to supply themselves with the meats or fatty animal substances necessary for the heat and life of the body. The Canadian teamsters live almost exclusively upon bread and fat, which, in a temperate climate, would produce nausea and skin eruptions.

In warm climates, as in China, Hindoostan, Africa, and the tropics, the food of the natives is principally composed of vegetables and fruits—rice being the general diet, with only animal or other food enough to amount to a condiment or seasoning. Though the amount of food consumed by some of the nations is very small, and their habits very temperate, we do not find that even they are any the less liable to many of the diseases which afflict those who eat largely of a mixed diet. It is reasonable to suppose, however, that less food and lighter clothing are required in warm or hot climates than in those of the temperate and frigid.

The negroes on the plantations of Mississippi and Alabama grow sleek

and live to an advanced age by subsisting largely on fat pork and homi-
ny, corn bread, sweet potatoes, rice, etc.　In the pampas of Brazil and
Buenos Ayres, where immense herds of wild cattle are found, the hunters catch these bovines, strip them of their hides and horns, and, if hungry, will cut out a huge chunk of beef, half roast it, and eat it without
salt or bread.　In some parts of Brazil the natives feed on a flour made
from the roots of a certain plant or tree, moistening the same with the
juice of the orange or lemon.　Others find support in the yam, the ba-
nana, or plantain, etc., while they are hugely addicted to drinking a species of whiskey called aguardiente.

In Asia and Africa many of the natives derive their staple nutrition
from gum acacia, and among us many an invalid has derived healthy
nourishment from preparations containing gum acacia, when his stomach
would neither bear nor digest any other article in the shape of food.　In
Peru the Indians will subsist for a month at a time by chewing a plant
called erythroxylin coca, and in the mean time perform journeys of hundreds of miles.　The Hindoos live principally on rice, and are considered
a long-lived and a very docile people.　On the other hand, many of the
Indian tribes of North America, who live on roots, barks, berries, etc.,
are very savage and warlike in their habits.　The Chinese drink strong
tea, and the Turks coffee equally as strong, without apparent detriment
to their general health.　The laboring Scotch thrive partially on oatmeal
porridge, without using a particle of meat.　The Irish want nothing better than plenty of potatoes, cabbage, and buttermilk.　The English,
French, German, Italian, Spanish, and other civilized people of Europe
live upon mixed diet, though each have their peculiar likes and dislikes
in the shape of dishes, and the average health of each nation is about the
same.　So in America they eat everything and anything, without particular injury to the constitution, except when eating too fast and too much
at a time, which is a proverbial national error.

People are liable to eat what they have been taught or educated to eat,
without stopping to inquire concerning any physiological laws on the
subject.　Scrofula is the most prevalent of all diseases,—this fact being
justly attributed not to pork or food of any kind, but to the manner in
which the people are lodged, living in small or unventilated apartments,
crowded together and breathing foul air and the pestiferous effluvias of
their own bodies.

There can be no doubt that many of the maladies incident to the human race are produced through the agency of improper food, over-feed-
ing, etc., on the internal organs ; yet it can be readily shown that a far
greater amount of maladies are induced through the medium of atmospheric impressions and vicissitudes on the external surface of the body.
More diseases arise from breathing foul air, or from lack of the natural
atmospheric air, than from the worst or poorest kind of food.　Disease,

therefore, is not so much a result of the kind of food we eat, as it is in the quantity and quality. What may be excellent for one man may be very injurious for another; custom, habits, idiosyncrasies, temperaments, etc., having a great deal to do in the digestion of food, and converting it into wholesome or nutritious blood, capable of supplying all the tissues of the body with their natural needs or stimuli. Very few people seem to know what their stomachs were intended for, or even know where they are situated. All sorts of deleterious substances are crammed into the stomach by thousands of people. When any article of food is repulsive to any of the senses, it had better be avoided as an article of diet. This antipathy is so intense in some as to amount to actual idiosyncrasy. The sympathy and antipathy displayed by some persons with regard to alimentary food or drinks are extremely curious. Some notable instances are on record. BOYLE fainted when he heard the splashing of water or liquids. SCALIGER turned pale at the sight of water-cresses; ERASMUS became feverish when he saw a fish. ZIMMERMAN tells us of a lady who shuddered when touching the velvety skin of a peach. There are whole families who entertain a horror of cheese; on the other hand, there was a physician, Dr. STARKE, of Edinburgh, who lost his life by subsisting almost entirely upon it. Some people have been unable to take mutton even when administered in the microscopic form of pills. There is a case of a man falling down at the smell of mutton, as if bereaved of life, and in strong convulsions. Sir JAMES EYRE, in his well-known little book, mentions three curious instances of idiosyncrasy: the case of a gentleman who could not eat a single strawberry with impunity; the case of another, whose head would become frightfully swollen if he touched the smallest particle of hare; the case of a third, who would inevitably have an attack of gout a few hours after eating fish. We ourselves know of a lady in Connecticut who will turn pale and faint at the smell of an apple. She could certainly claim innocence with reference to tempting any Adam.

This ignorance of the uses of the stomach, or rather abuse of the functions, is sometimes the source of much suffering and disease. Besides the gastric tubes which supply the stomach with the gastric juice, which is necessary to dissolve the food before it can be converted into blood, it is extensively covered with a net-work of nerves and blood-vessels, rendering the stomach very sensitive and very liable to inflammation. This inflammation sometimes becomes very active, producing vomiting, pain, fever, etc., all caused by imprudence in diet. It is a warning. If the warning be not heeded, this inflammation becomes chronic; the nerves lose their sensibility; the stomach becomes inactive, and that most distressing of all diseases, dyspepsia (and often epilepsy or fits), takes up its abode as a permanent guest. Most frequently it comes on more slowly and without apparent warning.

The food we eat has to be properly digested. People are apt to suppose that digestion is performed in the stomach only. This is a mistake. The stomach performs the greater part of the work, but it is greatly assisted by other organs besides. Digestion really begins in the mouth. Besides the teeth, which are the true organs of digestion, there are situated in the cavity of the mouth three small bodies called salivary glands, which pour out a fluid called *saliva* (or spittle), which is just as necessary to the proper digestion of food as the gastric juice itself. The more thoroughly the food is mixed with saliva, the more perfect will be digestion. This should teach us to eat slowly, and to chew so well that every mouthful of food may contain a proper amount of it. It should also teach us that this saliva is too valuable a substance to be contaminated with tobacco-juice, or wasted in expectoration from smoking, especially where the temperament is nervous. Saliva is constantly being poured into the cavity of the mouth, whether we are asleep or awake. As a general thing, in a healthy person, about five wine-glasses full of saliva are secreted in a day.

We eat that the body may be supported with blood, for our food, before it can become a part of the body, must first be converted into blood. A full-grown, healthy working-man consumes in one year about twelve hundred pounds of victuals and drink—that is, about eight times his own weight; yet, if he should weigh himself at the end of the year, he would find that he weighs very little more or less than he did at the beginning. Now what has become of the twelve hundred pounds he has eaten? It has been wasted away. With every motion, every breath, every operation of the mind, the body has been wasted, and food has been required to support the waste.

The one great cause of the wasting of the body, and of the constant demand for food, is action. If the muscles could be kept from moving, our lungs from breathing, and our minds from thinking, then we might not require food, for there would be no waste. This condition of things, of course, could never exist without death speedily following.

Exercising violently excites hunger, since it makes us breathe faster, and therefore causes us to inhale more air. A man of sedentary habits does not require so much food as a laboring man, because he does not waste away as fast. Much of the wasted material of the body is carried off by the lungs, in the form of *carbonic acid*. The skin, too, does its share of the work. It not only assists in breathing, but it also carries out of the system a large portion of its dead particles.

Children require more food in proportion than adults, because they are growing, and therefore, so to speak, need more to build up their bodies. After we have attained our growth, we neither gain nor lose our weight, provided we are in health, for we consume as much food as the body wastes. This is called a state of equilibrium. As old age comes on the body begins to decline in weight, and then we waste more than we con-sume.

Food may be distinguished into two kinds, viz., nitrogenized and non-nitrogenized. The first class is called the plastic elements of nutrition, and is designed solely to make blood and to form the substance of the tissues in the general structure of man; while the non-nitrogenized kind is necessary to keep up the animal heat, by yielding hydrogen and car-bon, to be exhibited in the lungs. The elements of human nutrition and recuperation are vegetable fibrine, albumen, caseine, and animal flesh and blood; while the elements of respiration are fat, starch, gum, cane sugar, grape sugar, sugar of milk, wine, beer, and spirits. The elemen-tary principles or proximate elements of food consist in water, gum, su-gar, starch, lignin, jelly, fat, fibrine, albumen, caseine, gluten, gelatine, acids, salts, alcohol, etc. All these elements are found in sufficient abundance in either the vegetable or animal kingdoms, and are to be used according to the natural wants of man, or the supply of the waste. No precise rules, therefore, can be laid down to suit every particular state of either disease or health. Every one, accordingly, should eat and drink only those things which he may find by experience, habits, or pecu-liarities to best agree with his condition, and reject all substances which he may find injurious to his health and general well-being. It is the provocative variety, or the over-stimulation of the palate, that does the greater mischief to health. The plainer the food and the fewer the dishes, the greater will be the immunity from disease. Whether the diet be vegetable or animal substances, the result will be the same in rel-ative proportion to the nutriment yielded. Fish, for scrofulous and con-sumptive persons, is a most excellent diet, containing a principle called iodine.

Meats contain the most nitrogen, the nitrogenous portions of our food make flesh, and go to supply the wear and tear and wastes of the body; these are ultimately passed from the system in the urine. If more ni-trogenous food is eaten than is needed to supply these wastes, Nature converts it more rapidly into living tissues, which are, with correspond-ing rapidity, broken down and converted into urine. This is when the food is digested; but when so much is eaten that it cannot be digested, Nature takes alarm as it were, and endeavors to remedy the trouble in one of three ways. The stomach rebels and casts it off by vomiting, it is worked out of the system by attacks of diarrhœa, or the human crea-ture is made uncomfortable generally, and is restless both by day and by night; as a further punishment his appetite is more or less destroyed for several meals afterwards. Little or no nitrogen is poured off with the perspiration, breathing, or fæces.

Whatever diet we use, whether animal or vegetable, the secret of its utility lies not only in the quantity and quality, but in the manner in which either kind is cooked, when so prepared for food. Much ignorance prevails everywhere in this matter of cooking the substances that are requisite for the sustenance of our bodies. Let any person, unable to eat broccoli or greens cooked in a quart of water, try the effect of having them cooked in a gallon of water, or of having the quart of water changed three or four times during the process of cooking, and he will soon discover the difference. If good potatoes are "watery," it is because they are ill-cooked. Fried dishes, rich gravies, and pastry should be avoided because of their tendency to develop fatty acids in the stomach.

We may reasonably suppose that the physiology of digestion is yet too imperfectly understood to enable us to lay down any precise laws as to what to eat, drink, and avoid. With a little vigilance, however, each person can ascertain for himself what foods do and do not agree with him. As before intimated, the peculiarities in this respect are remarkable. Some cannot endure fat; others cannot get along without it. Some cannot touch mutton; others are made ill by eggs. Let each find out his own antipathy. Suppose the case of a healthy man—so healthy that he cannot be healthier. We will say the quantity of blood in his body is thirty pounds, and that he loses one pound of this in every twenty-four hours. Is it not plain enough that he must eat as much food in the same time as will supply the waste of blood he has lost? But if he should eat as much as will furnish a pound and a half of blood, he will have half a pound of blood too much in his system. Should he go on adding an extra half pound of blood daily more than is required to supply the tissues, what then will be the consequences? Bursting of the blood-vessels. But good Dame Nature has measurably guarded against any such plethoric catastrophe; for, after having supplied the waste of the body, the undue quantity of blood is converted into fat or adipose matter, thus restoring the blood's volume to a due standard. But this *quasi* fat is of no use to the body. It does not give it strength; on the contrary, it is an encumbrance to the machinery, and, in more ways than one, is an evil. He, therefore, who eats too much, even though he digests or assimilates what he eats, and should be fortunate enough to escape apoplexy, or some other disease, does not add a single particle to his strength. He only accumulates fat, and incurs the evils thereunto appertaining—one among many of which I will mention—I mean the accumulation of fat about the heart, and interfering, to a most dangerous degree, with the heart's action. A man's strength resides in his arterial blood—in his muscles and bones and tendons and ligatures—in his brawn and sinew; and his degree of strength depends upon the vigor, size, and substance of these; and if he were to eat without ceasing, he could not add to their size and substance one atom, nor alter their original healthy dimensions. Therefore it is a most mischievous fallacy to suppose that the more a man eats the stronger he grows.

8*

The quantity of food taken daily should just be sufficient to restore to the blood what the blood has lost in restoring the waste of the body, and that should always be proportioned to the degree of bodily exertion undergone.   But how are we to know the exact amount of the waste that is daily going on in our system, in order to apportion the quantity of food thereto?   Nature tells us not only when, but how much we ought to eat and drink.

For instance, when you are excessively thirsty, and when you are in the act of quenching your thirst with a draught of cold water, you know when you have drunk enough by the cessation of thirst; but there is another token, which not only informs you when you have drunk enough, but which also prevents you from drinking more, that is, if you drink water only.   While you are in the act of drinking, and before your thirst has been allayed, how rich, how sweet, how delicious is the draught, though it be but water!   But no sooner has thirst been quenched, than behold, in an instant all its deliciousness has vanished!   It is now distasteful to the palate.   To him, then, who requires drink, water is delicious; for him who does not require drink, water not only has no relish, but impresses the palate disagreeably.   To a man laboring under the very last degree of thirst, even foul ditch water would be a delicious draught; but his thirst having been quenched, he would turn from it with disgust.   In this instance of water-drinking, then, it is clear that the relish depends not on any flavor residing in the water, but on some certain condition of the body.   It is absurd to say that you cannot drink water because you do not like it, for this only proves that you do not want it; since the relish with which you enjoy drink depends upon the fact of your requiring drink, and not at all upon the nature of the drink itself.

Now apply this to eating instead of drinking.   Place before a hungry workman stale bread and fat pork, flanked by a jug of cold water. While his hunger remains unappeased, he will eat and drink with an eager relish; but when his hunger has been appeased, the bread and meat and water have lost what he supposed to be their delicious flavor.

If we ate only simple and natural food, plainly cooked, there would be no danger of eating too much—the loss of relish and the feeling of disgust, consequent upon satisfied hunger, would make it impossible.   Indeed, this sense of satiety is as much and as truly a natural token, intended to warn us that we have eaten enough, as the sense of hunger is a token that we require food.

As hunger instructs us when to eat, so disrelish teaches us when we should desist.   It would seem that the very *ne plus ultra* of the cook's art is to destroy the sensation of disrelish, which is almost as necessary to our health as hunger itself.   Thus it appears the object of modern cookery is to make the stomach bear a large quantity of food without nausea—to cram into the stomach as much as it can possibly hold without being sick.

The rule which should regulate the quantity of food to be used is found in that sensation of disrelish which invariably succeeds to satisfied appetites. If you be content to live plainly and temperately, you will never eat too much, but you will always eat enough ; but if you would rather incur the penalty of disease than forego the pleasure of dining daintily, all I can say is, you are welcome to do so—but do not plead ignorance—blame only yourself.

I have stated already that certain people have been known to eat from seven to forty pounds of meat or food in a single day. On the other hand, persons have lived on twelve ounces of food a day, and were actually exempt from disease. Dr. Franklin, in his younger days, confined himself solely to ten pounds of bread a week, drinking water only in the mean time. Rev. John Wesley lived to a great age on sixteen ounces a day, although he led a very active life as a preacher of the gospel; and a celebrated Italian nobleman, who led a dissipated life till near fifty years of age, suddenly reformed his habits, and lived on twelve ounces a day with a single glass of wine, until he had reached the hundredth year of his age. Was the wine one of the means by which he prolonged his life? It no doubt served to cheer his spirits. And this leads me to consider somewhat the nature of stimulants. By stimulants I mean ardent spirits, wines, and strong ales. Are they necessary as articles of diet? They are not always, but have their uses. They are pernicious to the general organism, if too freely indulged in. Liquids which contain or make solids are better than wines, etc., yet both have their uses. Milk, the moment it reaches the stomach, is converted into curds and whey. The whey passes off by the kidneys—the solid curd nourishes the body. Now, if we evaporate a glass of wine on a shallow plate, whatever solid matter it contains will be left dry upon the plate, and this will be found to amount to about as much as may be laid on the extreme point of a penknife blade ; and a portion, by no means all—but a portion of this solid matter I will readily concede is capable of nourishing the body—and this portion is only equal to one-third of the flour contained in a single grain of wheat! If we want nourishment merely, why not eat a grain of wheat instead of drinking a glass of wine? Yet wine has its uses as an exhilarant to the mind and body.

Once placed beyond the reach of the seductions of the palate, the simple rule of drink what you want and as much as you want will of itself suggest the needful limitation. Physiology tells us plainly enough, not only why liquids are necessary, but how all superfluous quantities are rapidly got rid of.

An interdict has been placed against hot drinks, which, if directed against tea and coffee so hot as to scald the mucous membrane, is rational enough, but is simply absurd when directed against hot in favor of cold drinks; the aroma of tea and coffee is produced by heat, consequently the pleasant, stimulating effect is considerably diminished when they are allowed to get cold.

Great diversity prevails as to the kinds of drinks which should be used. Some interdict tea, others only *green* tea; some will not hear of coffee; others allow mild beer, but protest against the bitter. Whoever very closely examines the evidence will probably admit that the excessive variations in the conclusions prove that no unexceptionable evidence has yet been offered. By this I mean that the evil effects severally attributed to the various liquids were no direct consequences of the action of such liquids, but were due to some other condition. We often lay the blame of a restless night on the tea or coffee, which would have been quite inoffensive taken after a simpler dinner, or at another hour.

When a man uniformly finds a cup of tea produce discomfort, no matter what his dinner may have been, nor at what hour he drinks it, he is justified in the inference that tea disagrees with him; if he finds that the same effect follow whether he take milk or sugar with his tea, then he has a strong case against the tea itself, and his experience is evidence as far as it goes. But we should require a great deal of evidence as precise as this, before impugning the wide and massive induction in favor of tea, which is drawn from the practice of millions. Had tea in itself been injurious, had it been other than positively beneficial, the discovery would long ago have been made on a grand scale.

The same may be said of coffee. Both tea and coffee may be hurtful when taken at improper times, or by bilious persons; and a little vigilance will enable each person to decide for himself when he can, and when he cannot, take them with benefit.

I may briefly state my opinion that the great objection against wines is its pleasantness, which is apt to lure us into drinking more than is needful. Wine is quite unnecessary for robust men living under healthy conditions; but to them it is also, when moderately taken, quite harmless. For many delicate men and women, living under certain unhealthy conditions, it is often indispensable. The physician must decide in all such cases.

Many think they cannot do without something to drink at regular meals. Cold milk at meals has the disadvantage, if used freely, of engendering constipation, biliousness, and the long train of minor symptoms which inevitably follow these conditions.

Warm drinks are preferable in moderate quantities. Field hands on cotton and sugar plantations find a wholesome drink in a mixture of molasses, ginger, and water. This is a safe drink for harvesters, as are many other temperate household preparations. A recipe for many of these will be found in the proper department of this work.

Whatever we eat or whatever we drink, let it be only enough barely to appease the instincts of hunger and thirst. If we rigidly do this, we shall seldom or never be afflicted with dyspepsia, liver complaints, heart disease, and the thousand ills to which flesh is heir, but will continue to enjoy unceasing rubicund health and vigorous old age.

CLOTHING.

Clothing must be adapted to the climate in which a person lives. Warm or heavy clothing is rendered imperative in a northern climate, while the lightest and thinnest can only be tolerated in the torrid zones. It is, however, a physiological fact that the more the whole surface of the body is exposed to the external air, within certain limits, the more vigorously is its functional action performed, and the better is it enabled to preserve its own proper temperature, as well as to resist all unwholesome impressions from vicissitudes of weather, or the extremes of heat and cold. It should always be as light and loose as possible without bodily discomfort.

The substances principally employed for clothing are linen, cotton, silk, wool, hair, or down. Woollens or flannels, being bad conductors of heat, afford the greatest immediate protection from cold ; and for the same reason are less debilitating to the cutaneous function than is generally supposed. The most healthy clothing for a cold climate, especially the year round, is undoubtedly that made of wool. If worn next to the skin by all classes in summer and winter, an incalculable amount of coughs, colds, diarrhœas, dysenteries, and fevers would be prevented, as also many sudden and premature deaths from croup, diphtheria, and inflammation of the lungs and bladder. Of course, the clothing should be regulated in amount according to the degree of the heat of the weather at the time prevailing. In a very hot day, for instance, a single garment might be sufficient, but on a colder day an additional garment should be added, and in this way keep the equilibrium of the temperature of the body uniform as possible day by day, the year round. Winter maladies would be prevented by the ability of a woollen garment to keep the natural heat about the body, instead of conveying it away as fast as generated, as is done by linen, flaxen, cotton, and silken garments. Indeed, the laboring classes, or those compelled to toil in the sun, would enjoy better health by wearing light woollen clothing, than by wearing linen or cotton fabrics. Among the Irish emigrants and others who arrive in the United States during the summer season, we find many clothed entirely in woollen garments, frequently wearing heavy cloaks or coats, and actually feeling less discomfort from the heat than those of our native-born citizens who are in the habit of wearing linen or cotton next to their skin, and similar fabrics over these for outer clothing.   It is more healthful to wear woollen next to the skin, especially in summer, for the reason that woollen textures absorb the moisture of perspiration so rapidly as to keep the skin measurably dry all the time.   It is curious to notice that the water is conveyed by a woollen garment from the surface of the body to the outer side of the garment, where the microscope shows it condensed in millions of pearly drops; while it is in the experience of all observant people, that if a linen shirt becomes damp by perspiration, it remains cold and clammy for a long time afterwards, and, unless removed at once, will certainly cause some bodily ailment, as palsy, rheumatism, etc.   To sit down, or remain inactive with a linen or cotton shirt wet with perspiration, will speedily cause a chill to the whole body, leading not unfrequently to some sudden and fatal disease.   In the night-sweats of consumption, especially, or of any debilitated condition of the system a woollen or flannel night-dress (light for warm weather) is immeasurably more comfortable than cotton or linen, because it prevents that sepulchral dampness and chilliness of feeling which are otherwise inevitable.   The British government make it imperative that every sailor in the navy shall wear flannel shirts in the hottest climates, a rule that should be adopted by all persons everywhere exposed to variable weather, to extreme heats and colds, merely regulating the amount of woollen garments worn to suit the variable temperatures of climates and seasons.   In saying all this, however, we must remember that comfort is very much a matter of habit; and therefore we should make due discrimination between the natural sensation of health and the morbid sensitiveness produced by false customs.   For instance, some keep their whole bodies constantly covered by many layers of woollen garments, and yet go into a shivering fit at every unusual breath of cold air.   The reason is, they never adapt their habiliments gradually to the degree of the heat or cold of the season.   If it be deemed advisable to wear woollen clothing all the year round, whether summer or winter, it does not follow that we are to wear more than one or two extra folds of clothing in addition to the under garments.   The true rule is not to cover all parts of the body equally with the same amount of clothing.   The fleshy parts require the least clothing, and the limbs and feet, or less muscular parts, the most.   Yet we often wear, in addition to under clothing, a thick vest, coat, and overcoat; and to these will add heavy scarfs of fur or wool to the neck, etc., while the legs and feet are seldom clad in more than a single additional garment to the drawers and stockings. These parts require more clothing, especially in the winter season, than any other parts of the body.   Furs are worn in the United States more for ornament than benefit.   They are the warmest clothing materials known; yet are not adapted for general wear, inasmuch as they are apt to overheat the body, and thus render it keenly susceptible to colds and other afflictions. By consequence, fur neck cloths, caps, etc., are very pernicious for the head and throat, inducing catarrhs, quinsy sore throat, and similar afflictions. On the contrary, a light woollen waist-coat worn constantly over the breast, summer and winter, would guard against these and other evils, and insure vigorous strength to the lungs or respiratory apparatus, and thus should not be dispensed with even in dog-days. The simple rule is to keep the head cool and the feet warm at all seasons of the year. Cheap and pretty silks, of which there are many varieties, are materials which are admirable for ladies' evening, dinner, or walking dresses, and cost less in the end than other fabrics.

While I contend that woollen or flannel clothing is the most suitable for the colder or even the more temperate climates, it is not for me to object to the use of linen or cotton clothing for those living in the torrid or tropical climes. Indeed, cotton and linen would seem best adapted to such climes. In the north, many persons cannot wear flannel next to the skin, on account of inducing some peculiar cutaneous affection; while others prefer such fabrics from choice, although exposed to all vicissitudes, never experiencing any evil effects from such a course. Such persons usually lead an active, out-door life, or are accustomed to exposing their bodies frequently, especially their chests, to atmospheric influences.

In a strictly hygienic regulation of dress, however, the color of the clothing is not to be disregarded. White color reflects the rays of the sun; black absorbs them. Light colored clothing is, therefore, more comfortable and sanitary in warm weather than dark colored, because the former repels the heat, while it is readily received and retained by the latter. The heat-reflecting or heat-retaining property of different fabrics varies exactly with their lighter or darker shades of color. This difference, however, is much greater in the luminous rays of light than in the non-luminous. When, therefore, we are not exposed to the sun, the subject of color is of very little importance. The absorbing power of dark surfaces renders the skins of dark-colored animals, as well as the darker persons or races of the human family, less liable to be scorched or blistered by the direct rays of the sun than are those of a lighter color.

As to the cut or fashion of garments, that is a matter to be decided by the taste or habits of the wearer. Fashion, however, is very arbi-trary, and seldom consults hygiene in matters of dress. Of late years she has really much improved, as to the regulation of attire with regard to both health and elegance. The hooped skirt, which at the outset of its career was so mercilessly ridiculed, has proved to be a great blessing to the ladies, as it enables them to dispense with a heavy drag of solid skirts, and gives their lower limbs free and easy play and motion. The hats or head-coverings now worn by both sexes are, in a sanitary point of view, far superior to those worn by our immediate ancestors, being very light, and affording free ventilation, which is indispensable for the avoidance of headaches, rushing of blood to the head, and many other afflictions.

I can therefore only say that the first physiological rule for dress is to have all garments as light in texture and as loose in fashion as is consistent with bodily comfort, or such as will admit of the most perfect freedom in the exercise of every muscle in the body. Inequality of clothing, as before remarked, is a far more frequent cause of colds than deficient clothing. For instance, if a person exposes a part of the body usually protected by clothing to a strong current of cold air, he will take cold sooner than by an equal exposure of the whole body. A great safeguard against disease is to regulate the texture and quantity of clothing according to the temperature of the climate in which a person lives, avoiding extreme colds or extreme heats; keeping the clothing always fresh and clean (especially that of the feet), and wearing a different garment at night from that worn during the day, not omitting the cleanliness of the whole body in the general hygiene of wearing apparel.

SLEEP.

Sleep is as much a necessity to the existence of all animal organizations as light, air, or any other element incident to their maintenance and healthful development. The constitutional relation of man to the changes of the seasons, and the succession of days and nights, implies the necessity of sleep. Natural or functional sleep is a complete cessation of the operations of the brain and sensory nervous ganglia, and is, therefore, attended with entire unconsciousness. Thoroughly healthy people, it is believed, never dream. Dreaming implies imperfect rest—some disturbing cause, usually gastric irritation, exciting the brain to feeble and disordered functional action. Individuals of very studious habits, and those whose labors are disproportionately intellectual, require more sleep than those whose duties or pursuits require more manual and less mental exertion. The waste of nervous influence in the brain of literary or studious persons requires a longer time to be repaired or supplied than in those even who endure the largest amount of physical toil, without particular necessity for active thought while engaged in their daily manual pursuits. But no avocation or habit affects this question so much as the quality of the ingesta. Those who subsist principally upon a vegetable diet, it is said, require less sleep than those who subsist on both animal and vegetable food. It seems certain that herbivorous animals sleep less than the carnivorous ; while the omnivora require more sleep than the herbivora and less than the carnivora. Man, therefore, partaking most of the omnivorous, living on a mixed diet of animal and vegetable food, requires more sleep than the ox, the horse, or the sheep, but much less than the lion, the tiger, or the bear.

Physiologists are not well agreed respecting the natural duration of sleep. Indeed, no positive rule can be laid down on this subject; the statute of Nature, however, appears to read: Retire soon after dark, and arise with the first rays of morning light; and this is equally applicable to all climates and all seasons, at least in all parts of the globe proper for human habitations, for in the cold season, when the nights are longer, more sleep is required.

History shows that those who have lived the longest were the longest sleepers, the average duration of sleep being about eight hours. The time of sleep of each individual must depend on his temperament, manner of life, and dietetic habits. For instance, John Wesley, with an active nervous temperament and a rigidly plain vegetable diet, and who performed an immense amount of mental and bodily labor, slept but four or five hours out of the twenty-four; while Daniel Webster, with a more powerful frame but less active organization, and living on a mixed diet, had a "talent for sleeping" eight or nine hours. Benjamin Franklin used to say that seven hours sleep was enough for any man, eight hours for a woman, and nine hours for a fool! Nevertheless, the invariable rule for all whose habits are correct, is to retire early in the evening, and sleep as long as the slumber is quiet, be the time six, seven, eight, or nine hours. Those who indulge in late suppers, or eat heartily before retiring, are usually troubled with unpleasant dreams, nightmare, and are oftentimes found dead in the morning. Restless dozing in the morning is exceedingly debilitating to the constitution. Persons addicted to spirituous liquors and tobacco, in connection with high-seasoned food, are in danger of oversleeping even to the extent of very considerably increasing the stupidity and imbecility of mind, and indolence and debility of body naturally and necessarily consequent upon those habits. Sleeping in the daytime, or after meals, is not a natural law of the physiology of man. No one requires to sleep after a meal unless he has eaten more food than his system required. Sleep may be indulged in during the day when sufficient sleep is not had at night; but this sleeplessness at night need seldom occur were our habits made conformable to the general hygienic requirements of Nature. Children may sleep all they are inclined to. The position of the body is of some importance. It should be perfectly flat or horizontal with the head, a little varied by a small pillow. Sleeping with the head elevated by two or three pillows or bolsters is certainly a bad habit. The neck is bent, the chest is compressed, and the body unnaturally crooked. Children are made round-shouldered from their heads being placed on high pillows. The beds should be made of straw, corn-husks, hair, various palms and grasses, never of feathers, which can only be mentioned in reprehension. The bed-clothing should always be kept scrupulously clean, and adapted to the season of the year, while the bed-rooms should always be sufficiently large and airy as best conducive to sound sleep and general vigorous health.

BATHING.

Were all to follow the natural laws of their organization in respect to eating, drinking, clothing, exercise, and temperature, an occasional bath or washing would be sufficient; but as the laws of life and health are transgressed in a thousand ways, the sum total of all the unphysiological habits of civilized life is a condition of body characterized by deficient external circulation, capillary obstruction, and internal congestion or engorgement. To counteract this morbid condition of the system, bathing of the whole body, on regular occasions, cannot, or should not, be omitted. For hygienic purposes, the particular process is merely a matter of convenience. You may bathe in a river if you like, or may employ the shower-bath; but these modes are no more beneficial than the towel or sponge-bath. After the ablution, in whatever manner performed, care should be taken to thoroughly rub the body with a crash towel. The best time for such purification of the body is on rising from bed in the morning. The temperature of the water should be adapted to suit different circumstances of constitutional health and disease. Cold or cool baths are best for those in robust health; but those who are deficient in blood, or have a low vitality, should use tepid water. Extremely feeble persons should commence with warm water, and gradually reduce the temperature as reaction improves. Sponging the body with spirits or vinegar may prove highly beneficial in many cases of debility, where water would be injurious. Excessive bathing tends to make the skin harsh and scaly by diluting the secretions of the sebaceous glands, the oil of which is intended to be regularly and naturally poured out to the surface of the skin in order to keep it smooth, glossy, and soft. Bathe as often as may be necessary to keep the skin clean, and you will then have fulfilled the requirements of hygienic bathing.

EXERCISE.—PHYSICAL AND MENTAL DEVELOPMENT.

Everything tends to prove that man was destined to lead a life of bodily action. His formation—his physical structure generally, and that of his joints particularly – his great capacity for speed and laborious exertion—the Divine injunction, that "he shall live by the sweat of his brow"—the bodily imbecility and enfeebled health invariably consequent upon sedentary habit—all go to prove that he was destined to lead a life of physical activity. Most people are apt to despise many of the aids to health, because of their very simplicity. A sensible Dervish, in the Eastern allegory, well aware of this weakness of human nature to despise simple things, and venerate those they do not understand, when called to the Sultan to cure him of a disease, did not dare to simply advise him to take exercise; but he said to him :—" Here is a ball which I have stuffed with certain rare and precious medicines. And here is a bat, the handle of which I have also stuffed with similar medicines. Your Higness must take this bat and with it beat about this ball, until you perspire very freely. You must do this every day." His Highness did so ; and, in a short time the exercise of playing at bat and ball with the Dervish cured the Sultan's malady. But it should be remembered that there are a great many cases where medicines must be given to assist nature, besides the employment of exercise to facilitate the recovery of the patient.

Nevertheless, exercise is one of the chief aids of all others I must recommend to be adopted as eminently essential for the remedying of bad health, and of preserving that which is already good. It is impossible for a healthy adult to be otherwise than active in body or mind, or both ; while it may be asserted, with abundant reason, that laziness is actually a disease, dependent on some abnormal condition of the organism. A variety of social circumstances may operate to produce an indolent disposition of mind and inactive habit of body, but these also produce a primary condition of ill-health.

The function of respiration, by which the blood is vitalized, and the nutrition of the muscular structure, on which depend all the motive power or strength of the system, are intimately connected with the circulation of the blood, and this with active exercise. Without this, there must be unhealthy accumulation somewhere ; and, as the larger arteries are not permanently dilatable, while the veins and capillary arteries are so, this accumulation or congestion must take place in the veins and capillary or hair-like arteries.

When the circulation is feeble from lack of bodily exercise, or other cause, the blood creeps sluggishly along the minute vessels composing the elementary tissue of the body ; these veins and capillaries become gorged, which engorgement operates as a still further impediment to the free flow of the blood. The blood, when not circulated with due energy through the ultimate tissues, becomes deteriorated in quality, and so, in turn, fails to supply that proper nutrition upon which, according to its degree of purity, all the tissues and functions of the body depend. If the propelling power arising from breathing pure air and using active bodily exercise is not sufficiently energetic, the circulation through the elementary tissue is so slow that the blood loses its healthful arterial hue before it has reached the extremities of the hair-like arteries ; and thus that part of the tissue which ought to be filled with arterial blood is gorged only with black venous blood, from which the proper secretion necessary to the nutrition of the body, cannot be separated, either in due abundance or of a healthy quality. Hence, if this state of congestion be permitted to exist from lack of active exercise and consequent free respiration, so as to vitalize the blood, there must needs be a speedy wasting of flesh, and all the other phenomena of consumption or any other disease. The strength of the system is intimately connected with the circulation of the blood, as stimulated in its flow by means of active bodily exercise and pure air.

This principle is well illustrated in the effects of gymnastics and training, by which the muscles of any part of the body are remarkably invigorated by regular systematic exercise. People of all trades and occupations find those parts of the muscular system which are habitually the most exercised to be the most powerful.

For healthful purposes all that is necessary is, any way, to exercise all parts of the body to a degree of fatigue without exhaustion ; that is, to a degree which will insure an energetic circulation of the blood throughout the entire economy. All exercises, however, to secure their full benefit, should be coupled either with some object of utility or amusement, otherwise the mind is apt to labor adversely to the body.

When I say that exercise is what is wanted to restore to health the weak and languid, I mean that it is not so much exercise that is wanted as the exhilarating effect which the enjoyment of exercise produces. A man who exercises half an hour unwillingly in his wood-shed, is not benefited in the degree one is who takes an hour's walk for pleasure through a beautiful country.

It is the enjoyment of exercise in which consists its chiefest excellence. It is the diversion of the mind from the ailments of the body. The invalid is by this drawn away from himself.

What can better accomplish this object than amusement? Laughter and lively talk may be said to be a species of exercise—mental exercise —which is very often as beneficial to an invalid as physical exercise. Anything that will induce a fit of laughter must have an influence in promoting an active circulation of blood, and, as we have seen, it is necessary to health that the blood should be duly aërated and flow with energy through the system. Whatever means may be employed to give rapid circulation to the blood must be conducive to health. I believe, then, most fully in using all proper means of amusement which will cheer the invalid, and thus be a mental stimulus or auxiliary to the preservation and restoration of health.

So, not only are amusements which afford exercise to the mental faculties useful, but occupation—some useful business pursuit, which requires, and hence secures, attention and labor during several hours of each day —is absolutely essential to the high sanitary condition of the body, for

nothing else will insure so constant, regular, and equally divided exercise for *both* mind and body.

Walking, running, leaping, hopping, dancing, rowing boats, etc., are
physiologically adapted to strengthen the whole muscular system. Even
boxing and fencing are to be advised when properly regulated. Wres-
tling is a dangerous method of developing muscular power. Ten-pins,
billiards, etc., are excellent exercises, but useful employment is better.
Singing, declaiming, reading, etc., are admirable methods of cultivating the vocal powers, and increasing the capacity of the respiratory apparatus. Riding on horseback, hunting, fishing, etc., are all more or less
beneficial in the prevention of disease and promoting good health. Riding in easy carriages, sailing in boats, swinging, and other passive exercises, are all to be duly considered as remedial expedients for invalids.

Amid the many vicissitudes of fortune and the moral crosses to which
female life is doomed, I recommend healthful exercise of the body, in
order that the material fabric may be fortified against the thousand
causes of disease continually assailing the sex.

Woman comes earlier to maturity by several years than man. The
tree of life blossoms and bears fruit sooner in the one sex than in the
other. It also sooner withers and sheds its leaves,—but does not sooner
die. Female life at any period is fully as good,—perhaps a little better
in respect to probable duration,—than that of the male. It is during the
period of from fourteen to twenty-one years that the seeds of female
diseases are chiefly sown—or, at least, that the soil is specially prepared
for their reception and growth. The predisposition to infirmities and
disorders of various kinds is affected by acts of omission and commission. In the first class need I mention the deficiency of healthy exercise of the body in the open air, and of intellectual exercise in judicious
studies. The hoop and the skip-rope, even in city homes, might useful-
ly supersede the piano, the harp, and guitar, for one hour in the day, at
least. In schools and seminaries there is no excuse—and, indeed, in
many of them this salutary point of hygiene is well attended to. In
others, however, gymnastic exercises have been hastily thrown aside—
partly because some enthusiasts have carried them to excess—partly because they were supposed to be inimical to the effeminacy of shape and
features so much prized by parents and progeny,—but chiefly, I suspect,
from that languor and disinclination to exertion which characterize the
higher and even the middle classes of female youth. This deficiency of
exercise in the open air may be considered the parent of one-half of female disorders. The pallid complexions, the languid movements, the
torpid secretions, the flaccid muscles and disordered functions (including
glandular swellings), and consumption itself, attest the truth of this assertion.

The exercises of small children consist in giving them the largest liberty and plenty of room. The cradle is a most pernicious method of exercising a child to sleep, and should be discarded from every family. For the ordinary or wakeful exercises of a child, the modern "baby jumper" will be found a preferable contrivance. Among the poorer classes, the children, for want of room to stir in, are apt to become sickly, puny, peevish, and often idiotic.

The best time for exercise is in the morning, an hour or so before breakfast, when the stomach is partially empty. If it should happen to be entirely empty, or nearly so, it should be fortified with a cracker or two, or some other light aliment. Vigorous evening exercises may also be employed by persons of sedentary habits with great advantage. "Night work," when mental or physical, is at once a violation of the natural order of things.

Thus, if you would preserve your health, you must take exercise, but not exercise exceeding your strength. Remember, the body must be induced to throw off its waste by action before it can be nourished. Nevertheless, it should also be remembered, that exercises of extreme severity are never required in ordinary cases of health, while in disease it must be incompatible with the strength and circumstances which surround the patient. With plentiful bodily exercise you can scarcely be ill,—without bodily exertion you cannot possibly be well. By "well," I mean the enjoyment of as much strength as may be consistent with your natural physique.

Exercise should be taken to the extent of quickened breathing and sensible perspiration. If in health, walk, when possible, at least from one to two miles every morning before breakfast. The invalid should go out into the open air, and ramble to the degree of strength he may possess, avoiding fatigue.

Exercise gives health, vigor, and cheerfulness, sound sleep and a keen appetite. Indeed, the effects of sedentary thoughtfulness are diseases that embitter and shorten life—interrupt rest—give tasteless meals, perpetual languor, and ceaseless anxiety.

Cheerful exercise, when at all practicable to be taken, whether active or passive, is absolutely an indispensable means to prevent or guard against disease, and to assist in the recuperative action of medicine when the body has become diseased.

AIR AND SUNSHINE.

As air may be said to be the very pabulum of life, it is highly essential that it should be pure,—inasmuch as any deterioration of it never fails to render the blood impure, and thus ultimately to affect both mind and body.

Air covers the entire globe, pressing alike upon land and water, having a depth of about forty-five miles. This vast ocean of air we call an atmosphere, from two Greek words, signifying vapor and space,—it being an immense fluid sphere or globe. This atmosphere presses upon man, and upon every object on the surface of the earth, with a force equal to fifteen pounds to every square inch. A man of average size has a surface of two thousand five hundred square inches; accordingly, the air in which he lives presses upon him with a weight of eighteen tons. This would of course crush every bone in his body, but for the fluids within him, which establish an equilibrium, and leave him unoppressed.

Pure air contains seventy-nine parts of nitrogen and twenty-one parts of oxygen. If we add a single part more of oxygen to the air, it would no longer be atmospheric air, but *aqua fortis*, an element capable of destroying everything coming beneath its terrible power.

The quantity of air consumed by a man of average size at each inspiration, is from fifteen to forty cubic inches, according to the capacity of the lungs. Thus, in about an hour, a person consumes about six thousand and sixty-six pints, or two hogsheads of air. This air meets in the lungs in one hour, about one half of that amount of blood, or twenty-four in twenty-four hours. In other words, the quantity of blood which circulates through the system is estimated to be about one-eighth of the weight of the body. So that a man weighing one hundred and fifty pounds will have in his circulation about eighteen and three-quarter pounds of blood. The whole of this large quantity of blood has been proved, by careful experiment, to circulate through the blood-vessels in the almost incredible brief period of sixty-five and seventy-six one-hundredths seconds of time, and that is very little over one minute! This indeed seems wonderful, when we consider the vast extent of vessels it has to travel through; the arteries, the veins, and the minute capillaries through which it must be urged with no little force.

The physiology of the respiratory functions explains the relation of an abundant supply of air to the maintenance of health and the attainment of longevity. Fresh air in the lungs is so immediately essential to life, that most animals in less than one minute, when deprived of it, suffocate, become unconscious, and appear to be dead,—real death occurring in a few minutes if air is not supplied.

There are at least three objects to be accomplished by breathing, namely: the renewal of the blood and the taking of impurities out of it; the warming of the body; and the finishing up of the process of digestion, and the change of chyle into nutritive blood. That carbonic acid and water are borne out of the lungs with every breath may be easily proved. If we breathe into lime-water, it will become white. This is owing to the carbonic acid in the breath uniting with the lime, and producing carbonate of lime. Then if we breathe upon a piece of glass, it becomes wet, showing that there is watery vapor in the breath. That the blood receives oxygen from the air we breathe, is proved by the fact that the in-going breath has one-fourth more oxygen in it than the out-going.   The lungs, then, take out of all the air we breathe one-fourth of its oxygen.   If we breathe it over a second, a third, or a fourth time, it not only has less oxygen each time, and is less useful for the purposes of respiration, but it becomes positively more hurtful by reason of the poisonous carbonic acid which, at every out-going breath, it carries with it from the lungs.

Equal in importance with the quantity of air we breathe is its purity. The supply of air for an ordinary man to breathe each minute, is from seven to ten cubic feet.   Now, suppose a hundred persons to be confined in a room thirty feet in length, breadth, and height, the room containing nearly thirty thousand cubic feet, it follows that the whole air of the room would be rendered unfit for respiration on account of the vast volume of carbonic acid thrown out of the lungs and skin of the one hundred persons thus crowded together.   This proves the importance of always having an abundant supply of pure atmospheric air always kept in circulation in crowded assemblies, churches, school-rooms, theatres, factories, workshops, and dwellings.

Consider the effect of sleeping in a small room, seven feet by nine, not furnished with the means of ventilation.   If a person sleeps eight hours in such a room, he will spoil during the time one thousand nine hundred and twenty cubic feet of air, rendering the air of the room positively dangerous to breathe.   Every disease is aggravated by the breathing of bad air!   Yet it is common to close all the doors and windows where sick persons are confined, lest the patients should take cold.   This is a bad practice.   The sick should have plenty of fresh air.   Their comfort is promoted by it, and their recovery hastened.   It it utterly impossible for the lungs to be expanded in an impure atmosphere, because the air-passages, irritated by the extraneous particles, spasmodically contract to keep them out.   The consequence of this is, those persons who reside permanently in an atmosphere charged with foreign ingredients or miasms, find their lungs continually contracting.

All sedentary habits weaken the abdominal muscles, and thereby lessen the activity of the breathing process.   Intense mental application, if long continued, powerfully diminishes the respiratory functions. Persons habitually in deep thought, with the brain laboring at its utmost capacity, do not breathe deep and free, and are consequently short-lived.   All crooked or constrained bodily positions affect respiration injuriously.   Reading, writing, sitting, standing, speaking, or laboring, with the trunk of the body bent forward, is extremely hurtful.   In all mechanical or manual labor, the body should be bent or lean on the hip joints.   The trunk should always be kept straight.   Dispense with bed-curtains, if you can.   In sleep the head should never be raised very high, as that position oppresses the lungs; nor should the sleeper incline toward the face with the shoulders thrown forward.

Grates and fire-places secure much better ventilation than stoves. No stove, especially furnaces, should be used without the means of the free admission of external air into the room. Lamps, candles, gas-burners, etc., are so many methods of consuming oxygen and rendering the air irrespirable. Smoking lamps are a very common source of vitiated air. The bad air of steamboats, railroad cars, stages, omnibuses, etc., are a source of constant suffering to many. I may here remark that the general misapprehension of the theory of catching cold frequently produces the evil sought to be avoided. More colds are taken in over-heated than in too cold places, and still more are owing to vitiated or foul air. In sleeping and other apartments, where thorough ventilation is impossible, the air may be rapidly changed and materially freshened, by opening all the doors and windows, and then swinging one door violently forward and backward. The rules of ventilation apply to all rooms and apartments alike, whether in dwelling-houses or travelling vehicles. There is no necessity for breathing air which has lost a part of its oxygen and acquired a portion of carbonic acid. The supply of good air is ample.

In connection with a full supply of atmospheric air to every human being, the importance of plenty of sunshine is not to be overlooked. Pure air for the lungs and bright sunlight for the eyes, is a physiological maxim which should never be forgotten. The nutritive process is materially checked in all vegetable and animal life when deprived of light for a considerable time. In the case of vegetables, they become etiolated or blanched. Almost the entire population of our large cities who occupy back rooms and rear buildings where the sun never shines, and cellars and vaults below the level of the ground, on the shaded side of narrow streets, is more or less diseased. Of those who do not die of acute diseases a majority exhibit unmistakable marks of imperfect development and deficient vitality. During the prevalence of epidemics, as the cholera, the shaded side of a narrow street invariably exhibits the greatest ratio of fatal cases. A certain amount of shade is essential to comfort, but when it reaches the point of excluding sunshine to a large degree, it becomes a positive evil. Let us always welcome the visits of the healthful air and glowing sunshine, and look out continually for the essential conditions of vigor and cheerfulness.

OLD AGE, OR LONGEVITY.

The true philosophy of life is to live and enjoy—to use and not abuse the essentials to human longevity and happiness. As we read in Holy Writ, in the earlier history of man, when the air was free from infection, the soil exempt from pollution, and man's food was plain and natural, individuals lived on the average four or five hundred years; the maximum point of longevity recorded—that in the case of Methuselah—being nine hundred and sixty-nine years. Without speculating upon the problem whether the years of the early historians included the same period of time as the years of our present almanac, it is sufficient for all practical purposes to know the general law, that human lives may be lengthened to one or two hundred years, or dwindled to the "shortest span," by our voluntary or individual habits. If it can be proved that any one man has lived one hundred, two hundred, or even three hundred years, under favorable hygienic circumstances, it will be sufficient evidence of a physiological principle that most men may attain to similar extreme longevity, by a mere simple obedience to the natural laws of his being.

The examples of extreme longevity are too numerous to be detailed even in a book of many pages, but a few examples may be cited on this point. Haller, the celebrated English physician, during his time collected more than one thousand cases of persons in Europe who attained the ages of from one hundred to one hundred and seventy years. In Baker's "Curse of England," we find a list of one hundred individuals whose ages ranged from ninety-five to three hundred and seventy! Twenty-two of these reached the age of one hundred and fifty and upwards, and thirty exceeded one hundred and twenty years. Modern statistics exhibit numerous examples of persons in the United States and all parts of the world attaining more than one hundred years. Indeed, it was common to the American Indians, previous to the introduction of "fire-water" among them, to live to one hundred years of age; although, as a general rule, the duration of life among savage races is much shorter than among the civilized and cultivated people of the globe.

In our present artificial state of society, it is not probable that one in a thousand persons dies a natural death. Alas! disease and violence sweep, with few exceptions, the entire human family to an untimely grave. Even the celebrated Thomas Parr, who died at one hundred and fifty-two years of age, came to an unnatural death by eating too heartily at a feast given in his honor by an English king; while Richard Lloyd, who was in full health and vigor at one hundred and thirty-two years, died soon after from being persuaded to eat flesh meat and drink malt liquor, to which he had never been accustomed in all his life before.

On physiological principles, natural death results from a gradual consolidation of the structures of the body. In infancy the fluids are in much larger proportion than the solids, but as we grow older the fluids decrease and the solids increase—thus gradually changing the flexibility and elasticity of youth to the stiffness and immobility of age. Thus in a perfectly normal condition of the organism, all the functions, powers and senses decline in the same harmonious relations in which they were developed. As the process of condensation goes on equally and imperceptibly, the motive powers grow torpid, the nutritive functions are enfeebled, the sensibility becomes dull, the external senses are obtunded, and lastly, the mental manifestations disappear—death occurs without a struggle or a groan.

Certain political and social economists have attempted to prove that old age and a vast population are not desirable things, on the ground that, while population increases geometrically, the alimentary productions of the earth only increase arithmetically ; hence, that some scheme of death or destruction is requisite or indispensable to kill off, or clear the ground of existing human beings as fast as the coming generations demand their places. In other words, that it is necessary that disease, violence, pestilence, murder, wars, and death should prevail, because of the earth's incapacity to produce sufficient food for the whole race of human beings, were all permitted to live out their natural lives and die a natural death. A small amount of rational investigation will show the fallacies of all such theories. Indeed, under existing governments and social arrangements, more than three-fourths of all the lands and all the labor, so far as the production of the means of human sustenance is concerned, is literally wasted, or worse than wasted ; while a large extent of the earth's surface has never yet been brought under cultivation, and that part which is cultivated the best admits of vast improvement.

Casting all speculation aside, it will not be denied that this earth was made the residence of man, and that God expressly enjoined upon him to be fruitful, and to occupy and replenish the earth, giving him at the same time dominion over all the vegetable and animal kingdoms, as a means for subsistence and happiness, while progressing through the gradual stages of his natural or terrestrial existence. Hence, the Creator did not bring man into existence without first furnishing him with the means of an abundant supply of all the elements requisite for a long life of health and joy. Man, however, has grossly violated the laws of nature, and blundered on in his perversity, till life has actually become a grievous burden, and extreme old age a great and moral curse instead of a divine and special blessing.

Were it necessary, a thousand reasons might be given for believing that the earth now has, and always will have, room and food enough for all the population that can be produced by human beings who live agreeably to the laws of their natural organism. Indeed, it is a philosophical maxim that "intensive life cannot be extensive." The races of man have now a hurried, stimulated, forced and disorderly existence, marrying at too early an age, bringing myriads of children into the world, "scarce half made up," only to perish by thousands in the earliest infancy, or to drawl out a miserable and unhealthy existence, if their lives are prolonged to manhood's estate, and sink at last, even then, into premature graves, from continued and perverse abuses of the hygienic and dietetic rules of life.

As already said, if the body develops itself slowly and healthfully (as it always will in its natural state), it is only reasonable to suppose that the periods of infancy, childhood, and adolescence or maturity would be greatly prolonged by the more simple conformity to the original laws of our being; the period of youth might and would be extended to what we now call "old age," say "threescore and ten," and "threescore and ten" would be but the beginning of vigorous manhood to be indefinitely prolonged, reaching on to a hundred, or even two hundred years!

The special means to insure sound health and a long life are to avoid all errors in diet and personal habits. As the fluids and solids of the human organism are formed from the materials taken into the stomach as food and drink, it follows that we all ought to abstain more than we do from concentrated materials of aliment, and live more on fruits and vegetable substances, and fret ourselves less with the cares of the world; so all individuals would be able to maintain the juices of the body, and reduce, in a large degree, the solid elements which induce rigidity of muscles, thickening of membrane, contraction of organs, all leading to disease, premature debility, old age, and death.

Let us all then strive to return to the elementary principles of organic or human life. Let our diet be plain, simple, and of a juicy nature. Let us refrain from excesses of all kinds, whether connected with our mental or physical powers, and thereby secure a long lease on life, attended with a thousand blessings unknown to those who lead "fast lives," eat and drink immoderately, and indulge in the various forms of intemperate or luxurious habits. It is never too late to commence a reform in all these things. The oldest person now living might prolong his life to an indefinite period, by avoiding the errors named, and submitting himself to the prior-ordeal mandates of nature. To assist Nature in her work of regeneration and recuperation of the human organism, my "Renovating Pills" will be found of most wonderful efficacy in connection with the hygienic and dietetic requirements already indicated. They will thus prolong the period of youth to vigorous manhood, and vigorous manhood to the extremest limit of life ever yet vouchsafed to the human being. The already "old and feeble," so called, may be sure of having their lives greatly prolonged, and finally, in the inevitable ordinances of Heaven, or the laws of gradual progress and decay, passing away with cheerful resignation and peace to that mysterious bourne from which no mortal traveller ever has returned.

LIFE, HEALTH, AND DISEASE.

What is life? In general terms life may be said to be a subtle emanation of Deity—a principle that pervades all the works of creation, whether organic or inorganic. It is a sort of ENTITY, whose nature is as mysterious and unfathomable as that of Divinity himself. Many scientific men have contended that life is *electricity*, and arguments and experiments have been adduced to show that such is the fact. For instance, a scientific body of France pulverized stone, and by the use of electricity produced from the atoms living insects. But this and similar experiments are accepted as evidence that electricity is not life, but is a leading phenomenon of its actuality. Life is something neither physical nor spiritual. It is allied to both, but is neither. It is not soul, for soul is something infinitely higher than life—a something of which life itself is but an inadequate, visible manifestation.

Health is perhaps a subtle thing, yet most importantly palpable to our senses and perceptions. It is that state of the human body in which the structure of all the parts is sound, and their functions regularly and actively performed, rendering the individual fit for all the duties and enjoyments of life. Or, in other words, it is that condition of the animal economy when the functions of all the organs, beginning with the heart and lungs, act in natural and harmonious relation, the one with the other, and the whole together, rendering existence not only a state of completeness, but a pleasure, a beauty, and a charm, and therefore the chiefest cause and leading feature of all from which the human being derives that phase of joy called bliss. In the various temperaments the phenomena of health are somewhat different; hence, what would at once preserve it in one, might not preserve it in or restore it to another, until some reasonable period of time had elapsed. Health varies much in people of the many occupations which necessity and circumstances compel them to adopt for a livelihood or for pleasure, and the acuteness of the senses which would be necessary in some recreative or productive occupations, would be morbid in persons otherwise engaged. But the general symptoms of health are, in all temperaments, a sparkling eye, a clean skin, a white and rose-blended complexion (unless where the temperament naturally prescribes a rich and glowing olive), ruby lips, pearly teeth, untainted breath, glossy hair, expanded chest, elastic spine, muscular limbs, symmetrical waist, well built and firm pelvis, fleshy thighs and calves, and a buoyant grace of the whole body. Added to these we have a rich and melodious voice (wherever the slightest hoarseness or discordance of tone is noticed look for danger), and a calm and cultivated spirit in the old, a joyous spirit in the young. What munificent gifts are these, and who should fail, by every means in his power, to secure them? Disease is the opposite of health, and means any departure from the normal condition of the general organism, or any impairment or derangement of any function by which the regular action of any other one or of the whole are made or forced to work in an irregular or unnatural manner—producing and entailing disorder, pain, misery, and death! We see disease in the lustreless and phrenzied eye, in the pallid and sunken cheeks, in the parched lips, in the jaundiced or yellow skin, in the contracted chest, in the difficult respiration, in the racking cough, in the expectoration of tubercles and sputa from the lungs, in the palpitating heart, in the scrofulous sores and ulcers, in the bloated or attenuated abdomen, in the disabled legs and arms, in decayed teeth and toothless jaws, in fetid breath, in crooked spine, in the deformed pelvis, in all derangements of the sexual organs, in baldness, in disordered stomach and bowels, in neuralgias, rheumatisms, leprosies, spasms, epilepsies, palsies, loss of the senses of sight, hearing, smelling, taste and touch, hypochondrias, manias, drunkenness, pains, aches, wounds, bruises, maimings, and in innumerable other agonies! With the simple methods by which health can be preserved by those who were born to health, how astonishing it is that disease and misery are the general rule, and health and pleasure the exception! Who of all the human race may now say, "I have health! I am actually living in a state of nature, or in that perfect mental and physical condition in which I was or ought to have been born." Not one, is my reply. We may therefore regard life as a negative rather than a positive quality of existence. Occasionally there may be freedom from the slightest degree of actual suffering, and yet that pleasurable condition which would be natural to the regular co-operative work of all the organs of the body will be wanting.

In health our moments fly on lightning wing, and we are scarcely conscious of their rapid exit; in sickness, on the contrary, our moments are clogged with leaden heels, and pass in that lingering manner as to render our sufferings seemingly the more acute by reason of the slow or tardy march of time. To the sick, time does not pass lightly, but with the heavy tread of a giant.

How inestimable is that state of being comprehended under the name of health!—yet how few are ever led to consider its priceless value and importance. Health, perfect health, is not to be found in our present age among the races of men; yet even in its negative aspect, its most deteriorated quality, what were all the joys, all the riches, all the advantages of this world without its possession? Unless all, from the highest to the lowest, from the king to the beggar, learn to prize health and avoid disease,—death, who is no respecter of persons, will continue to reap his rich harvests among them all. Cæsar could not escape, nor could the renown of a thousand victories diffuse an anodynic or soporific influence over the pillow of the great Napoleon, nor save the laurels of

Marengo from the blighting mists of St. Helena! Intellectual cultivation oftentimes sows the seeds of physical deterioration. When we see that the prince is equally liable to the same physical and mental miseries as the vagrant, it becomes everybody to bear in remembrance the axiom that a sound body is the natural basis of a sound mind, and *vice versa*, and that every rational method should be adopted to preserve them. I have shown briefly that there is no condition or state of man that is exempt from disease and death. It may now be asked, Are there no means of preventing the ravages of the one, and postponing the sad triumph of the other? No means of restoring lost health, or of rendering sickness compatible with contentment, or even happiness itself? Yes. The severest diseases are and may be prevented; and are curable and cured—even consumption itself when judicious treatment is applied. All right-thinking persons will admit that sickness may be obviated, disease mitigated, and even death robbed of his prey for years, by approved remedies rightly employed.

REGULATING THE PASSIONS.

It has been truly said that we may religiously observe all the laws of hygiene in relation to air, light, drink, food, temperature, exercise, clothing, sleep, bathing, and the excretions, and yet lack one thing—one grand essential to human health and happiness. Yes, if our passions are our masters and not our slaves, they will rule and ruin us instead of obeying and serving our behests. There is, therefore, no single hygienic influence more conducive to health, happiness, and long life, than a cheerful, equitable temper of mind; and there is nothing that will more surely disorder the bodily functions, exhaust the vital energies, and stamp premature infirmities on the constitution, and hurry us on to an early grave, than an uneven, irritable, fretful, or passionate mental habit.

Medical men, at least, well know that a violent fit of passion will suddenly arrest, alter, or modify the various organic secretions. Excessive mental emotion will deprave and vitiate the secretions as readily as a deadly poison taken into the stomach. A paroxysm of anger will render the bile as acid and irritating as a full dose of calomel; excessive fear will relax the bowels equal to a strong infusion of tobacco; intense grief will arrest the secretions of gastric juice as effectually as belladonna; and violent rage will make the saliva as poisonous as will a mercurial salivation. There are many persons whose rage, either thoroughly real or exaggerated, is so violent that they froth at the mouth, and are thrown into spasms or violent convulsions. These fits of anger are often assumed, however, by designing parties for the purpose of frightening stern parents and guardians and others into the support of their own views and wishes. Such persons, finding their displays copied from nature of no avail, will suddenly become tame as lambs, but the effect upon their general health is found in the appearance of many nervous disorganizations, which, if the cause be often repeated, become permanent.

Thousands of facts of the above kind could be mentioned, but enough has been presented to demonstrate the law that a sound body cannot exist unless connected with a well-balanced mind. A vigorous exercise of the higher mental powers, a lively cultivation of the intellectual faculties and the moral affections, will never fail to sustain and elevate the human character, while, on the other hand, the violent indulgence of the animal propensities and the lower order of the passions, will wear out the mental machinery and enervate all the physiological powers. Will not the inspiration of love exalt the soul to the realms of " bliss, exquisite bliss ? " Will not the influence of hatred depress the soul, and sink it to the nethermost depth of misery and despair ? Contrast the emotions of benevolence, or gratitude, or veneration, or conscientiousness, or mirthfulness, or faith, or hope, with that of envy, revenge, jealousy, fear, grief, remorse, or despair ! The first are as refreshing to the soul as the gentle dews of morn to the tender blades of grass ; the other as withering as the fiery blasts of a crater to the verdant vales. The one energizes the mind and reanimates the body—the other sinks, chills, and enfeebles both ; one manufactures, creates as it were, vital power—the other wastes and destroys body and soul.

Those who would maintain permanent and uniform health and live to an old age, will perceive the necessity for cultivating all the nobler impulses of our nature with unremitting care and judgment. When we " nourish wrath to keep it warm," we only add to the venom of a malicious heart. That anger which " dwells only in the bosom of fools," should have no inheritance in the bosom of the wise and thoughtful of our race. The " evils of life," whatever they may be. are often " blessings in disguise," and therefore should be met with a brave fortitude and courage, instead of wailing, complaining and lamentation. Fretting, scolding, and fault-finding, not only aggravate all the necessary evils of life, but greatly multiply them. When we indulge in these faults, we but sow the dragon's teeth to reap a harvest of greater sorrows. More than this, we dissipate unwisely our best talents and energies, and render life a curse instead of a blessing. The grand essential, therefore, of a cheerful mind is self-control. This is the great law of mental hygiene. Before any one can acquire self-government, he must learn to govern the animal propensities, and make them subservient to the intellectual faculties and moral sentiments. It may require long, patient, and thorough discipline ; it may cost much self-denial, and appear to demand great temporary sacrifices, but it is worth all it may cost. Occasionally it is acquired through long years of bitter experience ; and sometimes the greater part of a life is spent in suffering disappointments, troubles, and crosses, ere the mind is found at peace with itself, and in right relations to all surrounding nature. Happy are they who can, even in such expensive schools, learn the art of adapting themselves to the invariable laws of the universe, which they cannot successfully oppose or in any respect alter ! Indeed, the only guarantee a man can have for a long life of health and happiness is to constantly cherish and maintain an even, cheerful, and hopeful spirit.

THINGS FOR THE SICK-ROOM.

BARLEY WATER.—Pearl barley, two ounces ; boiling water, two quarts. Boil to one quart and strain. If desirable, a little lemon-juice and sugar may be added. This may be taken freely in all inflammatory and eruptive diseases : Measles, Scarlet Fever, Small-Pox, etc.

RICE WATER.—Rice, two ounces ; water, two quarts. Boil one hour and a half, and add sugar and nutmeg to suit the taste. When milk is added to this it makes a very excellent diet for children. Should the bowels be too loose, boil the milk before adding.

SAGE TEA.—Dried leaves of Sage, half an ounce ; boiling water, one quart. Infuse for half an hour and strain ; may add sugar if desired. Balm, Peppermint, Spearmint, and other teas are made in the same manner.

A REFRESHING DRINK IN FEVERS.—Boil an ounce and a half of tamarinds, two ounces of stoned raisins, and three ounces of cranberries in three pints of water until two pints remain. Strain, and add a small piece of fresh lemon-peel, which must be removed in half an hour.

ARROW ROOT JELLY.—Stir a tablespoonful of arrow root powder into half a cupful of cold water, pour in a pint of boiling water, let it stand five or ten minutes, and then sweeten and flavor it to suit the taste.

IRISH MOSS JELLY.—Irish Moss, half an ounce ; fresh milk, one and a half pints. Boil down to a pint. Strain and add sugar and lemon-juice sufficient to give it an agreeable flavor.

ISINGLASS JELLY.—Isinglass, two ounces ; water, two pints. Boil to one point. Strain, and add one pint milk and one ounce of white sugar. This is excellent for persons recovering from sickness, and for children who have bowel complaints.

TAPIOCA JELLY.—Tapioca, two large spoonfuls ; water, one pint. Boil gently for an hour, or until it appears like a jelly ; add sugar, wine, and nutmeg, with lemon-juice to flavor.

RICE JELLY.—Mix a quarter of a pound of rice, picked and washed, with half a pound of loaf sugar, and just sufficient water to cover it.

Boil until it assumes a jelly-like appearance.   Strain, and season to suit
the taste and condition of the patient.

GRAPES.—In all cases of fever, very ripe grapes of any kind are a
beneficial article of diet, acting as both food and drink, and possessing
cooling and soothing properties.   They are also extremely grateful to
every plate.

TOAST.—To make a most excellent toast for a reduced or convalescent
patient, take bread twenty-four or thirty-six hours old, which has been
made of a mixture of fine wheat flour and Indian meal, and a pure yeast
batter mixed with eggs.   Toast it until of a delicate brown, and then
(if the patient be not inclined to fever) immerse it in boiled milk and
butter.   If the patient be feverish, spread it lightly with cranberry jam
or calves'-foot jelly.

RICE.—In all cases where a light and nice diet for parties who have
been or are afflicted with diarrhœa or dysentery is required, rice, in
almost any cooked form, is most agreeable and advantageous.   It may
be given with benefit to dyspeptics, unless costiveness accompanies the
dyspepsia.   To make rice-pudding, take a teacupful of rice, and as
much sugar, two quarts of milk, and a teaspoonful of salt.   Bake, with
a moderate heat, for two hours.   Rice flour made in a batter, and
baked upon a griddle, makes a superb cake ; and rice-flour gruel, seasoned
to the taste, is most excellent for the sick-room.

BREAD JELLY.—Boil a quart of water and let it cool.   Take one-
third of a common loaf of wheat bread, slice it, pare off the crust, and
toast it to a light brown.   Put it in the water in a covered vessel, and
boil gently, till you find, on putting some in a spoon to cool, the liquid
has become a jelly.   Strain and cool.   When used, warm a cupful,
sweeten with sugar, and add a little grated lemon-peel.

RICE GRUEL.—Ground rice, one heaping table-spoonful ; water, one
quart.   Boil gently for twenty minutes, adding, a few minutes before it
is done, one table-spoonful of ground cinnamon.   Strain and sweeten.
Wine may be added when the case demands it.

WATER GRUEL.—Oat or corn meal, two table-spoonfuls ; water, one
quart.   Boil for ten minutes, and strain, adding salt and sugar if desired by the patient.

SAGO GRUEL.—Sago, two table-spoonfuls ; water, one pint.   Boil
gently until it thickens ; stir frequently.   May add wine, sugar, and
nutmeg, according to circumstances.

ARROW-ROOT GRUEL.—Arrow root, one table-spoonful ; sweet milk
and boiling water, each one half pint.   Sweeten with loaf-sugar.   This
is very good for children whose bowels are irritable.

DECOCTION OF BRAN.—New wheat bran, one pint ; water, three
quarts.   Boil down to two quarts, strain off the liquor, and add sugar,
honey or molasses, according to the taste of the patient.

TAPIOCA.—Tapioca is a very delightful food for invalids. Make an ordinary pudding of it, and improve the flavor agreeably to the desire of the patient or convalescent, by adding raisins, sugar, prunes, lemon-juice, wine, spices, etc.

BEEF LIQUID.—When the stomach is very weak, take fresh lean beef, cut it into strips, and place the strips into a bottle, with a little salt. Place into a kettle of boiling water and let it remain one hour. Pour off the liquid and add some water. Begin with a small quantity, and use in the same manner and under similar circumstances as beef tea. This is even more nourishing than beef tea.

BEEF TEA.—Cut one pound of lean beef into shreds, and boil for twenty minutes in one quart of water, being particular to remove the scum as often as any rises. When it is cool, strain. This is very nourishing and palatable, and is of great value in all cases of extreme debility where no inflammatory action exists, or after the inflammation is subdued. In very low cases, a small tea-spoonful may be administered every fifteen or twenty minutes, gradually increasing the amount given as the powers of life return. In cases of complete prostration, after the cessation of long exhausting fever, it may be used as directed above, either alone or in conjunction with a little wine.

PANADO.—Put a little water on the fire with a glass of wine, some sugar, and a little grated nutmeg; boil all together a few seconds, and add pounded crackers or crumbs of bread; and again boil for a few minutes.

FRENCH MILK PORRIDGE.—Stir some oatmeal and water together, let the mixture stand to clear, and pour off the water. Then put more water to the meal, stir it well, and let it stand till the next day. Strain through a fine sieve, and boil the water, adding milk while so doing. The proportion of water must be small. With toast this is admirable.

COMMON MILK PORRIDGE will be found very palatable in ordinary cases. Everybody knows how to make it.

BUTTERMILK PAP.—Fresh buttermilk, four parts; water, one part; mix, boil, and thicken with Indian meal. Eat with butter, sugar, or molasses.

COFFEE MILK.—Put a dessert-spoonful of ground coffee into a pint of milk; boil it a quarter of an hour with a shaving or two of isinglass; let it stand ten minutes, and then pour off.

RESTORATIVE JELLY.—Take a leg of well-fed pork, just as cut up, beat it, and break the bone. Set it over a gentle fire, with three gallons of water, and simmer to one. Let half an ounce of mace and the same of nutmegs stew in it. Strain through a fine sieve. When cold, take off the fat. Give a chocolate-cup the first and last thing, and at noon, adding salt to suit the taste. This is very valuable in all cases of debility where animal food is admissible.

DRINK IN DYSENTERY.—Sheep's suet, two ounces ; milk, one pint ; starch, half an ounce. Boil gently for thirty minutes. Use as a common drink. This is excellent for sustaining the strength in bad cases of dysentery.

CRUST COFFEE.—Toast slowly a thick piece of bread cut from the outside of a loaf, until it is well browned, but not blackened. Then turn upon it boiling water of a sufficient quantity, and keep it from half an hour to an hour before using. Be sure that the liquid is of a rich brown color before you use it. It is a most excellent drink in all cases of sickness and convalescence.

CRANBERRY WATER.—Put a tea-spoonful of cranberries into a cup of water and mash them. In the mean time boil two quarts of water with one large spoonful of corn or oatmeal, and a bit of lemon-peel ; then add the cranberries and as much fine sugar as will leave a smart flavor of the fruit--also a wine-glassful of sherry. Boil the whole gently for a quarter of an hour, then strain.

WINE WHEY.—Heat a pint of new milk until it boils, at which moment pour in as much good wine as will curdle and clarify it. Boil and set it aside until the curd subsides. Do not stir it, but pour the whey off carefully, and add two pints of boiling water, with loaf-sugar.

ORANGE WHEY.—Milk, one pint ; the juice of an orange, with a portion of the peel. Boil the milk, then put the orange to it, and let stand till it coagulates. Strain.

MUSTARD WHEY.—Bruised mustard seed, two table-spoonfuls ; milk, one quart. Boil together for a few minutes until it coagulates, and strain to separate the curd. This is a very useful drink in dropsy. A tea-cupful may be taken at a dose, three times a day.

SIPPETS.—On an extremely hot plate put two or three slices of bread, and pour over them some of the juices of boiled beef, mutton, or veal. If there be no butter in the dish, sprinkle over them a little salt.

CHICKEN BROTH.—Take half a chicken, divested of all fat, and break the bones ; add to this half a gallon of water, and boil for half an hour. Season with salt.

VEGETABLE SOUP.—Take one potato, one turnip and one onion, with a little celery or celery seed. Slice and boil for an hour in one quart of water. Salt to the taste, and pour the whole upon a piece of dry toast. This forms a good substitute for animal food, and may be used when the latter would be improper.

CALVES'-FOOT JELLY.—Boil two calves' feet in one gallon of water, until reduced to one quart. Strain, and when cool, skim carefully. Add the white of six or eight eggs, well beaten, a pint of wine, half pound of loaf sugar, and the juice of four lemons. Mix them well, boil for a few minutes, stirring constantly, and pass through a flannel strainer. In some cases the wine should be omitted.

SLIPPERY ELM JELLY.—Take of the flour of slippery elm one or two tea-spoonfuls; cold water, one pint. Stir, until a jelly is formed. Sweeten with loaf sugar or honey. This is excellent for all diseases of the throat, chest, and lungs, coughs, colds, bronchitis, inflammation of lungs, etc. It is very nutritious and soothing.

NUTRITIVE FLUIDS.—Below will be found directions for preparing three nutritious fluids, which are of great value in all diseases, either acute or chronic, that are attended or followed by prostration,—debility, whether general, or of certain organs only, derangement of the digestive organs, weak stomach, indigestion, heartburn, or sour stomach, constipated bowels, torpidity or want of activity of the liver, thin or poor blood. They are highly nutritious, supplying to the blood in such a form that they are most easily assimilated, the various elements which are needed to enrich it, and thus enable it to reproduce the various tissues of the body that have been wasted by disease. In cases where the stomach has become so weakened and sensitive that the lightest food or drinks cannot be taken without causing much uneasiness and distress, these fluids are invaluable. They strengthen the stomach and neutralize all undue acidity, while, at the same time, they soothe the irritation by their bland and demulcent qualities. When carefully and properly prepared, according to the direction following, they very nearly resemble rich new milk in color and consistency, while their taste is remarkably pleasant. Care should be taken that all the ingredients are of the best quality. Soft water must be used in all cases. Fresh rain-water is to be preferred, but spring water may be used if perfectly soft. Hard water will cause the fluids to be of a yellow color, and if the milk is old, they are apt to separate.

Fluid No. 1.—Put one pint of new milk (the fresher the better) and two pints of soft water in a vessel perfectly free from all greasy matter, over a slow fire. Rub two even tea-spoonfuls of superfine wheat flour and two tea-spoonfuls of carbonate of magnesia, together with a little milk, into a soft batter, free from lumps; add this to the milk and water as soon as they begin to boil. Boil gently for five minutes—*no longer*, stirring constantly. Pour into an earthen or glass dish to cool, adding, at the same time, two tea-spoonfuls of loaf sugar, and one tea-spoonful each of saleratus and table salt, rubbed fine; stir until cold. The fluid must not be allowed to remain in a metallic vessel of any kind, and it must be kept in a cool place.

Fluid No. 2.—Put one pint of fresh milk and two pints of soft water in a vessel over a slow fire. Rub together with a little fresh cream into a soft batter, free from lumps, one table-spoonful each of good sweet rye flour, ground rice, and pure starch—which add to the milk and water as soon as they begin to boil. Boil for five minutes, stirring con-

stantly. Remove from the fire, and add three tea-spoonfuls of loaf sugar and one tea-spoonful each of saleratus and table salt. Observe the
same precautions as in No. 1.

Fluid No. 3.—Put in a vessel, over a slow fire, one pint of fresh
milk and two pints of soft water. When they begin to boil, add one
table-spoonful of wheat flour, two table-spoonfuls pure starch, and two
tea-spoonfuls of carbonate of magnesia, rubbed together with a little
milk into a soft batter, free from lumps. Boil gently for five minutes,
stirring constantly. Pour into an earthen vessel to cool, and add one
tea-spoonful of the best gum arabic, dissolved in a little warm water, one
tea-spoonful each of saleratus and table salt, and one table-spoonful of
pure strained honey. Stir until cold. The same precaution must be
observed as in preparing No. 1.

Directions.—One half pint or less of these fluids may be taken at a
dose, and at least three pints should be taken during the day, and the
amount gradually increased to two or three quarts. Commence with
No. 1, and use two weeks : then use No. 2 for the same length of time,
after which No. 3 is to be used for two weeks. Continue their use as
long as necessary, taking each for two weeks before changing. In all the
diseases enumerated above, the use of these fluids, in connection with
proper herbal remedies, will ensure a speedy restoration to health.

GUM ACACIA RESTORATIVE.—Take two ounces of pure white gum
Arabic,—procure the lump, the powdered is very apt to be adulterated,
—pulverize it well, and dissolve by the aid of a gentle heat in a gill of
water, stirring constantly. When it is entirely dissolved, add three
table-spoonfuls of pure strained honey. Let it remain over the fire until
it becomes of the consistency of a jelly. The heat must be very gentle,
it must not boil. If desirable, flavor with lemon or vanilla. This will
be found a very pleasant article of diet for delicate stomachs. When
the articles used are pure it will be transparent and of a light golden
color. This will be borne by the weakest stomach, when everything else
is rejected. It is *highly nutritious.*

MALT INFUSION.—Infuse one pint of ground malt, for two hours, in
three pints of scalding water. The water should not be brought quite to
the boiling point. Strain, add sugar, if desired ; flavor with lemon-
juice. This is an excellent drink in inflammatory fevers, acute rheumatism, etc.

PEAS.—Take young and fresh shelled green peas, wash them clean,
put them into fresh water, just enough to cover them, and boil them till
they take up nearly all the water. Season with salt, pepper, and butter. This dish, if prepared according to directions, and eaten warm, will
not harm any invalid—not even one suffering from diarrhœa.

MILK.—In some cases where a milk diet is advisable, owing to the
peculiar condition of the patient's stomach, it will cause distress. This

is frequently the case when there is undue acidity. In such cases let it be prepared in the following manner, and it will be found to set well: — Take a tea-cupful of fresh milk, heat nearly to boiling; dissolve in it a tea-spoonful of loaf sugar; pour into a large-sized tumbler, and add sufficient plain soda-water to fill it. Prepared in the above directed manner it will be perfectly free from all unpleasant effects.

SOUPS FOR THE CONVALESCENT.—To extract the strength from meat, long and slow boiling is necessary; but care must be taken that the pot is never off the boil. All soups should be made the day before they are used, and they should then be strained into earthen pans. When soup has jellied in the pan, it should not be removed into another. When in danger of not keeping, it should be boiled up.

EGGS.—In cases of extreme debility, eggs are most excellent. They should never be boiled hard. The best way to prepare them is to beat them well with milk and sugar. Where it will be appropriate to the case, add some fine pale sherry wine.

MILK FOR INFANTS.—Fresh cow's milk, one part; water, two parts; sweeten with a very little loaf sugar. When children are raised by hand, it is always necessary to dilute the milk. As the child advances in age, the proportion of water stated above may be gradually lessened.

WATER GRUEL.— Corn or oatmeal, two table-spoonfuls; water, one quart. Boil ten or fifteen minutes, and strain. Add salt and sugar to suit the taste of the patient. This should be used freely, during and after the operation of cathartic medicines.

HOW TO ASSIST THE DOCTOR.

THE SICK-ROOM.

IF there is a choice of rooms, the patient's welfare demands that he should be placed in the one affording to a greater degree light, pure air, warmth, etc. The patient should not be put into the room which is dark and gloomy, but let it be one that is light and cheerful, and with a fire-place in it, if possible.

If the illness be fever, an ophthalmic affection, brain disease, or other disease requiring quiet, a back room away from the family should be selected, as quiet is absolutely necessary, and the patient will not care to look at anything or to speak much. If, however, he be suffering from an accident, he will be more contented and cheerful if he is placed near to the rest of the family, where he can assist in the conversation, watch your movements, and see you at your labors. It will greatly tend to make him forget to a greater extent his misfortune, and it will also save time in waiting upon him.

The room should be free from all unpleasant odors, and should not be exposed to disagreeable effluvia from water-closets, sinks, etc. The furniture of the room should be but very simple and plain, and, in infectious diseases, but very little should be placed in the room. If you have ever been in a hospital, you may have noticed the bare floors, the iron bedsteads, the absence of woollen bed-clothing, and the plain tables, and most probably pitied the inmates for their lack of comforts, and involuntarily the thought may have arisen in your mind that fortune is more propitious to you when sick, for your sick-room would have at least a good carpet, upholstered furniture, and your bed an easy one to repose upon, and plentifully supplied with woollen blankets, etc. But *you* and many more are also deluded in this respect. If you will bear in mind that woollen fabrics retain *smells* much longer than cotton and linen, and are therefore less sanitary, you would probably not consider them so advantageous. The room should have no upholstered chairs or sofas, canebottomed or plain wood are preferable, and it would be better if no carpet was on the floor, except perhaps a narrow strip for you to walk upon to prevent noise, but a clean boarded floor, kept clean and sweet by scrubbing and " elbow-grease " is infinitely better. It is better to have no curtains ; but if the room looks too cheerless without them, use light muslin or something which will easily wash.

The position of the bed is also very important. In case of accident the bed should be placed where the patient feels most comfortable, only it should be placed where there is a good light to see and dress the wound ; but in fever and small-pox the bed should occupy the position between the door and fire-place. The reason for this is, that as fire cannot burn without air, there must be a draft to feed it ; as this becomes heated and escapes up the chimney, it is replaced by a fresh supply drawn in through the door and window. This prevents a spread of the disease, as the chimney acts as a ventilating shaft, carrying away the impurities of the room. A stove will also do this, but to a much less extent. It is very apparent, therefore, that if a person stands between the bed and the fire-place, he must breathe air laden with the effluvia from the patient, whereas, on the other side, that is, between the bed and door, he inhales air that has not yet come in contact with the patient. If, from the form of the room, the bed cannot be placed in this position, the space between the window and the bed should always be sufficient to stand in.

The room should always be fully prepared before the patient is placed in it, as the setting it to rights is not only annoying, but may do positive harm to the patient. The fire, if any is wanted, should particularly be previously built, for very often the chimney refuses to draw well, and the poor patient is choked with the smoke. He may suffer from a chest complaint, and his difficulty of breathing be so aggravated as to put him in a miserable plight. The windows should not be so fastened that you cannot open them, especially from the top. An equable temperature should be kept up, neither too hot nor too cold, and extremes avoided.

The bed itself is very worthy of consideration. Unqualifiedly, the best is a hair mattrass, but, as this is so expensive, it cannot be expected to be found in every house, but, unless obliged, use no feather bed. It is too soft, and the patient sinks into holes, so that, in case of wounds or burns, you cannot get at them properly, and besides, if the feathers get wet, you cannot easily put them right again. Good clean straw or chaff, evenly packed, is far superior. It costs but little, to begin with, is more comfortable, far superior in a sanitary point of view, and has this advantage: that in case of being spoiled, it can be emptied, the cover washed, and refilled without loss of time, and at a very trifling expense.

The bed should not be too wide, for if the patient needs help, the attendant is obliged to move him kneeling on the bed, or at arms' length, should he be lying in the middle.

It is often a matter of much concern how to change the bed-clothing in case of fracture or low states of disease, where the patient cannot be moved from the bed. The following method should be pursued :—roll up the clothes to be changed tightly to the middle, lengthwise, not across the bed ; put on the clean things with half the width rolled up close to the other roll, lift the patient on the newly made part, slip off the soiled clothes, unroll the clean ones, and the bed is made.

Before the patient is put to bed scour the floor right well, and wash it with hot water with a few pennies' worth of chloride of lime, or, if you cannot get this, use a little quicklime, and rub it well into cracks and corners. The whole of the lime need not be removed, as the little particles left sticking in the cracks and pores of the wood will prevent insects, give a clean, sweet smell to the place, and tend to keep away infection. After the room is thoroughly dried, it is ready for the sick occupant.

If all this is done, you will have the *healthiest* sick-chamber possible, and rob the disease of its exciting causes. He must then be well nursed, and as this is so important, the author will next consider

NURSES AND NURSING.

Next to the physician, the nurse has responsibilities that must be faithfully discharged, as the life of the patient is not alone dependent upon the skill of the physician, but in a great measure also upon careful nursing. Every physician will tell you that he recollects cases in his practice where all his skill would have been unavailing had it not been for the excellent nursing that the patient received.

It is a common opinion that women only can nurse.   This is erroneous, as men are frequently met with, especially husbands and brothers, who are quite as gentle in their touch, quite as considerate about little wants, and far more tender and thoughtful than almost any woman.   A male nurse has, moreover, one great advantage—his strength.   Ask that wife who requires lifting from the bed, and she will tell how safe she feels in her husband's strong arms, and what a comfort it is to be lifted by him. It is a dreadful feeling for a patient not to have full confidence in the power of the person assisting, and the nervous shock induced by the fear of being let fall, may take days to recover from.   It is, therefore, not to be thought that nursing is peculiarly woman's work, but that men are just as capable.

A nurse should have five qualifications—*sobriety, cleanliness, firmness, gentleness,* and *patience.*

Sobriety.—The drunken nurse should not be allowed to cross the door-sill of the sick-room.   It is no place for her,—she cannot be trusted. Human life is too precious to be entrusted to the care of one who cannot resist the temptation to indulge in intoxicating drinks.

Cleanliness.—The nurse should not only keep the room clean, but always be clean herself.   A very little thing will spoil the appetite of a sick person, and nothing offensive, as dressings from wounds or burns, should be allowed to remain in the room.   All necessary vessels should be emptied as soon as done with, well washed out, and left in the open air.   It should be remembered that bad air is just as poisonous to a person as bad food, and hence it should be frequently changed by opening the window.   The dreaded draft will do no harm, but bears upon its wings the elements conducive to the health of both patient and attendants.   The fever-poison is weakened by admixture with pure air just in the same proportion as spirits are weakened by the addition of water. The food that the patient cannot eat should not be left in the room—it will breed distaste for it if always in the sight of the patient.   The drinking-water should be frequently changed, as it absorbs all the gases in the room, so that if the patient is allowed to drink it, it actually puts back into his stomach what his body exhaled.   Always give him fresh water, then, when he wants to drink.

Firmness.—The lesson that firmness is not rudeness should be learned first.   It is not to be expected that a suffering person knows as well what is best for him as those whose brains are clear.   If, therefore, a certain thing is best to be done, do it, do it kindly, but do it, and the patient will thank you afterwards.

Gentleness.—It should never be forgotten that gentleness is an absolute requirement of a nurse.   If the poor patient suffers from rheumatism or a broken limb, and the bed-clothes must be changed, it should be done gently, and all needless suffering avoided.   If his position in bed requires change, do not torture him, but gently move him, and avoid all jerks and knocks with great care.

Patience.—Need a word be said to the effect that of all beings nurses should especially be patient ? It should never be forgotten that the difference is a great one between the nurse and the person under his or her care, and it should be remembered that in their own experiences they have been cross and irritable even when they were well, that they were easily put out, and so peevish and fretful from the slightest causes. They should then consider how it must be with the person taken suddenly from active life and compelled to lie still in one position, or with one whose whole body is racked with pain. The one, therefore, who loses patience, however sorely tried, and who cannot bear with these trials for a while, should stay away from the sick-room in the capacity of nurse.

Nursing, in a great measure, is a natural gift either in man or woman, just as much as music, painting, and other things are. It is not every one, therefore, who is fit for a nurse, not because they wilfully do wrong, but they are not adapted for it. There are many good-hearted yet thoughtless people who would never make good, handy nurses with all the training in the world.

The *awkward* nurse is a queer creature, and she is everlastingly getting into some trouble. If she is going up stairs with her hands full, she is sure to step on the bottom of her dress, and either drops what she is carrying or falls herself. If the fire wants coal, she throws on a whole scuttleful, a good part of which falls upon the fender, and the poor patient is so terrified that he cannot rest for hours. If she has a hole in her dress, or a bit of braid is loose, it will be sure to catch a chair or the fire-irons, bringing them down with a rattle. If of matronly age and wears caps, she will have strings so long that when she stoops over to catch the patient's whisper, the ends will tickle his nose or other parts of his face. At least one of her fingers is sure to be enveloped in a rag tied on with black cotton. If the patient wants a little bread and butter, the knife that has been used for cutting cheese or peeling onions is unerringly used. If she is cooking cabbage or frying bacon in the next room, she always forgets to close the door leading to the patient's room, fills it with a strong smell which sickens him, and then says that it is *too bad* that the patient cannot eat a morsel of food. If the patient thirsts, she will fill the glass full to the brim, put her hand under his head, bend his neck till his chin touches his breast, then puts the glass to his lips, spills a good part of it on his clothes, and thinks he is very awkward to choke over a mouthful of water. If a candle is to be lighted, she sticks it in between the bars of the grate, which soon fills the room with the rank smell of burning tallow, and when she finally succeeds in lighting it, she finds she has a wick several inches long,

gained at the expense of the melted tallow; or if it be gas, she takes a
short bit of paper, turns the gas full on, makes a sudden blaze like a
flash of lightning, forgets the bit of paper in her hand while she is regulating the blaze, burns her fingers, throws the lighted paper on the
floor, and puts her foot on it. All this does not escape the patient's
notice, and he gets so nervous and frightened that he loses his night's
rest. If the patient is so far convalescent as to be able to sit up in bed
to take his food, she will, of course, put the tray on his knees, then
assist him into the sitting posture, and ten chances to one the things
are upset all over the counterpane.

Then there is the *fussy nurse*, and there are many of this sort. Her
zeal to benefit the patient is so great, that she sadly overdoes it : she
bustles in and out of the room every few minutes, wearies the patient
by persistently asking him if he cannot eat something, which she would
willingly walk miles to get if wanted, raising him up, tucking in the
bed clothes, drawing up and lowering the blinds ; one, in fact, who is
perfectly miserable if she is not constantly on the move. The fussy
nurse is generally a kind-hearted, loving creature, and it is her very
goodness which makes her weary the patient, who congratulates himself on the relief gained whenever she vacates the room.

Then we have the *careless, slovenly nurse.* Doctors are always suspicious of this person ; they can never feel sure that their patients really
had the right quantity of medicine ; if she happened to remember it
they would get it, but if not, she would make up for it by giving a
double dose next time. There is no clean glass or cup when wanted.
Food is taken to the patient, and if he cannot eat it, it is left there for
hours. There are so many crumbs of bread in the bed that it feels to
the patient like lying on a gravel walk. Cinders cover the hearth all
over, and the fire is black. The slops, which should have been removed
in the evening, are hid under the bed, filling the room with bad smells.
Those bits of meat, crumbs of bread, and other matters which have
fallen on the floor are left there ; the consequence is, that being winter,
the mice and perhaps rats finding a warm room and something to eat,
think it a comfortable place, and use it accordingly. No one can im-
agine the degree of comfort these scampering animals afford to the
helpless creature in bed.

Next we have the *cruel nurse*, who does her duty, but not from love ;
she carries out the doctor's orders exactly. In matter of duty she is
inflexible ; if the medicine has to be taken at a certain time, she brings
it to the minute, and worries the patient into taking it on the instant.
Her law in all things is like that of the Medes and Persians, which
altereth not. She may be perfectly honest in her dealings, but the
utter absence of tenderness and compassion makes her an undesirable
nurse.

And lastly, we have what I trust is a very rare character, the *dishonest nurse*. She drinks all the wine, and partakes pretty freely of the food intended for the patient, and tells the doctor that the patient ought to get better according to the quantity of nourishment he gets through. She is also dishonest in another way : she finds it a great deal of trouble to make the patient take his medicine, so she just empties it away, a regular dose at a time, so that when the doctor calls, he may see that the bottle is gradually emptying.

All these characters are to be met with, and doctors find one or more of them in various sick-rooms every day. Now, it is not well to be too exacting in such matters, but as a good nurse is, next to a good physician, necessary to properly combat disease, it is well to object to what are positive faults.

A good nurse should be tender and compassionate, and ought to have all her five senses in a healthy, active condition. *Sight*, that she may be able to read directions, or read aloud to the patient, and watch the change of countenance. A quick-sighted nurse will not need to wait for the sufferer to make his demands ; she will see in a moment what is wanted from the motion of the eye, or the lips, or a finger. *Hearing*, that she may be able to catch the faintest whisper, and not oblige a weak patient to exert the voice or repeat his requests. *Feeling*, that she may readily detect the temperature of the skin of the patient, and not use any application which will either scald with heat or chill with cold. *Smell*, that all impurities in the atmosphere of the room may be readily detected. *Taste*, that she may not offer food unfit to be used, or improperly cooked if good in itself.

She need not be highly educated, but she should be able to read writing, so that she can fully understand the directions on the labels. She ought to have a knowledge of common and every-day affairs, and possess the qualification of "common sense." But she must not place too high a valuation on her own opinion or skill, as that may cause her to use either in opposition to the wishes of the doctor. She must do everything for the patient that she can, and deal with the doctor fairly.

PART II.

DISEASES.

THE great difficulty of treating disease, by those who are not physicians, is the liability to mistake the character of the affection, being unable through obscurity of the symptoms to ascertain the organ or tissue affected.   Without entering minutely into diagnosis, the author will endeavor to simplify the study of morbid conditions of the human body, so that the unscientific may more readily ascertain the disease and apply the appropriate remedy or treatment.

  1. General condition pertaining to :
    a. Temperature and dryness of skin.
    b. Condition of pulse—full and quick, or slow and weak.
    c. Appearance of tongue.
    d. State of bowels and kidneys.
    e. Desire for food and drink.
  2. The general appearance of the patient.
    a. Size—emaciation or increase, general or local.
    b. Aspect of face or expression.
    c. Changes of color of skin.
  3. The position or posture.
    a. In bed—the manner of lying, on the back or either side, quiet, restless, etc.
    b. Out of bed—posture, gait, stiffness, loss of power of limbs, etc.
  4. The sensations of the patient.

Whenever any of these conditions are at variance with the normal state, the presumption, or rather certainty, is that some organ or tissue is assailed by disease.   Some of the general indications of the patient in many cases often make known the character of the affection, when not suggested by other symptoms.   For instance, the skin is remarkably moist and soft in delirium tremens; the perspiration profuse and sour in acute rheumatism; exhausting sweats in the latter stages of consumption or profuse suppuration; the crackling feeling of emphysema, and the pitting under pressure in dropsy.

The pulse is hard and wiry in abdominal inflammations; in acute hydrocephalus its frequency is very great, slow and labored in brain diseases, irregular in disease of the heart, almost imperceptible in cholera or in the latter stages of the low fevers.

The tongue covered with a thin white layer is indicative of disorder of the stomach; when patchy, the stomach is considerably irritated; when yellow, the patient is bilious; when shining, glazed, and chapped, it indicates long-continued inflammation or ulceration of the bowels; aphthous patches indicate imperfect nutrition, etc.

In cholera the stools resemble rice-water; when clay-colored, it denotes a deficiency of bile; when yeast-like, fermentation takes place instead of digestion.

The urine is dark-colored in fevers, very limpid and abundant in hysteria, scanty in dropsies, acid in rheumatism.

The *aspect* is often very significant. In scrofula the corners of the nose and lips are swollen, in chlorosis a waxy pallor is observed, in malignant diseases a sallow hue, in heart-diseases a blue color of the lips, in pneumonia a dusky flush, in phthisis a hectic flush. When the expression is anxious, it indicates disease of the heart and dyspnœa; when pinched and contracted, there is much suffering, as in the low forms of fever; the skin is white in anæmia, yellow in jaundice and malignant cases; it has a muddy hue in splenic diseases, blue in cholera, and livid in commencing mortification.

If the patient's head is elevated by choice in bed, it denotes heart-disease; when he is very feeble he lies on his back; in peritonitis the knees are drawn up; in cramps or pain of the abdomen, he lies on his side.

In order that the reader may not have a confused idea of what is meant by inflammation, I will describe it insomuch as to give its phenomena. These are *redness, heat, swelling,* and *pain.* When all these are present it constitutes *inflammation.* When a fever or disease partakes of this character, it is inflammatory. Chronic inflammation is characterized by all the essential conditions of the acute form, differing, however, in this, by being preceded through all its changes with symptoms so mild that it is only after a certain time that the patient is much inconvenienced constitutionally. Inflammation always denotes increase of activity of the vascular system. When of a localized character, the increase is noticed in the capillary circulation; when general, as in fevers, or of some important organ, the whole circulatory apparatus is abnormally active.

MIASMATIC FEVERS.

These, as signified by name, owe their origin to, or are caused by, a peculiar principle to which the name of *malaria* or *miasm* has been given. Of the chemical nature of miasm we literally know nothing; but we have abundant evidence that it is a specific cause of disease. There are, practically, two kinds of malaria: First, *koino-miasmata,* the product of vegetable decomposition, or terrestrial emanations; second, *Idio-miasmata,* the deleterous effluvia originating from the decomposition of matter derived from the human body. Both of these are prolific causes of disease, yet the profession, owing to the subtile nature of the miasms, are in a great degree ignorant as to the manner of operation. These two causes may act separately, and produce their different symptoms, or they may operate together, causing a confusion of morbid phenomena.

"Marsh gas," or the product of vegetable decomposition, owing to its diversification, is of course the greater cause of disease. Two requisites, heat and moisture, are necessary for its production; and hence, where these abound in any quantity, so proportionably is the miasm evolved. For this reason, low, marshy lands are at certain seasons very unhealthy, while those regions at a greater elevation are peculiarly healthy in this respect. Wherever vegetation is profuse, and to which abundant heat and moisture are contributed, there we may reasonably expect a plentiful product of miasm and consequent disease. Experiments have proved that in decomposition of vegetable matter, animal matter—infusoria—is produced in very rapid succession, having an exceedingly short-lived existence. These infusoria are inhaled at every breath, as the air contains swarms of them, but which are imperceptible to any of the senses. It is reasonable to suppose that they, in a great measure, contribute largely to periodic fevers. The diseases generally classed as Malarial are Intermittent, Remittent, Yellow, and Typhus Fevers.

INTERMITTENT FEVER.

This is commonly called *Fever and Ague*, or *Chills and Fever*. As the name implies, the fever is not constant, as in the continual fevers, but *intermits*, so that in its career there are well-marked periods of absence of febrile symptoms. It is a fever characterized by a succession of attacks, with equal *intervals* and *intermissions*, that are complete, but irregular, owing to the paroxysms being of uncertain duration. By *interval* is meant the time from the beginning of one paroxysm to the beginning of the next, and by *intermission* the period of time between the close of one paroxysm to the beginning of the next. The length of the interval determines the variety of ague. When the interval is twenty-four hours, it is called *quotidian*; thirty-six hours, *tertian*; and when seventy-two hours, it is called *quartan*. These varieties duplicate, and are then called double quotidian, etc.

The disease is announced by a paroxysm which has three stages, the cold, the hot, and the sweating. The cold stage is well marked; the patient yawns, has a feeling of weakness, stretches, no appetite, and no inclination to move. Paleness is observed in the face and extremities; the patient shakes, the teeth chatter, and the skin shrinks, causing *horripilation* or "goose-flesh."

When this stage declines, the hot stage comes on, which is characterized by a high fever. This is followed by the sweating stage, which increases from a mere moisture at first to a profuse perspiration. After this the body returns to its natural temperature, and apparent health returns.

During the cold stage the circulation is thrown upon the internal organs, the spleen becomes congested, which organ is enlarged, causing what is known as the *ague cake.*

A quotidian begins generally in the morning, a tertian at noon, and a quartan in the afternoon. The cold stage is shortest in the quotidian, and longest in the quartan. Intermittent fever is more common in the spring and autumn than at other seasons of the year, and in fall more severe and dangerous.

TREATMENT.—Commence treatment with a cathartic, as senna or the Renovating Pill. In the cold stage give hot drinks, and even stimulants may be of service. Induce warmth and comfort by extra covering, foot-baths, bottles filled with hot water applied to the surface, etc. In the hot stage, cooling drinks and anything that mollifies febrile action.

When an intermission ensues, administer Peruvian bark, or, preferably, one of its active principles, quinine. This can be given in a large dose, or smaller doses repeated. Fifteen grains may be given at once or in successive doses. It may be taken in pills or in solution with elixir of vitriol. Quinine is a specific in this disease, and it rarely ever fails in curing every case, if the patient be placed under its influence. Peculiar head symptoms and buzzing in the ears denote the influence of this admirable remedy. My experience has not taught me that there is much danger in an overdose, and I consider it more or less harmless; yet, like every other remedy, it must be judiciously and intelligently administered. The web of the black spider rolled up in five-grain pills, and taken, one pill at a time every two hours, is a valuable domestic remedy. Decoctions of dogwood bark are successful in many cases; so also of the bark of the tulip tree.

REMITTENT FEVER.

This is commonly called *Bilious* Fever. It is a disease whose attack is generally sudden and well marked, without prominent premonitory symptoms, if any, at all times. There is sense of languor and debility for a few days previous to the onset; slight headache, lack of appetite, furred tongue, bitter taste in the mouth in the morning, pain in the joints, and a feeling of uneasiness.

The first onset is announced by a rigor or chill, distinct in character. though generally brief and sometimes slight, but at times severe and prolonged. Sometimes the chill is first felt in the feet; at other times commences at the shoulder-blades, or in the back, running from thence

10

through the whole body. Usually there is but one well-marked chill; the paroxysms of fever returning subsequently, and seldom preceded by a cold stage.

The symptoms of this disease intensify at certain periods of the day; preceded occasionally, but not generally, by a chill. Between this period of severity in the febrile symptoms and a similar period following there is generally a decrease in the violence of the symptoms, during which the fever moderates, but does not, as in intermittent fever, totally disappear. It remits in severity, and hence the name. The pulse in the hot stage ranges from one hundred to one hundred and thirty. The pains in the head, back, and limbs are almost insufferable. The covering of the tongue is yellowish or dirty white, and in severe cases, in the advanced stage, the tongue is parched, brown or nearly black in the centre, and red at the edges. Food is distasteful, and nausea and vomiting ensue, with frequently pain, upon pressure, in the epigastrium. The bowels are at first costive, but become loose, and the fæces are dark and offensive.

TREATMENT.—Give an emetic or cathartic in the formative stage. When the disease is fully developed, sponge the body all over several times a day with cold or tepid water, whichever is most grateful to the patient, and give cooling drinks, as the effervescing draught. When the fever is high, moderate it with tincture or fluid extract of green hellebore, in doses of from three to ten drops. Dover's powder should be given as a diaphoretic. Ice-water can be drunk at pleasure. A mustard poultice should be placed over the pit of the stomach whenever tenderness exists.

Quinine is the great remedy in this disease also, and should be administered in the same manner as advised in fever and ague. It is to be given in a remission. Whenever the fever has been subdued by large doses of quinine, its administration should not be abruptly ceased, but be continued in smaller or tonic doses for several weeks afterward.

There is a form of fever called *Congestive.* It is also called *pernicious fever.* It is not essentially remittent, but may also be intermittent in character. The congestion may only operate upon one of the internal organs, or upon all of them. Congestion may ensue in the earlier or later stage of the disease. There is usually congestion of the brain, and profound stupor follows. It assumes all types of periodic fevers, but is more frequently quotidian or tertian. The first attack generally simulates a simple attack of intermittent, and excites but little attention. The second attack is severe, producing great coldness, and the patient has a deathlike hue of face and extremities. As the disease advances, the heat of the skin becomes pungent. The skin also becomes dry, husky, and parched, followed, after a time, by a cold, clammy sensation. The eyes are dull and watery, and at times glassy:

the countenance dull, sleepy, and distressed ; the tongue trembles upon protrusion, indicating weakness, and is at first covered with whitish fur, which changes to either brown or black ; the breathing is difficult, and inspirations often thirty to the minute.   Pressure over the liver, stomach, or bowels occasions pain ; and the mind is often disturbed, and falls into lethargy and stupor, or is delirious.

The treatment is the same as in remittent fever.   Quinine and the other remedies are of the some signal service.   In stupor friction is to be made along the course of the spine with spirits of turpentine or ammonia.

In convalescence the diet must be light and nutritious, and as strength returns may be increased.   Exercise out of doors should be encouraged. If recovery be slow, it should be hastened by wine, ale, or brandy, and the usual vegetable tonics.

Any person who is suffering from almost a continuity of the disease, or the so-called chronic form of malarial fever, desirous of corresponding with me on the subject, I should be most happy to reply to, for in the vast and beneficent domain of Herbalism there are many remedies that can be advised as curative, to mention which would occupy too much space in a volume of this size.   We can be eclectic in Nature's laboratory.

YELLOW-FEVER.

The first symptoms of this fever seem identical with remittent, often well marked by periodicity, but finally reaction occurs, and it assumes a typhoid character.   The disease is ushered in generally with a chill, severe at times, though usually moderate, of short duration, and rarely repeated.   The chill is followed by slight fever, with increased heat of surface ; but this rarely rises to any considerable height, and continues only for two or three days, when, in cases likely to prove fatal, it is succeeded by coldness of surface, etc.   Sweating exists in many cases. The pulse is singular in character, but rarely rises above a hundred ; the tongue is moist and white for the first few days, but as the disease advances it becomes red, smooth, shining, and dry, having a black streak in the middle.   The most prominent symptoms are nausea and vomiting.   In fatal cases the vomiting is persistent, and towards the termination the green biliary matter thrown up changes to a thin black fluid, having a sediment like the grounds of coffee.   This is the terrible *black vomit* (vomita-nigra) of yellow-fever.   The bowels are generally costive, and the abdomen tender upon pressure.   Severe headache generally exists, and the countenance bears a singular expression, in which a smile seems to play upon the lips, but the rest of the face bears a wild or sad look.   Restlessness is common to this disease night and day.   Blood often escapes from the nose, gums, ears, stomach, bowels, and urinary passages. The skin bears a tinged color similar to that in jaundice. The disease appears both endemically and epidemically. At first the disease is hard to recognize, presenting but the usual symptoms of fevers in their incipient stage, with no symptoms to distinguish the disease, or, if any, very obscure; but when the severe pain in the back and loins exists, the conjunctiva injected, and a red flush of the face and forehead is present, the identity of the disease is no longer in doubt, especially when extraneous circumstances, calculated to suggest the probability of an attack of yellow-fever, are also present.

TREATMENT.—In the early stage of the attack it should be treated, as regards medicines, the same as a case of malarial fever. If any derangement of the stomach exists, a gentle emetic is proper; this rouses the nervous system from its lethargy, promotes the action of the liver, and, by determining the blood to the surface, restores the capillary circulation. The best emetic for this purpose is lobelia combined with boneset. The febrile stage requires a thorough bath with tepid water and whiskey over the entire surface, with friction by rubbing with a towel or the hand. Large mustard-poultices should be placed over the spine and abdomen. Immediately upon the decline of fever, if the symptoms denote urgency, administer the antiperiodic remedies advised in intermittent and remittent fever. The sulphate of quinia may be combined with tannin, because the astringent properties of the tannin have a beneficial effect in subduing inflammatory action of the mucous membranes. This remedy should not be delayed a moment if the patient is in a period of prostration, and its retention by the stomach should be favored by anodynes, carminatives, or stimulants, as the case may require. Oil of turpentine and Cayenne pepper can also be combined with advantage in this disease. The strength of the patient must be supported by every means that can be employed—gruel and weak animal broths, bread-water, my nutritive fluids, milk and water, etc , are important means for this object. The revulsive influence of a blister over the stomach is of great service in this stage. If reaction is induced and convalescence established, the remaining strength of the patient must be carefully husbanded by proper tonics and wholesome and digestible diet, increasing the quantity as the patient gains strength.

All exposed to yellow-fever should avoid the night-air and sudden changes of temperature; they should sleep in the highest part of the house; be moderate in taking exercise; they should take nutritious but not stimulating food, and never expose themselves to infected air with empty stomachs or when fatigued.

TYPHUS FEVER.

This is also called *Hospital, Jail, Camp, Putrid,* and *Ship* Fever. It is usually preceded by lassitude, debility, and loss of appetite, and ushered in by rigors and chills, and characterized by frequent exacerbations and declines during its progress. It generally presents itself as an epidemic, and runs a uniform course. From the third to the seventh day of the fever the peculiar *petechial* eruption occurs. It is of a florid, reddish, or reddish-pink color, disappearing on pressure, which distinguishes it from the petechiæ of typhoid. The breathing is hurried, the skin dry and hot, the tongue thickly coated, and the thirst urgent. There is great distress about the head, which often results in delirium. This stage of excitement continues generally, with little increase or abatement in the symptoms, for some time. The fever is greatest towards evening, least in the morning. The bowels are generally costive, and if it continues for some time, all the secretions become vitiated, the body exhaling a nauseous odor, and the tongue, gums, and teeth become coated with a dark-brown slime. Collapse generally follows, voluntary powers depressed, surface relaxed, and diminished in temperature, often covered with a clammy sweat; pulse small and tremulous. The tongue becomes black and dry, voice faint, breathing short, feeble, and very anxious. The mental functions become greatly disordered, the patient is restless and fearful, his delirium is low-muttering, and he lies in a state of stupor from which he can be scarcely aroused. Often an irritating cough is present, coming on as if in convulsive paroxysms. In this stage of collapse the patient is disposed to lie on his back, with his feet drawn up, and there is a great tendency in his body to slide towards the foot of the bed. As the disease progresses, all the symp·toms of prostration increase. A convulsive motion of the tendons, as as in typhoid, is observed; his stupor becomes fixed; hiccough, involuntary discharges from the bowels, a cadaverous smell of the body, generally occur towards the close of the disease. Death, in violent cases, is generally preceded by extreme prostration, cold, clammy sweats, involuntary fecal discharges, and a discharge of grumous blood from the mouth, nose, and anus; or by convulsions.

This is a contagious disease, and emphatically one of poverty and low life.

TREATMENT.—Place the patient in a well-ventilated apartment, wash the body with soap and water, and give an emetic and cathartic, if the patient's condition requires it. Then give quinine in two or three grain doses every two or three hours, until its effects are observable. Control the fever with veratrum, as advised in typhoid cases. If great prostration is present, add capsicum or prickly-ash to the quinine, which should be continued in regular doses throughout the greater part of the course of the disease. A decoction of ladies'-slipper, or, preferably, cypripedin, in two or three grain doses every two hours, should be given in delirium or tendinous convulsions. Support the strength with iced-milk, chicken-broth, beef-tea, milk-punch, etc. The bladder should receive attention, and, if distended, should be evacuated by the influence of a sitz-bath, or by a catheter. In cases of cerebro-spinal congestions, make counter-irritations along the course of the spine, apply cold water to the head, and bottles of hot water to the feet. Convalescence is to be aided by the proper tonics, as golden-seal, columbo, etc., and complete repose should be allowed to the convalescent.

ERUPTIVE OR EXANTHEMATOUS FEVERS.

These are all characterized by fever and the usual constitutional disturbances, together with an eruption or exanthem distinguishing each variety. They owe their origin to animal or vegetable malaria, or both combined, and the peculiarities of this class are, that they, when once affecting the system, render the patient comparatively exempt from any future attack of the disease.

TYPHOID FEVER.

This is a very insidious disease, its commencement being scarcely perceptible. The patient has a sense of indisposition, but is unable to describe his condition. He feels slight debility, a dull and heavy feeling in the head, which increases and terminates in violent frontal headache. At full development of the disease, the limbs are weak, accompanied by lameness, and sometimes rheumatic pain. The bowels may at first be constipated, but in a few days the tendency is to diarrhœa. The pulse is quickened, a creeping, chilly sensation is felt, and the skin is dry and warm. The tongue is but slightly coated, and the appetite often remains until the disease is fully developed. After the full development, a number of small vesicles, called *sudaminæ*, may be observed on the abdomen. They are small, and may escape notice unless carefully observed. On the fifth day after the occurrence of these, another eruption occurs, which consists of small red or purple spots, resembling flea-bites. These spots are called *petechiæ*. If these are observed, the disease is unmistakably typhoid fever. When the abdomen is percussed, it yields a drum-like resonance, and a gurgling may be heard on the right side, a little below the navel. Nervous symptoms arise, frequently delirium, great pain in different parts of the body, stupor, and a buzzing noise in the head are often complained of. The tongue becomes red, and is protruded with much difficulty, pulse increases, eyes have a watery appearance, and remain partly open when asleep. The breathing becomes difficult, mouth half open, and a black substance (*sordes*) collects on the teeth. The urine becomes nearly suppressed, and has a dark-red appearance. The bowels bloat, and evacuations of frothy and watery excrement are frequent. If the disease is about to terminate unfavorably, the patient becomes stupid, with low, muttering delirium, his muscles jerk, hiccoughs, picks at bed-clothes, and labors under profound coma. The anatomical character of this disease is ulceration of certain glands, called *Peyerian*, of the intestines, which are sometimes perforated by the process, when, of course, death inevitably follows. The course of the disease is from 11 to 21 days.

TREATMENT.—If the disease is suspected, the patient should be placed in bed, and his bowels evacuated by warm-water injections, if costive. If indigestible food is contained in his stomach, an emetic of lobelia should be administered. Rice-gruel should then be given. The tincture of American Hellebore should, on the approach of the febrile paroxysm, be given until the pulse becomes less frequent, and perspiration ensues. Lye and slippery-elm poultices should be applied to the abdomen as long as bowel symptoms prove troublesome. Quinine and Hydrastin should be exhibited, with a view to overcome the periodicity of the fever. At the same time a cold infusion of marsh mallow, acacia, and flax-seed, should be taken. Apply cold water to the head, and keep the feet warm. Control the fever throughout its whole course with the veratrum or aconite. If the patient is restless and unable to sleep, give a little morphine in a decoction of Ladies'-slipper. If the diarrhœa is persistent, let the patient take a decoction of rhus and cranes-bill. When the red tongue is noticed, administer the spirits of turpentine, in from six to ten drop doses, three or four times a day. Beef-tea, brandy, etc., should be given to support the strength through the course of the disease. During convalescence care should be taken that the patient does not eat hearty food. Convalescence should be assisted by goldenseal and other tonics. The danger in the treatment of this disease is over-medication, and hence only such agents as are chemically called for should be given, and the patient's strength well supported throughout the course of the fever.

DIPHTHERIA.

Diphtheria is scarcely more than a modification of scarlet fever. The patient first complains of lassitude, headache, loss of appetite, has rigors and chills, active and quick pulse, a light furred tongue, redness of the back of mouth, enlargement of the glands about the neck, a hot, dry, and pungent skin, and in most cases an exudation upon the mucous surfaces of the upper air-passages. This soon becomes organized into a tough, white membrane, covering the soft palate and tonsils. These sometimes degenerate into ulcers. The breathing in consequence of this membrane becomes hurried and difficult, pulse quick, and frequently the asphyxia ensuing ends in death; it generally reigns as an epidemic and is regarded as contagious.

TREATMENT.—The first step in the treatment should be a thorough emetic and an active cathartic; free perspiration should be produced by aconite or veratrum, and the kidneys should be kept in vigorous

operation. Flannel cloths, wet with the compound tincture of capsicum, myrrh, and lobelia, should be applied to the neck, changed every
half hour, and applied as hot as the patient can bear it. Jugs of hot
water should be applied to the feet. The inflammation of the throat
should be subdued by a gargle of a hot decoction of golden-seal. If
the disease assumes an unfavorable aspect, give a powder containing
one grain of quinine, one-half grain of capsicum, and one grain of hydrastin every two hours. If the patches ulcerate, use a gargle of sumach and wild indigo. For the difficulty of breathing give sanguinaria
and lobelia in emetic doses for the purpose of dislodging the membrane.
The secretions should be increased even to ptyalism by irisin, the effect
of which will be to overcome the adhesiveness of the membrane. The
" Herbal Ointment " used for this purpose, and also to subdue the local
inflammation, acts specifically and should be used in all cases.

During convalescence the diet should be nutritious, and baths, fresh
air, and a liberal amount of fresh fruits ordered.

SMALL-POX (*Variola*).

The symptoms are divided into four periods. The period of invasion occupies about three days, and is marked by languor, lassitude, restlessness,
stretching, gaping, petulance, sullen mood ; these are followed by chills
and rigors. Towards evening the skin becomes hot and dry, pain attacks
the head, loss of appetite, nausea, and frequently lumbago. On the
third day, heat, fever, flushed face, headache, and in children sometimes convulsions. The period of eruption commences on the fourth day
(often on the third), with the appearance of a series of small red circular
points (papulæ). They do not rise above the surface then, but can be
seen in it, and felt by the finger. They are situated in the substance
of the skin, and roll about under the finger, the size that of a small pin's
head. These gradually enlarge, the patient in the mean time suffering
severely, until the period of suppuration arrives. The fever is now
great, the hands, feet, and face swell, and salivation is profuse and constant. There is hoarseness and pain, and the saliva emits a most disagreeable odor. Then comes the period of recovery. The pustules
scab, the fever and other unpleasant symptoms gradually disappear,
and, if all goes right, the danger is over from the twelfth to the fifteenth day after the eruption.

What is known as *confluent* small-pox is when the pustulus are very
numerous and running together ; and when all the symptoms are very
severe, the disease is known as *malignant*. Variola patients emit a
peculiar fetid odor, which is characteristic, and distinguishes it from
Varioloid.

TREATMENT.—An active purge should be given at the outset. For
this purpose a combination like the " Renovating Pills " should be

selected, as the catharsis produced is thorough and unattended with subsequent debility or costiveness. Diaphoretics should be given to promote early appearance of the eruption. The patient should be placed in a cool and well-ventilated room, and frequently sponged with tepid water. Not much treatment of a medicinal character is required. The fever should be controlled by aconite or veratrum, as in all active fevers. If complicated with pneumonia, pleurisy, etc., the treatment necessary is such as is advised in those diseases. Pitting to a great extent may be avoided by sweet-oil applied to hands and face.

Varioloid is but modified small-pox. It has all the essential characteristics of the disease except its virulence. The treatment is the same as advised for small pox.

The utility of vaccination is a mooted question. It has unquestionably done great harm, as in many cases scrofulous and syphilitic taints have been implanted. Aside from this, however, it has been the means of almost banishing the dreadful plague from existence, and its practice should be encouraged. Great care, however, should be exercised in the selection of the vaccine virus, so that its purity is unquestionably established before being used as an agent of prevention.

CHICKEN POX (*Varicella*).

This is a very mild eruptive disease, characterized by a slight fever of short duration, and followed by vesicles which desquamate about the fifth or sixth day. The fever is sometimes ushered in by slight rigors, though there is seldom any chill. There is often headache, and vomiting occasionally. The eruption appears in one or two days after the inauguration of the fever. It consists of red spots at first, which quickly become vesicular, and are frequently attended with itching.

TREATMENT.—Very little treatment is required, except in cases of feeble vitality, when the disease often assumes a severe character. In such cases the stomach and bowels should be well cleansed, the surface sponged with hot water, and the fever controlled with arterial sedatives. Tonics should be given if the patient is enfeebled. The diet should be nutritious, but composed of easily digested articles.

MEASLES (*Rubeola*).

This is an acute inflammation of the entire skin, of an infectious and contagious nature. It is ushered in with chills, followed by heat, drowsiness, pain in head, back, and limbs, sore throat, dry cough, and other symptoms common to febrile action, growing in violence until the fourth day. Then the eruption appears, producing heat and itching. The breaking out appears in patches of half-moon shape, which distinguishes this disease from the other eruptive diseases. They reach their height at the fifth day on the face and neck, and on the legs about the seventh

10*

day. Their decline is in the same order as appearance, disappearing about the tenth day, when the scarfskin peals off in the shape of scurf.

TREATMENT.—If the attack be a mild one, all the treatment necessary consists in light diet, acid and demulcent drinks, as flaxseed-tea decoction of slippery-elm, etc. Sponging with tepid water is very grateful to the sufferer in all cases. If during the first stage the eruption should be tardy in its coming, it should be hastened by a warm bath, and sweating drinks made from saffron, mullein, pennyroyal, summer savory, etc. If tardy on account of excessive fever, give tincture of green hellebore, ipecac, lobelia, snake-root, etc. In enfeebled constitutions stimulants are necessary.

SCARLET FEVER (*Scarlatina*).

Also a contagious disease. The eruption is in the shape of pimples of a scarlet hue, displayed in patches over the whole surface. The fever is usually more intense than in measles, and accompanied by sore throat, swollen face, and coated tongue. The greatest degree of redness is attained at the third or fourth day. The decline is the same as in measles. Scarlet fever is distinguished from other diseases by the swollen condition of the flesh, which spreads out the fingers peculiarly. The throat becomes ulcerated, and swallowing is attended with pain and difficulty. There is no cough, which also distinguishes it from measles.

The following will show the difference between scarlet fever and measles :—

In Scarlet Fever.	*In Measles.*
The eruption is bright scarlet.	The eruption is dark-red color.
It appears on the second day.	Does not appear till the fourth day.
Is quite smooth to the touch.	Is raised.
Is in small round spots.	Is larger and crescent-shaped.
Disappears on pressure.	Does not disappear.
The face is quite dry.	Face swelled ; running from the eyes and and nose.

TREATMENT.—This should be cooling in its nature, cooling drinks, sponging with cold water, etc. In ordinary cases little more is required, excepting a few drops of tincture of belladonna may be given several times per day. When high fever exists, give the remedies advised in measles. Hot foot-baths are advisable. As this is a prostrative disease, beef-tea and the ordinary stimulants should be given from the first. What is called malignant scarlet fever is only a severer form than the above. Gargles of sage and Cayenne pepper are used to allay the throat affections. The abscesses in the region of the ear, and consequent deafness, can be obviated by subduing the inflammation of that part by the usual methods.

NETTLE RASH.

This commences with fever, lasting two or three days; then itching
pimples, diversified in shape, appear, which go off during the day and
come again at night.   Teething causes it sometimes, while at other
times it is due to improper diet.

TREATMENT.—This is indicated by the cause.   If due to indigestible
food, the stomach must be unloaded by an emetic of blood-root or
ipecacuanha.   A lotion of vinegar and water is of service.   Tonics and
simple diet will complete the cure.

ERYSIPELAS.

This disease commences with languor, aching or soreness of the
limbs, chilliness, alternating with flushes of heat.   The pulse is quick,
skin hot, tongue foul, appetite gone, thirst, nausea sometimes; vomiting, headache, restlessness, sore throat, swelling and tenderness of
the glands of the neck, arm-pits, or groin, according to the seat of the
cutaneous inflammation.   The eruption usually makes its appearance,
about the third day of the fever, in the form of a small reddish spot,
somewhat elevated, painful or tender to the touch.   This occurs most
frequently upon the face, especially on the side of the nose, cheek, or
rim of the ear.   In some instances the inflammation advances slowly,
in others it spreads quickly over large portions of the body, accompanied by tumefaction, and a burning and stinging pain in all cases.
About the third day of the inflammation small blisters, filled with yellow serum, appear, which break about three days afterward.   On the
fifth or sixth day they begin to dry, and on the seventh or eighth form
crusts or scabs, which desquamate, and a new skin forms.   In phlegmonous erysipelas the inflammation involves not only the skin, but the subcutaneous tissues also, and the symptoms are all severer.   It often
assumes a very malignant type, and is then a disease of a most fatal
character.   It is liable to attack wounds; and those who are nursing
patients suffering with erysipelas should never wait upon a woman who
has been but recently confined, as she will be very liable to contract
puerperal peritonitis, a very fatal disease.

TREATMENT.—Give a lobelia emetic, a mild purge, and a hot bath
at the commencement.   In the mild form cover the inflamed patch
with collodion, and renew every two or three hours.   The emetic and
purge should be followed with quinine in two or three grain doses every
three hours.   The inflamed surface should also be washed with a decoction of the bark, or a solution of quinine.   Bruised cranberries are a
good application.   Cloths wrung out of a hot decoction of white-oak
bark and golden-seal should be applied to the inflamed part to prevent spreading.   In wounds apply lint saturated with compound tincture of myrrh and capsicum.   If the fever is violent, treat it as in all

other febrile cases. A nutritive diet should follow medical treatment as soon as the disease has passed its active career.

ROSE RASH (*Roseola*).

This is an eruptive disease of little importance. The febrile symptoms are slight, more or less attended with gastric derangement, which continues two or three days before the rash appears and subsides with it. The eruption generally commences upon the face, is of uniform redness, and causes itching or tingling. The rash continues from one to five days, and is followed by a slight scaling off of the skin. It is often the accompaniment of dentition and is not contagious.

TREATMENT.—Little more is necessary than a warm bath and a few drops of veratrum. If the eruption is troublesome, two or three drops of tincture of Belladonna should be added to a tumbler of water, and a teaspoonful given occasionally.

ERYTHEMA.

The eruption of this disease is of superficial redness, generally in irregular patches, slightly elevated, and attended with heat, tingling, and sometimes slight pain. It may be local or owing to constitutional disturbance. It may be caused by friction of contiguous surfaces, as in the groin and arm-pits, in fat infants, particularly when not frequently washed. When owing to constitutional causes, it usually appears on the face, breast or limbs. It lasts from a few days to a week or longer.

TREATMENT.—If the cause can be ascertained, it should be removed by the proper remedies. Anoint the affected part with a little lime-water and sweet-oil, or bathe with a strong decoction of golden-seal. Glycerine may also be applied, but if you can procure the "Herbal Ointment" (see page 472) I advise its application, as it is a specific for this and kindred affections.

GLANDERS.

This may be contracted from the horse, and is a very malignant disease. It is characterized by a purulent and sometimes bloody discharge from the nose, a peculiar pustular eruption, and by tumors in different parts of the body. Its initial stage is the same as in all eruptive fevers, attended with neuralgic pains in the limbs. In the course of four or five days the eruption makes its appearance in different parts of the body, usually most abundant upon the face and limbs. The discharge from the nose ensues in the course of a week or ten days, being at first yellowish, afterwards bloody, and very offensive. The body finally exhales a fetid odor, the mind wanders, delirium and coma follow, and by the end of the second week, or during the third, it generally proves fatal, if not arrested sooner in its course. It is fortunately very rare;

and attendants upon a horse affected with glanders should be very careful that they do not come in contact with the virus. The affected horse should be shot, as the disease is very seldom cured.

TREATMENT.—Support the strength of the patient, and stimulate the emunctories. This can be best achieved by a thorough alcoholic vapor bath, followed by an active lobelia emetic and a brisk cathartic. After this give quinine, three grains, and baptisin, two grains, every two or three hours, for a day or two. The nostrils should be syringed with warm water, to which a few drops of creosote has been added, three or four times a day. The throat may be gargled with the same preparation. Support the strength with chicken-broth, rice-gruel, cream, punch, porter, ale, etc. If this course is not effectual, repeat every three or four days.

DANDY FEVER (*Dengue*).

This disease occasionally prevails as an epidemic in the southern seacoast towns. There is pain, stiffness of the neck, back, and loins, and swelling of the muscles of the limbs and joints. Intolerance of light, restlessness, chilliness, fever, headache, a full and quick pulse, red eyes, a hot and dry skin, and an intense thirst prevail. The fever usually lasts from one to two days, when a gradual remission occurs, and the patient feels quite comfortable. After an interval of two or three days the fever returns, the pains are increased, the tongue is thickly coated, the stomach irritable, and the patient becomes dejected and fretful. Nausea is a prominent symptom, but seldom any vomiting occurs. About the sixth or seventh day an eruption, resembling scarlatina, appears, and gives relief to the distressing symptoms. It disappears after two or three days, the color of the skin gradually fading, with slight desquamation. The duration of the disease is about eight days. The causes are evidently miasmatic poison, in concert with epidemic influence.

TREATMENT.—Essentially the same as in scarlatina, accompanied with such remedies as advised in rheumatism. Quinine, in antiperiodic doses, should also be administered, and the anodynes should be given if the pains are severe. Tonics may be required in some cases; and in convalescence, frequent baths, a generous diet, and out-door exercises should be prescribed.

PURPURA.

This affection is characterized by a greater or lesser number of livid spots on the skin, from extravasated blood. In simple cases the effusion is confined to the skin and cellular tissues, mostly occurring on the arms, legs, and breasts. The spots at first are small, and resemble fleabites. The countenance is pale, and the patient complains of debility, loss of appetite, irregularity of the bowels, and periodic fever. If allowed to progress, it will assume a form known as *purpura hemorrhagica*, in which the spots are longer, and resemble whip-marks or violent bruises. They are bright red at first, but become purple or livid. A great variety of symptoms are presented by each case, and the disease is a very singular one.

TREATMENT.— In the simple form a very liberal diet of fresh vegetables, out-door exercise, and some simple tonic, are all that is necessary. In the hemorrhagic character, quinine, in one or two grain doses, should be given every three hours. Diet should consist of green vegetables, salt meats, eggs, and the free use of lemonade. A liniment of camphor, whiskey, and turpentine should be externally applied. If internal hemorrhage occurs, give oil of erigeron, in five-drop doses, every half hour; or matico, in from five to ten grain doses, may be administered every twenty minutes until it ceases.

ANATOMY OF THE ORGANS OF DIGESTION.

Mouth.—The mouth is separated from the nose by the hard and soft palate, and communicates. It is bounded in front by the lips, and its sides by the cheeks. The space between the lips and teeth is called the vestibule. The mouth is lined by a mucous membrane, which is covered by numerous glands, some being mucous and some salivary. The mouth contains a double row of teeth, thirty-two in the aggregate, performing the first process in digestion, the *mastication* of food.

Tongue.—The tongue is an oblong, flattened, muscular body, which varies in size and shape ; it is the organ of taste, and also of importance in speech and mastication. Its posterior extremity or root is attached to a bone, called the *hyoid*, by yellow fibrous tissue. Its anterior extremity is called the *tip ;* its intervening portion its *body.* The mucous covering of the tongue is very thick upon its upper surface, and very thin upon its under surface. Upon its upper surface are a number of projections, of various sizes and shapes, called *papillæ.* The largest are eight or nine in number, called *papillæ maximæ*, and are situated at the posterior portion of the tongue, in two convergent lines. The smallest papillæ are fine and pointed, and are found near the middle of the tongue, and are termed *filiform.* The intermediate papillæ are most abundant, some of which are *conical*, others *fungiform.* The tongue assists in the process of deglutition.

Palate.—The palate separates the back portion of the nose from the mouth, and is divided into two parts. The *hard palate*, of a bony base, covered by mucous membrane, which is continuous with that of the mouth ; the soft palate is the membranous separation between the back portion of the mouth and nose. From the middle the *uvula* projects, about three-quarters of an inch in length ; from each side of the uvula there are two divergent crescentic folds of mucous membrane, which are called *lateral half-arches;* the space between which constitutes the *fauces.*

Between the anterior and posterior arches of each side is the *tonsil gland.* The tonsils are about the size of an almond, and consist of a collection of large mucous follicles.

Salivary Glands.—The salivary glands are of light pink color, and their secretion is of great service in mastication and digestion. These are three in number — the parotid, submaxillary, and sublingual. The *parotid* is the largest; it lies on the side of the face in front of the ear, and beneath the skin. The submaxillary lies in a depression on the internal face of the lower jaw-bone. The *sublingual* is the smallest of the three; it is situated under the tongue.

Pharynx.—The pharynx is a muscular and membranous sac, communicating with the mouth, nose, œsophagus, larynx, and the tube (Eustachian) leading to the ear. Its length is about five inches, although this varies by extension and contraction. Its uses are for deglutition, respiration, and modulation of the voice.

Œsophagus.—This is the canal that conveys the food from the pharynx to the stomach. Its length is about nine or ten inches, and its diameter is not uniform, gradually increasing (as it descends). Its upper portion is the narrowest part of the alimentary canal; and hence foreign bodies which are too large to pass through the alimentary canal are generally arrested in the neck. It never contains air. Deglutition is performed by the contraction of the longitudinal fibres of the œsophagus, which shorten the passage, and by contraction of its circular fibres successively from above downward.

Stomach.—The stomach is a conoidal sac, somewhat bent or curved, and situated below the breast-bone or in the epigastric region. The left[3] extremity is much the larger, and terminates in a rounded sac; at the upper portions of this extremity is the *cardiac* orifice[2] where the œsophagus is

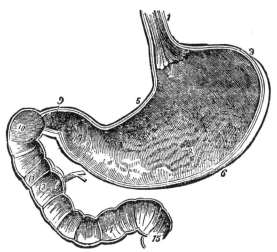

The Stomach.

continued into the stomach, immediately below the diaphragm. The right extremity is continuous with the intestines, and its orifice is called the *pyloric*. The structure of the pylorus is much thicker than that of any other portion. The stomach is held in its position by the œsophagus[1] and the duodenum,[10] as well as by reflexions of the peritoneum. The upper and lower curvatures of the stomach are called the greater and lesser cuvatures.[5][6] Near the pyloric extremity of the stomach is a small dilatation[7] called the *antrum pylori*. The dimensions of the stomach are variable, depending upon the mode of life. It has four coats; the peritoneal, muscular, cellular and mucous.

In the stomach the food receives the admixture of the gastric juice, which is the solvent agent of digestion. The fluids taken into the stomach are for the most part absorbed from it; the solids, with the exception of the insoluble parts, are by the action of the gastric juice reduced to a substance called *chyme*, which in general is grayish, semifluid, homogeneous, with a slightly acid taste and smell. The chyme is then poured into the duodenum through the pyloric orifice for the subsequent action of the intestines.

Intestines.—The intestinal canal is from thirty to thirty-five feet in length, and is divided into *large* and *small* intestines. The small intestine is four-fifths of the length of the whole canal, reaching from the pylorus to the large intestine; it is cylindrical, and about one inch in diameter; there is a gradual diminution in calibre as it descends. Its coats are the same as those of the stomach. The mucous coat is very vascular, and its absorbents are very numerous. The glands are the crypts or follicles of Lieberkühn, the glands of Peyer, the solitary glands, and Brunner's glands.

The small intestine is divided into duodenum, jejunum, and ileum.

The *Duodenum* commences at the pylorus, and is about twelve inches long. The common duct formed by the junction of the bile and gall ducts opens into it about four or five inches from the pylorus. The *Jejunum* (from jejunus, *empty*) constitutes the upper two-fifths of the small intestine, and the *ileum* the remaining three-fifths.

The large intestine reaches from the ileum to the anus, and is one-fifth in length of the whole canal; it differs much from the small intestine, and has a sacculated appearance. It likewise has four coats. It is divided into cæcum, colon, and rectum.

The *Cœcum* is a cul-de-sac or blind sac, and the commencement of the large intestine, and hence often called the *caput coli*. At the inferior portion is a worm-like process called *the appendix vermiformis*. On the side of the cæcum is the *ileo-cœcal* valve, an elliptical opening whereby the small intestine empties into the large.

The *Colon* is the largest portion of the large intestine; gradually diminishes in diameter until it terminates in the sigmoid or S-like flexure on the left side. It ascends on the right side, and forming an arch transversely, descends upon the left side. The *Rectum* is the terminating portion of the large intestine, and reaches from the sigmoid flexure to the *anus*. It is somewhat barrel-shaped, being larger in the middle than at either end.

DISEASES OF THE DIGESTIVE ORGANS.

STOMATITIS.

This is characterized by inflammation of the mouth. It may involve the whole membrane, or be confined to isolated portions. The first prominent symptom is a loss of taste, and a sensation similar to that produced by scalding liquids. The surface is red, very tender, and painful. The inflammation may extend to the fauces, nasal passages, and Eustachian tube. The stomach often becomes irritable, bowels loose, and the patient debilitated and emaciated. When caused by vitiated secretions, produced by the disturbed condition of the lymphatics while suckling, it is known as "*nursing sore-mouth*," or technically, *follicular stomatitis*. It may then extend to the stomach and bowels, causing ulceration, diarrhœa, dyspepsia, dysentery, and great prostration of the nervous system; and if not arrested, the mucous membranes of the air passages are involved, producing cough, expectoration, tuberculous degeneration and death. The teeth may fall out, and the gums be absorbed.

Aphthæ or Thrush is another form of stomatitis. It is generally characterized by small ulcers scattered over the surface, or in patches of white exudation, which may become thick and absorbed, and leave a raw-looking surface, or a foul spot. Children are very liable to it, and it is generally caused by acidity of the stomach, or general derangement of that organ by improper diet or unhealthy milk.

TREATMENT.—This depends upon the cause, which, if ascertained, should be removed. If due to carious teeth, they should be removed, and if owing to dyspepsia, the proper remedies should be given. The mouth should be frequently washed with a warm decoction of golden seal. The system should be supported with tonics, a generous diet, and a liberal use of fresh succulent vegetables, as grapes, etc., should be prescribed. Sage-tea gargles are very useful. The mother should also pay attention to her diet, so as not to supply the babe with improper milk. If due to acidity of the stomach, the necessary absorbents should be administered.

GLOSSITIS.

This is inflammation of the substance of the tongue, involving its muscular structure. It usually commences with a throbbing pain in the tongue, followed soon after with redness and swelling. In the course of a few hours the tongue enlarges so much as to fill the whole mouth, forces open the jaws, and protrudes from the mouth. Some fever usually accompanies it. Swallowing is usually almost impossible, speech gone, abscesses may form, and the tongue may even become mortified.

TREATMENT.—If due to a disordered state of the stomach, an active lobelia emetic should be given, and followed with an anti-bilious purge, like the Renovating Pill. If due to scalds or burns, the mouth should be washed with mucilage of flaxseed and slippery elm. If due to mercury, vapor baths should be taken, a free use of the syrup of stillingia resorted to, and equal parts of charcoal and yeast used as a gargle.

QUINSY (*Tonsillitis*).

This consists of inflammation of the tonsils, which may in many cases extend to the adjacent tissues. It usually commences with a slight chill, followed by much febrile excitement, uneasy feeling in the throat, and difficulty of swallowing, which increases in severity very rapidly, until at last deglutition becomes almost impossible. There is a constant disposition to swallow, in order to free the fauces from a tenacious, colorless mucus which adheres to that part. The respiration is not much affected unless in bad cases. From the commencement there is fever, severe headache, and a rapid pulse. The termination is usually an abscess, which at length opens, and a discharge of very fetid pus ensues, which affords relief. The duration of the disease is usually about a week, and is scarcely ever fatal.

TREATMENT.—Administer a free lobelia emetic, and anoint the throat thoroughly with the Herbal Ointment. In ordinary forms this will be sufficient. If an abscess, however, forms, it should be evacuated by an incision. In malarial districts, quinine in anti-periodic doses may be necessary, and if the fever is severe, veratrum should be given. The throat should be gargled with a decoction of golden seal, and to prevent termination into induration and permanent enlargement, alteratives should be given, especially in strumous habits.

PHARYNGITIS.

This is characterized either by acute, sub-acute, or chronic inflammation of the pharynx. There is slight pain upon pressure, or in the act of swallowing. It is seldom attended with fever, but in severe cases abscesses may form, causing great difficulty in swallowing and breathing. In the acute form the inflammation is usually limited to the mucous membrane, and simply constitutes an erythematic affection. The chronic form is known as " *clergyman's sore throat*," and is attended with a dry, hacking cough, hoarseness, and a sense of fatigue of the vocal organs after a slight exercise.

TREATMENT.—The treatment of simple pharyngitis is but little more than merely to regulate the stomach and bowels, the external application of cold packs, and a few days' rest. In the chronic form an invigorating and tonic course of treatment should be pursued, in connection with rest, baths, and pure air. To relieve the local difficulty, one grain of stillingia may be mixed with a drachm of sugar, divided into ten powders, of which one should be taken every two hours. The inhalation of hot vapor from bitter herbs is to be recommended. Blood-root in connection with constitutional treatment is highly beneficial. Patients will find that my "Acacian Balsam" in the chronic form is a virtual specific; the Herbal Ointment should also be outwardly applied. If owing to a complicated constitutional disorder, or if it exists in association with catarrh, it constitutes an affection requiring the most skilful treatment, and those who may wish my advice in such cases may refer to page 590 for general directions for consultation.

PAROTITIS (*Mumps*).

Mumps is an inflammatory affection of the salivary glands, especially the parotids. It generally commences with slight fever, stiffness of the jaws, and a slight pain or swelling in one or both parotid glands. The parts are hot, painful, and very tender upon pressure. Mastication and swallowing become painful, which causes considerable nervous irritability. Metastasis to the breasts of the female and to testicles of the male is liable to occur, especially if the patient is subjected to undue exposure. Inflammation of the brain may occur in some cases. It reaches its height in about four days, disappearing entirely about the seventh.

TREATMENT.—Keep the patient quiet, and give a mild purge. For external application a liniment of goose-fat and camphor is very beneficial. If there be much fever, resort to the usual anti-febrile treatment. If inflammation of the brain should ensue, resort to active cathartics, and give small doses of macrotin and quinine. The "Herbal Ointment" will be found a superior remedy, see page 472

ŒSOPHAGITIS.

This is an inflammation of the œsophagus, or that portion of the alimentary canal which conveys the food from the pharynx to the stomach. Heat and pain, increased by swallowing, at some point along the tube, are the earliest symptoms. Occasionally there is pain between the shoulders, and, perhaps, tenderness on pressure, with more or less difficulty in swallowing. Hiccough, an eructation of glairy mucus, and vomiting, are sometimes present. There is also more or less constitutional disturbance. Ulcers and abscesses may form. It may become chronic, and stricture of the canal at any part of its passage may result,

which may so effectually prevent deglutition as to cause death by
starvation.

TREATMENT.—In the acute form, the stomach should be cleansed by
a lobelia emetic, and the bowels opened by a purge. The surface
should be sponged with hot water, and sufficient tincture of veratrum
given to maintain a gentle diaphoresis. In the chronic form the alteratives are to be administered, and the bowels occasionally purged. The
patient should be confined mostly to a vegetable diet of fluid character.
Frequent sips from a decoction of golden seal and slippery elm should
be taken. Stricture of the œsophagus should only be treated by a
competent physician, as the means employed for its cure might do more
harm in improper hands than any possible good.

INFLAMMATION OF THE STOMACH (*Gastritis*).

This usually commences in the acute form with violent vomiting and
a burning pain in the region of the stomach. Swallowing becomes difficult, thirst is intense, tongue is dry and smooth, headache often violent,
delirium and prostration are present. If the stomach only is inflamed,
there is constipation; but if the bowels also are affected, there is
diarrhœa. The attendant fever is as common, and the disease may
assume such a gravity that death inevitably ensues, especially in perforation of the stomach. Chronic gastritis is a common disorder. It is
generally of a mild character, unless of long continuance, when it may
occasion considerable organic disorder. Its approach is gradual, presenting a variety of symptoms, but may be known from dyspepsia in there
being more pain at some particular point, and more frequent vomiting
after taking food.

TREATMENT.—Give an emetic, and cleanse the stomach by means of
large draughts of warm water. Counter-irritation should be resorted to
over the stomach. The vomiting may be checked by opium, and the
tincture of crawley may be given to control the fever. If produced by
a corrosive poison, the necessary antidotes will, of course, be required.
All solid foods should be withheld, and the drinks should be mucilaginous, as marshmallow, slippery elm, gum-water, etc.

The treatment of chronic gastritis is not so easily stated. It depends
greatly upon associated conditions and complications. Diet is an important element in the treatment. My " Restorative Assimilant" internally,
and " Herbal Ointment" externally, generally cure each case; but
some cases are of such a serious character that a cure can only be
effected by special symptomatic treatment. Those desiring to consult
me are referred to questions, page 390.

CANCER OF THE STOMACH.

The early symptoms of cancer of the stomach are usually similar to
chronic gastritis. The appetite is impaired, and frequent nausea and

vomiting supervene. The pain in the stomach is of a lancinating character. The gastric functions are impaired, and the mucous discharges become sour and purulent, finally bloody, and if subjected to microscopical examination, cancer cells are found. The complexion has a yellowish-white, waxen appearance, which distinguishes cancer from other diseases of the stomach.

TREATMENT.—The treatment consists chiefly in combating the symptoms as they occur. Cundurango should be given a fair trial in all cases. If the disease has reached a certain stage, no remedy will produce a radical impression; but I have the assurance that I have cured many cases of well-defined cancer of the stomach, in more or less advanced stages of the disease, by the employment of consistent and energetic chemical treatment.

HEART-BURN (*Gastralgia*).

Two forms of heart-burn are commonly observed: one, attended by acid eructations, causing irritation of the throat and fauces; and in the other, the ejections from the stomach are rancid and alkaline, and connected with a gnawing pain and distention of the stomach. It principally occurs during digestion, and may be of every grade of severity. It is caused by excess of acid, or an accumulation of gas, in the stomach.

TREATMENT.—This depends upon the cause. If acid, administer pulverized charcoal, with a little magnesia, or, what is just as good, compound spirits of lavender. If alkaline, give lemon-juice as often as required.

GASTRALGIA, OR GASTRODYNIA.

This is a neuralgic affection of the stomach, and is often a symptom of dyspepsia. The appetite is generally impaired, though sometimes remains good. There is a gnawing pain in the stomach, and a strong disposition to vomit. The tongue is usually foul, the skin cool, and pulse quite disturbed.

TREATMENT.—If owing to long-continued use of indigestible or improper food, abandon it, and change to other articles. Take quinine, and a little cherry laurel water, to subdue the neuralgic affection, and tonics to restore the tonicity of the stomach.

SPASM OF THE STOMACH.

This consists of a sense of pain, stricture, or contraction, occurring in paroxysms. The stomach feels as if rolled into a ball, or drawn towards the back. It assumes different degrees of violence, being often exceedingly painful.

TREATMENT.—It is instantly relieved by a dose of some preparation of wild gum, in combination with a fourth of a grain of gelsemin. External application of the "Herbal Ointment" acts equally as specifically.

WATER-BRASH (*Pyrosis*).

This also occurs generally in paroxysms. The pain is intense, and of a burning character. An eructation of a thin, insipid, watery liquid occurs, and, when discharged, affords momentary relief.

TREATMENT.—Quinine and the general tonics will remove this difficulty. Certain habits, as inebriety, anxiety of mind, etc., are to be overcome, and a generous diet indulged in.

DYSPEPSIA, OR INDIGESTION.

This is one of the most common affections in the whole catalogue of diseases. Scarcely a human being lives that has not or will not be a victim to this harassing disease. In simple indigestion, the symptoms vary much in nature and severity. One may suffer severely, while another has merely slight depression of spirits. Loss of appetite, nausea, vomiting, constipation alternating with diarrhœa, furred tongue, foulness of breath, palpitation of the heart, pains in various parts, dull headache, hypochondriasis, etc., are present in all cases. The patient's appetite may at one time be wholly lost; at other times it is morbid and ravenous, which, if indulged in, will only add to his misery. There is seldom any healthy feeling of hunger, but, in place of this, the patient has a most miserable sensation of hollowness or sinking at the region of the stomach. Nausea and vomiting are the most distressing symptoms of dyspepsia; the former may occur soon after the food is swallowed, or it may be deferred for an hour or two. The matter ejected is most frequently sour, and mixed with bile, often having the flavor of rotten eggs, which is due to a gas known as sulphuretted hydrogen. This gas, in ascending, often brings the solid food into the throat and mouth, making the patient almost a ruminant animal. Suffering is experienced when the stomach is full or empty, though it differs in various cases. Sometimes not much uneasiness is felt until several hours after eating, when all its attendant horrors are manifested. This is due to fermentation of the food. Water-brash, gastralgia, spasm of the stomach, etc., are constant companions of the dyspeptic, and his days are most miserably spent, while his nights are not much better, because his sleep is not refreshing; the body is not reposed, and he is the frequent victim of horrible nightmares. A dyspeptic patient suffers from every variety of indisposition, and it is easy to learn from his dejected countenance and woe-begone look that he yearns for that comfortable human existence that only a healthy digestive apparatus affords to man. He is fretful and peevish, dissatisfied with others and with himself; has individually no comfort, and allows but little to those around him; everything that was formerly bright and cheerful now bears a gloomy aspect; his smiles are derisive, his opinions cynical; and everything that is bright, cheerful, and lovable has gone with the enjoyment of good health. The disease is in fact a malady that embraces in its symptoms and consequences nearly every physical and mental torture known to mankind.

TREATMENT.—When it arises from inertia of the stomach, it may be removed by stomachics. If produced by bad habits, it can only be corrected by strict adherence to the physiological laws controlling the digestive functions. When it occurs from softening of the mucous membranes and a deficiency of the gastric secretion, alnuin is a good remedy; and chelonin acts well in chronic inflammation of the organ. When dependent upon nervous debility, herbal phosphorus and cyprepedin act well. Constipation should be relieved by leptandrin and similar cathartics. Diet and hygiene form a very important part in the treatment, and these should receive very careful attention. Fresh air, baths, friction, out-door exercise, careful avoidance of overloading the stomach, are indispensable adjuncts to all treatment. It is but just to myself, and eminently due to my readers, to acquaint them with my mode of treating dyspepsia, and which, I confidently assert, is attended with as specific results as can be expected from any medicinal agents. It is my sincere belief that failure is impossible if the remedies are taken faithfully, for a reasonable length of time. I advise in all cases and in all forms of the disease, my "Restorative Assimilant," "Renovating Pills," and "Herbal Ointment." The Assimilant is taken internally, in prescribed doses, three times a day; the pills are taken as occasion requires, to keep bowels regular, and the Herbal Ointment is rubbed externally, once or twice a day, over the region of the stomach and bowels. The philosophy of this treatment is obvious; the Assimilant restores the tonicity of the digestive organs, increases secretion of gastric juice, promotes chymification, stimulates the accessory organs of digestion, and, by its assimilative properties, increases the functional action of the absorbents, and restores the chemical process of digestion to its healthy state. The pills increase the peristaltic motion of the bowels, augment biliary discharges, stimulate the mesenteric glands, while, at the same time, they give tonic power to the whole alimentary canal. The ointment, by its discutient properties, removes all inflammation, localizes healthy blood to the organs and tissues, and prevents centralization of morbific agents.

These remedies at once assert their value, and gain complete mastery over the disease in a short time; and should any of my dyspeptic readers, though faithless in medicinal relief from repeated failures, be pleased to give them a trial, the author is confident that the medicines will cure them and restore them to vigorous health, so that they may once more enjoy the boon of healthy digestive organs. (See page 469.)

ANATOMY OF THE LIVER.

The liver is the largest glandular organ in the body; its office is to secrete bile. It is oblong and oval in shape, and occupies the position on the right side, under the lower ribs. It weighs from four to five pounds; it measures from ten to twelve inches transversely, and from six to seven antero-posteriorly; its greatest thickness is from four to five inches. On the upper surface it is convex, and on the lower concave. Its *color* is of a reddish-brown, with occasional spots of black.

The under surface of the liver presents a deep fissure, called umbilical or longitudinal, reaching from the anterior[16] to the posterior[17] notch,

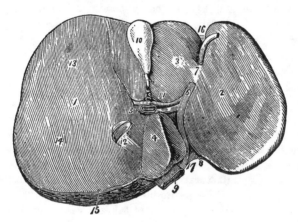

containing the remains of the umbilical vein of foetal life. Sometimes this fissure is converted into a foramen,[7] or opening, the right and left lobes being connected. At right angles to this fissure is another, called the *transverse*[11] fissure, containing the portal vein, hepatic artery, and hepatic duct, bound together by the *capsule of Glisson*, a membrane of cellular tissue. The *gall-bladder*[10] lies in a deep depression upon the under surface of the right lobe of the liver. The *lobulus quadratus*[3] is that portion of the liver included between the depression occupied by the gall-bladder and the longitudinal and transverse fissures. At the posterior and inferior portion of the liver is a triangular lobe called the *lobulus Spigelii*.[4] The elongated ridge running from the lobulus Spigelii outwardly is the *lobulus caudatus*.[5] These lobules are, however, all contained in the two lobes of the liver. The *right lobe*[1] is the largest and thickest, and the *left*[2] terminates in a thin cutting edge. The *structure* of the liver may be seen by tearing the liver of any animal. This will show a granulated arrangement, and each of these granules is usually called an *acinus*. These acini consist of a terminal branch of the portal vein and hepatic artery, together with the incipient radicles of the hepatic duct and hepatic vein, and in the capillary network thus constituted are numerous cells, which secrete the bile.

The liver is liable to a variety of disorders, and, when affected, exerts a marked influence on the organs and tissues of the body. The functions of the organ are so important that impairment arising from any organic cause quickly disturbs the harmony and health of the whole economy. Its office is to eliminate the superfluous carbon from the blood. This carbon enters into chemical combination with other substances, forming the compound known as bile, and which is poured into the duodenum, or upper bowel, where it assists greatly in the process of digestion.

DISEASES OF THE LIVER.

HEPATITIS.

Inflammation may be confined to its outside covering, or involve the entire substance of the liver. It usually makes its appearance with sympathetic fever, pain, a sense of tension on the right side, inability to lie on the left side, difficulty of breathing, a dry cough, vomiting, and a troublesome cough. As the morbid action increases, high fever, with hot skin, thirst, and scanty urine is observed. The pain is acute and lancinating, and is apt to run up to the right collar-bone, and to the top of the shoulder. The pain is increased by coughing, breathing, and lying on the left side. A soreness is felt by pressing over the liver, and usually, when enlarged, is readily recognized by the touch. The pulse is full and hard, bowels costive, stools clay-colored, and the tongue is covered with a dark-brown, or even black coat, and there is a bitter taste in the mouth.

TREATMENT.—Evacuate the stomach and bowels, and apply hot packs, rubefacients, or even vesicants in some cases, to the region of the liver. The purges should be such that will thoroughly evacuate the bowels with watery discharges, as jalap, elaterium, etc. Promote perspiration by a spirit vapor bath, or by American hellebore, or other diaphoretics. When the urine is red and scanty, an infusion of marshmallow, pumpkin-seeds, or trailing arbutus should be given. Quinine, gelsemin, and irisin may be necessary in some cases.

CHRONIC HEPATITIS.

Chronic inflammation of the liver usually involves the entire organ, and may be the result of the acute form, although it exists independently of it. It is a disease very common in the South and West, and is evidently owing to malarial poison, in connection with heat and atmospheric vicissitudes. It is a very insidious disease, and the whole organ may assume a pathological condition before attracting any special attention. The most common symptoms are a disordered stomach, occasional vomiting, a sense of fulness and weight in the right side, ir

11

regular bowels, pains in one or both shoulders, unhealthy stools, yellowness of skin, eyes, and urine, a short dry cough, disturbed appetite, febrile exacerbations towards night, and general emaciation. The patient is generally despondent, his temper is irritable and peevish, and he is frequently the prey to the dread of some impending evil. The exercise of his mental faculties is often impossible in a literary or argumentative direction, and the loss of the cherished attribute of manhood is most frequently added to his misery. If the patient be a female, sexual congress becomes to her a revolting union, and her husband's approaches create in her only a feeling of disgust and scorn.

TREATMENT.—The diet should be regulated, outdoor exercise should be taken, baths liberally used, and chafing liniments applied over the liver; keep the bowels open with leptandrin, or decoction of the plant, and give one-tenth of a grain of gelsemin with two grains of quinine, every three or four hours, until about twenty doses have been taken. This may be followed by dandelion and blackroot in small doses four or five times a day. An alterative like irisin may also be given. I also most strongly advise my "Restorative Assimilant," "Herbal Ointment," and "Renovating Pills;" to be used about the same as ordered in dyspepsia. The pills, especially, exercise specific control over morbid conditions of the liver, and frequently cure the disease, unaided by other remedies.

It is frequently the case that chronic inflammation of the liver is so complicated that it will not respond to any ordinary treatment. In such cases a careful analysis of the symptoms and general condition of the patient must be made, and the treatment so modified and varied as to suit all the conditions of the case. In these cases it is difficult to designate the required treatment, as each individual case is characterized by its own pathological phenomena, and requires essentially particular treatment. My success in the treatment of these stubborn cases has exceeded even my own anticipations in many instances, and I now like to combat the "bilious" foe with my herbal weapons — and the laurels generally rest on my brow. Those who wish to consult me are referred to page 390.

CIRRHOSIS.

The result of chronic inflammation of the areolar tissue of the entire organ is often induration or cirrhosis of the liver. The tissues become so firm, and ultimately so constricted, as to diminish the caliber of the portal vein, hepatic artery, and duct, resulting in the wasting away or atrophy of the lobular structure, and the hepatic cells become studded with fat. This condition sadly interferes with the circulation of the blood through the portal vein, producing inflammation of gastric and intestinal linings. It is the *hob-nailed* liver of some writers. The usual symptoms are constipation, a dry skin, high-colored urine, fickle appetite, and derangement of the nervous system. The spleen often becomes enlarged, while the liver diminishes in size, the pain becomes more intense, and frequently the kidneys are also involved. Digestion is feeble, chills, hectic fever, and night-sweats are often present, and frequently a dropsical condition of the lower limbs and abdomen is observed.

TREATMENT.—All alcoholic stimulants should be avoided, and the action of the liver aroused by prickly ash, leptandrin, dandelion, emetics, etc. The tonics should be given, and Indian hemp should be administered in sufficient quantities to maintain a gentle influence upon the bowels and kidneys The alteratives, if indicated, should be exhibited, and continued as long as required.

This disease is certainly an unfavorable one for treatment in its advanced stages, but my treatment in well-defined cases has been attended with the most favorable results, and I hope ere long that the result of my investigations into the morbid character of the disease in all its phases, that I have made for many years, will enable me to still more rob the disease of its formidable nature.

GALL-STONES.

These concretions are generally oval or pear-shaped, and formed in the gall-bladder or hepatic ducts. They vary in size, from that of a small pea to a fowl's egg, and in chemical composition present cholesterine, coloring matter, and the salts of lime, magnesia, etc. They occur oftener in females than in males, from the fact that their inactive life is more conducive to their formation. They give rise to a dull, heavy pain in the region of the liver, and more or less febrile excitement. In their passage through the duct they cause the most excruciating pain, which is accordingly intensified in proportion to the size of the stone. Impaction of the cystic duct, with complete obstruction and inflammation, ulceration, and perforation of the duct and bladder may occur, giving rise to great difficulties.

TREATMENT.—To reduce the spasm, Dover's powder, or other anodynes, should be given, and hot packs or fomentations should be applied externally. A vapor bath and lobelia emetic often afford great relief. Belladonna plasters should be applied over the region of the liver, as they dilate the cystic duct, and alleviate the pains. Thoroughwort is a good remedy, and should be freely taken. If the stones can be found in the alvine discharges, their chemical character should be definitely ascertained, and the proper chemical treatment resorted to in order to prevent their re-formation. Those who may desire my services in this respect can forward to me the stones, and on receipt I will carefully analyze them, and suggest the proper treatment.

JAUNDICE (*Icterus*).

The most prominent symptoms are yellowness of the skin, eyes, and urine, owing to the deposit of the coloring matter of the bile in the blood. The appetite is impaired, the food is loathed, an uncomfortable feeling of a load at the pit of the stomach is felt. The stomach is sour, sometimes there is sickness and .vomiting, a bitter taste in the mouth, a dull pain at the right side, sleepiness, and an uncomfortable feeling of lassitude at all times distresses the patient. The urine is heavily tinged with bile, and the stools clay colored. It is usually idiopathic, but may be a concomitant of other diseases. Torpidity of the liver is the chief cause, yet any functional disorder of the organs may cause it.

TREATMENT.—If caused by inactivity of the liver, the organ should be aroused by a lobelia emetic and active antibilious purges. I can certainly advise no better cathartic for this purpose than my Renovating Pill. The liver should be further stimulated to,action by the application of an irritating plaster over the region of the liver. Tonics, like quinine, poplar, and liriodendron, may be necessary in some cases. The diet should consist of fresh vegetables, and as much out-door exercise should be taken as the patient can bear.

The liver is the seat of many other diseases, but as they are more or less rare, of difficult detection, and treatment difficult, I deemed it prudent not to enter upon any consideration of them. The organ may hypertrophy or atrophy, its blood-vessels may become diseased, it may be affected by syphilitic taint, it may become fatty, it may degenerate into a waxy or albuminous mass ; disease may change it into a pigment or nutmeg liver ; it may be the seat of hydatids or parasites, tumors or cancer may assail it, and finally it may be the seat of tuberculous matter of a miliary character. The symptoms produced by these morbid conditions are so obscure, and many of them the common property of all, that none but a skilful physician is capable of recognizing the identity of the affection ; and I advise all patients who are suffering from any liver disease that presents phenomena, not recognizable in the simpler affections of the organ, to intrust his case to a competent physician.

I have devoted nearly a lifetime to the study of liver diseases, and I am ready to maintain that my success in their treatment is greater than by any other system of medication. I am daily consulted with reference to some chronic disease of the liver, both in person or by letter, and patients under treatment are scattered in all sections of the country. Constant communication by correspondence enables me to treat such cases as satisfactorily as by personal interview, as is attested by the gratifying success achieved in all cases. (See page 390.)

ANATOMY OF THE SPLEEN.

The organ [213], occupying the right of the following cut, is the spleen. It is a soft vascular organ, of a purplish color. It is not a true gland, as it has no duct.

The shape of the spleen is irregular and variable, but it is generally the section of an ovoid, with a convex surface resting against the dia-

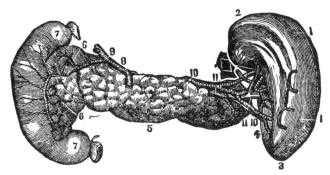

Spleen and Pancreas.

phragm, opposite the ninth, tenth, and eleventh ribs, and a convex surface directed towards the stomach.

It varies in size more than any other organ in the body. It is generally five inches long and three wide, and weighs from five to seven ounces. The proper substance of the spleen is a soft, pulpy mass, of a reddish-brown color, resembling grumous blood. Its office in the economy is not well understood, but· is evidently concerned in the blood-depurating process. It is numerously supplied with lymphatics. The long and flat gland lying between the spleen and duodenum, in the left of the cut, is the *Pancreas*, or *sweet-bread*. It is of a light-pink color, and is about seven inches long. Its right extremity [6], or *head* is much the thickest part, and is often called the *lesser pancreas*. Its left extremity gradually diminishes in breadth until it touches the spleen [8][9][10]. The superior edge has a groove for the passage of the splenic artery. Its structure is conglomerate. Its excretory duct is called the *duct of Wirsungius*.

Its secretion is somewhat similar to saliva, hence it is often called the *abdominal* salivary gland. Its secretion contains a larger amount of solid matter than the saliva, and assists in the process of digestion.

SPLENITIS.

The functions of the spleen have formerly been the cause of much controversy, nor are they better understood at the present day ; but the organ is evidently concerned somewhat in the blood-making process but that it performs a very important part is doubtful, as the whole organ has been removed without affecting the health in the least. In some countries, the practice of removing the spleen in pigs, for the purpose of facilitating the fattening practice, has been resorted to, which fact has suggested to some over-confident analogists the propriety of removing the spleen in the human subject as a remedy for debility.

Splenitis prevails most in malarious districts, and is a frequent result of chills and fever. A feeling of weight, tightness, sometimes pain in the left side, which is increased by pressure, or an attempt to lie on the left side, are the earliest symptoms. The organ enlarges—sometimes so much that it can readily be felt by the hand. It is known by the name of "ague-cake," and causes numbness and weakness of the legs, difficulty of breathing, palpitation of the heart, obstinate constipation, vomiting of food, piles, dry skin, and occasionally dropsical affections.

TREATMENT.—This does not differ much with the treatment advised for acute and chronic inflammation of the liver. Quinine, in combination with leptandrin and irisin, is indicated in all cases. Counter-irritation should also be made over the splenic region, and, when complicated with dropsy, the required directions should be administered. My "Restorative Assimilant," "Herbal Ointment," and "Renovating Pills" cure every case, if taken for a reasonable length of time.

The spleen may also be affected with dropsy, or become studded with tuberculous matter. In such events the treatment is the same as for dropsy and tubercular depositions of any other internal organ.

DISEASES OF THE PANCREAS.

The pancreas is rarely the seat of disease. The symptoms of its morbid conditions are usually obscure. It may be affected by inflammation, passive or acute. In typhoid, typhus, and puerperal fevers, it occasionally becomes involved in inflammation. The symptoms of disease of this gland are usually pain in the epigastrium, enlargement and tenderness, a sensation of heat and constriction, salivation, nausea and vomiting, diarrhœa, loss of appetite, despondency, chills, alternated with flushes of heat, and debility, with great emaciation. The vomiting in some instances is very obstinate ; the matters ejected are thin, ropy, and of a sour or saltish taste. Jaundice is often observed.

TREATMENT.—Control the disease by equalizing the circulation with hot packs, veratrum, aconite, mild purges, etc. In the chronic form, administer mandrake, blue flag, and poke-root, as these remedies are known to increase the functions of this gland. Lobelia and capsicum, in some cases of chronic congestion and inflammation, act with decided benefit. In all diseases of this gland it would be well, however, to intrust the treatment to a competent herbal physician.

DISEASES OF THE BOWELS.

The intestinal tube is very seldom affected throughout its whole extent, but inflammation may involve any portion of it at one time. If the duodenum is affected it is called *Duodenitis*, if the cæcum or blind gut is inflamed, it receives the name of *Typhilitis*, if it involves the small intestine, it is called *Enteritis*. These diseases are very rare, however, and their consideration as separate affections is of not much importance, except to the nosologist. The treatment is upon general principles and corresponds withthat given in all inflammatory affections of the intestinal mucous membrane. Dysentery is a typical case of enteric inflammation, hence we will commence with the consideration of it.

DYSENTERY (*Colitis*).

This is also known as bloody flux, and consists of an inflammation of the membrane of the colon and rectum, and characterized by small mucous or bloody evacuations, griping, and straining. The disease comes on with loss of appetite, costiveness, lassitude, shivering, heat of skin and quick pulse. These are followed by griping pain in the bowels and a constant desire to go to stool. The passages are mostly small in quantity, and composed of mucus mixed with blood. These passages are attended with severe griping and straining, technically known as *tormina* and *tenesmus*. Nausea and vomiting sometimes attend the early stages. When the natural fæces pass off, they are usually formed in round compact balls, called *scybala*. Fever is commonly present, with a feeble, almost thread-like pulse. The discharges have but little odor at first, but become exceedingly offensive as the disease advances. The chronic form is characterized by frequent small evacuations, consisting mostly of mucus, but sometimes mixed with pus, bile, fæces and blood. The symptoms are the same, but less intense than in the acute form. Emaciation, debility, dropsy, and consumption result, if not arrested. When the liver and stomach become disordered at the commencement, it is called *bilious* dysentery. Various forms of the disease are known as adynamic, intermittent and remittent, typhous, rheumatic and epidemic dysentery ; but it is not necessary to classify the disease under these heads.

TREATMENT.—A free lobelia emetic may be given at the outset, and the bowels evacuated by a purge ; castor-oil with laudanum is the best for this purpose. After the purge, take twenty grains of quinine and one drachm of leptandrin, divide into six powders and take one every hour until all are taken. The tenesmus should be relieved by injecting into the rectum five or six ounces of starch water, containing about twenty drops of laudanum, as often as is necessary. Ipecacuanha is a superior remedy. Gelsemin may be given afterwards, and if required the fever should be controlled by veratrum. The patient should lie quietly in bed, and his diet should consist of grapes, baked apples, flour porridge, bread, rice, coffee, beef-tea and ripe fruit. The astringents are of course necessary, and for this purpose tannic and gallic acids, kino, rhatany, opium, capsicum, cranesbill, etc., can be given. Tonics should be combined when the patient is weak, and if the debility is very great the alcoholic stimulants should be administered. I can with safety recommend my "Restorative Assimilant" as a sure cure for both acute and chronic dysentery, as well as for all bowel complaints. The Herbal Ointment should be rubbed externally on the whole abdomen to relieve the inflammation. In the chronic form, the astringents, with such other remedies as may be indicated by the symptoms, are all that is necessary.

DIARRHŒA.

This common disorder is characterized by frequent and urgent demands to evacuate the bowels. It is usually preceded by a sense of indigestion, fulness of stomach, flatulency, and more or less colic pains. The pain generally subsides after an evacuation, and returns as an indication of another discharge. The discharges may be thick, consisting of ingesta, or they may be serous, or of a rice-water appearance. Sometimes they consist of disintegrated mucous membranes, blood, and bile. There is usually a disagreeable sinking sensation in the abdomen along with the discharge, with exhaustion, a cool skin, and a feeble irregular pulse. It may be attended with fever, indicating extensive irritation of the mucous coat. The urine is usually scanty. When the discharges are composed of serum, and highly colored with either yellow or green bile, it is called *bilious* diarrhœa; when composed principally of mucus, it is known as *mucous* diarrhœa, and when of a thin, watery character, the name of *serous* diarrhœa is given to it. The disease may become chronic.

TREATMENT.—If it occurs in children, a little paregoric, or essence of peppermint or spearmint, usually cures in a short time. Opium in combination with ipecac, as in the Dover's powder, is an excellent remedy. The astringents are all indicated. Starch injections, as advised in dysentery, should also be resorted to, and counter-irritation of the abdomen is also serviceable. In the chronic form the tonics should be combined with the astringents. I cannot recommend my "Restorative Assimilant" (see page 469) too strongly. It is certainly an admirable remedy for this complaint, relieving it most instantly.

Chronic diarrhœa may often be so dependent upon a vitiated condition of the system that it becomes quite difficult to cure. In such cases the most careful treatment is necessary to overcome the disease. During the war, and also afterwards, the author was consulted for this affection by those who contracted it in the army in thousands of cases; but under proper treatment all recovered.

CONSTIPATION.

By this is understood a collection of excrementitious matters in some part of the intestinal tube. It is marked by unfrequency of stool, and by the recurrence of fulness and tension in parts of the abdomen. It occurs in patients of a lax and weak habit of body, or it may arise from rigidity of the muscles. It may also be due to imperfect functional action of the stomach, liver, pancreas, etc., in which case the intellectual faculties are dull, the complexion is sallow, the skin dry, urine scanty, acidity of the stomach, and headache. Sometimes the accumulation of fæcal matter is so great that the masses can be felt through the abdominal walls. It is frequently caused by an atonic condition of the muscular structure of the intestines, and in very many cases it results from neglect to attend to the calls of nature. These calls should be imperative, and whenever the desire arises they should not be disregarded, but obeyed as quickly as opportunity allows. I once knew a sea-captain who only evacuated his bowels when in port, and who remarked to me that when he " battened down the hatches of his vessel, he also battened down the hatches of his body, and no matter how long the voyages, no stools are made." The consequences were, that whenever he came to port he had a hard time to be relieved of his fæcal accumulations. In many other cases no movement of the bowels was observed for ten or twelve weeks. Constipation is attended with various sympathetic affections, and finally deranges the blood, impairs the health, tone, and vigor of the whole system. It is frequently the cause of piles, strangury, dysmenorrhœa, amenorrhœa, leucorrhœa, apoplexy, epilepsy, dyspepsia, insanity, etc.

TREATMENT.—The cause of the difficulty should be carefully studied, and the proper treatment resorted to. The diet should be composed of laxative articles of food, as fresh fruits, unbolted-flour bread, etc. If dependent upon a lax state of the muscular fibres, golden seal, in combination with mandrake and blackroot are the proper remedies, and when due to vitiated secretions of the stomach, liver, etc., the American Columbo should be given. In atony of the bowels, nux vomica should be carefully administered with the cathartics. Cathartics and enemas are of course indicated for present relief in all cases, and those should be selected which operate sufficiently, without causing irritation of the mucous membranes. Kneading the bowels often overcomes habitual constipation. There exists no better remedy than my " Renovating Pills," they cure every case of habitual constipation. The bowels may become obstructed from other causes, *Intussusception*, or invagination of the bowels, or when one part of the bowel is drawn into another portion, produces complete closure of the canal. The bowels also become twisted. These conditions may be known by the vomiting of stercora-

11*

ceous or fæcal matter, and when this is observed, instant medical aid should be called for, as the condition is one of great danger, and requires intelligent treatment.

INTESTINAL WORMS.

Every animal seems to be a nest for other animals, and man is no exception to the rule. There are five varieties of intestinal worms, all more or less familiar to every one of my readers.

1. *Ascaris lumbricoides.*—This worm resembles the common earthworm, and is supposed to belong to the same species. It varies in size from four to eighteen inches in length; it also varies in color, having in some instances a whitish pink hue, and in others a dull, dirty-yellow color. It feeds on the chyme found in the intestines, upon absorption from which the growth of the human system depends. They are generally found in the smaller intestines.

2. *Ascaris vermicularis*—This worm is sometimes improperly called the thread-worm, for there is another variety more like a thread than this. It is commonly called the maw-worm, and is the smallest known. The male is exceedingly small, but the female is about half an inch long. It is very slender, and about the size of small sewing-thread. From the fact that it inhabits the rectum chiefly, it is often called the *seat-worm*. This is the animal so troublesome and annoying to children, but is occasionally also found in adults. The child infested with them runs about during the day apparently well, but when night comes it complains of itching in the rectum, which is sometimes excessively annoying.

3. *Tricocephalus dispar.*—This is the long thread-worm, from one to two inches in length, but sometimes reaches a length of four inches. It is like a small thread, except at the posterior extremity, where it is enlarged. It is not so often found as the others. It is of light color. The male is smaller than the female, and differs little in shape. It is common to all parts of the intestinal canal.

4. *Tænia solium* or *vulgaris.*—This is the common tape-worm. Of this family there is but one variety in the United States, though there is another peculiar to other parts of the world. It varies greatly in length and size. The ordinary length is from seven to fifteen feet, but it sometimes arrives at the enormous length of one hundred feet. It is of a flat, ribbon-like shape, about one-quarter of an inch in breadth in the largest places, and tapers to almost a mere thread at the caudal extremity. Its color is whitish or yellowish; and it is made up of numerous segments or joints, which are most distinct and perfect at a distance from the head. These segments resemble a gourd-seed, and are four-sided. The head is smaller than most of the body, with a small point in the centre with openings. It is supposed that this animal can exist or reproduce itself if but a single joint exists, but this is doubtful

unless the head exists. When the head is evacuated the remainder will decay and be also expelled. This animal is hermaphrodite, and impregnates itself. It inhabits the small intestines. Persons affected with this worm frequently pass joints, but it often remains in the body for a long time without its presence being thus revealed.

5. *Tænia lata*, or *bothriocephalus latus.*—This is the broad tape-worm, and does not exist in this country unless imported. It is found in Central and Western Europe. It is much broader, and the joints are shorter than in the common long tape-worm. The joints are more per-

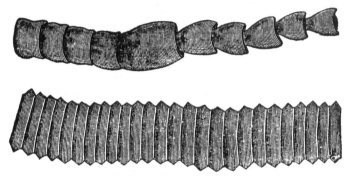

Sections of the Tape Worm.

fect, well developed, and thrown off in connected rows, and by a cavity in the centre, and not in the border of the joint. It varies in length from one to twenty feet.

Almost every variety of symptoms is found to result from the irritation that worms produce in the human system. The symptoms, however, occur mostly in children, and are generally produced by the long, round, or common worms. The abdomen is prominent, full or bloated; the appetite variable and capricious; sometimes deficient and sometimes voracious. The breath is usually offensive, the tongue has a white-coated appearance, and often the upper lip will be much swollen. The eyelids also swell often, sometimes so much that the child can barely see; and occasionally swollen patches will present themselves in other parts of the body. Children troubled with worms are apt to pass restless nights, and frequently start in their sleep. Paleness around the mouth, extending up the sides of the nose, is another common symptom. Itching of the anus is the most common and only particular effect produced by the small worms. St. Vitus' dance and epilepsy often result from verminous irritation, but the latter is usually harmless when properly treated. A dry, choking cough is a symptom peculiar of worms. Itching of the nose is a common symptom, and the child is almost incessantly rubbing that member.

The symptoms of tape-worm are somewhat peculiar, and deserve a brief notice. Persons of all ages are subject to them, but they are most common to middle age. The disturbance they occasion is that of great uneasiness and distress, which often, sooner or later, destroys the general health. Uneasiness in the head, sometimes pain, slight giddiness and ringing in the ears, are the symptoms most complained of. The countenance changes frequently from a flushed to a pale condition; twitching of the muscles, especially those at the mouth, and a pinched, contracted appearance of the nostrils, accompanied with itching, are peculiar symptoms of tape-worm. The appetite is variable, the eyelids swollen, the breath offensive, etc., and other symptoms common to other worms are present also in tape-worm. Nausea occurs at times, with ejections of frothy mucus. The patient grits his teeth in sleep; and the abdomen seems full, with contraction of the navel. After a night's sleep there is a sensation of an animal moving about in the bowels, accompanied by darting pains, which subside after eating. The patient becomes weak and nervous, and finally, worn out with excitement, gets hypochondriacal and even deranged. Of course, the most unequivocal symptom is a discharge of joints of the worm.

TREATMENT.—This varies with the symptoms of each case. If convulsions exist, the first step should be to subdue these by brisk friction and warm applications along the spine and abdomen. Anti-spasmodics in these cases should be given; also sweating drinks. If these symptoms are relieved, the compound powder of senna and jalap may be given with pink and wormwood in sufficient doses to produce free evacuations of the bowels. This is to be repeated for two or three days, and is usually successful. It is equally reliable in the treatment of the long thread-worm. The powder is composed of three drachms each of the above herbs decocted in a pint of water; dose, a tablespoonful. It produces sometimes alarming symptoms, but these, however, are harmless and of short duration. Pinkroot and wormwood are good remedies, however, given in any form. The melia azedarach, or the Pride of China, given in decoction, is a favorite remedy; so also is the burr of the red cedar, the efficacy depending upon the turpentine it contains. Santonine in doses of three or five grains is efficacious, and very serviceable because it is tasteless, and therefore readily administered. Blue vervain is a good remedy, and for this reason my " Restorative Assimilant " is so efficient for the expulsion of worms. Seat, or maw-worms, are best expelled by injections of moderately strong salt and water, or soap-suds. Turpentine in emulsion also makes an efficient injection.

For tape-worm various remedies are used. Kousso, pumpkin-seeds, and turpentine have each a good reputation. Male Fern, however, is the most specific remedy that can be used. It is certain to dislodge the distressing enemy.

My "Male Fern Vermifuge" is without doubt the best vermifuge ever compounded and offered to the public. It instantly expels the minor worms, and the tape-worm is quickly dislodged by it. It is com· posed of such articles as make it applicable to every variety of worms, and it is veritably infallible in its effect. (See page 471.)

I admonish all persons to avoid eating pork that is not well cooked, for it is an established and indisputable fact that tape-worm is caused by eating raw pork, provided that it is not in a healthy condition. That which is commonly known as "measly pork" contains the germs of tape-worm, and should not be eaten unless thoroughly cooked. Tape-worm is most prevalent among the peasants of Central Europe, being they subsist largely on raw pork.

PERITONITIS.

This is an inflammation of the serous membrane lining the abdominal cavity, and investing the viscera, and may be either acute or chronic. During the early stages of the disease there is a feeling of lassitude, pain in the back and limbs, chills alternating with flushes of heat, headache and a feeling of uneasiness about the abdomen. As soon as the febrile action is established, the pain becomes sharp and severe. The abdomen is very tender, the slightest pressure by the hand causing most intense pain. The patient lies on his back, with his knees drawn up and shoulders elevated, finding that this relaxes the abdominal muscles, and prevents pressure by the bedclothes. Nausea, vomiting, thirst, constipation and suppression of urine, are frequent symptoms. The face is pale and contracted, respiration is oppressed, each inspiration aggravates the pain; pulse is frequent and small, tongue moist, and the patient is generally wakeful. The abdomen becomes tympanitic, and when a fatal termination is approached it becomes very much distended. The pulse also becomes feeble and quick, and the countenance assumes a ghastly appearance. It is very rapid in its course, death sometimes occurring within twenty-four hours. Puerperal peritonitis is only another variety of this disease, and attacks women in child-bed. It may arise idiopathi-cally, or it may be caused by wounds, blows, falls, etc.

TREATMENT.—The stomach and bowels should be evacuated by an emetic and purge. If associated with malarial influence quinine should be given. The fever should be controlled by veratrum. A large mustard plaster or turpentine stupe should be applied to the abdomen. Large doses of opium to allay the pain are also indicated. The patient should drink freely of marsh-mallow or flaxseed tea, and be supported by tonics, beef-tea, etc.

SUMMER COMPLAINT (*Cholera Infantum*).

This is a complaint which usually attacks children between the ages of two months and three years; it occurs in the warm season, and is chiefly

confined to cities. It is very fatal. It commences with a profuse diarrhœa, stools thin and variously colored. The stomach becomes irritable,
and rejects everything. Loss of flesh, languor, and prostration follow.
and stools become colorless and odorless, skin is dry and harsh, head and
belly hot, thirst is great, and fever at night-fall. Delirium is present in
many cases, indicated by violent tossing of the head, etc.

TREATMENT.—The child should be removed to a vicinity abounding in
pure air, if possible ; otherwise, in a large and airy room, and may even
be taken into the open air occasionally. Its food should consist of the
farinaceous articles of diet, if weaned ; otherwise, of its mother's milk ;
mucilaginous drinks can also be given. If the vomiting be obstinate,
give camphor, or a little opium, or combined, as in paregoric. The
astringents, as turmeric and cranesbill, must be given to check the diarrhœa. Rhubarb is a good remedy, also leptandrin, prepared chalk, etc.
Lime-water is grateful, and should be given. Charcoal is the proper
remedy when the stools are very offensive.

CHOLERA MORBUS.

This is characterized by violent purging and vomiting of bilious matter,
attended with griping, sickness and a constant desire to go to stool. The
attack is usually abrupt, but it is sometimes preceded by loss of appetite, nausea, headache, chilliness, colicky pains, etc. It occurs generally at night, and the vomiting and purging occur in quick succession.
The evacuations are usually copious, consisting of the ingesta first, but
afterwards of a sour, acrid, serous liquid, causing a scalding sensation in
the throat ; there is slight tenderness over the abdomen, hiccough, anxiety, restlessness and exhaustion. The pulse is quick, small and feeble,
the skin cool and moist, or bathed in clammy perspiration. It is quite
a serious disease and runs a rapid course—death often occurring within
twenty-four hours.

TREATMENT.—If the stomach is overloaded with indigestible food a lobelia emetic should be given in connection with warm ginger tea. Hot
packs or mustard plasters should be placed on the abdomen, and bottles
of hot water to the feet. Lumps of ice should be placed in the mouth to
allay the patient's thirst. Opium is a very good remedy, and may be
given by mouth or by injection. A tea made of chamomile flowers or
columbo often succeeds well. Where great exhaustion is felt, a brandy
toddy should be given.

ASIATIC CHOLERA.

This is an endemic disease of India, and visits other lands by travelling in what is called the cholera cycle. The Hindoos call it *purrhee
morlii* (rapid death) ; the Mahometans, *euncrum vaudi* (diarrhœa and
vomiting) ; and the Arabs, *el houwah* (hurricane). It is evidently

caused by a noxious malaria arising from human or animal decomposition. It is characterized by three stages. The first is marked by derangement of the digestive organs, rumbling in the bowels, pain in the loins or knees, twitching of the calves of the legs, impaired appetite, thirst, and especially a slight diarrhœa. These symptoms continue from a few hours to several days. The pulse is frequently very slow, the tongue is furred, and a sense of great debility is present in all cases. In the second stage vomiting occurs, and the characteristic rice-water stools make their appearance. These stools are thin and watery, and have a peculiar spermatic odor. The cramps become excessively severe, drawing the muscles into knots. The tongue is pale and moist, pulse feeble, the breathing hurried, with distress about the heart, great thirst, and the secretion of urine nearly stopped. The thin, colorless fluid discharged by vomiting and purging is the watery portion of the blood, and when so much has been discharged that the blood cannot circulate freely, the patient sinks into the third, or stage of *collapse.* This is characterized by great prostration, the pulse being hardly perceptible, skin cold and clammy, face blue or purple, eyes much sunken, hands dark-colored, looking like a washerwoman's, breathing short and laborious, a sense of great heat in the stomach, intense thirst, inanition, and death. Recoveries from the third stage seldom occur.

TREATMENT.—In the first place the diarrhœa should receive prompt attention. The patient should lie in bed, and from five to ten drops of laudanum every two or three hours should be given. The astringents should also be administered. Morphine can also be given. The diet should be carefully regulated, and every symptom promptly met with an appropriate remedy. In the second stage the treatment should be energetic, quinine should be given, and the sinking powers sustained with tonics, beef-tea, etc. A pill containing opium, camphor, and cayenne pepper should also be administered. Brandy may also be given freely. I also advise my "Restorative Assimilant" as a good remedy; it should be taken in full doses. Its success has been very gratifying wherever it has been used.

In the third stage the above remedies are to be pursued with increased energy, especially the stimulants, and every effort should be made to promote the warmth of the body.

PROLAPSUS OF THE RECTUM.

This is more common to children than to adults, and is frequently a sequel to protracted diarrhœa, the falling caused by the debility occasioned thereby. It is also associated with disease of the digestive organs, and is peculiar to persons of feeble habit, or of a scrofulous or tuberculous diathesis. It causes pain in the lumbar region, constipation, sometimes diarrhœa, cardiac irritation, and general prostration.

TREATMENT.—The bowels should be replaced as soon as possible to prevent inflammation, that would naturally follow. The bowel can be replaced with the finger, well greased with sweet oil, gently pressing the tumor within the fundament. Cold water should be applied to the parts, and a decoction of white oak bark should be injected. A T-bandage should be applied to restrain the bowel from protrusion.

ANAL FISTULA.

This consists of an abscess occurring in some portion of the cellular tissue around the anus. As suppuration occurs the pus can be detected by the touch, and which sooner or later makes its way to the surface, and is discharged. While the abscess is forming the patient is considerably feverish, and feels a tenderness about the anal region. At first the discharge is a bloody pus, which in time becomes watery and acrid, or sanious. The channel through which it passes is called the fistula. If it communicates with the rectum, the fistula is said to be *complete ;* but if it does not perforate the mucous membrane, it is said to be *incomplete* or *blind.* Fistula is more liable to occur in scrofulous and consumptive persons than in others, though it may be caused by piles, habitual constipation, or the presence of foreign bodies in the rectum.

TREATMENT.—During the active inflammatory state the bowels should be evacuated by a mild purge, and if the pain is severe, an opiate may be given. Flaxseed poultices, or hot fomentations, should be applied, and as soon as fluctuation is quite evident, an incision should be made, and the pus evacuated. A weak decoction of white oak bark may then be injected, and the parts drawn together by adhesive straps. The poultices should be continued as long as there is any hope to prevent a fistulous opening. If the fistula does occur, it gives great annoyance, and is quite difficult to cure. The surgical treatment consists in introducing a ligature through the fistulous opening into the bowels and out the anus, securing it to a small piece of cork, and twisting it once or twice a day until it cuts through, or by dividing the septum by a knife, and healing it from the bottom. Others cauterize the fistula, and attempt to stimulate adhesive granulations in that way. I grant that success attends all these surgical operations, but I do not see the propriety of subjecting the patient to all the attendant pain and confinement to bed when a cure can be as radically effected in as short a space of time by purely medicinal treatment. I have cured very many cases, and in no instance have resorted to cauterization or the knife. Consultation, either in person or by letter, is free with reference to such cases. (See page 390).

PILES (*Hemorrhoids*).

By these are understood the existence of small excrescences within the rectum and around the anus, which are characterized by a varicose condition of the hemorrhoidal veins. They may be situated either internally or externally, and when blood is discharged they are called *bleeding* piles, if not, *blind* piles. The tumors vary in size from a pea to a hen's egg. They are more common in women than men, owing to the sedentary habits of the former. They are caused by obstruction of the portal circulation, drastic purgatives, habitual constipation, pregnancy, uterine misplacement, etc.

TREATMENT.—If costiveness exists, give some mild purgative, as senna and leptandrin, or the "Renovating Pill," and keep bowels gently open, so as to secure one passage a day. Thoroughwort, in decoction, is also very useful. A compound decoction, or an ointment made of witch-hazel, white oak bark, and sweet-apple tree, applied to the tumors, very often cures them. In congestion of the liver, or derangement of the portal circulation, resort to the treatment advised in chronic hepatitis. If there is much inflammation, apply a slippery elm, stramonium, or poke-leaf poultice. Daily injections of cold water are also very useful. The diet should be regulated, and fatigue should be avoided. As a remedy for either internal or external piles, I can recommend nothing better than my "Herbal Ointment." If thoroughly applied to the tumors about twice a day, it gives instant relief, and cures them in a short time.

DISEASES OF THE ABSORBENT SYSTEM.

These are diseases affecting the lymphatic glands. The lymphatic system is that particular system of organs inservient to the formation and circulation of lymph, and consists of glands and vessels. When any of these glands become inflamed, the affection is *lymphangeitis, angeioleucitis,* or *lymphadenitis.*

SCROFULA.

This is commonly known as "King's Evil," and derives its name from the Latin *scrofa,* a sow, because it was supposed that it also affects swine. It is most apt to occur in persons of sanguine temperament, with thick upper lip. When fully developed, it gives rise to a deposit of tuberculous matter. It is characterized by a morbid state of the system, manifested by glandular swellings, chiefly in the neck, suppurating slowly, and healing with difficulty. At first there appear small, hard, movable kernels about the neck, just under the skin. These are the affected lymphatic glands. No redness or soreness is perceptible at first, but when in course of time they reach the size from a filbert to a hen's egg, or even larger, they come to a head and break, discharging a watery fluid, or a mixture like whey and curd. No great pain is seldom if ever felt. When the ulcers heal, they are apt to leave a puckered condition of the skin, and ugly scars. There is scarcely any tissue or organ in the body that scrofula does not assail, and it forms the basis, in many cases of disease, of all their virulence and stubbornness. Strumous habits are very common, being mostly hereditary; but they may also be contracted by bad habits, or be the sequel to low vitality or prostrating diseases. The taint is apt to become universal if in marriage the health of either party is not considered of equal importance with affection, etc., etc. It impairs the functions of all the organs; it renders the mental faculties more or less imbecile; it gives to the patient a heavy, sullen, and forbidding appearance, and is destructive of all beauty of form or sprightliness of character. It is so serious a disease that no one affected with the taint, however slight it may be, should defer such rational treatment as will cure him of one of the greatest enemies of mankind.

TREATMENT.—How lamentable it is that we have no Kings now a days, whose "sacred touch" will cure the prevalent scrofula. In olden times persons believed that if the scrofulous patient could get into the presence of the King, and be touched by his royal hand, his disease would vanish in nothingness. Hence the name of "King's Evil." This folly reached its height in the reign of Charles II. and after the Restoration; the number who flocked to the royal palaces to receive the "touch" is said to have been immense—no less than *ninety-two thousand* in twelve years. If Kings are no longer divine, and whose sacred touch no longer cures, we are not left hopeless, for the products made by a divine hand as manifested in the herbal world afford us abundant agents of cure, if we but have the wisdom not to ignore them, and the intelligence to use them properly.

Rational treatment should be preventive and curative. The preventive treatment consists in regulating the diet and to supply all the chemical material lacking in the histogenic character of the tissues. The habits should be conformed to well-established hygienic laws, and the digestive and assimilative organs should especially be elevated in tonicity and healthfulness. Exercise and bathing are very important, and must not be neglected. When it manifests itself by its characteristic features, tumors, ulcers, etc., the herbal alteratives alone will effect the cure. The best of these are rock-rose, stillingia, corydalis formosa, yellow-dock, fig-wort, sarsaparilla, etc. If the system is debilitated the tonics should also be given to give tone to the various organs of the body. The ulcers should be treated as all chronic indolent ulcers—the best application to them being my "Herbal Ointment." My "Blood Purifier." (see page 471) is composed of the choicest alteratives known, and acts specifically in the cure of this disease, and ever since it has been given to the public, its success was asserted in every case in which it received a competent trial.

Certain cases of scrofula, in which nearly all the tissues and organs are involved, and where the vitality of the system is at a low point, energetic special treatment is necessary. In such cases the author can be consulted, according to directions given on page 390.

TABES MESENTERICA.

This consists of an engorgement and tubercular degeneration of the mesenteric glands, followed by emaciation and general disorder of the nutritive functions. It occurs particularly in children of a scrofulous diathesis, and in those who are weaned too soon, or fed on indigestible substances. The disease is often owing to irritation in inflammation of the lining membrane of the intestines, giving occasion to enlargment of the glands of the mesentery, or duplicature of the peritoneum. Diarrhœa, emaciation, loss of appetite, or sometimes immoderate appetite, hardness and swelling of the abdomen, and toward the end hectic fever, are the chief symptoms of this disease. Recovery is seldom from this disease, if it has attained such a stage in which the glands have become extensively disorganized.

TREATMENT.—Digestible food, fresh air, etc. must be provided for the patient, and the bowels should be kept soluble. The treatment advised in scrofula should be resorted to in this disease. The patient's strength is especially to be well supported by good food, tonics and stimulants. This disease is commonly known as "*opneme*" in certain localities, which literally means *taking of* or wasting away, and persons can yet be found who ascribe the miserable condition of the child to the power of witchcraft, and the celebrated "witch doctors" do yet find employment and supply their amulets or engage in heathenish incantations. I advise every mother when the first symptoms of this disease are recognized to at once engage skilful medical aid, and her child may oftentimes be saved.

ANATOMY OF THE RESPIRATORY ORGANS.

LARYNX.

The *larynx* is a canal formed of cartilages, whose various movements regulate the voice. It is situated in the median line in the upper and anterior part of the neck. It can readily be felt from the exterior, and is commonly called "Adam's Apple." It forms the commencement of the wind-pipe, and in shape is cylindrical below and prismatic above. It is larger in males than in females, which accounts in a measure for the different quality of the voice between the sexes.

It is composed of five cartilages; viz., thyroid, cricoid, two arytenoid, and epiglottis. The *thyroid* is the largest; it occupies the upper anterior portion of the larynx. The *cricoid* is next in size, and situated at the base of the larynx. Its form is that of a laterally-compressed thick ring. The *arytenoid cartilages* are two in number, pyramidal in shape, and situated at the upper and back portion of the larynx. The *epiglottis* is a thin, oval, cartilaginous plate, behind the root of the tongue, and attached to the angle of the larynx ; it resembles a leaf in shape, and is perforated with numerous foramina or holes. During deglutition it is pressed over the *rima glottidis*, thus preventing either solids or liquids from entering the respiratory tract.

Within the larynx are two ligaments on either side. The *inferior* ligaments are usually called the *vocal chords*, though they are more properly ligaments. The space between them is called the *rima glottidis*, and the space between the *superior* ligaments is the *glottis*. The larynx is lined with mucous membrane, inflammation of which constitutes laryngitis.

TRACHEA.

The *trachea* [7] (see figure) is a cylindrical tube, four or five inches long, reaching from the larynx to the point of division into the bronchial tubes. It is formed of from sixteen to twenty cartilaginous rings, united by elastic ligamentous tissue. It is lined with mucous membrane continuous with that of the larynx, which is extremely vascular, and covered with numerous follicles.

The *bronchi* [8] [9] or bronchial tubes are essentially of the same structure and arrangement as the trachea ; the right bronchus is shorter and of larger diameter than the left. The bronchial tubes ramify into numerous sub-divisions, which finally terminate in the lobules of the lungs.

In front of the first two rings of the trachea and upon the sides of the larynx is the *thyroid gland*. It is sometimes much enlarged, constituting *goitre*.

THE LUNGS.

The lungs are the organs of respiration properly ; they are two in number, and situated in the chest, placed side by side, being separated from the abdomen by the diaphragm.

The size varies with the capacity and condition of the chest, age, inspiration, expiration, and disease. They are conical in shape, are longer posteriorly than anteriorly, and have concave bases. The color of the lungs is of a pinkish gray, mottled with black ; these black spots are more numerous in adult life than in infancy. The right lung is shorter but larger than the left, whose transverse diameter is somewhat diminished by the position of the heart. It has three lobes, the left having but two.

The structure of the lungs is spongy, and its compression between the fingers produces a crackling sound called *crepitation*. It consists of air-vesicles [20], held together by cellular tissue, called *parenchyma*, through which blood-vessels and air-vessels are ramified. A certain number of air-cells communicate with each other, and with a single branch of the bronchial tube ; these are separated from neighboring cells by partitions of parenchyma, and thus are formed the *lobules* in which the aëration of the blood is performed.

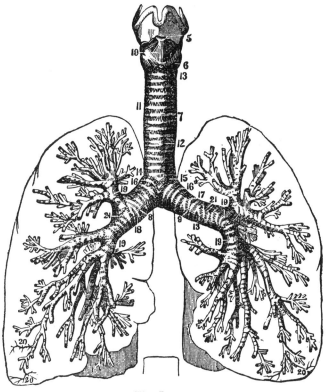

The Lungs.

PLEURÆ.

The pleura is a serous membrane investing each lung, and then reflected upon the walls of the chest. That portion in contact with the chest is called the *pleura costalis ;* that covering the lungs, the *pleura pulmonalis.*

DISEASES OF THE RESPIRATORY AND CIRCULATORY SYSTEMS.

CORYZA.

This is the " running at the nose " or " cold in the head," so frequently contracted. It consists of acute inflammation of the Schneiderian or mucous membrane of the nose, and the sinuses connecting with it. It causes considerable annoyance, and often creates some constitutional disturbance. It is caused by the partial application of cold, as to the back of the head or neck, to the feet, etc., and the effect is especially apt to be produced after perspiration from heat or exertion.   When it reigns epidemically it is called *influenza*.

TREATMENT.—It will usually subside without any treatment, but the subsidence can be greatly hastened by hot baths, a draught of ginger tea upon retiring, and the inhalation of some hot aromatic vapors, such as of balm, water-pepper, etc.

OZŒNA.

This consists of chronic inflammation of the nostrils, with an uneasy feeling, heat, and stiffness of the nose, swelling of the mucous membrane, and an offensive discharge. The nostrils are sometimes closed, owing to the thickness of the membrane. The discharge is often quite purulent, of a yellowish or greenish color, or sanious, and tinged with blood. It is very frequently associated with ulceration, and caries or necrosis of the bone. The breath is usually extremely offensive, and the sense of smell is occasionally lost. It is frequently the result of scrofulous, scorbutic, or syphilitic taint, and is a serious and disgusting disease.

TREATMENT.—The constitutional symptoms should receive special attention, and if owing to or connected with scrofulous or syphilitic taint the general treatment for those diseases should be given. The stomach and bowels should receive careful attention, the digestion being invigorated by alnuin, viburnin, etc. A salt water bath should be taken every morning to stimulate the emunctories. The vapors of tar, naphtha, astringent and narcotic herbs are very beneficial; an inhaling of mecca oil through an atomizer is successful and necessary in obstinate cases. Tonics, as quinine, etc., are necessary in some cases. Those persons who may wish the treatment to be directed by a competent physician, and who desire prompt relief and cure, may consult me, as I have given special attention to this disease, and have cured the most obstinate cases.

CATARRH.

We now come to a disease that is a bane to the existence of many a person. The catarrhal patient is never happy, for he knows that he is inseparably connected with a disease that is excessively annoying to himself and no less disagreeable to those with whom he comes in contact. It consists of inflammation of the mucous membrane lining the nose and sinuses or cavities connecting with it. It is a very common affection, arising from repeated colds, damp apartments, wet feet, insufficient clothing, hot rooms, a sudden check of perspiration, and a rheumatic or scrofulous disposition predisposes to an attack. The symptoms are weariness, pains in the back and limbs, frontal headache, increased discharge from the nose, hoarseness, sore throat, impaired vision, fever, constant hawking, cough, and, if the disease continues, partial or complete deafness. By the constant dropping of the secretions into the throat, the catarrhal inflammation is made to extend to the mucous membrane of the throat and larynx, causing gastritis, tonsillitis, laryngitis, pharyngitis, and bronchitis. Consumption is not an unfrequent sequel to catarrh, and it may so undermine the vitality of the system that the most energetic and rational treatment will only re-establish it. A case that illustrates the ravages of catarrh in its ordinary severe forms is given in the following letter:—

WASHINGTON, D. C., April 3, 1871. ·

Dr. O. PHELPS BROWN.

RESPECTED SIR:—My catarrh, which had almost destroyed my power of speech, had nearly lost me the senses of smell and taste, and was rapidly extending to the lungs, by dropping down, has disappeared. I owe this great blessing to your course of treatment. I applied to you by advice of acquaintances, with many doubts; but a "drowning man catches at a straw," and I wrote you a full description of my sufferings. I cannot be too grateful to Providence for having directed me to do this. Use my name in any way you please for the benefit of others afflicted as I was, etc.

S. BROWN MILLS.

This patient describes the effect of nasal catarrh, as developed in himself, but partially. He has omitted to say that his breath was so offensive that people could not sit in the room with him; that the matter was discharged so copiously that it descended into the stomach, causing vomiting, reducing him in strength and flesh to a comparative skeleton; that he had inflammation and elongation of the soft palate (uvula); had lost his appetite, and was troubled with hectic fever.

He was subject to the usual despondency and hopelessness of patients suffering from long-standing catarrh, and it required every effort to arouse his drooping spirits to anything like natural vivacity. In fact, the symptomatic hopelessness and great depression of the spirits in catarrhal patients is often a greater barrier to speedy cure than the pathological condition of the disease itself.

TREATMENT.—In simple acute catarrh, a hot bath and a large draught of ginger tea will usually cure. The inhalation of the vapor of hops, water-pepper, etc., is also serviceable. The febrile excitement should be controlled by veratrum, the bowels evacuated by a mild purge. It is only in the chronic form that catarrh presents difficulties that require the most patient and skilful treatment to remove. Its condition should be thoroughly understood before treatment is attempted. It is not merely a local disease, but dependent upon a vitiated condition of the blood, hence merely local treatment will prove ineffectual. The blood must in all cases be depurated of morbid elements, and enriched in its constituents. The English daisy, Virginia thyme, etc., and the tonics, are all required. Astringents and local alteratives should be topically applied, and such remedies administered whose virtues are expended upon diseased mucous membranes. Of these, matico is unquestionably the best. From my success with this plant, I confidently believe that it is a virtual specific for catarrh of every degree of severity. It should be combined with such other remedies as each individual case presents. An air-bath, to relieve the congested state of the mucous membrane, is very necessary in the treatment.

The only effectual mode of treating catarrh is by combining appropriate local treatment with the required constitutional medication. The local treatment consists in cleansing the nasal passages, and the sinuses communicating with them, of the vitiated secretions, and afterwards applying astringents, saline solutions, or topical alteratives, as respectively required. For this purpose a syringe may be used, but that instrument but poorly accomplishes the desired purpose. I have invented an apparatus that serves the purpose admirably. This is the "Nasal Douche Apparatus" shown in the cut. This useful instrument is the most valuable inprovement yet made upon the various contrivances employed for cleansing the nasal cavities, or for carrying medicated liquids to the afflicted membranes. Any quantity of liquids can be thrown by a gentle current to any part of nasal passage or sinuses. Warm water should be employed in preference to cold for a nasal douche, as the latter has a tendency to produce irritation or spasmodic action. The usual medicated liquids are those containing the vegetable astringents, common salt, carbolate of iodine, etc., etc.

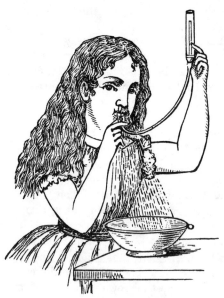

Dr. O. Phelps Brown's
Nasal Douche Apparatus.

The disease can only be mastered in such a manner— all other methods of treatment invariably fail; but if judicious constitutional treatment is employed to overcome the vitiated condition of the blood, and such local treatment as will stimulate the Schneiderian membrane to healthy functional action, the disease can always be cured, no matter how virulent its character may be.

Sufferers from this disease should not fail to possess the "Nasal Douche Apparatus," as by its use the nasal cavities can only be effectively and harmlessly cleansed or medicated; syringes, being for this purpose positively injurious, in consequence of the unavoidable force of the current produced by them, which invariably irritates the diseased membranes. Further particulars with reference to the apparatus may be had by addressing the author.

In my professional career thousands of cases have come under my observation and treatment. It does certainly present insurmountable obstacles to the treatment of those whose opportunity of investigating and treating the disease has not been as extensive as mine, and hence you will find that the common practitioner generally pronounces it incurable, simply because *he* is unable to cure it. If rational treatment such as I advise and employ is engaged, and varied according to the requirements of each case, the disease is no more formidable than other chronic diseases, but is radically cured in a few months. Those desiring to consult me are referred to page 390.

LARYNGITIS.

This consists of an inflammation of the parts composing the larynx, especially the mucous membranes, and may be either acute or chronic. When it is known that in the larynx are situated the vocal organs, and that the aperture for the air to reach the lungs is situated at the apex, it can readily be conceived why inflammation impairs the voice or impedes the respiration. In the acute form there is hoarseness, a pain about the larynx or "Adam's apple," cough, and difficulty of swallowing. If the inflammation is violent the patient's life is in imminent danger from strangulation, caused by closure of the *rima glottidis*. The voice is often completely lost. In bad cases the patient starts up suddenly in bed begging for air; his lips assume a livid or purplish color, the surface becomes cold, the pulse frequent and feeble, the countenance ghastly, perspiration clammy, and finally death occurs from insufficient aëration of the blood. The chronic form is more common than the acute, and is generally associated with induration or ulceration of the mucous membrane. It causes great debility, emaciation, night-sweats, loss of appetite, vomiting and diarrhœa, and the patient often dies in a state of hectic exhaustion.

TREATMENT.—Control the circulation with veratrum, administer an emetic and purge, and apply hot packs to the throat. Hot water should be used frequently as a gargle. The inhalation of hot vapors, as that of belladonna, lobelia, stramonium, mullein, sweet fern, etc.,

12

gives great relief. Some practitioners use ice-bags in place of hot packs to the throat. They seem to answer the same purpose. In case of impending strangulation, no objection should be made to laryngotomy, if in the opinion of the physician or surgeon it is deemed necessary. In the chronic form the disease demands the same treatment, though modified to suit the conditions of the case. A gargle of golden seal, and a syrup of Ceanothus Americanus, or frost-wort, taken internally, are very beneficial. Mecca oil is also used with great advantage. Tonics and stimulants become necessary if the strength is failing. I can offer to the patient an almost sure cure in my "Acacian Balsam," which is to be taken internally, and my "Herbal Ointment," applied externally.

If complicated, or owing to syphilitic contaminátion, special treatment (see page 390) is advised.

BRONCHITIS.

Inflammation of the bronchial mucous membrane is of common occurrence. Its severity is proportionate to the size of the tube involved. The disease may exist independently, but is often associated with lung diseases. It may exist either in the acute or chronic form. In the former variety, affecting the large and middle-sized tubes, coryza, sore throat, hoarseness, and slight chills are the first symptoms; lassitude and pain in the limbs are also present, and as the disease progresses there is a sensation of heat, soreness, and rawness of the bronchial surface, oppressed breathing, and a spasmodic cough and pain. The cough in the early stage is followed by a clear, frothy expectoration, with a saline taste, which changes to yellowish or greenish sputa, or it may be streaked with blood. If the small tubes are involved, the pulse is extremely frequent, great difficulty of breathing, blue appearance of the countenance, coldness of surface, and a tendency to asphyxia is noted. As soon as the disease becomes chronic the febrile symptoms disappear, but the pulse remains frequent, and the cough and dyspnœa are persistent, though to some extent relieved by free expectoration. The sleep is irregular, and night-sweats frequent, occasioning great debility. The cough becomes croupy, and diarrhœa often attests approaching dissolution.

TREATMENT.—A hot bath, hot packs, and veratrum will often terminate the career of the acute form at the outset. In the more severe forms an emetic should be given, and the hot packs or chafing liniments to the chest and throat frequently renewed. Blood-root and other expectorants should be given, and quinine should be administered if the disease is associated with malarial influence. The tonics may become necessary to sustain the strength. The vapors of mecca oil, goose-grease, and bitter herbs are beneficial. In the chronic form the treatment varies with the cause. If owing to syphilitic taint the treatment for that disease should be given, and if rheumatic in origin, colchicum, in connection with tonics, is the treatment indicated. The inhalation of the various vapors before alluded to should also be instituted, and the strength of the patient carefully husbanded by tonics, beef-tea, wine whey, etc. A remedy that combines both tonic and expectorant qualities is found in my "Acacian Balsam," which generally cures the worst cases very quickly. The "Herbal Ointment" should at the same time be thoroughly rubbed upon the chest, throat, and back. Consultations, either in person or by letter, will receive careful and prompt attention.

CROUP.

Croup is an inflammation of the mucous membrane of the larynx and trachea, or windpipe. It is one of the scourges of childhood. False membranous croup is owing to an oozing of a peculiar fluid, which thickens into apparent membranes, and adheres to the surface of the windpipe. In membranous croup, there is much greater danger than in the simpler form.

The symptoms are, difficult breathing, hoarseness, loud and shrill cough, with fever. When the symptoms are violent at first, the disease will be in all probability not fatal, as the membranous croup comes on insidiously, and is scarcely ever ushered in by high inflammation.

TREATMENT.— An early and effective emetic is indicated in all cases. Some mechanical emetic, as ipecacuanha, alum, etc., should be preferred. Flaxseed poultices, my "Herbal Ointment," and irritating liniments should be applied to the neck. The Dover's powder should be given to promote perspiration and rest. Inhalation of vapor from hot water and mullein leaves is of great service. The bowels should be kept regular. In membranous croup, if the membrane cannot be dislodged by emetics, and suffocation is imminent, tracheotomy becomes necessary. Croup may often be prevented by tying a bag containing powdered rosin, which is electro-negative, around the throat at night.

PNEUMONIA.

This is commonly called *lung fever*. It is characterized by inflammation of the parenchyma or texture of the lungs. The patient is generally found lying on his back, complains of pain in his side, has more or less difficulty of breathing, a cough at first dry, but soon accompanied by bloody phlegm. As the disease becomes severe, the phlegm becomes very tenacious, so that it will adhere to the spit-cup if turned upside down. Three characteristic stages are observed in this disease, viz., *congestion*, *hepatization*, and *softening*. In the first stage the lungs become engorged with blood or congested, and if the lungs are percussed a dull sound is elicited, and if the ears are applied to the chest a minute crackling sound is heard, similar to that produced by rubbing fine hair between the fingers and thumb. It is only heard during inspiration, and is caused by the air breaking up the mucous adhesions. The urine is scanty and high colored. In the second stage the lungs become solid, or hepatized, resembling the liver. Some writers call it *red softening.* The dulness becomes more distinct upon percussion, and a whistling sound is heard if the ear is placed to the chest. The cough is more or less dry, but the fever is aggravated. There is great prostration, rest-lessness, complete loss of appetite, constipation, a loaded brown tongue, and the respiration is hurried and imperfect. In the third stage the lung softens and becomes filled with matter, and portions of the lung are apt to give way. The cavities may be detected by increased reso-nance at some parts by percussion, and the cavernous breathing by aus-cultation. There is also a metallic tinkling heard, and the sputum be-comes more liquid, looking like prune-juice, and the general condition of the patient worse in every respect. If the disease advances into this stage, recovery is not very probable.

Pneumonia may be double or single ; the right lung suffers, however, more frequently than the left. If pleurisy is associated with it, it is called *pleuro-pneumonia.* When characterized by great debility and prostration, and is of a low type, it is called *typhoid pneumonia.* The pneumonia of children is called *lobular,* as it is generally confined to one or two lobes of the lung.

TREATMENT.—Bleeding formerly was done in each case, and is again receiving attention by some physicians, but I deem it injudicious, as a general thing, though it may be of benefit in some plethoric cases. The treatment should be commenced with a mild cathartic, and the fever should be controlled with veratrum. The expectorants should be ad-ministered, and in cases of great prostration, beef-tea and alcoholic stimulants must be given. The chest should be blistered, and a cloth smeared with lard should be placed on the raw surface. Sleep should be promoted by lupulin or the opiates, and if great difficulty of breath-ing exists, turpentine should be poured on hot water, and the patient allowed to breathe the vapor. Fresh air, quietude, and rest, with frequent sponging of the body with tepid water, should not be neglected.

ASTHMA.

This is characterized by difficult breathing, occurring in paroxysms, accompanied by a wheezing sound, a great desire for fresh air, and un-attended by fever or organic disease of the lungs or heart. It is evi-dently caused by an irritable condition of the cerebro-spinal system or medulla-oblongata, which deranges the nervous influence through the cervical and pneumogastric nerves. It is also called *Phthisic.* The attack generally comes on suddenly, but in some cases for a few days before the onset there is loss of appetite, flatulence, belching of wind, languor, chilliness, and drowsiness. The attack generally occurs at night, when the nervous system is at its lowest ebb. At first a sense of tightness, with a feeling of constriction about the chest, is felt, which intensifies into a fearful struggle for breath. The patient assumes various postures to facilitate in emptying and filling the lungs, and the feeling that he must have fresh air, induces him to rush to the window and put his head far out to catch the stirring breeze. The hands and feet are cold, the expression haggard and anxious, the body wet with perspiration, and the pulse irregular. The paroxysms usually last for some hours, when breathing becomes more easy. If the symptoms subside without expectoration it is called *dry asthma*, but when any phlegm is raised it is known as *humoral asthma*. The paroxysms may recur every night, remitting gradually in severity, before a final subsidence takes place. The very troublesome complaint, which seems to combine the peculiarities of asthma and coryza, occurring in some persons during hay-making, or even later, is called *hay asthma*. This complaint is often a distressing one.

TREATMENT.—During the paroxysm the inhalation of vapor of hot water, or that arising from a decoction of anti-spasmodic herbs, such as conium, belladonna, etc., lessens the severity of the spasm. The following preparation is a very good remedy : Ethereal Tincture of Lobelia ℥ ij ; Tincture of assafœtida, ℥ i ; laudanum, ℥ ss ; fluid extract of stillingia, ℥ ij ; simple syrup, ℥ iv ; mix, and take a tablespoonful every two hours. Electro-magnetism, smoking stramonium leaves, inhaling the smoke from burning paper, dipped in a solution of saltpetre, are all beneficial. The anti-spasmodics, especially cherry-laurel water, should be taken to prevent the occurrence of frequent attacks. In hay asthma, changes of locality will often save the patient from an attack. The tincture of lobelia is a very good remedy. Quinine and nux vomica carefully administered are good remedies. Chloride of lime placed in a saucer in the sleeping-room often gives relief. My "Acacian Balsam" internally, and the "Herbal Ointment" rubbed externally on the chest, and up and down the spine, have cured many cases. Many interesting cases have come under my notice and treatment, but space forbids any allusion to them. By special treatment I think every case can be cured.

PLEURISY.

This is characterized by inflammation of the pleura or serous membrane enclosing the lungs. The disease usually commences with a chill, which is succeeded by a sharp, lancinating pain in the side ; cough, short and quick breathing, and fever. The pain is usually called a *stitch* in the side, and is felt somewhere in the mammary region. It is increased by inspiration, cough, and motion, lying on the affected side, or by pressure. As the pain subsides, the effusion of a serous liquid occurs into the pleural cavity. The cough is usually short and dry, though a little frothy mucus may be expectorated. Severe pain often attends, and the patient tries to suppress the cough as much as possible. The breathing is more or less difficult in most cases, and the patient is said to have a catch in his breath. When the effusion is both sudden and copious, the function of one lung may be more or less suspended. The fever is usually considerable, and presents the usual phenomena of febrile affections. At some stages the patient's voice is said to be *ægophonous*, or similar to a goat's.

TREATMENT.—Commence with a mild cathartic, and though opposed to bleeding, yet if there is a human ailment requiring bleeding it is pleurisy, as it often gives prompt relief from pain. Sweating should be encouraged at the outset, and for this purpose the tincture of Virginia snake-root, in teaspoonful doses, every half-hour, is the best. It may be given in an infusion of catnip, balm, or pleurisy root. The affected side may be fomented with hops, tansy, wormwood, etc., applied very hot, or it may be blistered. The fever is to be controlled and the perspiration kept up with full doses of veratrum. Dover's powder may be given to procure sleep. The diet should be of the very lightest kind. The alteratives may be given if the effusion is not absorbed, and should these fail, the surgeon may perform *paracentesis*, or tapping of the side.

APNŒA, OR ASPHYXIA.

Literally the word asphyxia means pulseless, and was for a long time only used in that sense, but is now applied generally to all cases of *suspended animation*. It is produced by the non-conversion of venous or blue blood of the lungs into arterial, or red blood. Death is caused in all cases from want of oxygenized blood, and the stagnation that results in the pulmonary capillaries. There are several varieties of asphyxia; and as life can in many cases be revived, I shall state the procedure of resuscitation in each case.

ASPHYXIA BY EXTREME COLD.

When a person is subjected to extreme cold, the first symptoms are painful feelings, followed by sensations similar to those produced by inhalation of carbonic acid gas. He becomes benumbed, indifferent to the danger of his situation; the muscular system becomes enervated, step grows tottering, speech imperfect; and as these influences increase, the breathing becomes irregular and slow, the muscular powers fail, and he sinks into a state of insensibility and death.

TREATMENT.—Rub the person with snow if practicable, or the whole body may be submerged in cold water for a short time. These applications should be gradually increased in temperature until the surface approaches a natural state, or the muscles and joints are sufficiently relaxed to admit of free motion. Then resort to artificial respiration as in drowning.

ASPHYXIA BY INHALATION OF GASES.

Some gases cause death by spasmodic closure of the glottis, others by want of oxygen. Carbonic acid gas is the most common noxious gas.

TREATMENT.—Place the patient in a region where pure air abounds, and then practise artificial respiration.

ASPHYXIA BY SUBMERSION, DROWNING.

Death in this case is not caused by the stomach and air passages being filled with water, but ensues in consequence of the person being plunged in a medium unfit for respiration. In no case where the body is recovered immediately after drowning, should the means of resuscitation be left unemployed. Life has been revived even in cases that were submerged half an hour.

TREATMENT.—1st. Treat the patient *instantly, on the spot*, in the open air, freely exposing the face, neck, and chest to the breeze, except in severe weather.

2d. Send for the nearest medical aid, and for clothing, blankets, etc.

3d. Place the patient gently on the face, the forehead resting on his wrist. This empties the mouth of fluids, and allows the tongue to fall forward, which leaves the entrance to the pipe free.

4th. Turn the patient slightly on his side, and apply ammonia, snuff, or other irritating substances, to the nostrils; then dash cold water on the face, previously rubbed briskly until it is warm. If there be no success, instantly—

5th. Replace the patient on his face, and turn the body gently, but completely, *on the side and a little beyond*, and then on the face, alternately; repeating these measures with deliberation, efficiency, and perseverance, fifteen times to the minute. When the patient reposes on the chest, this cavity is compressed and expiration takes place; the pressure is removed when turned on the side, and inspiration occurs.

6th. When in the *prone* position, make equable but efficient *pressure along* the spine, augment expiration, and remove it before rotation on the side, to facilitate inspiration.

7th. Induce circulation and warmth, while continuing these measures, by rubbing the limbs *upward* with *firm pressure* and with *energy*, using handkerchiefs, etc.

8th. Replace the patient's wet clothing by such other covering as can be instantly procured, each bystander furnishing a coat or waist-coat. Meantime, and from time to time, let the surface of the body be *slapped* freely with the hand, or let cold water be *dashed briskly* over the surface, previously rubbed dry and warm.

Let the patient often inhale diluted pure hartshorn, as this stimulates the respiratory organs.

CONSUMPTION (PHTHISIS).

This is a constitutional affection manifesting itself in most essential changes in the tissue of the lungs. It may be acute or chronic. The acute form, or *galloping consumption*, commences with chills, fever, rapid pulse, cough, pain and difficulty of breathing, which are soon followed by night-sweats, hectic fever, great emaciation, exhaustion, and if its course is not arrested, death. The chronic variety is, however, that which we usually meet with.

For the sake of convenience, I will class the symptoms of consumption into four general stages, viz., *the Incipient stage; the Solidification stage; the Maturation or Softening stage; and the Ulceration and Suppuration stage.*

The first stage of Tubercular Phthisis is generally stated to be that to which the *physical* signs indicate a *deposit* in the lungs. Evidently, however, there is, and must be, an antecedent state of disordered health before the most skilful observer can detect the *sound* which indicates the least shade or degree of solidification of the lungs, whether by means of the stethoscope, or other methods usually resorted to by the profession for such purpose. When the physical signs are observed, the use of the stethoscope, etc., may be regarded as little more than professional display, without a particle of advantage, except as developing in some degree the actual amount of lesion or injury then sustained by the tissues of the lungs. There must be a causative agent that originates the predisposition or tendency to the deposit of tubercles in the tissues, or which elaborates or prepares the material in the system, from which only tubercle is formed. *But we should not wait to see the physical signs developed if we would expect uniform and hopeful treatment of tubercular consumption.*

From my own long experience in the *specialty* of thoracic diseases, I do not hesitate to say that the *actual first set of symptoms* of consumption consists simply in the *wasting of flesh*, particularly if this is attended with, or by, a low scale of health and strength. Such loss of muscle, plumpness, as well as juices and fat, is first noticed in three principal places. The first region of flesh-consuming is usually the face; the second, the hands; the third, over the sacral or hip bones. The sacral region, where it first gives out, is lame and sore. The hands look poor and "scrawny;" the muscles of the arms and legs are soft and flabby.

If the face shows it first, the eyes stare; the brow, temples, and scalp look lean; the muscular tissues of all the limbs soon waste, and the pectoral muscles, as also all the chest muscles, waste away, and then the breathing is already become imperfect and weak.

The diminished respiration is soon attended with cough; then pains are felt through the breast or thorax.

The patient next is sensible of something wrong, and is conscious of a sense of general debility. The fact is, nutrition is lost. The vital powers are flagging, for the *wasting of the body*, in *spite of eating*, is *more rapid than the repair*.

Then comes a state of *spirit* depression—not the *cause* of consumption, but caused by the already deficient vitality, and all the more helping on the grand catastrophe; for it is a law of our being, that where *nerve* structure is not itself nourished, it, too, will fail in its work, just as surely as muscle fibre fails of power from the same cause. To recapitulate:—

1.—*Incipient stage.* This may present itself at a very early age, or may appear in middle age, and the first indications are, generally, a subdued and saddened feeling, the former buoyancy of spirits subsides, and the person becomes languid. The face begins to assume a sickly hue, and, to a practised eye, tells a sad tale. The skin becomes whiter, and a nervousness and sometimes irritable disposition of mind appears; and if any hint be given about consumption threatening, the person rebels against it, and will not tolerate such an idea. The appetite and digestion frequently become impaired, and may manifest itself in capricious fancies for certain sorts of food. A slight cold or any excitement will bring on diarrhœa. The breath is short, and the breathing hurried; running or walking up an incline, or ascending a flight of stairs, is unpleasant, and attended by a fluttering and palpitation of the heart. The strength and weight of the body diminish, but this varies. The sleep is disturbed, the skin becomes hot, there are burnings of the palms of the hands, and cold feet; a short, dry, teasing cough, or tickling, or hawking up of mucus from the throat appears. There is also a feeling of *feverishness* and uneasiness after meals, which are unfavorable symptoms, indicating the first *mal*-assimilation of the food, which, if not rectified, will inevitably deposit the germ of tubercles, and hence no time should now be lost in opposing the disease, before it lays siege to the citadel of the body.

2.—*Solidification.* The cough, which at first appeared very trifling, now begins to assume an anxious aspect, and becomes troublesome. It may not as yet be attended with expectoration, and if it be, the matter expectorated is of a ropy and viscid nature. The breathing becomes more impeded; hectic fever sets in, with chills and heats, while the weakness of both body and mind increases, although the intellect is

12 *

sometimes extremely bright or sound to the very last. Pains, like those of *pleurisy*, are felt about the chest, and are indications of those *inflammatory* effusions and adhesions which attest the *progress* of the disease, and the infraction of the lung structure, and the impeding of the access of air to the cells of the lungs. The blocking up of the air-cells constitutes the stage of *Solidification*, and thus interferes with the due motives or functions of the chest, and, if not arrested, creates an afflux of fluid to the parts, thus promoting congestion and fresh deposits in the lungs.

3.—*Maturation and Softening*. In this stage, all the former symptoms are aggravated, and consumption is now confirmed. Fresh deposits in the lungs occur, and hasten the maturation and softening. These *local* lesions in their turn re-act on the system at large, aggravating the general infection and depressing the vital powers. Hence the advancing inertia of all the *vital* powers—the universal languor, loss of flesh, and strength, and weight. The cheeks and lips become blanched —painfully contrasting with the circumscribed *hectic* patch of the former. The expectoration is changed, and becomes more copious, opaque, and viscid, more massive, and frequently streaked with blood, or mixed with flocculent, wool-like, or curdy particles. It is most troublesome in the mornings, and when going to bed. The feverishness and general exhaustion increase; restless nights, with perspirations, hurried breathing, change in voice, and emaciation also increases. The appetite fails —either constipation or diarrhœa, more frequently the latter, comes on, with great increase of cough and vomiting after meals. If the disease advance to this stage, it will require much vigilance and judgment to arrest its progress, as the mischief in the lungs is now very great, and *ulcers*, rapidly forming, constitute what is called tubercles.

4.—*Ulceration and Suppuration*. The disease now assumes a totally different aspect, and becomes exceeding formidable in its nature and results. The cough becomes more severe, and the expectoration greenish, yellow, or even sometimes like tufts of wood chewed, appearing, when viewed in water, like jagged round balls. Hemorrhage, or bleeding from the lungs, is likely to come on, and the difficulty of breathing is very great. The patient can scarcely lie down; many times he must be kept with his head bolstered up in a chair, or in his bed, when sleep is desired. Sometimes the voice is reduced to a mere whisper, while in others it remains quite strong to the last. The perspiration, or night-sweats, are very copious, and very exhaustive of the vitality of the organism. The *ulcers* or tubercles in the lungs increase, causing large excavations, from which issue copious expectorations, sapping and undermining the foundation of the entire system.

The most unpractised eye can now at once detect the ravages of this disease in the altered appearance of the whole frame; the body is reduced to a mere skeleton; the eyes are sunken; cheek bones prominent, with sunken cheeks; the head bends forward; the chest is wasted, and the breathing becomes distressingly painful. The mental faculties generally become impaired; yet a gracious God, amid all this suffering, frequently permits the faculties to remain intact until the last ember burns out.

TREATMENT.—This resolves itself into such a management of the case as will tend to prevent the development of the disease, or its removal when it exists. It will be seen that consumption has its origin in a vitiated and defective condition of the general organism. This may occur as the result of hereditary predisposition, or from defective nutrition, or from imperfect development of either a part or the whole of the organic structure, and general disobedience to the physiological law of the general organism. Whenever this predisposition exists, the defective organization, as far as practicable, should be remedied by a faithful adherence to the laws of physiology and dietetics. Children possessing this organization should not be confined too closely in schools or to study, but should be reared in the country, and be exposed to fresh air and out-door exercise. Both boys and girls should be allowed to ramble through the fields, and indulge in those gymnastic exercises which tend to give strength and vigor to the system generally, such as jumping the rope, rolling the hoop, flying the kite, hoeing, wheeling, riding on horseback, etc., and not be studiously confined in-doors, because it is a " delicate child." Tidy mothers should not be horrified if they find their child of frail organization making mud-pies, or that he has torn his frock in climbing an apple-tree. Their diet should be plain and nutritious, consisting of bread and milk, oatmeal porridge, baked apples and milk, vegetables, and a liberal amount of meat once or twice a day. Their sleeping apartments should be well ventilated, and they should be warmly clad in all seasons. Misses, upon the approach of the catamenial flow, should be well instructed that the feet should be kept warm and dry, that washing and bathing in cold water should be avoided, and all exposure to cold and moisture is hurtful.

The medicinal treatment of consumption has been extensive, and to enumerate all that has been tried and recommended would fill a volume. Some recommend inhalations; these answer their purpose well for temporary relief. The disease must be treated upon general principles. The cough should be allayed by appropriate remedies, the occasional diarrhœa checked by the astringents, the debility removed by tonics, and vitality stimulated by alcoholic liquors. It is beyond question, that spirit-drinking has been beneficial in a number of cases, if taken rgugularly and moderately. Phosphorus is a good remedy, especially if given in a form as it exists in *erythroxylon coca*. External irritants, as Croton oil to the chest, answer very well. The blood of the consumptive con-

tains too much oxygen, and too little carbon ; hence to supply this deficiency cod-liver oil, which is a highly carbonaceous food, is excellent.
It gives warmth to the body, and supplies the disease with material for
destruction, without expense to the body. The chalybeates may also be
given to give strength and enrich the blood in its red particles. Change
of climate is rarely beneficial. The diet must be highly nutritious ; fresh
air, occasional baths, and plenty of friction, should not be neglected.
While investigating the best means of treating this disease, I deemed
that if a combination could be made that would prove remedial to all
the morbid characters of consumption, that would antagonize each
pathological condition as they arose, thus holding the disease in abey-
ance, and allow the forces of reparation and recuperation to mend the
ravages of the disease, that such a combination would most surely cure
the disease. After various experiments, I, finally, by intimate knowledge of the chemical elements of plants and the pathology of the disease, was led to compound the "Acacian Balsam," which has stood the
test for years, and the thousands of testimonials of the permanent cure
of many bad cases of consumption attest its virtues.

It is a superior exhilarant. It purifies all the fluids and secretions in
the shortest reasonable period. It nourishes the patient who is too
much reduced to partake of ordinary food. It will supply the place of
food for a month at a time. It strengthens, braces, and vitalizes the
brain. It heals all internal sores, tubercles, ulcers, and inflammations.
It stimulates, but is not followed by reaction. It at once obviates emaciation, building up wasted flesh and muscle, as the rain vivifies and
enhances the growth of the grass. It is without a rival as a tonic, and
it immediately supplies electricity or magnetic force (as if it were a bat-
tery) to every part of the enfeebled and prostrate body. In conjunction with the balsam, I also advise external application of the " Herbal
Ointment" (which answers all the purposes of counter-irritants) to the
chest, throat and back, and the bowels regulated with the "Renovating Pill" (see page 469).

ANATOMY OF THE HEART.

The heart is a hollow muscular organ, surrounded by a membranous
sac called the pericardium. It lies between the two pleuræ of the
lungs, and rests upon the cord-like tendon of the midriff, in the cavity
of the chest.

Its *shape* is conoidal, though it is somewhat flattened upon that side
that rests upon the tendon of the diaphragm. Its apex inclines to the
left side, touching the walls of the thorax between the fifth and sixth
ribs. It *measures* about five inches and a half from its apex to its base,
three and a half inches in the diameter of its base, and *weighs* about six
or eight ounces. It contains *four cavities*, which perform two functions :

that of receiving the blood and emptying the blood into the lungs, and that of receiving it again after it has been oxygenated, and distributing it throughout the vascular system. The receptacles are *auricles*, and the *ventricles* propel the blood to the lungs and through the body.

The auricle and ventricle of the *right side* receive and propel the venous blood into the lungs. The auricle and ventricle of the *left side* receive and propel the arterial blood throughout the system.

The blood *circulates* as follows : The ascending and descending vena cavæ empty the blood (venous) into the right auricle ; from here it passes to the right ventricle, through an opening protected by a valve, downwards ; from the right ventricle it is propelled through the pulmonary artery, which divides into two branches, to the lungs ; in the lungs it is oxygenated by the inspired air ; it is then brought from the lungs, by four pulmonary veins, into the left auricle. The left auricle has an opening communicating with the left ventricle, protected by a valve opening downwards, and from the left ventricle it passes into the aorta, thence to be distributed throughout the body.

The *right auricle* is a cavity of irregular shape, somewhat oblong, and like a cube ; anteriorly it has a convexity which is called its *sinus ;* superiorly there is an elongated process resembling the ear of an animal, whence the term auricle. Its walls are thin, and composed of muscular fibres, which are called *musculi pectinati*, on account of their parallel arrangement, resembling the teeth of a comb. The superior [5], and inferior vena cavæ enter the auricle from behind. The elevation between the orifices is called the *tuberculum Loweri*. The *coronary* veins open into this cavity, and their orifices are protected by the *valves of Thebesius*. The opening to the ventricle is circular, and surrounded by a dense white line.

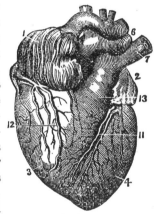

The Heart.

The *right ventricle* [3], is a triangular cavity, with thick walls, and of greater capacity than any other cavity of the heart. Its muscular structure is in the form of large fleshy bundles, called *columnæ carneæ*, from which proceed thin, white cords, called *chordæ tendineæ*, which are attached to the edge of the *tricuspid valve*. This valve is circular, having at its lower edge three spear-pointed processes, whence its name. It closes downwards, and prevents the blood from returning into the auricle, and, therefore, it passes out by the *pulmonary artery* [7]. The valves protecting the orifice of the pulmonary artery open outwards, and are called the *semi-lunar valves*. They are formed by three half-moon-shaped folds of the lining membranes, and their use is to prevent the blood returning from the artery to the ventricle, when it dilates. Behind each valve is a pouch or dilatation, called the *Sinus of Valsalva*, into which the blood flows by its reflux tendency upon the dilatation of the ventricle, and thus these valves are closed. The pulmonary artery is of the same diameter as the aorta, but its walls are thinner. After its origin it curves upwards and backwards, and divides into two branches, the right of which is larger than the left [7], and passes under the arch of the aorta.

The *left auricle* [2], is more concealed from its natural position than the right. The four pulmonary veins enter into it, which give it a quadrangular shape. Its walls are muscular and somewhat thicker than those of the right auricle. The partition between the auricles is not always perfect even in adult life.

The *left ventricle* [4], forms by its cavity the apex of the heart; it is like a cone in shape. Its walls are thick, and its *columnæ carneæ* numerous, strong and projecting ; the *chordæ tendineæ* are well developed, and attached to the *bicuspid* or *mitral valve*. This valve consists of two leaflets, one of which is much larger than the other. The contraction of the ventricle closes the valve, and the blood passes out by the aorta [6]. The heart is supplied with blood by the right and left *coronary* arteries [11] [12]; the veins which accompany them empty by a common trunk into the right auricle.

It will thus be seen what a complex piece of machinery the human heart is, and how vital the organ must be. It will be apparent to every reader that the least interruption or derangement of its functional action is sure to be manifested upon the integrity of the general system. Any valvular derangement or breaking down of the septum between the auricles and ventricles will allow the commingling of arterial with venous blood, threatening death with asphyxia. Atrophy and hypertrophy interfere with the muscular action of the walls of the heart, and, in fact, it will be obvious from the complex character of the structural anatomy and the importance of the functional actions of the heart, that any disease assailing the organ is attended with danger.

In circulation the contraction of all the cavities is followed by their dilatation. The contraction is called the *systole ;* the dilatation, the *diastole*. What is called the *impulse* of the heart occurs during the *diastole*. The heart's impulse is the shock communicated by its apex to the walls of the thorax, in the neighborhood of the fifth and sixth ribs. The impulse is not the same as the arterial pulse. The heart emits two sounds, *first* and *second*, followed by an *interval*. The first are the longest. The following table shows the connection of the sounds of the heart with its movements :—

First Sound.—Second stage of ventricular diastole. Ventricular systole, and auricular diastole. Impulse against the chest. Pulse in the arteries.

Second Sound.—First stage of ventricular diastole.

Interval.—Short repose, then auricular systole, and second stage of ventricular diastole, etc.

Each cavity of the heart will hold about two fluid ounces, but it is probable that the ventricles do not entirely empty themselves at each stroke ; they will therefore discharge about one and one-half ounces at each pulsation. Reckoning 75 pulsations to the minute, there will pass through the heart in this time 112 ounces or 7 lbs. of blood. The whole quantity of blood in the human body is equal to about one-fifth of its weight, or 28 lbs. in a person weighing 140 lbs. This quantity would therefore pass through the heart once in four minutes, or about fifteen or twenty times an hour. It is very probable that circulation is much more rapid than this estimate. The number of contractions of the heart in a minute is about 70 or 75. The frequency of its action gradually diminishes from the commencement to the end of life. Just after birth it ranges from 140 to 130, in old age 65 to 50. Age, sex, muscular exertion, emotions, and temperament exert a controlling influence over the heart's action. In persons of sanguine temperament the heart beats more frequently than in those of the phlegmatic, and in the female sex more frequently than in the male. Its action is also increased after a meal, and by rising from a recumbent to a sitting or standing posture. The time of day also affects it ; the pulse is more frequent in the morning, and becomes gradually slower as the day advances.

The pulse is always a sure index of health or disease. In inflammation and fevers the pulse is much more frequent than during health. When the vital powers decline it becomes frequent and feeble. In nervous affections with more oppression than exhaustion of the forces, the pulse is often remarkably slow.

The membrane lining the interior of the heart is called the *endocardium*, and the enveloping membrane on the exterior the *pericardium*.

DISEASES OF THE HEART AND CIRCULATORY SYSTEM.

PALPITATION.

This is the most common disease of the heart, and may be connected with various structural changes of the organ, yet it frequently exists independently of any organic lesion, and is often sympathetically dependent upon dyspepsia, hypochondria, hysterics, mental agitation, venereal excesses, masturbation, etc. It may also be due to a low and deficient state of the blood, or *anæmia*. The impulse is weak, fluttering, or tumultuous, generally increased by trifling causes. The beats are increased in frequency, sometimes marked by intermission, and occasionally accompanied by a bellows murmur. The complexion is generally pallid and bloodless, the lips and inside of mouth also pale, the pulse quick and jerking, and the patient complains of breathlessness and fainting. He dislikes animal food, but relishes acids. In females the deficiency of menstrual flow is superseded by the whites, or sometimes the flow becomes very profuse.

TREATMENT.—During the paroxysm a compound of yellow jessamine, scull-cap, and ladies'-slipper should be given, in sufficient doses every hour, until relieved. The feet should be bathed in warm water and the patient avoid all exertion or excitement. If due to anæmia, the proper remedies as well as nourishing diet should be prescribed. If co-existent with dyspepsia, hypochondria, etc., the proper treatment for those affections should be instituted.

ANGINA PECTORIS.

This disease presents rather difficult pathological features. By some writers it is called *neuralgia of the heart*. The principal symptoms are, violent pain about the breast bone, extending towards the arms, anxiety, difficulty of breathing, and sense of suffocation. The paroxysm may be brought on by fast walking, over-eating, or violent exercise, but they may also come on when the patient lies quietly in bed. If connected with ossification, or other morbid conditions, it is an affection of great danger.

TREATMENT.—During the paroxysm the most powerful stimulating and narcotic anti-spasmodics are required. The feet should be placed in warm water, a large mustard plaster should be applied over the cardiac region, and one drop of the tincture of aconite may be given every minute or two, until the spasm is relieved. If it is associated with any organic disease of the heart, the proper treatment for such disease should be instituted, and if due to a neuralgic affection of the organ, the proper remedies for neuralgia should be given. Patients suffering from this dangerous disease should lose no time in consulting some well-skilled physician.

PERICARDITIS.

This consists of inflammation of the sac in which the heart is contained. It does not essentially differ from other serous inflammations, as there may be exudation and liquid effusion, the quantity varying from a few ounces to a few pints. The disease is usually ushered in with a slight chill, followed with fever, or it may commence with fainting. Pain, oppression, weight, palpitation, cough, hurried and difficult respiration, frequent and irregular pulse, inability to lie on the left side, headache, delirium, faintness, anxiety, debility, restlessness, and great nervous irritability usually attend the attack. The face and extremities are swollen, and the urine scanty and high-colored. The essential conditions of fever are always present, the pulse sometimes attaining 120 to the minute. If the acute form advances for several weeks it becomes chronic, or may by insidious advances be chronic from the first. The symptoms are nearly the same as in the acute form.

TREATMENT.—The treatment should be commenced by a lobelia emetic, an active purge, and the application of hot packs to the chest. The tincture of veratrum should be given in sufficient quantities to control the inflammation and lessen the action of the heart. Usually, from two to five drops every half hour is sufficient. If associated with rheumatism, colchicum, cannabis sativa, or macrotys racemosa, should be given. In malarial districts, quinine becomes necessary. Blistering or local depletion may be necessary in some cases.

ENDOCARDITIS.

This is an inflammation of the internal lining of the heart. There is at first pain about the heart, whose disordered action may be violent, or else feeble, irregular, and intermitting. There is more or less difficulty of breathing, and the organ gives forth some abnormal sounds, such as the bellows murmur, the rasping and sawing murmur, arising from thickening of, or deposit on, some of the valves. One or more of the above symptoms occurring during the course of acute rheumatism, may be considered a sign of endocarditis. The patient generally lies on his back, and his pain may sometimes be so slight as scarcely to be noticed, but in dangerous cases there is extreme anguish, liable to be followed by orthopnœa, or necessity of being in the erect posture to be able to breathe, followed by restlessness, delirium, and death. The murmurs may occur at any stage of the disease, from the very beginning towards the close.

TREATMENT.—The treatment is essentially the same as for pericarditis in the commencement of the attack, with the exception that it may be necessary to administer stimulants in some cases. Leeches may be applied to the cardiac region, and between the shoulders. Digitalis and veratrum should be cautiously administered to control the heart's action. If associated with rheumatism, colchicum should be given. Mustard poultices, blisters or hot packs may be applied to the chest to hasten the absorption of the deposit of lymph.

If *myocarditis*, or inflammation of the entire substance of the heart, complicates either pericarditis or endocarditis, the active treatment advised in the latter diseases will remove it.

CHRONIC VALVULAR DISEASE OF THE HEART.

This frequently results from chronic endocarditis. They may either be contracted or distorted, preventing accurate closure, or ulceration may occur through the valves. Vegetations and a peculiar deposit may take place under the tissue of the valves, and occasionally there is a deposition of cartilaginous or osseous matter, and in rheumatic or gouty subjects, of the urate of soda, or the valves may become atrophied or wasted away. The effects in slight cases may occasion but little difficulty, but in severe it is apt to produce hypertrophy and dilatation, dropsy, local inflammations, and ultimately death. These results are owing to an impediment in the forward movement of the blood, and to the regurgitation of the same, producing an accumulation behind. This is plainly illustrated in an affection of the mitral valve. If its orifice is contracted by deposits, the blood accumulates in the left auricle by the impediment, and distends it; congestion of the pulmonary veins is the consequence; the lungs share in the congestion, and pulmonary apoplexy may be the result. This of course occasions an insufficient supply of blood to the general system, which the heart is willing to relieve, and, therefore, makes greater efforts, but becomes hypertrophied or enlarged in so doing. Again, suppose some insufficiency in the mitral valve, owing to ulceration, for example, the blood will regurgitate into the left auricle at each pulsation, it produces the same effects. If the *semilunar* valves are contracted, a less supply of blood is sent to the general system, but congestion of the heart and consequent enlargement and dilatation of the left ventricle may occur. The general symptoms of valvular disease is difficulty of breathing, increased by muscular efforts, or emotion, palpitations, the pulse intermittent or jerky. Distinctive murmurs accompany these affections; in mitral deficiency we hear a prolonged murmur in a low key, like whispering the word "*who;*" in contraction of the aortic valves we have a comparatively superficial sound like whispering the letter "z;" in regurgitations we hear squashing sounds.

TREATMENT.—The mitigation of the urgent symptoms may be accomplished by ladies'-slipper, hops, or henbane. In violent action of the heart cherry laurel water may be given with the henbane. Hot footbaths and mustard plasters may also be necessary. In sudden palpitation and difficulty of breathing, the compound spirits of lavender should be given. Collinsonia is the proper remedy if hypertrophy of the valves is suspected. In valvular insufficiency the tonics and a liberal diet should be prescribed. Conium, belladonna, digitalis, irisin, veratrum, stramonium, and cannabis sativa, are also extensively used in various combination, if they are indicated.

ATROPHY OF THE HEART.

This may result from various causes. When it exists, greater resonance accompanies percussion, and the two sounds of the heart will be more feeble, but more distinctly heard. The symptoms are pallor, coldness and dropsy of the extremities, cough, irregular respiration, palpitation, oppression; in females, irregularity or vicarious menstruation. It may occur with the exhausting diseases, as cancer, consumption, diabetes, etc.

TREATMENT.—The patient should avoid all excesses in mental and bodily exercise. The diet should consist of rich animal broth, with a liberal amount of fats and sugar, cod-liver oil, and the tonics should be administered.

HYPERTROPHY AND DILATATION OF THE HEART

As these are generally coexistent, they should be considered together. The dimensions of the heart may be increased either by augmentation of its muscular walls, or enlargement of its cavities. The former is hypertrophy, the latter dilatation. The most prominent symptom is difficulty of breathing, produced by any exertion; also palpitations, which are sometimes so violent as to shake the whole body. The secondary signs are violent headache, vertigo, buzzing in the ears, flashes of light, pulmonary congestion, pneumonia, apoplexy of the lungs, congestion of the liver, bilious disorders, and general and local dropsy. The patient's suffering is often extreme, and, unable to lie in bed, he is forced to assume constantly a sitting posture, with the body bent forward. Death usually occurs suddenly in syncope or fainting. Valvular disease is the most frequent cause, though they may be caused by rheumatic irritation, excessive exertion of the organs from any cause, as violent exercise, playing on wind instruments, violent passions, intemperance, etc.

TREATMENT.—The exciting cause should be removed, especially valvular disease. The patient's habits of life and occupation should be regulated, and his diet moderated. Mild cathartics should occasionally be given and passive exercise engaged in. Digitalis is the special medicine; cherry laurel water is also used for the same purpose. These should be carefully administered. The tincture of aconite and colchicum should be given where it has resulted from rheumatism. In dilatation the tonics, cod-liver oil, and animal food should be prescribed. Digitalis is also specially required. Wild cherry bark is an excellent tonic, and as nervous symptoms are very apt to be present in females, opium, belladonna, valerian, etc., may be given with advantage. Every effort should be made to enrich the blood.

CYANOSIS, OR BLUE DISEASE.

In this disease the skin bears a leaden or purple tinge over the whole body. There is a reduction of warmth, and labored breathing. It is due to the admixture of blue or venous blood with arterial or red blood, and caused by the right and left sides of the heart remaining open after birth, or by obstruction of the pulmonary artery, thereby withholding the blood from the lungs and preventing arterialization. It is a disease confined to infants, and is almost necessarily fatal.

TREATMENT.—The circulation must be sedated by allowing the child complete rest, or by the careful administration of veratrum ; good food, fresh air, and protection from extremes of heat and cold are necessary. Apply friction to the head and body by some soft cloth. If syncope occurs, the child should be placed in a warm bath, and camphor applied to its nostrils.

The heart is liable to be assailed by other diseases. *Softening* of the heart may take place without inflammation ; it may result in rupture of the heart. Various *indurations* of the heart may occur, as of the fibrous, cartilaginous and osseous character. *Fatty degeneration* is a rare disease. *Tubercle, cancer,* and *polypi* are also noticed.

The heart is the most important organ in the body ; hence its diseases to the physician are full of interest. Nothing gives to a person greater anxiety than the suspicion or knowledge that he is affected with heart disease. The dread of sudden death is universal, and so it generally occurs in cardiac diseases. The most important requisite in the treatment is its early application, as most of the diseases can be cured if treatment is bestowed in time, and hence it behooves every one who feels some abnormal action or uneasiness about the heart to engage treatment, or seek competent medical aid as soon as possible. Those who desire to consult me are referred to page 390. My experience in the treatment of heart diseases has been in extent second to none in this country, and the success has been most gratifying:

DISEASES OF THE BLOOD-VESSELS.

ARTERITIS.

Inflammation of the arteries is rare in the acute form. The symptoms are pain and tenderness along the course of the vessel, attended with a thrill or throbbing. Lymph is effused within the vessel, often producing a complete arrest of the circulation, and resulting in gangrene. It is highly probable that in spontaneous senile gangrene the cause is arteritis. Chronic arteritis is more common, but difficult to discover. Deposits occur in the arteries, exciting ulceration, or ossification may occur in old age.

TREATMENT.—Give a mild purge, a hot bath, and sufficient veratrum to control the circulation. The inflamed part should be fomented, blistered, or stimulating liniments and counter-irritation may be applied. The alteratives are always indicated.

ANEURISM.

This is a pulsating sac, filled with blood, which communicates with an artery. *True* aneurism consists of a sac formed by one or more of the arterial coats. *False* aneurism is owing to a complete division of the arteria¹ coats, either from a wound or external ulceration; the sac formed of cellular tissue. Every artery may be affected with any aneurism, but the aorta, carotids, axillary, brachial, iliacs, femorals, and popliteals are the arteries most commonly affected. The tumor at first is small, gradually increasing, soft and quite compressible, being filled only with fluid blood. It pulsates synchronously with the heart, and is increased by pressure on the side furthest from the heart. A peculiar thrill is imparted to the hand, and which can be heard if the ear is applied. The strength of the part is much impaired as the tumor enlarges, and the circulation in the extremity weaker. During the progress of the tumor the adjacent parts are displaced and absorbed, even bone is rendered carious and absorbed by constant pressure of the aneurism. The pain and numbness increase, and the general health fails, and at length the tumor may burst, opening upon the skin or some internal cavity, and prove fatal.

TREATMENT.—Complete rest, and the frequent application of hot-packs to the tumor should at first be prescribed. A stimulating lini-ment may be rubbed over the part. One composed of the compound tincture of myrrh and the oil of origanum answers the purpose well. The "Herbal Ointment" is an excellent application. The gentle appli-cation of electro-galvanism should be resorted to if the above treatment does not suffice. Pressure by well-secured pads, or by the thumbs and fingers, continued for a long time, is often tried and successful in some cases. If the above treatment fails, some competent surgeon should be consulted, who will in practicable cases ligate the artery. Valsalva had a curious plan of treatment for aneurism. It consisted of repeated blood-letting, with food enough merely to support life. A cure worse than the disease.

PHLEBITIS AND VARICOSE VEINS.

This is an inflammation of the veins. The signs are pain and tender-ness in the course of the vessel, which soon becomes cord-like and knotted, by which it may be distinguished from arteritis. There are swelling and redness of the adjacent parts, the redness being in streaks. The limb below the part is swollen, from obstruction of the circulation and effusion of serum. Pus is a frequent production of phlebitis, in which case perfect occlusion of the vein *above* occurs, with the forma-tion of an abscess, or the pus passes into the heart and produces excessive prostration. *Varicose veins* are the sequel generally to phlebitis.

TREATMENT.—The treatment consists in fomentations, leeching, and occasional purging. The alteratives should also be given. The topical application of tinctures of lobelia and arnica are also useful. Rest is enjoined. The abscesses and consequent ulceration should be treated upon general principles. If the veins become varicosed, astringent applications, and careful bandaging, should be resorted to.

The best method of curing varicose veins, however, is by elastic stockings. These give an equable pressure, which can be so regulated as to afford any compression desired, on every part of the leg where the varicose veins exist. If the veins are varicosed throughout the whole length of the limb, the full-length stocking should be worn ; if confined only to the leg, the stocking represented on the right-hand side of the cut is alone necessary, and in some cases the knee-caps and anklets are only required, depending upon the situation of the varicose veins. These elastic contrivances are not only radical cures, but patients suffering from varicose veins have no idea what ease and comfort they afford. They give a very agreeable support to the limb, prevent varicose ulcers, besides quickly reducing the enlarged veins to natural size. They are made of the

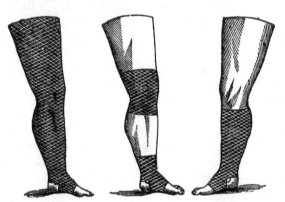

Elastic Stockings, Knee-Caps and Anklets.

best silk, are very durable, and not so expensive as not to be afforded by the poorest sufferer. All those desiring these admirable contrivances are requested to correspond with the author ;—preliminary correspondence as to size, measurement, etc., is in all cases essential to secure that perfect adaptation which is indispensably necessary in order to afford relief and cure. Great harm is done if the elastic appliance is not eligible in every respect, and therefore patients should hesitate before purchasing those inferior, half cotton articles, which are purchasable everywhere ; they do not fulfil the conditions required of them, and are capable of doing great injury, owing to the unequal compression they afford. Preliminary correspondence free.

MILK LEG (PHLEGMASIA DOLENS).

This is caused by inflammation of the crural veins, hence called *crural phlebitis*. The inflammation is owing to the pressure of the gravid womb. The popular idea that in this disease the woman's milk has fallen into her leg, and which has inflamed, is absurd. The disease begins in from two to seven weeks after delivery, with pain in the lower bowel, groin, or thigh. In several days the pain diminishes, and the limb begins to swell, in the calf first most frequently, and from thence extending upward. The skin becomes entirely white, smooth, and glossy, does not pit when pressed, is painful to the touch, and is hotter than the skin of the other limb. Fever is always present.

TREATMENT.—The patient should lie upon her back, with the swelled limb placed upon pillows, or a bolster, raised so that the foot shall be a little higher than the hip, and she should by no means endeavor to walk until the leg is nearly well. A narrow blister can be applied along the course of the vein, and digitalis may be carefully administered. Take an old flannel petticoat, with the hem cut off, and the gathers let out, and dip it in vinegar and hot water, equal parts, wring it out, and cover the whole limb with it. A blanket or oiled silk may be placed underneath to keep it from wetting the bed. Repeat this and keep it up for six hours, and when it becomes tedious to the patient, it should be removed, and the limb bathed with warm sweet oil, two parts, and laudanum, one part, and then covered with flannel. In two or three hours return to the hot water and vinegar, keep up for five or six hours, then resume the warm sweet oil and laudanum, and in this way alternate until the inflammation is subdued, or until the calf of the limb can be shaken. The bowels should be gently moved, and the diuretics administered, and in cases where the inflammation lasts, and the fever is considerable, veratrum should be given. If recovery does not take place after the active inflammation has subsided, the limb should be entirely enveloped by a spiral bandage, or, what is much better, the full-length elastic stocking represented on the foregoing page should be worn. This gives immediate relief, reduces the leg to natural size, and permits the patient to exercise without any injurious results following. Those desiring this indispensable article are requested to correspond with the author.

DISEASES OF THE BLOOD.

SCURVY (SCORBUTUS).

This disease was known to the ancients. The first distinct account of scurvy is contained in the history of the Crusades of Louis IX. against the Saracens of Egypt, during which the French army suffered greatly from it. Lord Anson's voyage, in which more than eighty of every hundred of the original crews perished from the disease, is familiar to every reader of history. This disease illustrates the importance of vegetable food to the human being, as it is a direct result of a diet free from vegetable substances. It used to be very prevalent in the English and American navies, but is now obviated by the ration of lime-juice in the former, and fresh or desiccated vegetables in the latter. It commences with a feeling of languor, or general debility and mental despondency ; a sense of fatigue is experienced on the slightest exertion ; the face is either pale or sallow, and presents an appearance of puffiness ; the gums are swollen, soft, and of a purplish color, and bleed easily ; the breath becomes offensive, and an eruption appears on the body.   The mucous surfaces frequently bleed, the feet become swollen and hard and painful, and a disposition is evinced to inflammation of a low grade of the viscera, and also to hemorrhagic effusions. The tongue and appetite remain unaffected, and death is produced either by debility or hemorrhage—the intellect remaining sound to the last.

TREATMENT.—Nothing will avail in the absence of fresh vegetable food, and hence the chief treatment consists in giving vegetable food, or the vegetable acid, as citric acid or lemon-juice.   Cabbage and potatoes are excellent, aud milk is a good article of diet.   If fresh vegetables cannot be obtained, dried fruits should be substituted.   If the disease has advanced, and there is sponginess of the gums, myricin, rhusin, and hydrastin may be given in combination with capsicum and cream. If active hemorrhage occurs, the oils of turpentine, solidago, and mecca oil may be used to advantage.   If chronic blood derangement follows, as is often the case, the alteratives should be given, of which my " Blood Purifier " (see page 471) is the best.

HEMORRHAGES.

BLEEDING FROM THE NOSE (EPISTAXIS).

There is no part of the body more disposed to hemorrhage than the mucous membrane of the nose.   The blood effused through this membrane escapes generally through the nostrils, but may enter the mouth through the posterior nares.   It is often symptomatic of diseases of the liver, spleen, and other organs, and generally attends the last stages of malignant and low fevers.   It may be slight or dangerously profuse. In plethoric or robust patients it constitutes often a means of relief to the vascular system.

TREATMENT.—When it becomes necessary to check the hemorrhage, the patient should be placed in a cool room, the head elevated or held upright, and the feet plunged in warm water containing mustard. The neck should be bared, and cold water aspersed over it and the face. Lemonade and cooling drinks may also be given.   When it becomes habitual, or periodic, and especially if it be vicarious of menstruation, it may be anticipated by local depletion on the nape of the neck.   In the passive states of the disease, the astringents should be injected into the nose.   Tannin, matico, Monsel's solution, etc., are the best.

If it will not stop, the nostrils should be plugged both anteriorly and posteriorly.

HÆMOPTYSIS.

This is a hemorrhage from the respiratory organs. The blood that is expectorated comes from three different sources. It may come from the mucous membrane of the bronchial tubes, from a vessel ulcerated in a tuberculous cavity as in consumption, and from an aneurism of the aorta, or from the large trunks arising from it, in which case it soon proves fatal. Some cases depend on suppression of the menses, and are habitual and not dangerous, but in the majority of cases it is caused by disease of the heart, or consequent to irritation of tubercles. It may be simple, the blood being all spit up, or it may be attended by an infiltration of blood into the minute tubes and air cells, rendering a portion of the lung solid. The symptoms are some degree of pain or oppression at the chest, with cough, which brings up mouthfuls of blood, fluid or clotted. The quantity may vary from a tea-spoonful to several pints, so that the patient may be suffocated by the abundance of the blood.

TREATMENT.—A free current of air should be allowed to pass over the patient, his covering should be light, and a mild purge should be given to him. The feet should be placed in hot water. If dependent upon derangement of the menses, the sitz-bath (hot) should be ordered, and matico or other astringents be given. Or it may be arrested by putting one drachm of the oil of origanum in a pint bottle, and allow the patient to inhale the vapor. If matico, tannin, or other vegetable astringents are not at hand, common salt, acetate of lead, sulphuric acid, and alum may be used in case of emergency. Small doses of digitalis should be given to control the circulation.

HÆMATEMESIS.

This is hemorrhage from the stomach. Whatever irritates the mucous surface of the stomach, or interrupts the return of blood from that organ is liable to cause this disease. Blows and injuries received by the abdomen, violent concussions of the trunk, pressure, intemperance, worms, powerful emetics, suppression of menstrual discharge, application of cold, or of cold and moisture to the lower extremities during perspiration, or the catamenial flow, prolonged constipation and pregnancy, are all liable to cause it. The blood is usually vomited profusely, is sometimes mixed with food, and generally of dark color. The premonitory symptoms are pain or tension about the stomach, with faintness or a sense of sinking, or of anxiety at this region, flatulent or acrid eructations, lassitude with irregular chills and flushes of heat.

13

TREATMENT.—Apply ice to the region of the stomach, and give a full dose of the oil of turpentine conjoined with castor oil, to be repeated if rejected.   Administer the astringents, in all cases the vegetable, but if not at hand, acetate of lead, creasote, tincture of iron, alum whey, sulphuric acid, etc., can be given.   During the discharge total absti- nence is to be observed, but afterwards, mild mucilaginous drinks and farinaceous food in small quantity may be given, and the transition to solid and more nutritious food should be carefully conducted.

HÆMATURIA.

The source of the blood voided through the urethra may be either from the kidney, bladder, or urethra.   When it proceeds from the kidneys, it is attended with a sense of heat and pain in the loins, and sometimes with coldness of the extremities, and the blood is intimately mixed with the urine.   When the disease is in the ureters, there is a sense of pain in their course, and fibrous shreds having the shape of the ureters are voided.   When the hemorrhage is from the bladder, it is usually preceded by heaviness and tension in that region, extending to the perineum, groins, and small of back ; the urine is passed with diffi- culty ; the blood is little, if at all, combined with the urine.   If from the urethra, the blood is red, liquid and pure, and comes away generally drop by drop.

TREATMENT.—This depends upon its seat and cause.   If from the kidneys, the oils of origanum, copaiba, cubebs and turpentine should be administered, and hot packs applied externally.   If the urine is alkaline, as in typhus fever and scurvy, the acids should be given.   If from the bladder or urethra, matico or other vegetable astringents should be injected.   The avoidance of stimulants and absolute rest should be insisted on in every case.

DROPSIES.

If in man a large venous trunk is compressed or obliterated, so that the blood no longer circulates through it, while the collateral vessels can relieve but imperfectly, dropsical effusion is sure to take place. The effusion is proportionate to the size and importance of the vein obliterated.   If, for instance, in the vena cava, or large vein in the abdomen, an obstacle should prevent the return of the blood, the two lower extremities and the scrotum will become filled with serum.   If the trunk of the portal vein is more or less obliterated, the serous col- lection takes place in the abdomen.   If the obstruction occurs at the very centre of circulation, namely the heart, and the return of blood everywhere embarrassed. the dropsy becomes general ; hence dropsy is one of the most common symptoms of heart diseases.   Dropsy is often caused by cold, applied in such a manner as to check the secretions of the skin; is often connected with eruptive diseases, as scarlatina; it may result from granular degeneration of the kidneys, debility, exhaustion from loss of blood, etc. ; or from obstruction to the return of venous blood, owing to tumors, hypertrophy of the liver, glandular enlargements, etc.

BRIGHT'S DISEASE OF THE KIDNEY.

This is a dropsy owing to a disease of the kidneys. Dr. Bright, of England, first pointed out, 1827, the frequent connection which exists between dropsy and what has since been called granular degeneration of the kidneys, or " Bright's Disease." This state of the kidneys is not an inflammation, but a slow degeneration of its structure, commencing by an abnormal deposit of fat in the cells lining the little tubes in the kidneys. It is a degeneration similar to the tubercular deposit, or the fatty liver common in consumption, and may properly receive the name of *fatty kidney*. It is a slow, insidious disease, beginning generally much further back than the patient is aware of. By degrees the tubes of the kidneys become blocked up with excessive fatty deposits; the result of this is, that the tubes become dilated, so as to press on the network of the portal veins which surround them. The veins being thus compressed, the capillaries which open into them are unable to discharge their contents, and so become distended with blood, and either allow serum to exude from their walls, or else burst and admit the escape of red particles and fibrine. This may be illustrated in a familiar way. If the mouth of all the little brooklets that flow into a brook be effectively dammed up, so that the brook received none of their supply, the brooklets by constant accession would naturally overflow their banks and inundate the adjacent land, and the brook go dry. So as the accumulation of the fat goes on, the portal networks of veins and the uriniferous tubes waste away or become atrophied, and hence shrinking of the kidney and deficiency of the kidney ensue. Albumen is always present in the urine in this disease. This can be discovered by boiling the urine in a small tube, the albumen becoming like the white of an egg boiled. Urea, a natural constituent of the urine, is deficient.

The symptoms in the first stage are weakness and dyspepsia, and the blood loses its red particles very rapidly, but there is little to call attention to the kidneys. In the second stage the symptoms are a pallid, pasty complexion, a dry hard skin, drowsiness, weakness, indigestion, and frequent nausea, often retching the first thing in the morning, and palpitation of the heart. A most characteristic symptom is that the patient is awakened several times in the night with desire to make water. In the third stage, if the patient is exposed to cold, the kidney becomes congested; anasarca or general dropsy with perhaps ascites, makes its appearance ; debility increases, the urinary secretion becomes more inefficient, urea and other excrementitious matter accu·mulate in the blood; a drowsiness and coma, signs of effusion of blood, are sure precursors of death. It is caused by intemperance, privation of air and light, and neglect of proper exercise ; frequent exposure to cold, and the other causes of scrofula and consumption.

TREATMENT.—This is one of those harassing complaints which physicians in family practice seldom have the patience to investigate and manage with sufficient care.

The condition of the stomach, bowels and skin should receive especial attention. Free action of the skin should be maintained, as in this way the kidneys are relieved and the blood purified. Stimulating diuretics should not be used. Mecca oil, tonic teas, etc., may be given. There is no better specific agent than helonin, from three to ten grains a day. Eupurpurin and populin may also be given with good effect. Vapor baths are beneficial, and counter-irritation should be made over the region of the kidneys.

It is my confident belief that this grave disease can be cured in nearly every instance if not too far advanced. I am induced to such a belief by the success that attends my treatment. I should be happy to correspond with any one of my readers who may suspect this affection, and shall cheerfully analyze any urine that may be sent to me for that purpose, as in my laboratory there are all conveniences for that purpose. (See page 390). For those under my treatment the analyses are gratuitously made, but to others a fee of $5 must in all instances be remitted.

ASCITES.

This is a collection of water in the belly, though sometimes the fluid is outside of the peritoneum and next to the muscles. There is a sense of distension and weight, especially on the side on which the patient lies. When the collection is large, the breathing becomes short and difficult, and the swelling is uniform over the whole abdomen. In some instances the fluctuation may be heard when the patient moves about. This sound distinguishes this complaint from pregnancy or peritonitis. There are generally loss of appetite, dry skin, costiveness, scanty urine, oppression of the chest, cough, colic pains, and variable pulse. A frequent cause of this complaint is chronic inflammation of the peritoneum ; it is also produced by scarlet fever, hob-nailed liver, and other diseases of that organ—in short, whatever obstructs the portal circulation.

TREATMENT.--The remedies for this disease are mainly diuretics and purgatives. Digitalis is an excellent remedy, but should be cautiously administered. The patient should have as a constant drink an infusion of two parts of hair-cap moss, and one each of juniper berries and dwarf-elder bark ; also an infusion of queen of the meadow. The purgatives that produce watery stools, such as elaterium, should be given. The compound infusion of parsley is about the best agent to promote the absorption of the fluid. The skin should be kept well open, and the strictest temperance both in eating and drinking must also be observed. If all medicinal treatment fails, the surgeon should be called, who will perform *paracentesis abdominis*, or tapping the abdomen ; but this should be deferred until all other means have failed.

HYDROTHORAX.

This is a dropsy of the pleura, rarely existing as an independent affection, but generally associated with a general dropsical condition of the system. It is particularly liable to be connected with organic heart disease. When the effusion is slight, only a slight uneasiness is felt in the lower part of the chest, but as it increases, the patient suffers uneasiness in assuming the recumbent posture, a cough and difficulty of breathing being the result. The latter often becomes very severe, the face swells, the cheeks assume a purple and the lips a livid hue, the skin is dry, urine scanty, bowels constipated, thirst, and more or less mental excitement ensues.

TREATMENT.—If owing to heart disease, that affection should receive special attention. The fluid may be evacuated by means of small doses of elaterium and podophyllum, followed by a free use of chimaphila, galium aparine, and aralia hispida. Other diuretics may also be used, and the general rules of treatment observed as advised in Ascites.

DROPSY OF THE HEART.

This consists of a collection of fluid within the pericardium. There is a feeling of uneasiness, or pressure in the cardiac region, a slight cough, difficult and irregular respiration, faintness, disinclination to lie down, a feeble pulse, capricious appetite, disturbed sleep and delirium. If there is stupor, cold extremities, the perspiration clammy, and the action of the heart very much disordered, it usually proves fatal.

TREATMENT.—Same as for Hydrothorax. Tapping may become necessary in both cases.

DROPSY OF THE OVARIES.

This consists of an accumulation of fluid in one or more cells within the ovary, or in a serous cyst connected with the uterine appendages. The ovary loses its original form and structure, and frequently attains an immense size, containing several gallons of water. The effusion sadly interferes with respiration, and it causes exhaustion and often peritonitis. The serum may exist within the cavity of the abdomen, or be confined within the cystic tumor. As the tumor enlarges, it ascends the pelvis and occupies more and more of the abdominal cavity, and may float loosely in the fluid within it, and form adhesions to the peritoneum, omentum, or neighboring viscera.

TREATMENT. - Galvanism is often very successful. The current should be passed through the tumor, and be as strong as the patient can bear it, and should be passed in all directions for half an hour several times a day. The hydragogue cathartics and diuretics should also be given, and the alteratives administered. The strength of the patient should be well supported.

This disease is curable by medicinal treatment alone in its early stages if properly treated, but may become so far advanced under improper management, that tapping becomes necessary, or, if the patient's strength will allow, the removal of the whole tumor.

The author would be pleased to correspond with any lady suffering from this serious disease.

DROPSY OF THE SCROTUM (HYDROCELE).

This is a collection of water in the membrane which surrounds the testicles. It is often caused by rheumatism, gout, scrofula, etc. In some cases the accumulation is very large. It may be distinguished from scrotal hernia by pressing the tumor towards the anus; if it bounds rapidly forward it is hydrocele.

TREATMENT.—The following is excellent. Take queen of the meadow, one ounce; colt's foot, one-fourth pound; yellow parilla, one-fourth pound. Make one quart of decoction or syrup, and take one table-spoonful three times a day. A suspensory bandage should be worn. These can be had from me at reasonable prices. In some cases the scrotum must be tapped, and the vinous tincture of hemlock bark injected to prevent the return of the effusions.

I have under my treatment at all times many dropsical patients, and if received under my care at a reasonable early stage, no necessity for tapping arises, and the patient is cured by medicinal treatment alone. Any one desirous of consulting me, may refer to page 390 for the necessary question to be answered.

ANATOMY OF THE URINARY ORGANS.

KIDNEYS.

The kidneys are two hard glands for the secretion of urine, placed in each lumbar region, just above the hips; they are outside of the peritoneum, or lining membrane of the abdomen, and surrounded with an abundance of fat. The *right kidney* is rather lower than the left, on account of the superposition of the liver. The *length* is about four inches, and the breadth two inches. The shape is oval, resembling a bean ; the position upright, and the fissure (or *hilum*) is directed to the spinal column. The upper end of the kidney is rather larger than the lower. It is covered by a strong *fibrous capsule*. The color is a reddish brown. Upon making a longitudinal section of the kidney, as represented in cut, two different structures are presented. The internal is of a darker color, and consists of about fifteen of what are called the *cones of Malpighi*,[3] which are arranged in three rows, the apex of each converging towards the hilum. This constitutes the *medullary* portion of the kidneys. The external structure is of lighter color usually, is extremely vascular, and of a granulated arrangement ; it constitutes the *cortical* portion. The urine is formed in the tortuous tubes of the cortical substance,[2] between whose walls are a number of small bodies called *corpuscles of Malpighi*. At the apex of each cone is the *papilla renalis*, and in the centre of each papilla is a slight depression, called *foveola*. Each papilla is surrounded

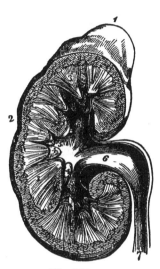

The Kidney.

by a small membranous cup, called *infundibulum*,[4] into which the urine is first received as it oozes from the orifices of the papillæ. Four or five of these infundibula join to form a common trunk, called *calyx*,[5] and the junction of about three calyces forms a common cavity, called the *pelvis*,[6] which is conoidal in shape, and from which proceeds the ureter,[7] the excretory tube of the kidney, which conveys the urine to the bladder. The ureter is a cylindrical tube of the size of a quill, with thin, extensible walls. It enters the inferior fundus of the bladder very obliquely, and opens by a very small orifice.

Just above the kidney, and reposing on its upper extremity, placed one on each side, are two small bodies, varying much in size, called the *supra-renal capsules*.[1] They have no secretion, consequently no duct, but evidently perform important functions in fœtal life, when they are much larger.

BLADDER.

The bladder is a musculo-membranous sac for the reception of urine. It is situated in the cavity of the pelvis, behind the pubic bones, and in front of the rectum in the male, but in the female the uterus and vagina are between the rectum and bladder. In shape the bladder is oval, the larger end being downwards ; in women it is more spheroidal ; in children it is pear-shaped. It is divided into a superior and inferior *fundus*, a *body*, and *neck*.

Its dimensions vary with health and disease. Ordinarily it will hold about a pint. At the neck of the bladder is a circular muscle, called the *sphincter*, which, in a state of contraction, retains the urine in the bladder until the necessity to voiding it arises. The *urethra* is described under anatomy of the sexual organs.

DISEASES OF THE URINARY ORGANS.

NEPHRITIS.

This is inflammation of the kidneys, and which may occur either in its substance, its lining membrane, or in its capsule. The symptoms are deep-seated pain in the small of the back, extending down the groins in one or both sides, increased by pressure; urination either increased or diminished, urine scanty and high-colored, and mixed with blood or gravelly matters. If both kidneys are affected the urine may be suppressed, and comatose symptoms present themselves. Chills, fever, deranged stomach, and constipation nearly always attend it. The testicle is retracted, which distinguishes this disease from lumbago, etc. It runs very rapidly into suppuration, the sign of which is the appearance of pus in the urine.

TREATMENT.—The disease should be controlled by the use of hot packs, vapor baths, lobelia emetics, mild purges, and the internal administration of aconite and veratrum. The mucilaginous drinks should be drunk, and the opiates given if the pain is very severe. In chronic nephritis, where there is debility of the organ, the best remedies are turpentine, copaiba, buchu, uva ursi, pareira brava, and pipsissewa.

DIURESIS.

This is the *diabetes insipidus* of some writers. By this term is understood the excessive secretion of pale, limpid urine, without sugar. The principal symptoms are insatiable thirst and the elimination of a large quantity of urine. These symptoms are usually preceded by a variable appetite, constipation, and derangement of the functions of the skin. The copious flow of urine may only be occasional, following over-mental or physical excitement. It may be distinguished from *diabetes mellitus* by the absence of sugar in the urine.

TREATMENT.—The skin should receive special attention, and excess of drinking should be avoided. The constitutional debility should be overcome with baths, and the general tonics; apocynin, from one-eighth to one-fourth of a grain, four or five times a day, is a specific for this disease.

DIABETES MELLITUS.

This is characterized by increase of urine, containing sugar. The first indications of this disease are languor, dry, and harsh skin, intense thirst, pain in the small of back, constipation, with alternate chill and fever. After a time the general health gives way, and there are muscular weakness, loss of sexual power, pain in the loins, coldness of extremities, a burning sensation in the hands and feet, loss of weight, and a chloroform odor of breath. The gums become spongy, the teeth decay, the mind becomes depressed and irritable, and the appetite voracious. Consumption is often a sequel to this disease. The urine has a sweetish taste, due to the presence of sugar, which can readily be discovered by adding yeast to the urine, which gives rise to various fermentation.

TREATMENT.—A healthy state of the general system should be maintained by fresh air, frequent baths, and a generous diet. No saccharine or starchy articles of food should be eaten. The bowels and liver should be gently stimulated by small doses of leptandrin and leontodin. Great success is obtained by the use of unicorn root. Mecca oil has also been successfully employed in this disease.

Diabetic patients who may desire the author to treat them, may consult him as directed on page 390.

GRAVEL (LITHIASIS).

This disorder consists in the deposition from the urine, within the body, of an insoluble sand-like matter. In health the urine carries off the results of the waste and disintegration of the tissues in a soluble state, but when these matters are in excess the urine frequently deposits them after being voided, on cooling. This often occurs after irregularities of diet, without actually being a morbid condition, but when the accumulation is excessive it causes a serious disease. The gravels are chemically either urates, lithates, phosphates, or oxalates, according to the diathesis of the patient. The passage of gravel or renal calculi from the kidneys to the bladder through the ureters, causes the most excruciating pain. When anything in the bladder, as a mucous shred or a large gravel, acts as a nucleus, the constant accessions to this nucleus form what is known as *stone in the bladder*, which may be of various sizes.

In gravel the patient has a dull aching pain in the back, attended with urgent and frequent desire to urinate, preceded by cutting or scalding pains in the urethra, neck of bladder, or in the course of the ureters. In stone we have the same symptoms, but the sudden stoppage of the stream during micturition is always suggestive of its presence in the bladder, and the patient has a constant desire to relieve the pain by pulling at the end of his penis.

TREATMENT.—Diluents should be freely used, and a strict attention

13*

paid to diet. Animal food should be sparingly eaten, and alcoholic drinks totally avoided. The chemical nature of the gravel should be ascertained, and when this is done the chemical opposites administered. No treatment will avail, if not in chemical opposition to the diathesis of the patient. If medicinal treatment is ineffectual after a stone has been formed, the surgeon should be consulted, who will remove it by an operation called *lithotrity* or another termed *lithontripsy*.

Unless the stone be too large, my experience is that solvent treatment will prove effectual in nearly every case. The solvent treatment consists, of course, of such herbal agents as are chemically opposed to the nature of the calculus. By such a course of medication my success has been most gratifying.

ISCHURIA, OR SUPPRESSION OF URINE.

This frequently attends inflammatory diseases, especially acute nephritis. It may either arise from an irritation of the kidney beyond the point of secretion, or from a torpor or paralysis of the kidneys. It is important to distinguish it from *retention of urine*. It is sometimes very dangerous, being attended with vomiting, drowsiness, coma and convulsions. A vicarious secretion from the skin, bowels, etc., is also often established. It is evidently due to a sort of paralysis of the nerve centres.

TREATMENT.—Leeches may be placed over the loins, and digitalis or squill administered. The demulcent drinks should be freely used. If uric acid is in excess, some carbonate may be given. If dependent upon torpor, the stimulating diuretics, as turpentine, should be used. Frequent hot sitz-baths are also beneficial.

INCONTINENCE OF URINE (ENURESIS).

This is often associated with some constitutional weakness. The bladder may be exclusively irritated and not be able to hold the urine, or the little circular muscle at the neck of the bladder may be debilitated or paralyzed, owing to acridity of the urine. In some cases it may be owing to debility of the kidneys.

TREATMENT.—A course of tonics, sea-bathing, cold baths, warm clothing, etc., together with astringents and stimulating diuretics, will usually cure it. Small doses of the extract of belladona will also afford relief. In case of paralysis of the bladder, nux vomica, electricity, counter-irritant application to the spine, and local irritants are necessary.

CYSTITIS.

This is an inflammation of the bladder. The symptoms are pain above the pubes, tenderness on pressure, the pain extending into the penis, scrotum, and perineum, producing straining and pain in urination ;

sometimes pain over the abdomen, which is swollen, or the inflammation may extend to the peritoneum, causing peritonitis. It may terminate in suppuration, the pus appearing in the urine, or, if the abscess occurs in the coats of the bladder, it may open suddenly. It is caused by direct irritation as by a catheter ; also by gonorrhœa, difficult labor, turpentine, cantharides, etc. When the inflammation becomes chronic it is called " *Catarrh of the Bladder.*"

TREATMENT.—Mucilaginous drinks should be freely used, such as decoctions of marsh-mallow, uva ursi, etc. Dover's powder may be given to relieve the pain. About three grains of populin and one-fourth of a grain of gelsemium given three or four times a day, exerts a marked beneficial influence in this disease ; linseed oil and essential tincture of hydrangea are also remedies of great value. The chronic form will require special treatment, in accordance to condition and nature of each case.

ANATOMY OF THE NERVOUS SYSTEM.

The principal divisions of the nervous system are the brain, spinal marrow, and nerves. The tissue of this system is included in membranes or sheaths, and consists of two differently colored pulpy materials, one of which is *white* or *medullary*, and the other *gray*, *cortical*, or *cineritious*. The sheath of the nerves is called the *neurilemma*, and the internal material *neurine*. All ganglia and nervous centres consist of a mixture of white fibres and gray globules.

An *anastomosis* is the interchange of fasciculi between two trunks, each fasciculus remaining unaltered, although in contact with another. A combination of anastomoses into a network is called a *plexus*.

SPINAL MARROW.

The spinal marrow is the medullary column included within the bones or vertebræ of the spinal column. It has three coverings : 1st, The *dura mater*, which is a white fibrous membrane, and forms the external ; 2d, The *arachnoid*, a serous membrane, forming the middle covering. It is extremely thin and transparent ; 3d, The *pia mater*, a cellular membrane, forming the immediate covering. It is very vascular, consisting almost entirely of vessels.

THE BRAIN.

The brain consists of four principal parts : medulla oblongata, pons varolii, cerebrum, and cerebellum. Like the spinal marrow it also has three coverings bearing the same names. The *dura mater* adheres very firmly to the bones of the cranium, and consists of two laminæ, which are divided into folds called *falx cerebri, tentorium,* and *falx cerebelli.*

The medulla oblongata is the upper part of the spinal cord ; it is conical in shape, and extends from the first bone of the spinal column to the pons varolii. Its divisions are the *corpori pyramidale, olivare* and *restiforme*.

The pons varolii is cuboidal in shape, and situated just in front of the medulla.

The cerebrum is the largest mass composing the brain. It is oval in shape, and weighs from three to four pounds. It is divided into two hemispheres, each hemisphere consisting of an anterior, middle, and posterior lobe. The surface presents a number of convolutions, or *gyri*, each separated by deep fissures, or *sulci*. The interior of each hemisphere is medullary in character, and the surface of each convolution is cineritious for the depth of about one-sixth of an inch.

The ventricles of the brain are five in number : they are called the *right* and *left lateral*, the *third, fourth*, and *fifth ventricles*.

The more minute anatomy of the cerebrum is exceeding complex, and not of special importance in a popular work of this kind.

The cerebellum constitutes about one-sixth of the brain, and is contained between the occiput and tentorium. It is oblong and flattened in shape, and composed of white and gray substances.

CRANIAL NERVES.

These are nine in number, and all emerge from the foramina, or opening at the base of the brain. They are designated by their function as well as numerically, viz. : 1st, olfactory ; 2d, optic ; 3d, motor oculi ; 4th, patheticus ; 5th, trifacial ; 6th, motor externus ; 7th, facial and auditory ; 8th, pneumogastric, glosso-pharyngeal, and spinal accessory ; 9th, hypoglossal.

According to function the cranial nerves may be divided into three classes, viz. : *nerves of special sense*, including the 1st, 2d, and the auditory branch of the 7th ; *nerves of motion*, including the 3d, 4th, 6th, facial branch of the 7th and 9th ; *compound nerves*, comprising the 8th and 5th.

The principal nerve of the arm is the *brachial ;* of the forearm, the *ulnar* and *radial ;* of the thigh, the *great sciatic*, which divides, about one-third above the knee, into two large branches, the *peroneal and popliteal ;* further on the popliteal is called the *posterior tibial*. In the pelvis there are the *pudic, gluteal*, and *lesser ischiatic*.

The *sympathetic nerve* is distributed with all the other nerves of the body, and by means of plexuses supplies all the internal organs.

The nervous system is a complex piece of machinery, and its anatomy requires much study before any competent familiarity with it can be gained. The physician, who has an inadequate knowledge of the anatomy of the nervous system, and philosophy of nervous phenomena, or the physiology pertaining thereto, cannot hope to treat diseases assailing the system with any material success. Competence in this respect is the reward only of a long devotion, and practical experience.

DISEASES OF THE NERVOUS SYSTEM.

INFLAMMATION OF THE BRAIN (CEREBRITIS).

This consists of inflammation of the cerebral substance, and due to long exposure to a vertical sun, the inordinate use of ardent spirits, cold, fright, external injury, the sudden disappearance of an old discharge, and it sometimes occurs as a consequent on small-pox, or erysipelas of the face and scalp, and fevers. The symptoms are violent inflammatory fever, hot and dry skin, flushed countenance, suffused eyes, quick and hard pulse, the arteries of the neck throb, and delirium. The senses are morbidly acute, there being intolerance of light and sound. The person is extremely restless, the muscles of the face are spasmodically contracted, the upper eye-lids hang down, and as the disease progresses, blindness and deafness ensue. The countenance is vacant or idiotic, the eye loses its lustre, the pupils become dilated, and the eyes often squint. In the still more advanced stage, the discharges pass off involuntarily, the countenance becomes pale and sunken, the pulse weak and irregular, the coma more profound, and death soon closes the scene. It is commonly called " Brain Fever."

TREATMENT.—This should be most energetic. Bleeding to fainting has been the practice of many physicians, but I deem it unnecessary, as revulsion can be made by other means. Leeches may, however, be applied to the scalp. The hair should be closely shaved from the head, and ice, alcohol or ether, with water, applied to the head. The decoction of ladies'-slipper should be given internally. At the outset purgatives should be given. Those that act thoroughly, such as gamboge, colocynth, etc., are the best. The bladder should be emptied every day. In the stage of collapse, stimulants may be given.

APOPLEXY.

This is a condition in which all the functions of animal life are suddenly stopped, except the pulse and the breathing. There is neither thought nor feeling, nor voluntary motion; and the patient suddenly falls down, and lies as if in a deep sleep. The disease assails in three different ways. The first form of attack is a sudden falling down into a state of insensibility and apparently deep sleep, the face being generally flushed, the breathing stertorous, or snoring, the pulse full and not frequent, with occasional convulsions. From this mode of attack death often occurs immediately, but in some cases recovery occurs, with the exception of paralysis of one side, or the loss of speech, or some of the senses. The second mode of attack begins with sudden pain in the head, and the patient becomes pale, faint, sick, and vomits. His pulse is feeble, has a cold skin, and occasionally some convulsions. He may fall down, or be only a little confused, but soon recovers from all the symptoms, except the headache; this will continue, and the patient will sooner or later become heavy, forgetful, unable to connect ideas, and finally sink into insensibility from which he never rises. This mode of invasion, though not so frightful as the first, is of much more serious import.

The third form of attack is where consciousness is retained, but power on one side of the body is suddenly lost. The patient retains his mind, and answers questions rationally, either by signs or words. He may either die soon, or live for years, with imperfect speech, or a leg dragging after him, or an arm hanging uselessly by his side.

Those persons who have large heads, red faces, short and thick necks, and a short, stout, square build, are more predisposed to this disease, than thin, pale and tall persons. Literary men, especially editors, lawyers, doctors, etc., are subject to this disease, owing to mental overwork.

The symptoms preceding an apoplectic attack are headache, vertigo, double vision, faltering speech, inability to remember certain words, sometimes forgetfulness of one's one name, a frequent losing of a train of ideas, and occasionally an unaccountable dread. It is caused by whatever hurries the circulation as strong bodily exercise, emotional excitement, exposure to the sun or severe cold, tight cravats, etc.

TREATMENT.—If the face is turgescent and red, and the temporal arteries throb, and the pulse full and hard, the patient should be placed in a semi-recumbent position, with his head raised, his clothes loosened, particularly his neck-band and shirt collar, and then quickly as possible, cold water or ice should be applied to the head, leeches to the nape of the neck, and mustard plasters to the calves of the leg. Tight ligatures may also be tied around the thighs, sufficiently tight to arrest the venous circulation; they should be removed gradually as consciousness returns. Administer a stimulating purgative, as a few drops of croton oil. Injections may also be given. If the patient is old, and the pulse feeble, the ice applications, ligature, etc., may be omitted, and instead apply warm flannels and warm bricks to the body, and administer camphor. To prevent future attacks, gentle tonics should be given, and the skin kept healthy by daily bathing and friction. The bowels must not be permitted to become costive. The diet should be well regulated. The mind should be kept cheerful and hopeful, and free from all excitement. Intoxicating drinks should be totally avoided, and sexual congress should be of rare occurrence. In fact every thing that might provoke an attack should be avoided.

CONGESTION OF THE BRAIN.

This consists of an accumulation of blood in the cerebral vessels. The countenance is flushed, the eyes suffused, light becomes intolerable, and there is singing in the ears, vertigo, momentary loss of speech, and sometimes delirium. Simple congestion is merely a functional affection, and in a slight or moderate degree involves no immediate danger. It may, however, produce apoplexy and sudden death. It is caused by any mechanical impediment to the return of blood from the head, as tumor of the neck, heart disease, etc. It is a concomitant to nearly every inflammatory cerebral affection.

TREATMENT.—The treatment consists in diverting the blood from the head by hot mustard foot baths, and an active cathartic. Ice or cold water may also be applied to the head, and the circulation reduced by veratrum. The treatment is the same as advised in apoplexy, in all essential particulars.

SUNSTROKE.

The injury done to the brain in this case is the same as in apoplexy, with the exception of the clot. It is essentially congestion of the brain. Persons who are exposed by necessity of pursuit to the extreme heat of the sun, should be protected by a wet cloth or cabbage-leaves placed on the head and under a light hat. The symptoms are first dizziness, followed by intense headache. Thirst becomes excessive, the pulse indistinct at the wrist, violent throbbing of the carotid and temporal arteries, and insensibility ensues by a convulsive shivering of the body.

TREATMENT.—Place the patient immediately in a cool and shady place, and instantly apply, copiously, cold water, or, what is better, pounded ice in a bag, to the head. Make friction over his legs to relieve the congested state of the brain. Application of turpentine by friction on the spine is also of service. Inhalation of ammonia or hartshorn is beneficial, and a small quantity of the carbonate of that substance may be given internally. Continue this treatment until the patient is out of danger, or until death ensues. In plethoric patients, bleeding from the arm is required, and in this instance only is bleeding advisable. After the patient becomes conscious and apparently out of danger, he is to be removed to his home, and a brisk cathartic administered, to effect revulsion. In no case should he be allowed again to expose himself to sun during the first four or five days after the occurrence of the sunstroke. The application of water or ice to the head should be abandoned by gradual increase of temperature, to prevent any reaction

INSANITY.

This is an unsound manifestation of intellectual power. The indications which should excite alarm are headache, vertigo, mental confusion, fretful temper, inaptitude for usual occupations, defective articulations, dimness of vision, and flightiness of manner. The patient is also aware that he is not right, he shuns his old friends, has frightful dreams, is tortured with wicked thoughts. If it exists with general paralysis it is frequently incurable. Derangement is manifested in various ways, viz :—

1st. *Mania.*—This is characterized by general delirium, in which the reasoning faculty is disturbed and confused, if not lost, ideas absurd, wandering, or erroneous ; conduct violent, excited, and extremely mischievous. The maniac's hair is crisped, he neglects his family and business, suspects his friends, dislikes the light, and certain colors horrify him, his ears are sometimes very red, noise excites and disturbs him, and he has frequent fits of anger and melancholy, without any cause. His delirium extends to all subjects, and the entire intellect, affections and will are in a chaotic wreck.

In *puerperal mania* occurring after delivery, the delirium is frequently extreme, there being a tendency to suicide or child-murder. Maniacs in general have a disposition to murder or suicide.

2d. *Monomania.* This is characterized by mental aberration on one subject. The patient seizes upon a false principle, and draws from it injurious conclusions, which modify and change his whole life and character. In other cases the intellect is sound, but the affections and disposition being perverted, their acts are strange and inconsistent. Attempt is made to justify their hallucinations by plausible reasoning.

3d. *Dementia.* This is a condition in which the weakness of intellect is induced by accident or old age. The ideas are numerous, but vague, confused and wandering; the memory is impaired, and the manners childish, silly and undecided.

4th. *Moral Mania.* Moral insanity is a condition in which there is a perversion of the natural feelings, affections, temper, habits, and moral dispositions. The conduct is eccentric, and an uncontrolable destructive tendency, or a propensity to every species of mischief, are frequently the leading features. A slight insanity is popularly called "a kink in the head;" in Scotland, "a bee in the bonnet."

If insanity is characterized by fear, moroseness and prolonged sadness, it is called *lypemania* or *melancholia.* If religion is the theme of delirium, it is termed *theomania.* If amatory delusions rule, it is called *erotomania.* If the suicidal tendency is strong, it is designated *autophomania,* and if characterized by aversion to man and society, it is called *misanthropia.* If the tendency is to stealing, it constitutes *kleptomania.* *Close confinement,* and *low diet,* such conveniences as prisons afford, are the best cures for this species of mania.

It is a pitiful sight to see the thousand fancies in regard to themselves of the insane. One imagines himself as an inspired individual, and charged with the conversion of the world, while another sincerely believes that the devil has entered into him, and he curses God, himself and the universe. Still another believes that he controls the world, and directs the movements of the planets. One believes that all the wisdom is concentrated in him, and offers to teach the wisest. Another imagines himself some grand king, is proud, withdraws from his fellows, and will allow no one to come in his presence without proper acts of homage. Yet another is Napoleon, or some other great general, and he fights his battles anew, and majestically marshals his imaginary army. *Idiocy* is owing to a congenital deficiency of mind, and in consequence the idiot may often be a deaf-mute, and be governed by insane passions.

The cause of insanity is hereditary predisposition, constant revolution in the mind of some painful thought, injured feelings which cannot be resented, mortified pride, perplexity in business, disappointed affections or ambition, political or religious excitement, loss of friends or property, and in general, whatever worries the mind or creates a deep distress. Another prolific cause is masturbation.

TREATMENT.—The real character of the malady should be ascertained, and, if possible, the pathological condition giving rise to the disorder corrected. Out-door exercise, lively amusements, fresh air and daily bathing, contribute largely to establish a cure. The exciting cause should be removed. The stomach and bowels should receive due attention. The tonics should be given to improve the general health of the patient. Ladies'-slipper, scullcap, cannabis indica, gelsemium, aconite, veratrum, belladonna, quinine, opium and lupulin, stand in good repute for this disorder. The moral treatment should be such as is best adapted to the condition of the patient. It is probably best, when practicable, to place the patient in some well-conducted insane asylum, where he will have proper attendance and treatment. If this is not feasible, the physician should make such arrangements as will best secure the patient, if of vicious disposition, from harming himself or others, but in no case should unnecessary restraint be placed upon the patient.

I have conducted the treatment in many cases of insanity, many of whom I had never seen, and wherever my instructions were faithfully carried out, a cure was generally effected. If any of my readers have relatives or friends who may have become insane, and who may desire to know my opinion of the case, or its chances for cure, and will describe the case to me fully, I will cheerfully state them. (See page 390 for address.)

DELIRIUM TREMENS.

This is also called *mania a potu*, and in common parlance it is the "horrors" or "jim-jams." It is caused by the sudden withdrawal from the habitual or prolonged use of alcoholic stimulation. Its most prominent characteristics are delirious hallucinations, fear, muscular tremors, weak-ness, watchfulness, and the want of sleep. The symptoms are incessant talking, fidgeting with the hands, trembling of the limbs, a rapid pulse, profuse sweating, and a mingling of the real with the imaginary. The patient's face is pale and sallow, his eye is rolling, quick and expressive, and is busy day and night, and can scarcely be confined to his room. He is unwilling to admit that anything ails him, answers questions ration-ally, and does whatever he is bidden at the time. Then he begins to wander again, the expression becomes wild, the eyes vacant or staring, and becomes the victim of pitiful and ludicrous illusions of senses, phan-tasms and hallucinations of every kind; he sees imaginary objects, such as rats, mice, lice, dogs, cats, snakes, and hears and imagines the most extraordinary and absurd delusions. In favorable cases, sleep ends the crisis about the third or fourth day; where death occurs, the delirium is active until sudden suspension of breath ensues.

TREATMENT.—Sleep is the cure for this disease, and opium and its preparations are the sovereign remedies. Give one-third or one-half of a grain of morphia; if this does not produce sleep, give thirty drops of laudanum every two hours till sleep is produced. A draught or two of the patient's accustomed drink may also be given, and large doses of opium may be dispensed with if cold applications are made to the head, and the use of a tepid bath, prolonged for a few hours. Lupulin is also a good remedy.

HEADACHE (CEPHALALGIA).

This, in its widest acceptation, includes all uneasy sensations of the head. It may be confined to one spot, or embrace one side, as in hemi-crania; or it may be diffused, and of indefinite extent. It may be felt in the depths of the brain, or only in the scalp and cranium, and con-tinue for an instant, or last for days and weeks. It is usually paroxysmal, and the pain may be simple or very violent. It is a constant attendant to the different forms of inflammation of the brain. It is caused by various conditions; decayed teeth may cause it. When confined to one side, the pain is of a lancinating character; when due to a disordered stomach, it occurs in the forehead and temples; when it occurs from a congestive state of the brain, it is of a dull, heavy, aching character; when due to spinal irritation, there is a protracted pain in the top or back part of the head; and when it is accompanied by nausea and vomit-ing, it is called "sick-headache."

TREATMENT.—Immediate relief may frequently be obtained by thoroughly evacuating the stomach, and drinking hot tea or coffee, followed by adding ten drops of tincture of belladonna to a tumblerful of water, and taking one tea-spoonful every ten or fifteen minutes. A hot foot-bath and bathing the head in stimulating liniments also afford relief in some cases. If it is due to a full habit, the diet must be regulated. In some bad cases cold applications to the head, leeches to the temples, and hot sinapisms to the spine may be required. Rubbing my "Herbal Ointment" on the forehead, temples, and nape of neck gives instant relief.

HYPOCHONDRIA.

Among the causes of this distressing complaint are disappointment, misfortunes of a heavy character, care, masturbation, excessive mental labor, undue anxiety, costiveness, neglect of cleanliness, indigestion, sedentary occupations, living in close and gloomy apartments, or wet and marshy localities, excessive indulgence in sexual pleasures, or anything which tends to weaken and disturb the nervous system, or over-stimulate the brain. The mental symptoms are countless. The chief one is a constant dread of some unexplainable evil; the patient fears that his wife, if he has one, is unfaithful, or hates him, or that his business is going to ruin, and he will be reduced to beggary, or that his friends despise him, or that he will be charged with the commission of some monstrous crime, or that he has all, or a majority of the worst physical diseases that surgeon or physician was ever summoned to treat. These are the lightest symptoms, and if not immediately attended to, will become aggravated, and go on increasing in violence and extent until the sufferer dies naturally from exhaustion and misery, gets hopelessly insane, or perhaps commits suicide. The organs of sense are more or less deranged, and external sensations are magnified and corrupted even as those of the mind are. Thus, the eye appears to see all sorts of forms which it *does not see;* the smell detects odors which do not exist; the touch demonstrates to the brain objects with which it does not come in contact; the taste is perverted and disordered to an extent which seems, to an uninterested observer, impossible; and the ears convey imaginary sounds of the most perplexing and terrific character. The queer fancies of the hypochondriac are often of such a character as to obliterate pity for the unhappy individual, and provoke both disgust and laughter. Cases have been known where the victim imagined that he was a teapot, or had glass legs which would break upon the lightest exertion, or was made of jelly, and could not move without dissolving into an undistinguishable mass of gelatinous matter, or was as large as an elephant, or as small as a pipe-stem; or had horns growing from the head, or a bottle attached to the end of the nose, or was covered with creeping and venomous insects. Hypochondria is also productive of fainting spells, cold surface of the body, an eye either glassy and unnaturally brilliant, or without any lustre, palpitations, pains in the stomach, pale and livid countenance, and occasional paroxysms of fever.

TREATMENT.—A cure may be effected by the employment of such medicines as will restore tone to the stomach and nervous system, and also by removing, as far as is possible, all the causes which lead to the origin and perpetuation of the malady. Where it is within the scope of the patient's, means he should be kept continually on the move (without fatigue), a constant change of scene being one of the most desirable of self-acting remedies. All allusions to his real or fancied miseries should be avoided, or, if found necessary, of the kindest and most consoling description. It is always the case that the hypochondriac will be the harshest, the most suspicious, and the most ungenerous in every way, towards his best friends. This is an unfailing type of the disease. The friends must bear these annoyances patiently and self-denyingly. To lose one's temper with such a sufferer is to commit a great crime; out-of-door exercise must be as constant as is consistent with the weather and the patient's circumstances. Leave the hypochondriac alone as little as possible. Let him eat and drink but moderately of nourishing but easily-digested food, and above all things keep him from the use of stimulating drinks and tobacco. Music has been found highly beneficial in these cases—anything is good, in fact, which affords lively amusement. A cold or tepid sponge bath should be taken morning and evening, and the rule of "early to bed and early to rise," should never be violated. The bowels must always be kept open—a good passage every twenty-four hours being required—and where the patient is extremely weak, a good substantial tonic, such as "Restorative Assimilant," should be administered three times a day. When the patient has a fainting smell, and thinks he is dying, give him motherwort tea, with spirits of camphor in it, if no other assistance happens to be at hand. This is only general treatment for temporary benefit. To eradicate the disease thoroughly it is necessary to know all about the individual case, and the chief causes of its origin and development. Nature's remedies may then be applied without fear of failure.

NEURALGIA.

This disease affects one tissue only—the nervous, and pain is the only symptom. The pain is of every degree of intensity. It may affect every nerve, but is more commonly confined to the most important. The tearing pain comes on suddenly and in paroxysms. It may be so agonizing as to cause a temporary loss of reason.

When the fifth pair of nerves is affected it is called *tic douleureux;* and *face ache* when confined to the facial nerve and branches. It is called *sciatica* when the pain begins at the hip and follows the course of the sciatic nerve. It may also occur in the female breasts, the womb, in the stomach and bowels, hands and feet, etc.

TREATMENT.—This is palliative and radical. The palliative treatment consists in the administration of aconite, hyoscyamus, ladies'-slipper, belladonna, opium, morphine, lupulin, cicuta, etc. These can either be applied locally, or taken internally. Morphine and aconitin should be injected subcutaneously, and immediate relief follows. In sciatica, blistering along the course of the nerve often cures. Ten grains each of aconitin and extract of belladonna and one drachm of lard, form an excellent ointment for external application. The " Herbal Ointment " (page 472) arrests the pain almost instantly. The radical treatment consists in removing the cause. If due to malarial influence, quinine should be given. If associated with kidney disease, that organ should receive attention. The alteratives are serviceable in many cases.

BILIOUS COLIC.

This is neuralgia of the mesenteric net-work of nerves, or rather hyperæsthesia of the plexus. By hyperæsthesia is meant excessive sensibility or passability. It is characterized by sharp twisting pain extending from the navel to the lower portion of the abdomen. It occurs in paroxysms, and is of a most excruciating character. The patient is restless, hands, feet and cheeks are cold, and the pulse is small and hard. The abdomen is tense and distended ; obstinate constipation, and usually nausea and vomiting occur. The fits usually last from a few moments to several hours. The matter vomited up is generally bilious matter.

TREATMENT.—Administer an active purgative injection immediately, and give internally wild yam, camphor, etc., every fifteen minutes until the pain is relieved. A strong decoction of wild yam root is a specific cure for this affection. Scull-cap and high-cranberry bark are also good. The latter is called *cramp bark* on account of its excellence in spasmodic affections. The vomiting may be checked by laudanum. Hot baths, fomentations, etc., are also useful.

HICCOUGH.

This consists in spasmodic contraction of the midriff, and a certain degree of constriction, which arrests the air in the wind-pipe, thus producing sudden, short, convulsive inspirations, attended by slight sound. and followed immediately by expiration. It is often a symptom of low forms of fever and inflammatory diseases, or caused by the excessive use of alcohol or tobacco.

TREATMENT.—When purely nervous, suddenly attracting the mind will cure it. Hence the common advice to the hiccoughing patient, " think of your sweetheart " is so often effectual, because the fond object absorbs the whole mind. · When dependent upon a disordered state of the stomach, an emetic will relieve it. In fevers it denotes debility, indicating the need of stimulants.

WHOOPING COUGH (PERTUSSIS).

This is a hyperæsthesia of the pneumo-gastric nerve, and not due to inflammation, as may be supposed. It is a contagious disease. It consists of a convulsive cough, attended by hissing and rattling in the windpipe, and ineffectual efforts to expel the breath. This is repeated until a quantity of thick, tenacious mucus is expectorated, when the breathing again becomes free. The paroxysms apparently threaten suffocation, and the agitation affects the whole body. Blood is sometimes started from the nostrils, but, notwithstanding the violence of the symptoms, it is rarely ever dangerous.

TREATMENT.—An emetic may be given at first. Liniments of olive oil or the "Herbal Ointment" should be applied to the spine. The antispasmodics are or course indicated, such as belladonna, a decoction of bitter almond, or of cherry seed, etc. Lobelia is a good remedy, as is also skunk cabbage; daily vapor inhalations are also serviceable; cochineal has a good reputation; it should be used with stillingia.

SPASM OF THE GLOTTIS.

This is also called the *crowing disease* or *false croup*. It is common to children, and rarely occurs in adults. It is a spasmodic disease, and distinguishable from croup by the absence of fever. The child is suddenly taken with an impossibility of taking breath, and struggles convulsively for a time, its head thrown back, face pale, legs and arms stiff, and when it begins to breathe it is of a crowing character.

TREATMENT.—In the paroxysm set the child in an upright position, exposed to a full draught of cool and fresh air, and sprinkle cold water in its face. Loosen all its clothes around the neck, slap it slightly on the back, and apply friction along the spine. If not successful, place it in a warm bath, and then sprinkle cold water in its face. If due to teething, use the proper remedies, and give some gentle physic.

EPILEPSY.

This is characterized by the sudden loss of consciousness and sensibility, accompanied with spasms and convulsions. It comes on suddenly, and epileptics, by the sudden attacks, are at all times in danger. They may be taken while descending a flight of stairs, while traversing the bank of a precipice, while crossing a street crowded with vehicles drawn at full speed, or while in a throng of people whose feet would trample them to death, especially in case of an alarm of fire, a great public meeting or pageant, or other sudden danger. But all those afflicted in this terrible way are actually alive to the dangers of which they are the constant expectants. Epilepsy, in its severer forms, is a terrible disease to witness. It is productive of great distress and misery, and liable to terminate in worse than death, as it is apt, in many cases, to end in fatuity or insanity, and so carrying perpetual anxiety and dismay into all of those families which it has once visited.

The leading symptoms of Epilepsy are, a temporary suspension of consciousness, with clonic spasms, recurring at intervals; but so various are its forms, and so numerous its modifications, that no general description of the disease can be given. I will first describe the most ordinary type of the disease, and then note some of the several variations which occur from the standard type.

A man in the apparent enjoyment of perfect health suddenly utters a loud cry, and falls instantly to the ground, senseless and convulsed. He strains and struggles violently. His breathing is embarrassed and suspended; his face is turgid and livid; he foams at the mouth; a choking sound is heard in his wind-pipe, and he appears to be at the point of death from apnœa, or suspension of breath. By degrees, however, these alarming phenomena diminish, and finally cease, leaving the patient exhausted, heavy, stupid, comatose, or in a death-like condition. His life, however, is no longer threatened, and soon, to all appearances, he is perfectly well. The same train of morbid phenomena recur, again and again, at different, and mostly at irregular intervals, perhaps through a long course of years, notwithstanding the best medical science has been exercised to prevent and cure the distressing malady. This is the most ordinary form of Epilepsy.

The suddenness of the attack is remarkable: in an instant, when it is least expected by himself, or by those around him, in the middle of a sentence or of a gesture, the change takes place, and the unfortunate sufferer is stretched foaming, struggling, and insensible on the earth.

In this country, Epilepsy is commonly called the "*Falling Sickness*," or more vaguely, "*Fits*." The cry, which is frequently, but not always uttered, is a piercing and terrifying scream. Women have often been thrown into hysterics upon hearing it, and frequently it has caused pregnant females to miscarry. Even the lower animals are often startled, and appalled by a scream so harsh and unnatural, and parrots and other birds have been known to drop from their perch, apparently frightened to death by the appalling sound.

In most of the cases of fits, which have come under my notice and treatment, the first effect of the spasms has been a twisting of the neck, the chin being raised and brought round by a succession of jerks towards the shoulder, while one side of the body is usually more strongly agitated than the other. The features are greatly distorted, the brows knit, the eyes sometimes quiver and roll about, sometimes are fixed and staring, and sometimes are turned up beneath the lids, so that the cornea cannot be seen, but leaving visible the white sclerotica alone; at the same time the mouth is twisted awry, the tongue thrust between the teeth, and, caught by the violent closure of the jaws, is often severely bitten, reddening by blood the foam which issues from the mouth.   The hands are firmly clenched and the thumbs bent inwards on the palms, the arms are generally thrown about, striking the chest of the patient with great force.   Sometimes he will bruise himself against surrounding objects, or inflict hard knocks on the friends and neighbors who have hastened to his assistance.   It frequently happens that the urine and excrements are expelled during the violence of the spasms, and seminal emissions sometimes take place.   The spasmodic contraction of the muscles is occasionally so powerful as to dislocate the bones to which they are attached.   The teeth have thus been fractured, and the joints of the jaw and of the shoulder put out or dislocated.

This is the most *severe*, yet the most *common* form in which an epileptic attack occurs.   Fortunately, there is a large class of cases in which the symptoms are milder.   Sometimes there is no convulsion at all, or, at least, is very slight and transient ; no turgescence of the face ; no foaming of the mouth ; no cry ; but a sudden suspension of consciousness, a short period of insensibility, a fixed gaze, a totter, perhaps, a look of confusion, but the patient does not fall.   This is but momentary.   Presently consciousness returns, and the patient resumes the action in which he had been previously engaged, without always being aware that it has been interrupted.

Between these two extremes of epilepsy there are many links or grades.   Sometimes the sufferer sinks or slides down quietly without noise ; is pale ; is not convulsed ; but is insensible, much like one in a state of syncope, or fainting.

As it is impossible to give any single description of epilepsy which will include all its varieties, of course it is still more difficult to offer a strict definition of the disease.   We can only say it is a malady that causes a sudden loss of sensation and consciousness, with spasmodic contraction of the voluntary muscles, quickly passing into violent convulsive distortions, attended and followed by stupor or sleep, recurring in paroxysms, often more or less regular.   Yet all these circumstances may in turn be wanting.   There may be no convulsion, no interruption of consciousness, no subsequent coma or stupor, or even a recurrence of the attack.

The duration of the attacks is variable.   They seldom continue longer than half an hour ; the average duration may be said to be from five to ten minutes.   Attacks that spread over three or four hours generally consist of a succession of paroxysms, with indistinct intervals of comatose exhaustion.   In the long-continued fits, or in the protracted succession of fits, the patient often dies.

The periods at which the paroxysms return are extremely variable. Most commonly they visit the sufferer at irregular periods of a few months or weeks; sometimes are repeated at intervals of a few days; sometimes every day or every night, and very frequently many times in the twenty-four hours.

The epileptic attack may come on for the first time at *any age.* It may begin in infancy during the first dentition, or teething; more commonly about the age of seven or eight years, during the time of the second dentition; more frequently still, from fourteen to sixteen, shortly before the age of puberty. It is apt to occur for a few years subsequently to this. The first fit may not occur till between thirty and forty; or it may occur at sixty, or even at a later period of life.

TREATMENT.—There is perhaps no disease where a greater diversity of medical treatment has been instituted than in Epilepsy. The whole pharmacopœia has been exhausted, and each remedy extolled for its virtues. One medical man says he cures the disease by trephining; another thinks the oil of turpentine the best remedy; still another recommends the vapor of chloroform. This doctor applies ice, the other cauterizes the back with a hot iron, and yet another speaks highly of a compound of camphor, valerian, assafœtida, naphtha, and oil of cajeput.

Unless rational treatment is employed, the disease cannot be cured. If occurring in infants, it should be ascertained if it is not due to teething or worms, and the proper treatment instituted, if so caused. If connected with derangement of the catamenia, masturbation, or spermatorrhœa, the treatment for these complaints is necessary. The antispasmodics are indicated in every case, the best of which is blue vervian, although valerian, belladonna, scullcap, etc., are also good. The general condition of the system should receive strict attention.

On page 469 I have given a remedy which will prove in eight cases out of ten a simple and certain cure. I make no secret of its composition. I have sent the prescription to many thousands gratuitously. A fair trial will convince every one that it is one of the most potent remedies ever discovered for the cure of epilepsy, falling sickness, or fits. When this medicine is taken, the spasms gradually grow lighter and lighter, and finally disappear altogether, restoring the patient to the most perfect normal health. Its effect is truly wonderful. The time to accomplish a cure is usually from two to three months.

HYSTERICS.

This is a nervous condition confined to females, though well marked cases of hysteria are occasionally met with in males. The invasion of the disease is sudden and irregular, but in many cases decidedly periodical. The principal characteristics consist in alternate fits of weeping and laughing, with a sensation as if a ball was rolling towards the stomach, chest, and neck, producing a sense of strangulation. Consciousness is lost in violent cases, but it remains clear as a general thing, which dis-

14

tinguishes it from epilepsy. It is dependent upon irregularity of nervous distribution in very impressible persons.

TREATMENT.—During the paroxysms, the feet should be placed in warm water, and a hot mustard plaster applied to the lower part of the abdomen. A decoction of equal parts of ladies'-slipper and scullcap should be given until the spasm subsides. A tea made of ginger and bayberry, the tincture of castor, and assafœtida, are also good. The state of the womb should receive attention, and if dependent upon indigestion and constipation, tonics and laxatives are the proper remedies. I have never met with the annoyance or difficulty in the treatment of this disease that so many practitioners speak of, but regard the disease as easy of cure.

CATALEPSY.

This is an affliction of rare occurrence, and appears to be constitutional, or dependent upon some derangement of the nervous and muscular system which baffles inquiry. The sufferer is suddenly seized by it, and, although powerless to move, or speak, and to all appearance dead, is partially sensible of all that is going on around. In some cases, however, the senses are suspended. The body and limbs are not generally rigid, but will remain in the positions in which the bystanders may place them. Many years ago, when the light of science was not so bright, or shed so extensively as it is now, men and women were buried alive while cataleptic. The catalepsy, or trance, often lasts for weeks, the sufferer, in the meantime, partaking of no nourishment whatever.

"Absence of mind" is a slight form of catalepsy.

TREATMENT.—During the paroxysms the head should be showered with cold water, followed by hot foot-baths and stimulating liniments, with friction to the abdomen and spine. Some aromatic stimulant, as peppermint sling or compound spirits of lavender, should also be administered. For the toning of the nervous system and preventing recurrence of the trance, the "Restorative Assimilant" answers all purposes admirably.

ST. VITUS'S DANCE (CHOREA).

This is characterized by irregular contractions of the voluntary muscles, especially of the face and limbs, there being incomplete subserviency of these muscles to the will. It is a disease which usually occurs before puberty, and is generally connected with torpor of the system and of the digestive organs in particular. The spasms do not continue during sleep, and often, by a strong effort of the will, they can in a measure be controlled. Its duration is long, but usually devoid of danger, unless it merges into organic disease of the nervous centres, or of the heart, or into epilepsy.

TREATMENT.—The general system should be strengthened, and the intestinal canal stimulated. Purgatives once or twice a week, with appropriate regimen, will fulfil these. A mild purgative, like the "Renovating Pill," should be used. The decoction of scullcap and ladies'-slipper is very beneficial. It is cured in a short time by my "Restorative Assimilant."

LOCKED-JAW (TETANUS).

This is a disease of the true spinal system, and is manifested by spasm and rigidity of the voluntary muscles. When the muscles of the neck and face are affected, it is termed *Trismus*, or locked-jaw; when the muscles in front, *Emprosthotonos :* when the muscles of the back, *Opisthotonos ;* and when bending to either side, *Pleurosthotonos.*

Tetanus may be either acute or chronic; the former is the most frequent and most formidable; the latter, apt to be partial, milder, and more subject to treatment.

It is called *traumatic* when it follows a wound or injury, and *idiopathic* when of spontaneous origin.

Acute traumatic tetanus is more common in hot climates, and in military practice, and may follow a slight bruise or puncture, especially if some nerve has been injured. The symptoms may appear in a few hours, or in many days; at first, there is a stiffness and soreness about the neck and face, the contraction of the muscles causing a ghastly smile; chewing and swallowing are difficult, the forehead is wrinkled, eyeballs are distorted, nostrils dilated, and the grinning countenance is expressive of horror. Respiration is rapid, the tongue protrudes, and the saliva dribbles. The mind is clear until just before death, which generally takes place in a few days.

TREATMENT.—The indications are to remove all sources of irritation and diminish the spasm. The wound is to be cleansed from all foreign bodies, pus to be discharged by a free incision, if necessary, and warm anodyne poultices and fomentations are to be applied. Excision of the wound, or division of the nerve leading to it, may be done by the surgeon. Nutrition and opium are indispensable; the latter may be used either externally or internally. A lobelia emetic, if it can be administered, should be given, and a brisk purgative should be given. Tobacco, either by the mouth, or in enema, is an excellent relaxant. Camphor, assafœtida, etc., may also be used as antispasmodics. Cannabis indica internally, and ice to the spine, have been used advantageously in some cases. If, in opinion of the attending physician, it is necessary, chloroform or ether may be used as an anæsthetic.

PARALYSIS (PALSY).

The most characteristic symptom of cerebral hemorrhage is paralysis.

Very slight effusion produces this effect, and, in general, its intensity is in direct ratio of the extent of the effusion. It also arises from disease of the brain or its membranes, injuries of the brain and spinal cord, diseases of the cord or its membranes, or any injury of the large nervous networks, the action of lead, etc. The nerves of motion as well as those of sensation may be paralyzed, and when it exists on one side of the body it is called *hemiplegia*, and when confined to the lower limbs, *paraplegia*. When the muscles of the mouth or of an extremity are affected, it is called *partial* paralysis, and when both sides, whether in their extent or in some of their parts, are deprived of motion, it is termed *general* paralysis.

At the very moment of the effusion it acquires all at once its highest degree of intensity, then remains stationary or begins to diminish. Sometimes the paralyzed part has not previously experienced any disturbance with respect to either sensation or motion; sometimes, however, the patient has experienced in these parts pricking sensations, numbness, permanent or transient, an unusual feeling of cold, a sense of weight, and a certain degree of debility. The part paralyzed suggests the locality of the effusion or injury, but these are only of interest to the pathologist. When the affected muscles degenerate or atrophy, it is called *wasting palsy*, and when characterized by slow progress, and tremulousness increases to such extent that the agitation prevents sleep, all locomotion, difficulty of chewing and swallowing, etc., it is called *paralysis agitans*.

TREATMENT.—If dependent upon cerebral hemorrhage, the treatment of apoplexy should be instituted, and afterwards the use of derivatives such as purgatives, alteratives, diuretics, etc., and the use of local stimulants. The patient should be restricted in his diet, and all causes of cerebral excitement, whether physical or moral, should be avoided. The bowels should be well acted upon, and the condition of the bladder attended to. When the organic disease is removed, and all symptoms of vascular excitement have subsided, recourse should be had to nux vomica, or strychnine, tonics, and galvanism. In giving strychnine, the lowest dose should be given at first, and cautiously increased. Macrotin, viburnin, xanthoxylin, and rhusin are also good remedies. The local treatment consists in stimulating liniments, blisters to the spine, etc.

Those who may desire my counsel and opinion of their cases, as to nature and curableness, will please write as directed on page 390.

HYDROPHOBIA.

This is caused by the bite of a mad dog or other hydrophobic animals. The human subject is not as liable to hydrophobia as the lower animals, and it is consoling to know that only about one-tenth of those bitten are attacked by hydrophobia.

The interval of the bite and appearance of the disease varies from twelve days to two months. The wound heals like any other bite, but on approach of the disease the scar begins to have sharp pains, and the part feels cold, stiff, or numb. The patient feels a strange anxiety, is depressed in spirit, has an occasional chill, disturbed sleep, and spasmodic twitches. The appetite is lost, and, as the disease progresses, thirst appears, and he attempts to drink; but, the moment the water approaches his mouth, a spasmodic shudder comes over him, he pushes it back with horror, and the awful fact of his condition is known to him, and pitiful expressions escape him. His throat becomes full of glain, viscid mucus, which he continually tries to clear away. He strives to bite his attendants, suffers great depression of spirits, and finally dies from exhaustion, or in a horrible spasm.

TREATMENT.—The wound should be cut out, cups or suction applied to it, or thoroughly cauterized, and the patient should be kept quiet. Copious draughts of whiskey have been advised by some.

The red chickweed or scarlet pimpernel is said to be an absolute remedy. Four ounces of this should be boiled in two quarts of water until reduced to one quart, and a wine-glassful taken twice a day. The wound should also be bathed by the same. The common rose-beetle (*cetonia amata*), found so commonly on rose-bushes, is an effectual remedy. I desire in this connection to draw attention to a most absurd, ridiculous superstition which prevails; that is, if a person be bitten by a dog which is in perfect health, but afterwards goes mad, the person also will be affected, so they insist upon the dog being destroyed, for fear it should go mad at any future period. Instead of this the dog should be carefully taken care of. Patients would then have the satisfaction of knowing that there was nothing wrong with it, and their minds would be at rest.

DISEASES OF THE SKIN.

HUMID TETTER (ECZEMA).

This consists in the appearance of minute shining vesicles, not larger than the head of a small pin, on different portions of the body. They are usually clustered together, and surrounded by a red ring. The fluid in the vesicles becomes opaque in a few days, and finally forms light, thin scales, which fall off. In most cases a fresh crop appears as soon as the first crop is matured, in which case yellow crusts form over the diseased patch, and chronic tetter exists for weeks or months. The red eczema is the worst form of this disease.

TREATMENT.—Low diet, cooling drinks, gentle purgatives and warm baths should be prescribed. The acetic tincture of blood-root should be externally applied.   It speedily cures all cases.   Celandine, tar, slippery-elm poultices, etc., are also useful.

TETTER, SHINGLES (HERPES).

Tetter is a transient non-contagious eruption, consisting of circum-scribed red patches, upon each of which are situated clusters of vesicles, about the size of a pea.   After a few days the vesicles break, pour out a thin fluid, and form brown or yellow crusts, which fall off about the tenth day, leaving the surface red and irritable.   The eruption is attend-ed with heat, tingling, fever, and restlessness, especially at night. *Ringworm* is a curious form of tetter, the inflamed patches being ring-like in form.

TREATMENT.—Light diet, and gentle laxatives.   If the patient is old the tonics should be given.   The elder-flower ointment is an excellent external application.   The acetic tincture of lobelia is also good.   No-thing better, however, can be used than the "Herbal Ointment," men-tioned on page 472.

ITCH (SCABIES).

This annoying disease is caused by minute white insects, the *acarus scabei* or *sareoptis hominis*, which insinuate themselves beneath the skin.   It is said that these insects travel in pairs, male and female, hus-band and wife evidently, and that the female is very much the smaller. Under the microscope the animal appears as in the cut, which gives a

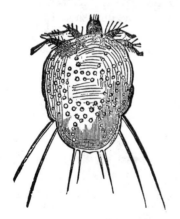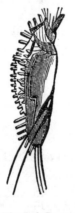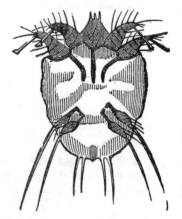

The Itch Insect.

front, back and side view of it.   The elegance of the animal is beyond question, and his mode of burrowing under the skin is sagacious.   When placed upon the skin he proceeds to make a hole through it, which he does by his head and fore-feet.   Into this he insinuates his whole body.

Like the mole, he makes a channel many times his own length, at the end excavating a chamber, where he takes his *siesta*, and from whence he saunters forth in quest of provender. As age approaches, tired of the home of his youth, he digs onward, scoops out another, in which he ends his days, beloved and respected by all his neighbors.

Itch is characterized by a vesicular eruption, and makes its appearance between the fingers and in other soft portions of the skin. If the pimples are scratched a watery fluid is poured out which forms small scabs, and if the disease is not cured, extensive sores occur. It is more common among the poor, but James I. of England said that it was only fitted for kings, so excellent is the enjoyment of scratching. It may be a royal luxury, but I am quite sure that persons having the itch would consent for it to be entirely monopolized by kings. A similar disease is caused by the *acarus sacchari*, an insect very common in brown sugar.

TREATMENT.—Whatever kills the little animal will cure the itch. This is best achieved by sulphur. It should be made into an ointment with lard, and thoroughly rubbed into the skin before the fire, morning and evening for a few days. This will put an end to the "squatter sovereignty" of whole colonies. An ointment made from veratrum also does well. Another method is equally if not more efficacious. Rub the entire surface of the body over with soft soap for half an hour—then a warm bath for half an hour, washing it thoroughly off, and exciting the skin to active circulation. Then an ointment, prepared as follows, should be rubbed over the entire surface: Take eight ounces of lard and into it thoroughly rub two ounces of flour of sulphur, and one ounce of carbonate of potash, making an even and uniform mixture, and it is ready for use. This, after it has remained on the skin for three hours, may be well washed off, and the disease is entirely annihilated. In persons of tender skin, or where considerable inflammation has been set up by continued scratching, it may be necessary to anoint with hard soap instead of soft, for it does not contain as much alkali, and leave out the carbonate of potash in the ointment—for reason of its being too stimulating. In these instances, it will take longer to cure the disease, but it is just as certain in its results. This mode of treating this disease is an entirely successful one—and no one need "to scratch" if these simple directions be attended to.

WATERY BLEBS (PEMPHIGUS).

This is characterized by loss of appetite, febrile symptoms, at first, followed by a bright red eruption of a smarting or burning sensation. In the centre of this eruption, minute vesicles appear, which gradually enlarge in blisters in the shape of bubbles and contain a watery fluid. They vary in size from a split pea to that of a hen's egg, and rise very rapidly.

and break in a few days, leaving a raw surface, which soon becomes covered with a crust.

TREATMENT.—The surface of the body should be bathed, and the bowels opened by a gentle purge. The inflamed surface should be covered by a slippery-elm poultice, and be kept moist with tincture of lobelia. When the constitution is feeble, quinine, alnuin, etc., should be given. The diet should receive especial attention, and out-door exercise enjoyed.

RUPIA.

This is a small blister, or vesicle, about the size of a chestnut, which at first contains a darkish fluid, which dries into a crust, falls off, and leaves an indolent ulcer. It is always connected with a vitiated constitution, and is dependent frequently upon imperfect diet, although chronic disease, such as syphilis, phthisis, dyspepsia, and poisonous mineral medicines, not unfrequently produce it.

TREATMENT.—The digestive organs should be corrected, and the blood nourished and enriched by wholesome diet and tonics. The local applications should consist of emollient poultices, and kept constantly moist with the tincture of hydrastin, baptisin, or myrrh. A poultice of equal parts of bayberry, white pond-lily and slippery-elm is very beneficial. The cause, however, is always to be ascertained before the treatment is interposed.

CRUSTED TETTER (IMPETIGO).

The eruption in this disease consists, at first, in slightly elevated pustules or pimples, closely collected together, with an inflamed edge. These break, and the surface becomes red, excoriated, shining, and full of pores, through which a thin, unhealthy fluid is poured out, which gradually hardens into dark, yellowish-green scabs. These scabs sometimes look like honey dried upon the skin, and hence the name of "honey disease." It is very common on the ears and lips of children. It is also called the *milk crust*, when it covers the whole face.

TREATMENT.—Give a purgative, and let the patient take a hot bath. As a local application equal parts of blood-root and white pond-lily, say one ounce, and cider vinegar, six ounces, mix, and let stand twenty-four hours, and apply as a wash with a sponge four or five times a day. The oxide of zinc ointment is also good, but the best and speediest cure is the "Herbal Ointment," described on page 472.

PAPULOUS SCALE (ECTHYMA).

This consists of mattery pimples developed on a highly inflamed skin, appearing chiefly on the extremities and rarely met with in children in the acute form. It is either acute or chronic. The eruption in the acute form is preceded by a slight fever, and in about thirty-six hours red spots appear on the skin, accompanied by heat and tingling. On the second day, the centres of these spots are raised by the pus con‑ tained, to which the name of *phlyzacious pustule* is given. This stage is accompanied by much pain. Maturation occurs from the fourth to the sixth day, and the disease usually terminates in two weeks. The chronic form is more common, and afflicts young children oftener than adults.

TREATMENT.—For the acute form, low diet, gentle laxatives, and the application of oxide of zinc ointment. The pustulated surface should also be covered with slippery-elm poultices, and kept constantly moist with tincture of lobelia. In the chronic form, in addition to the above, the tonics should be given, and the blood should be enriched by proper medication and nutritious diet.

LEPROSY.

The eruption in this disease makes its appearance as a small red spot, elevated a little above the general skin, usually occurring first on the limbs. The scales occurring on these patches occur in layers, one above the other, and have a bright silvery lustre. This is the *lepra alphoides*. The Hebrew leprosy was a variety of this form. What was known as the *Leuce* was generally not scaly, but consisted of smooth, shining patches, on which the hair turned white and silky, and was totally in‑ curable. When leprosy is of dark livid color, it is called *lepra nigricans*, and when copper-colored, it is due to syphilis, and is termed *lepra syphi‑ litica*. The leprosy of the Arabs is what is known as *Elephantiasis*, and the Greek leprosy includes the varieties met with at the present day. Leprosy is endemic in Egypt, in Java, and certain parts of Norway and Sweden.

TREATMENT.—The means best adapted for its removal, are, a mild, un‑ irritating diet, emollient fomentations, sulphureous baths, fumigations, etc., but often all treatment is ineffectual. A warm solution of the ses‑ quicarbonate of potash is effectual in some cases. An ointment of glyce‑ rine and hydrastin, and the acetic tincture of blood-root, are also service‑ able, but as a topical remedy, nothing could be superior to my "Herbal Ointment."

DRY TETTER (PSORIASIS).

This differs from leprosy in the eruption being more irregular. The spots sometimes come out in thick clusters, and blend in various ways. The eruption is not circular as in leprosy, but consists of irregular patches of every extent, and the surface is more tender and irritable than in leprosy. There are many varieties of this disease. The

14*

"Baker's Itch," "Grocer's Itch," and "Washerwoman's Scall," are only different varieties of psoriasis.

TREATMENT.—The acetic tincture of blood-root or oxide of zinc ointment, may be applied to the eruption, and the skin should be kept clean, and the pores open. The inflammations may be lessened by emollient and soothing applications. Sea bathing is very good. The general health should be attended to in all cases, and the tonics given in necessary cases.

PITYRIASIS.

This name is from the Greek *pityron*, signifying *bran*. It is characterized by patches of yellowish, or reddish yellow color, covered with fine branny scales, accompanied by smarting, itching, and burning. It may occur at any part of the body, under three or four varieties of form.

TREATMENT.—The treatment advised in psoriasis will answer in this disease

LUPUS.

This is the "Jacob's Ulcer" of common parlance, and from its rapacity it is named *Lupus*, which is the Latin name for *wolf*. It is also called "noli me tangere," *touch me not*. It occurs in a variety of forms, generally upon the face. It commences by slight thickening and elevation of the skin, usually not larger than a wheat grain. A thin, hard, brownish scab appears on its surface. The disease extends, usually slowly, but sometimes very rapidly, and cases have occurred where the whole nose has been destroyed in a month. It is very rapacious, destroying even the bones in its progress.

TREATMENT.—When it first makes its appearance it should be thoroughly destroyed with caustics, and healed by zinc ointment. At the same time, the alteratives should be given. My "Blood Purifier" (see page 471) is excellent for this purpose. Early institution of treatment will only prevent destruction of tissue.

ELEPHANTIASIS.

This is characterized by the development of tumors upon the skin, varying in size from the head of a pea to that of an apple, or even larger. Eventually these tumors ulcerate, and discharge an unhealthy pus, in some cases affecting the bone, and resulting in mortification and death. It is endemic in Lisbon. At first there is a discoloration of the skin of the face, the lobes of the ear lengthen, and the wings of the nose spread out; then the face becomes tuberculous, the features are puffed out, the lips thicken, the whiskers, eyebrows, and eyelashes fall out. The tubercles ulcerate after some years, there is ozœna, the fingers and toes mortify, and the body exhales a most loathsome odor. This is the leprosy of the ancient Egyptians.

TREATMENT.—The parts should be thoroughly bathed with a strong solution of the sesquicarbonate of potash, and stillingia and other alteratives administered. Where the parts become swollen, painting with the tincture of iron, followed by astringent poultices, has been found very beneficial. When confined to the extremities, amputation may become necessary.

ACNE.

This is a small pimple or tubercle which appears on various parts of the face. The disease leads to no particular evil results, save that it is unpleasant, slightly painful, and disfiguring. It commonly afflicts the young and robust of both sexes, and generally indicates strong passions, and too great an indulgence in animal food, or neglect of ablutions and out-of-door exercise. It is sometimes, in its more severe forms, the consequence of solitary practices. The common form of the disease is an eruption of hard, distinct, inflamed tubercles which remain unchanged for a long time, or else slowly advance to partial suppuration. They are to be seen on the forehead, cheeks, and chin, and sometimes on the nose. It is commonly known as the *brandy face* or *rum blots*.

TREATMENT.—Attention to the general health becomes necessary. It is not well to drive them in by lotions, as they are then liable to break out in some internal organ. Attention to diet, plenty of exercise, a pure imagination, and a clean body, together with open and regular bowels, will soon effect the disappearance of this troublesome enemy of good looks.

WARTS AND CORNS.

Warts consist of collections of hypertrophied cutaneous papillæ, or loops of veins, arteries and nerves. These loops, frequently, without any apparent cause, take on a disposition to grow, and by extending themselves upward, they carry the scarf-skin along with them, which thickens, and the whole forms the wart.

Corns consist in excrescences confined mostly to the toes and soles of the feet, resulting from wearing tight shoes. They occasionally form on the elbows and knees, or on the extremities of the fingers. When occurring between the toes, they are called *soft corns*.

Bunions consist of an enlargement, thickening, and inflammation of the mucous bursa at the side of the ball of the great toe. Occasionally the bursa suppurates, and a fistulous opening left after the pus has evacuated.

TREATMENT.—Corns may be cured by shaving them closely and

applying nitro-muriatic acid or chromic acid ointment. For soft corns
acetic acid is better. Warts should be clipped off with the scissors, and
chromic acid applied, or any other cauterizing agent will answer. The
tincture of thuja is also excellent. Bunions are cured by bathing them
frequently in the oil of erigeron.

PRURITIS.

This is dependent upon an altered condition of the nerves of the skin,
and consists in a painful sensation of itching. There is no perceptible
alteration in the appearance of the skin, and the itching is generally the
result of sympathy, through the nerves, with some diseased condition of
a distant part. It more frequently affects the fundament, the scrotum,
or the vulva of females.

TREATMENT.—The following is usually all the treatment that is required:—Take oleo-resin of lobelia, grs. xx; aconitin, grs. iij; sulphate of sanguinaria, grs. x; glycerine, ℥ ij. Mix. Apply the ointment
to the part three or four times a day. Lead-water and opium are
also beneficial.

MACULÆ, OR SPOTS.

This affection, which is characterized by an increased hue of the pigment of the skin, consists of freckles and moles. *Ephelis lenticularis,*
or common freckles, appears in small yellowish, brownish, or greenish-
yellow, irregular, rounded spots, caused particularly by the influence
of the sun's rays upon the parts. It occurs generally in females,
owing to their fine skin. *Ephelis hepatica* is observed in females
during pregnancy. *Ephelis violacea* is caused by the long use of
nitrate of silver. Moles are dark colored patches, usually covered
with hair. *Nævi* or *mother's marks* are called aneurisms by anastomosis, or an inter-connection and enlargement of the arterioles of
the skin. *Leucopathia,* or *Albinism,* consists of a diminution of the
coloring matter of the skin. It is found in all races, but is most striking in the black.

TREATMENT.—Freckles may be removed by keeping out of the sun,
and frequently washing the face in a solution of lactic acid. Fresh
buttermilk answers the same purpose. The best remedy, however,
is to be found in my "Floral Bloom." It quickly removes freckles,
moth patches, etc., and makes the skin clear and transparent. Moles
and mother's marks belong to surgery, and may in many instances be
removed. Albinism is incurable.

SCALLED HEAD (TINEA FAVOSA).

This is caused by an insect by the name of *achorion Schönleinii.* The
eruption takes the shape of large flattened pustules, which have an

irregular edge, and are surrounded by inflammation. Sometimes they appear first behind the ears, and at other times upon the face, spreading thence to the scalp. The face is usually involved to some extent wherever the eruption may originally show itself. Scalled head is mostly confined among children. In the outset of the disease the pustules on the scalp are generally distinct;—on the face they rise in irregular clusters. They are attended by much itching, and the efforts to relieve this torment hasten their breaking. When broken they discharge a viscid matter and run together, gradually forming sores of a vicious character. These sores are covered by yellowish-greenish scabs which present a revolting appearance.

TREATMENT.—The hair should be shaved close to the scalp, and the head thoroughly washed with soap and water, after which the zinc ointment should be applied in the morning and the tar ointment in the evening. Alteratives should also be given. This course, if persisted in, will remove the disease.

TINEA SYCOSIS.

This is commonly known as "Barber's Itch," and is confined to the face, especially to that portion covered by the beard. It is characterized by inflammation of the hair follicles, causing an eruption of small pustules forming incrustations eventually. It may be consoling to those who suffer with it to know that it is caused by a parasite with the humble name of *microsporon mentagraphytes.*

TREATMENT.—Shave the beard, and paint the part with a strong tincture of iodine for a few days. Follow this with a poultice, composed of equal parts of lobelia, blood-root, myrrh, and slippery-elm. Depilation, or pulling out the beard, may be necessary in some cases to effect the cure.

BALDNESS (ALOPECIA).

This may be partial or general, temporary or permanent, and occur at any period of life. Senile baldness usually takes place gradually, the hair first becoming thin on the crown, or on the temples and forehead. It is owing generally to the general loss of the nutritive functions of the hair, and of the follicular apparatus. Loss of color of the hair (canities) may depend upon advanced age, disease, or deep mental emotion. It usually occurs gradually, after the age of forty. Cases are recorded in which the loss of color was complete in eight days, while in others the hair was almost completely blanched in a single night.

TREATMENT.—If the hair follicles are not destroyed, baldness may be cured. The tincture of cantharides, lac sulphur, shampooing, etc., are each to be recommended. Tonics and strict cleanliness also promotes the growth of the hair. In my "Woodland Balm" (page 473) the bald or gray will find a remedy which has no superior for restoring the hair to a healthy growth and natural color.

ENTOZOA.

These grow in the body without forming attachments to its structures, have an independent life of their own, and possess the power of reproduction and generation. Several species infest the human body, some appearing always in the same organ and some in a particular tissue, and appearing oftenest where that tissue is plentiful. Scarcely any portion of the body is exempt from such growths. Their origin is a subject for two suppositions—that of generative reproduction, and of accidental or spontaneous development of germs that take on modes of life and development characterizing them afterwards. The first supposition is more philosophical, comports more with analogy, and is unquestionably the true theory. The interest attached to these growths, however, is their effect upon the system and cause of disease. Their presence in the system causes morbid phenomena, disordered functional action, and loss of health. The mischief they do in the system depends upon their number, size, rapidity of growth, and species. When numerous or large they imbibe so much nutriment as to rob the system of its necessary sustenance. Their habitation is generally a seat of irritation or inflammation, and more particularly when their location is in a cavity, and when they possess power of motion.

Psychodiara.—Hydatids.—These are organized beings, consisting of a globe-like bag of albuminous matter; the texture divided in layers, and containing a limpid, colorless fluid richer in gelatin than albumen. They live by imbibition, have no sensibility or power of motion, and appear more like a vegetable than an animal in their modes of life and reproduction. There are two kinds of hydatids, the *acephalocyst*, or cyst without a head, and the *echinococcus*, which is not different from the other in form but in containing minute animals (vermiculi echinococci) within it. The former is common to the human body, and generated between layers of membrane. The usual abode of hydatids is in the lungs, liver, ovaries, spleen, kidneys, etc. The hydatids occurring in the womb are often mistaken upon expulsion for products of conception, and their presence in that organ often produces similar signs as in pregnancy.

Sterelmintha.—These consist of solid porous texture, perforated by canals or cavities, which serve the purposes of digestion. These animals are hermaphrodite, *i. e.*, having both sexual organs on one individual. The varieties of tapeworm belong to this class. So also the *cysticercus*, which occurs in the muscular structure and in the watery portion of the eye. The liver-fluke—*distoma hepaticum*—also belongs to this class, but which rarely occurs in man, but is supposed to cause the well-known "rot" in sheep.

Cœlelmintha.—This class has a higher organic development than the preceding. It embraces several species of worms having hollow cylindrical bodies, distinct alimentary canals, with a mouth at one extremity and an anus at the other, a nervous system, and the sexual organs on different animals. The common intestinal worms belong to this class ; so also the *trichina spiralis*—causing the disease described below which is an animal which exists within the minute, white, ovate cysts imbedded in the muscles. The guinea-worm (*filaria medinensis*), so common to Africa and Asia, but unknown in this country, is a hair-like worm developed beneath the skin, especially in the scrotum and lower extremities It can be withdrawn when a pustule ensues, by care and patience, wrapping it around a stick until the end appears.

The *strongulus gigas* is an animal that locates itself exclusively in the kidney, and sometimes attains an enormous size. Its body is round, but tapers toward both ends. It sometimes attains a length of three feet, and a thickness of half an inch. It causes impairment of functions, waste of the renal structure, and sometimes inflammation, with pain and bloody urine. It is sometimes expelled through the water passages.

TREATMENT.—The treatment of parasites is indicated by their character or place of abode. If they exist in the alimentary canal, such remedies as are known to expel them should be employed. Anything is a good remedy that is harmless to the system but destructive of life to them. Various agents are poisonous, such as cherry-laurel water, camphor, oil of cubebs, oil of turpentine, copaiba, etc., but these must be employed at proper seasons and in such quantities that they will not harm the general system.

TRICHINIASIS.

This is a disease caused by the *trichina spiralis* which infests various animals, especially swine. If the meat of the hog affected is eaten raw or insufficiently cooked, it is most likely to cause this dangerous disease. Thorough cooking destroys the parasites. The symptoms are extensive gastric disturbance, with nausea and a tendency to vomit ; associated with rheumatic pains, stiffness of the muscles, irregular pulse, intermittent fever, which is violently aggravated in paroxysms, thirst, restlessness, nervous excitement, and utter wakefulness. The face generally swells, great prostration ensues, and the patient generally dies in a paralyzed condition.

TREATMENT.—In the early stage an active lobelia emetic should be given, and followed by a full dose of castor oil or spirits of turpentine. An alcoholic vapor bath should be taken, and sufficient veratrum to control the fever. If sleeplessness prevails, opium should be given. The above treatment may be repeated if not at first successful.

THE PROPER CARE OF CHILDREN.

The first requisite of an infant is plenty of pure and fresh air. It should be kept in open air as much as possible, and when in-doors in well-ventilated rooms. When carried in the open air, their heads should not be enveloped in blankets, and when sleeping, their faces should not be covered with the bed-clothes. The infant needs and should have all the oxygen a pure air affords, which is so essential to its proper growth.

The Skin.—The skin of infants should be kept clean, to render them less liable to cutaneous diseases. The unctuous covering of a new-born child should be removed as soon as possible. This can readily be done by smearing it with pure lard, and then washing with white Castile soap and water. Do not use the brown Castile soap, as it contains oxides of iron, which are irritating substances. Infants should be washed every day with warm water, to be followed in course of time with tepid water, then temperate, and finally, at an age of some months, with cold water.

Clothing.—The young child should be amply clothed, care being taken that they are sufficiently loose, to admit free motion in all directions. Flannels should be placed next to the skin in winter, and cotton in summer.

Food.—Proper regimen is of the utmost importance to the health of the young. Until the first teething, the proper and natural food is the mother's milk. If the mother is unable to nurse her child, a wet-nurse should be procured. If the mother's milk is insufficient, cow's milk, sufficiently diluted with water and sweetened with loaf sugar, should be taken in addition. This should be taken from a sucking-bottle, which, when not in use, should be kept in water, to prevent becoming sour. A nursing woman should pay the greatest attention to her health also, and, for obvious reasons, a scrofulous or consumptive mother should never suckle her offspring; she should also place a check upon her passions, as violent passion, grief, envy, hatred, fear, jealousy, etc., tend to derange the character of the milk, and often superinduce disorder of the infant's stomach, and throw it into convulsions. The diet of the mother should receive strict attention. Her drink should be simply water, or weak black tea, and her food plain and wholesome. Pastry and the richer articles of food should not be eaten. She should take daily moderate exercise to induce better assimilation of aliments. When her milk is scanty, a sufficiency can frequently be induced by placing a bread and milk poultice, over which a moderate quantity of mustard is sprinkled, on the breasts.

Weaning.—The child should be weaned after the appearance of its first teeth. Nature then designs it to have different food. Spring and fall are the proper seasons for weaning ; no child should be taken from the breast in the midst of summer. The weaning should be a gradual process, and the food to be given should be of the character of milk. Bread and milk, boiled rice and milk, soda-crackers and milk, soft boiled eggs, roasted potatoes and milk, preparations of sago, arrowroot, tapioca, oatmeal gruel, rice pudding, and similar substances are all indicated. My nutritive fluids, given on page 205, can also be given with good service. From these, in course of time, more solid articles of food can be given them. Sugar in moderate quantities is wholesome. Excessive eating should not be suffered. Water is the best drink.

Sleep.—A child should always sleep in a loose gown, to prevent restlessness. Nature should govern its sleep, and which should never be induced by opiates. It should be allowed to sleep to a natural awakening, and should not be aroused for any avoidable purpose. Its covering should be warm but *light*, thus avoiding pressure upon its tender limbs ; the infant should lie on its side, alternating at times from right to left, to prevent distortion of the spine. The body should be placed with the head to the north, and this rule applies to all, as the action of electric currents is to the north, thus allowing greater repose to the brain. Strong sunlight or moonshine should be excluded from their sleeping apartments. What I have thus far written is not only preservative of good health, but preventive of many species of illness to which infants are liable. Children are very liable to disease, necessitating great precaution in a variety of matters, the most important of which are the foregoing. When it is known that death destroys about one half of humanity before the age of five years, the physical life of children is of the utmost importance. While young, the moral, intellectual, and religious faculties should be shaped, as the child often indicates the man.

The baby exhibits indisposition by cries, struggles, etc., and if these are carefully noted, every mother may know what ails the baby.

A baby suffering from stomach-ache sheds tears *copiously*, and utters long and loud cries. As stomach-ache is paroxysmal in character, so will its cries remit, and enjoy repose, to be followed by movements up and down of the legs and the peculiar cry.

To cry in inflammation of the organs of the chest is painful ; it therefore does not cry or shed tears, but utters a muttering cry, abruptly completed, and coughs after long breaths.

In diseases of the brain, the child shrieks piercingly, followed by moaning and wailing. In extensive congestion, there is quiet dozing and probably snoring.

Loss of appetite, fretfulness, restlessness, thirst, great heat of skin, are all indications of disease, and require that solicitude and treatment that every fond mother should know how to bestow.

TEETHING.

Many children are lost from teething. The process of dentition often occasions fits. Its symptoms are, swollen and inflamed gums, fever, pain, and heat in the head, sore mouth, etc. Scarification of the gums is often resorted to; but if proper attention be paid to the case in its inception, no such barbarous and injurious method of palliation need be embraced. Bathing the head with diluted spirits, and the feet with warm mustard water; keeping the bowels free and regular by the simplest of herbal laxatives; and placing a plaster (composed of two-thirds flour mustard, one-third flour, and sufficient vinegar to produce the requisite moisture) between the shoulders, will generally obviate all danger and mitigate the pain and suffering. When the speckled sore mouth incidental to teething makes its appearance, treat the child as above, but wash the mouth with a mild solution of borax, and use for diet (if the child be weaned) gum-arabic water, and barley or rice water. If the stomach is acid, and the bowels are griping, administer mild doses of magnesia. Warm baths are always beneficial to children who are teething; but great care should be taken that the little ones do not catch cold after the baths.

The teeth should appear about the sixth month, though it is often later. The two incisors of the lower jaw are generally the first, and then those of the upper jaw follow. Between the twelfth and sixteenth months the grinders come, and next the eye teeth. The others soon follow, so that by the age of two years, the child has its full set of milk teeth, twenty in number. There are instances of children being born with full sets of teeth, as is recorded of Richard III. and Louis XIV.

GENERAL DISEASES.

GOUT.

This is due to the presence of lithic or uric acid in the blood. The attack usually makes its appearance in the night. The patient is first awakened by an intensely burning and wrenching pain in the ball of the great toe, or some other small joint. This pain continues for about twenty-four hours, and is accompanied by fever. It then remits, and the patient may get sleep, though for several successive days he suffers from the attacks. A similar visitation will likely result after a considerable interval. Recovery from the first attack may be complete —the skin peeling off from the red and swollen joint, and leaving it strong and supple as ever; but, after several repetitions of the attacks, the joint becomes stiff, owing to the deposit of lithic acid concretions or *chalk stones*. It is a disease entirely local in its character. It vitiates the blood, affects the general system, and the attack is generally preceded by general symptoms, irritability of temper, unpleasant sensations in the stomach and head, and uncomfortable feelings of body and mind are premonitory symptoms of this disorder. The pain is most excruciating. The stomach, heart, lungs, head, eyes, etc., may also be subject to gouty inflammation. It is caused by luxury and indolence, in the plurality of cases.

TREATMENT.—During the paroxysm the anodynes should be given and applied; subcutaneous injection of morphine is best. The constitutional treatment should be composed of chimaphilin and apocynin in combination; colchicum is also a very good remedy; chloroform liniment may also be externally applied. The patient's habits must be regulated, and his diet simplified, to prevent recurrence of the disease.

Those who may desire consultation with the author, in regard to this disease, are referred to page 390. Consultations, either in person or by letter, from those who may desire treatment, are carefully and gratuitously attended to.

RHEUMATISM.

This very painful affection is most frequently brought on by exposure to wet and cold after violent and fatiguing exercise of the muscles. The acute form is characterized by high fever, with a full bounding pulse, furred tongue, and a profuse sweat which has a sour smell. The urine is scanty and high colored; the joints swell and are slightly red and very tender. The pain is agonizing when the patient attempts to move. If the affection changes from one part to another it is called *metastatic*, and is very dangerous, as it may suddenly seize the lining membrane of the heart, and prove fatal.

The chronic form may follow the acute form, but is more often an independent disease. It differs from the acute form in the absence of fever. The fingers and limbs may frequently be rendered useless by rheumatism, by the great distortion ensuing. It is due to the presence of lactic acid in the blood.

TREATMENT.—The bowels should be evacuated by a purgative, and the tinctures of black cohosh and veratrum given until free perspiration is produced. The tincture of black cohosh, two parts, and tincture of colchicum, one part, in doses of from twenty to forty drops, is also a very valuable remedy. For articular rheumatism the alteratives should be given. My "Blood Purifier" is a sure and efficient cure, and the pain is almost instantly relieved by the application of the "Herbal Ointment" (see page 471).

Electricity may be resorted to in the chronic form. The treatment does not materially differ from that advised in the acute.

Fomentations of hops and cicuta, or stramonium leaves, placed upon the inflamed and swollen joints, will materially relieve the pain.

Rheumatism in the chronic form is often a very difficult disease to cure ; but if properly treated, by purely chemical medication, the acid condition of the blood will be negatived, and the patient relieved of his painful malady. Of the thousands of cases that have been under my care, I do not recall one failure.

Hip Disease (Morbus Coxarius).

This is a disease of the hip-joint, and common to scrofulous children. At first there is slight pain, commonly felt in the knee, lameness, and stumbling in walking, tenderness in the groin, and pain is produced by pressing the head of the bone suddenly against the socket. The limb is longer than the other, which is owing to a depression of the pelvis on the diseased side, the weight of the body being supported on the opposite limb. If the disease is not arrested, destruction of the head of the bone and socket results, and the thigh-bone is drawn up, constituting a spontaneous dislocation. Often an abscess forms and opens externally. The toes may be turned inward or outward.

This disease may be positively ascertained in the following way :— Remove the clothing of the patient and place him on any flat surface, as a bench, or table ; if he is placed so that the spine everywhere touches the table, the patient's knee on the affected side will be drawn up, the weight of the leg resting on the heel. If now his knee will be pressed down, the spine will be bent inwards, so that it no longer touches the table. This is an unerring diagnosis.

TREATMENT.—At the commencement of the disease a large irritating plaster should be placed over the entire hip, and caused to remain until a thorough counter-irritation is effected, and a discharge ensues. Perfect rest is necessary, and the limb should be confined in a carved splint. Iodine may also be externally applied, and the general health improved by tonics, alteratives, and nutritious food. Counter-extension as advised in cases of fracture is advisable in all cases. A competent surgeon should direct the treatment.

White Swelling (Hydrarthrus).

This disease occurs most frequently about the middle period of life, but is, however, very often seen in children. It will never appear before the age of puberty without a deviation from health, but not always so when it makes its appearance in after-life. It is a disease of the knee-joint characterized by swelling and white color, owing to the tension of the skin. It is of two varieties ; both, however, destroy the synovial or articular membrane of the joint. One begins with a trifling stiffness, slight swelling, and in effect reduces the membrane to a pulpy, degenerate mass. The swelling increases gradually, and when the part is touched, it reveals the presence of fluid. Finally the cartilages ulcerate, and the disease assumes such characters that amputation becomes absolutely necessary. The other form begins with pain in the joint, which is severe at one point, and attains its height in a week. It is characterized by inflammation of the synovial membrane, and in a few days the joint becomes swollen from a collection of water.

TREATMENT.—At the commencement bathe the parts with the following liniment :—oil of hemlock, ℥ iv. ; dissolve as much camphor in it as it will take up, and add twelve drops of croton oil, and three drachms of tincture of iodine. Bathe the limb thoroughly, after which apply hot cloths wrung from a strong infusion of arnica flowers and lobelia, and change as often as they grow cool ; with each change apply the liniment. This will arrest the disease if applied at the onset. The patient should be purged, and the compound syrup of chimaphila be administered to him. If the disease is farther advanced, and openings exist, they should be enlarged, and ointments and poultices applied, and the constitution supported by tonics and antiseptics. Splints and entire rest may be necessary in some cases, and when connected with a scrofulous diathesis, my " Blood Purifier " should be taken internally, and the " Herbal Ointment " applied externally. These will quickly eradicate the disease.

HECTIC FEVER.

Hectic fever is remittent, dependent upon local irritation, and rarely, if ever, idiopathic. It is attended by great and increasing debility, a weak, quick pulse, hurried respiration on any exertion, and increased heat of the skin. The febrile exacerbations are preceded by a slight chill, are slight at first, but soon become more evident, especially in the evening. The skin is at first dry, and the increased heat is more evident in the hands and face. The fever terminates in a free, profuse perspiration. The bowels are at first costive, but soon become relaxed, and an exhausting diarrhœa comes on; the urine is various, generally it is pale, and does not deposit; while there is generally a pallor of the surface, the cheeks present what is aptly termed the " hectic blush." As the disease advances, the whole frame becomes emaciated, the eyes sink in their orbits, but are brilliant and expressive ; the ankles and legs sometimes swell, and the sleep is feverish and disturbed. Finally the debility becomes so great that the patient expires while making some slight exertion.

Hectic fever accompanies nearly all forms of disease connected with great debility, especially scrofula and consumption. It may also be met with in surgical practice in disease or injury of the joints.

TREATMENT.—This depends much upon the cause or causes which give rise to it. If the digestive mucous membrane is diseased, the treatment consists in strict attention to diet, and in the administration of tonics, diaphoretics, and diuretics. The antiseptics should be given. Strychnine in doses of one-eighth of a grain is decidedly the best agent for this purpose. Cherry-laurel water should also be given. The fever is controlled, like other fevers, with veratrum. If associated with consumption, the " Acacian Balsam " (page 470) will cure it. Stimulants are very serviceable to counteract the debility. Generous diet and cleanliness are not to be neglected.

CURVATURE OF THE SPINE.

Curvature of the spine is due to caries or destruction of the bodies of the vertebræ. There are several varieties of curvature; what is known as lateral curvature consists in the distortion of the spinal column either to the one side or the other. In this case there may be no caries of the spine. It consists in depression of one shoulder, the body being thrown out of its axis, by the curvature. This affection is caused by occupations which keep the body in a laterally distorted position, and tax one side of the body more than the other. It is produced in children who study their lessons at school, with one elbow resting on a high desk, etc. In *Pott's Curvature of the Spine*, the angular curvature is produced by caries of the vertebræ, or ulceration of the substance between the vertebræ, followed by more or less loss of power over the lower extremity. In examining the spine, one or more of the spinous processes is found to project beyond the others. *Hump-backs* are usually caused by curvatures of the spine, but they may also be caused by projection of the sternum, or deviation of the ribs.

TREATMENT.—If associated with scrofula, the treatment for that disease should be instituted. In lateral distortion, calisthenic exercises should be engaged. In Pott's disease extensive counter-irritation should be made over the diseased part, and vigorous tonics given.

The treatment, however, best adapted to obviate all curvatures of the spine, is purely mechanical, and consists of braces, supporters, etc. Nothing else will achieve any satisfactory results. By mechanical appliances the spine is rendered straight, and compelled to maintain that position until a cure is effected. These mechanical appliances should be applied early, and be accurately adjusted and well fitted.

I am constantly applying such appliances in my office, and the results are excellent in nearly all cases. Those who cannot avail themselves of a personal consultation, may send age of patient, nature of curvature, height, and measure around the waist, and a suitable appliance will be sent. Preliminary correspondence free.

IMPERFECTIONS OF THE HUMAN FORM.

These embrace those only which are of slighter degree, and of idiopathic origin. They are usually acquired more or less early in life. Not unfrequently they result from bad management of the infant, having its head always too highly bolstered up, and the chest compressed by tight clothing. The school-room, however, is the arena where the human form is robbed the most of its symmetry. It is gratifying to know that greater attention is now paid to this evil, but still to a great extent the seats and desks provided for the pupils are perfect outrages upon their physical natures. The seats are invariably too high and the desks too low, obliging the pupil, for five or six hours, to sit with his head down, his spine curved backwards, and his feet dangling in space. This unnatural position soon causes a loss of erect carriage, and induces stooped shoulders, and incapacious chests. It is but rarely that we see persons having an erect posture in standing or walking, and but few have that prominent chest, so necessary to the perfection and elegance of the human form, and to the full breathing capacity for the lungs. The shoulders should be in the perfect form thrown backwards, and the body erect, the only curve in the spine being the natural inward one in the lumbar portion.

TREATMENT.—Elegance and symmetry of form can only be gained by proper gymnastic and calisthenic exercises. These should be of such a character as to be best adapted to overcome the particular deformity.

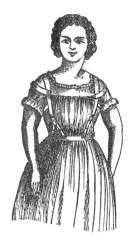

Lady's Shoulder Brace Applied.

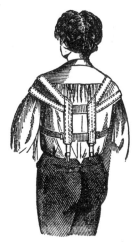

Gentleman's Shoulder Brace Applied.

In all cases suitable braces should be worn. These gently force back the shoulders, thereby increasing the volume and capacity of the chest, and enable the wearer to maintain the erect posture without fatiguing effort. In all pulmonary diseases, or where there exists an insufficient capacity of the chest, these braces should be worn. In the male they take the place of suspenders, and in the female they can be made to serve the purpose of sustaining the weight of the skirts. Nothing could be more conducive to health than these appliances; they often prevent the onset of consumption in those predisposed hereditarily to that disease. It is a well-known fact that the man or woman having an erect form and expanded chest is much less liable to disease, and at all events possesses greater vigor of health. The reason of this is obvious.

It is particularly advisable that every person having a defective form should wear a shoulder brace. The braces represented in the above cuts are of the author's own invention, and he does not hesitate to claim for them a decided superiority over all other braces for this purpose. They are worn with great comfort, gently obliging the wearer to maintain the erect posture, and enabling him to thoroughly inflate his lungs, which in course of time will lead to permanence of the upright stature with an expanded chest.

All persons desiring these superior braces can obtain them by addressing the author. (See page 389)

ABSCESS.

An abscess is a collection of pus or matter in the substance of some part of the body. When the matter is poured out from some part, the process is called *suppuration*, when it collects in a tissue, it is an abscess. It commences with all the symptoms of inflammation, fever, pain, redness, and swelling. The centre is firm, with swelling surrounding it. The formation of pus is indicated by rigors, an abatement of fever, and a feeling of weight, tension, and throbbing. The centre softens, which is termed *pointing*, and *fluctuation* is felt. There is a natural tendency to discharge the pus, which is more apt to be towards the skin. It is less apt to open into serous than into mucous tissues. The abscesses that form in scrofulous cases are called *cold*, because the conditions of inflammation are absent. They heal, after the discharge of pus, by a process called *granulation*.

TREATMENT.—The indication to be fulfilled in the treatment of abscess is to prevent the formation of pus, to evacuate it when formed, and to heal the parts so as to prevent further secretions. To prevent its formation cold applications and leeches should be applied to the part, the patient purged, and restricted to a low diet. When matter is formed warm fomentations and poultices should be applied, to hasten the progress of the pus to the surface. If abscesses distinctly *point* they need not be opened, but allowed to burst themselves, but if they occur in loose cellular tissue, under hard skin, and show a tendency to burrow, they should be evacuated by a free incision. After evacuation the poultices should be continued, or the parts be dressed with stimulating ointments, of which the "Herbal Ointment," page 472, is the best.

FELON (PARONYCHIA).

This is also called *whitlow*, and is an abscess of the fingers, of which there are three kinds, the first situated upon the surface of the skin, the second under the skin, the third within the sheath containing the tendons of the fingers, and sometimes involving the covering of the bone. The latter form is the most terrible, and begins with redness, swelling, and a deep-seated and throbbing pain, which becomes so excruciating as to banish all sleep, and nearly drive the patient to distraction. Relief is only secured by discharge of pus.

TREATMENT.—Carry the hand in a sling and use poultices. A poultice made of equal parts of slippery-elm, poke-root, flaxseed meal, and lobelia seeds, mixed with hot lye, and changed twice a day, is an admirable application. When the pain becomes great, the abscess should be laid open with a knife, cutting down to the bone. Nothing will insure loss of bone but a thorough and deep incision. This is most painful, but will give instant relief. After the evacuation, the treatment is to be followed as in ordinary abscess.

ULCERS.

Ulcers are breaches of continuity of surface, being caused by disease or unrepaired injury. A *simple* or *healthy* ulcer has its surface covered with a thick, creamy, yellow pus, not too profuse, and inodorous. The granulations are small, florid, pointed, sensitive, and vascular. A *scrofulous* ulcer is one occurring in debilitated constitutions, most frequently upon the neck and joints. They originate in the cellular tissue, beneath the skin, exist generally in clusters, and are characterized by imperfect and slow suppuration. An *indolent* ulcer occurs most frequently in the lower extremities of old persons, and is the most common of all ulcers. It is owing most frequently to a sore having been neglected or badly treated. Its surface is smooth, glassy, concave and pale. The discharge is thin and serous, and the surrounding tissue is swollen, hard, and of a dusky-red color. It is painless, and the patient is apt to let it go unnoticed, unless it by accident, exposure, or over exertion, it inflames and becomes painful. An *irritable* ulcer is one having an excess of organizing action, with a deficiency of organizable material. It is superficial, having an equal surface of a dark hue, and often covered with tenacious fibrin. It occurs most frequently near the ankle. It is very sensitive, and attended with great pain. A *phagedenic* ulcer is one of irregular form, with ragged, abrupt edges, and uneven brown surface, looking as if gnawed by an animal. It is attended with burning pain,

15

and great constitutional disturbance. A *varicose* ulcer is dependent upon a varicose condition of the veins, and usually occurs in the leg just above the ankle.   They are indolent, and mostly moist on the surface.

TREATMENT.—In the simple ulcer the treatment is simply protective. Water dressings are the best, as they keep the parts clean and remove the liquid pus. The "Herbal Ointment" is equally good. If the granulations become too luxuriant, an astringent wash, or slightly cauterizing them, becomes necessary.   In scrofulous ulcers constitutional treatment must be instituted.   The soft infiltrated tissues surrounding the ulcers should be destroyed by escharotics, and after the slough is removed, the healthy granulated surface treated as a simple ulcer.   In indolent ulcers the sore should at first be cleansed by poultices.   Healthy granulation should be aroused by lightly touching the ulcer with nitrate of silver, sulphate of copper, etc., or the same effect may be produced by strips of adhesive plaster being placed over the entire surface of the ulcer.   In irritable ulcer the treatment should first be constitutional, and tonics and stimulants administered.   The part should be relaxed, rested, and elevated.   This should be followed by a light poultice, or warm-water dressing, or if there is great pain, fomentations of the infusion of opium, conium, or belladonna should be applied.   In the treatment of phagedenic ulcers, fresh air and good diet are all-important.   The secretions must be corrected, and a Dover's powder given at night. The ulcer should be thoroughly destroyed by escharotics, followed by warm poultices.   In varicose ulcer cold water, rest, regular bandaging, or laced stocking, constitutes the treatment. *Strapping* with strips of adhesive plaster, by the support afforded, is excellent in all cases of ulcers.

My "Herbal Ointment" (page 472) acts most admirably as a local application in all cases of ulcer.   It causes healthy granulation, relieves the pain, and speedily causes union of the edges.

BOILS (FURUNCULUS).

Boils occur most frequently in the young, and in those of plethoric habit, in those parts where the skin is thickest.   They are usually gregarious, and depend upon derangement of the stomach and intestines, and frequently succeed eruptive diseases. The swelling is of a conical shape, having a hard, red, and painful base, and a yellow apex. If left to itself it bursts and discharges pus, and a core or slough of cellular tissue ; when completely emptied, the heat and pain subside.

TREATMENT.—Poultices and warm fomentations should be applied early, and as soon as pus has formed, the boil should be opened, after which the granulated wound should be dressed with basilicon ointment. If my "Herbal Ointment" is procurable, if may be applied from the first, as it speedily draws the boil to a head, and quickly heals it after discharge.

CARBUNCLE (ANTHRAX).

This is a serious disease ; it is a solitary inflammation of the cellular tissue and skin, presenting a flat, spongy swelling of a livid hue, and attended with dull heavy pain. It varies in size, and its progress is slow. Like the boil, it appears more often upon the neck, the shoulders, the back, buttocks, and thighs. The constitutional symptoms are low throughout, and the attendant fever is apt to be typhoid in character; prostration and delirium often terminate the case. It most frequently attacks high livers of an advanced age.

TREATMENT.—During the formation, apply either fomentations and poultices, or cold water dressing. An incision in the form of a cross should be made free and early, which may be followed by caustic applications, in order that the dying parts may thoroughly be removed. After this is done, the wound is to receive ordinary treatment.

CHILBLAIN'S (PERNIO).

This is an affection of the skin, produced by sudden alternations of cold and heat, most commonly affecting the toes, heels, ears, or fingers. It is attended with itching, swelling, pain, and slight redness at first ; it may afterwards become of a livid hue, with vesications and ulcerative fissures, which are difficult to heal.

TREATMENT.—Wash the parts thoroughly, and then apply tallow, and if on the hands, draw on a pair of old gloves, especially at night. The " Herbal Ointment " is a sure and rapid cure for chilblains.

BURNS AND SCALDS.

There are three principal divisions of these injuries, which may be produced by hot fluids, vapor, flame, or solids.

1st. Those which produce mere redness and inflammation, terminating in resolution, and perhaps desquamation.

2d. Those causing blisters on the skin, which often dry up and heal ; but if the true skin has been injured and inflamed, suppuration, and ulceration will result.

3d. Those causing the death of the part, in which there is not much pain, and which are followed by sloughs.

Extensive burns, even if superficial, are very dangerous, and those upon the trunk are more dangerous than those upon the extremities. The symptoms are paleness and shivering, with a feeble, quick pulse, often prostration, coma, and death. The greatest danger is during the first four or five days, from collapse ; subsequently from an affection of the head, chest, or abdomen, or from prostration.

TREATMENT.—Bathing the part in cold water will mitigate the pain, heat, and inflammation. Afterwards it must be protected from the air by raw cotton, or some bland unctuous substance. My "Herbal Ointment" gives instantaneous relief. Glycerine and carbolic acid are used by some, and linseed oil and lime water, or linseed oil, prepared chalk, and vinegar, by others. The indication is only to exclude the air. The blisters should be discharged of their contents, care being taken that the skin is not removed. The nervous excitement is to be calmed by opium, and sinking prevented by stimulants, but care is to be taken that over-stimulation does not result. The separation of sloughs is to be promoted by rest, poultices, and fomentations. In joints passive motion is to be made to prevent stiffness.

GOITRE (BRONCHOCELE).

This is an enlargement of the thyroid gland, an organ that if it performs any functions at all, does so only in foetal life. It generally commences by moderate increase of the gland, or thickening of the neck, and advances gradually until a portion or the whole gland becomes enormously swollen. It causes dyspnoea, and sometimes obstructs circulation to the brain, when the tumor acquires considerable magnitude. It is more common to females than males, and generally occurs before puberty. The species of idiocy sometimes associated with goitre is called *Cretinism*.

TREATMENT.—Alteratives and discutients. The alteratives, such as stillingia, rock-rose, etc., are to be preferred, and externally iodine may may be applied. Those who may desire my counsel in this disease are referred to page 390.

RUPTURE (HERNIA).

This signifies a protrusion of the abdominal viscera. The predisposing cause is a weakness of the abdominal walls, at the natural openings. This weakness may be increased by injury, disease, or pregnancy, or it may also be due to congenital difficulty. The exciting causes are muscular exertion, jumping, straining, playing on wind instruments, coughing, lifting weights, tight clothes, parturition, straining at stool, etc.

Hernia is divided, according to the site of the protusion, into *inguinal, ventro-inguinal, umbilical, ventral, perineal, vaginal, pudendal, thyroideal,* and *ischiatic ;* in condition, into *reducible, irreducible,* and *strangulated,* and if the contents are entirely intestinal it is called *enterocele,* but if it contains omentum it is termed *epiplocele.*

The symptoms of hernia are a painful swelling forming at some part of the abdomen, which is compressible and soft, and can be made to disappear by pressure in the proper direction, and it often disappears spontaneously. An enterocele is smooth, elastic, and globular, retires suddenly and with a gurgling noise. An epiplocele is more irregular in form, has a doughy feel, and retires slowly without noise.

Reducible hernia is one in which the contents of the sac can be reduced with proper manipulation. *Irreducible* hernia is owing to adhesions. or from membranous bands stretching across the sae, etc., when the contents cannot be replaced; and when the contents of the sac are incarcerated, with inflammation and an interruption to the passage of fæces, it is called *strangulated.* The more common forms are the inguinal and umbilical. Inguinal hernia is called *scrotal* when the intestine has descended from the groin into the scrotum.

TREATMENT.—The treatment consists in reduction and retention. This can only be achieved in the reducible hernia. Reduction is effected by a manipulation called *taxis*, the patient being placed in a recumbent position, and the muscles of the abdomen relaxed; gentle and steady pressure is made by the hand in the direction of the descent. Retention is effected by continued and suitable pressure by means of the pad of a well-fitting truss. By constant and careful use of a truss, a radical cure may be effected. A lobelia emetic, or the patient may be chloroformed, to relax the muscles, may be resorted to, if replacement cannot be performed without them. In irreducible hernia, the treatment consists in carefully regulating the bowels, avoiding great exertions, and wearing a suitable truss to prevent further protrusion. Strangulated hernia, if it cannot be reduced by taxis, becomes a subject for the surgeon. Radical cures may also be performed by the surgeon.

I have constantly manufactured for my patients a most excellent truss, which effects many cures. It is a light appliance, and occasions no pain or inconvenience to the wearer. It is the most comfortable truss that can be worn, is cleanly and durable, and easily adjusted. It is called the " Champion Truss "— a distinction to which it is clearly entitled. It is the greatest triumph of skill and genius ever attained in this or any other coun-

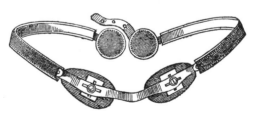

Dr. O Phelps Brown's Champion Truss.

try for the retention and radical cure of hernia or rupture. Its qualities may be briefly stated, as follows, viz. :—

It is worn with perfect ease and safety.
It keeps its place under all circumstances.
It never gets out of order.
Its pressure is equalized and gentle.
It makes no pressure on the spine.
It is applicable to single or double rupture.

These qualities are all that are required of a truss, either for retention or cure, and any truss lacking in any of them does not fulful its
purpose, and is capable of doing great injury.   Its perfect adjustment
is well represented in the following cuts.   The most violent paroxysms

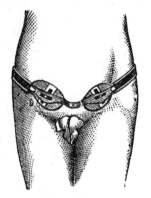   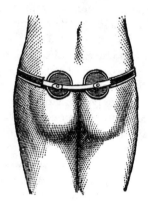

Front View.   Back View.

of coughing, muscular exertion, falls, etc., will not move it from its
properly applied position.   This indispensable quality of retention must
be possessed by every truss, otherwise it is useless.

Patients desiring the " Champion Truss," will please send the following measurement, viz., around the body where the truss is worn, and
state whether right, left, or double.   Trusses of the highest mechanical
perfection are also furnished for every other variety of rupture.   Preliminary correspondence *free* in all cases.

DISEASES OF THE EYE AND EAR.

The eye is one of the most delicate as well as the most complicated
organs of the body, and its diseases are but very imperfectly understood
by the ordinary practitioner.   A great deal of mischief has been done by
improper treatment of diseases of the eye, and I may also include the
ear, and many persons who now mourn the loss of sight and hearing,
partially or wholly so, might yet be in enjoyment of those senses if they
but had received the proper treatment.   Under this head I shall include
those diseases only which are capable of treatment in domestic practice.

CONJUNCTIVITIS.

This is an inflammation of the conjunctiva or mucous membrane of
the eyelids.   The sensation is as if particles of sand had insinuated
themselves beneath the lids, accompanied by heat, pain, and increased

lachrymal secretion, also intolerance of light. In severe cases, headache, nausea, constipation, loss of appetite, etc., are present. The causes of this form of inflammation are mostly local, as particles of sand, dust, insects, etc.

TREATMENT.—Remove the cause. If due to foreign particles in the eye, they should be removed. Bathe the eye thoroughly in water, rubbing towards the nose. If iron or steel is suspected, a vial cork, rubbed smooth with flannel, should be touched to all parts of the eye, which will remove the particles. When the eye is relieved, a mild purgative may be given, and cold water applications made to the eye. In severer cases, lotions of nitrate of silver, sulphate of zinc, etc., become necessary.

CATARRHAL OPHTHALMIA.

This is due to exposure to cold. The white of the eye becomes inflamed and very red, and generally there is a thin mucous discharge, which in severe cases becomes thick and purulent. This condition of the eye is accompanied by chilliness, aching of the bones, and some degree of fever.

TREATMENT.—Apply cold soft water to the eyes with little muslin packs, and give a purgative. If this will not relieve the inflammation, cold slippery-elm poultices, or the domestic practice of applying " smear case " to the eyes, may be resorted to. In obstinate or chronic cases a solution of four grains of sulphate of zinc to the ounce of water may be applied two or three times a day with a small brush. The eye should also be bathed with a decoction of golden seal. My " Herbal Ointment " (page 472) is excellent in all ophthalmic diseases.

PURULENT OPHTHALMIA.

The symptoms of this disease peculiar to children are similar to the Catarrhal Ophthalmia of adults. The eyes are kept constantly closed, the lids are red and swollen, and glued together by thick purulent matter becoming dry. The skin is dry and the bowels irregular. It is generally due to exposure to damp and cold, injuries in washing the child, acrid matter, or to a scrofulous constitution.

TREATMENT.—In the treatment of this affection the eyes should be thoroughly washed in a cold, weak solution of hydrastin, four or five times a day. Saturate packs with cold water, containing a little tincture of lobelia, and apply to the eyes and change when they grow warm. The bowels should be kept open with gentle laxatives. Some cases may need a solution of vegetable caustic, sulphate of zinc, or nitrate of silver. If caused by a scrofulous condition, use alteratives, of which the " Compound extract of Rock-rose and Stillingia " is the best (see page 471).

SCROFULOUS OPHTHALMIA.

This disease is chiefly confined to children. The child scarcely can bear the light, the lids are spasmodically closed, and the head constantly turned away from the light. The eye is not very red, but a few of the large vessels are considerable injected. It is very liable to recur, and may prove obstinate, and cause ulceration of the cornea.

TREATMENT.—In this disease it is very important that the general health should be looked after. The local treatment before advised should be resorted to, and the constitutional treatment should be very active and energetic.

STYE (HORDEOLUM).

This is a small painful pustule on the margin of the eyelid, having its origin in ciliary follicles.

TREATMENT.—It may usually be cured by applying spirits of hartshorn by means of a small steel needle, puncturing the tumor slightly. If this does not remove the inflammation, slippery-elm poultices should be applied, and tonics and alteratives given.

AMAUROSIS.

This complaint is due to anæsthesia of the optic nerve. The patient sees objects indistinctly, even when they are lit up by a bright light; they appear surrounded with a fog or mist, and no effort nor the employment of artificial means increase the distinctness. The outlines of objects appear not only indistinct, but also broken, and thus disfigured, the faculty of distinguishing colors is frequently lost, and double vision is not infrequent. This condition, as above described, is more properly *amblyopia*, it is only called *amaurosis* when the vision is entirely lost.

TREATMENT.—Electro-galvanism is one of the most promising remedies. Powdered bay-berry root, taken as snuff, is occasionally useful. Blisters behind the ear often afford relief. Nux vomica should also be given. The disease is often very obstinate, but I have cured some of the most unpromising cases.

FOREIGN BODIES IN THE EYES.

These should be sought for by inverting the lids, and having the patient turn the eyes in every direction. If it be found to adhere to the mucous membrane of the cornea or conjunctiva, it can usually be removed by a silk handkerchief wrapped around a probe. If lime, mortar, or lye should get into the eye, it should be removed, and the eye washed with a weak solution of vinegar and water. The ensuing inflammation should receive usual treatment. If the foreign bodies enter the interior chamber of the eye, the surgeon should only re-move it.

FOREIGN SUBSTANCES IN THE EAR.

Children frequently put peas, beans, kernels of corn, etc., into the ear, which, if allowed to remain, will produce active inflammation. Foreign bodies may also enter the ear by accident. These should all be quickly removed. It should be done by syringing the ear with warm water, or by means of forceps. Excessive accumulation of wax is to be removed by syringing with warm water frequently, and not by ear-scoops.

EAR ACHE (OTALGIA).

This is a neuralgic affection, and is caused by local inflammation, cold and exposure, and carious teeth.

TREATMENT.—If caused by inflammation, a warm poultice of slip-pery-elm, moistened with laudanum, should be applied, and frequently changed. If caused by carious teeth they should be removed; sweet oil and laudanum dropped in the ear often gives relief, and the common practice of blowing hot tobacco smoke into the ear is also useful.

Many of the eye and ear diseases are surgical in their character, such as strabismus, a few cases of cataract, etc., but a great many of them are amenable to medical treatment. Even cataract, which heretofore was considered eminently surgical, may in many cases be entirely cured by medicinal treatment alone. I have cured a case, in which there was total blindness for ten years, in the short space of two months. The patient ever since is in the full enjoyment of sight. My treatment has also been equally successful in cases of deafness. I regard all cases subject to relief or cure in which the tympanum or drum of the ear is not destroyed. If persons suffering from chronic diseases of the eye or ear will write and state their cases fully to me, I will cheerfully give my opinion by return mail.

MALIGNANT AND VENEREAL DISEASES.

CANCER (CARCINOMA).

This is a malignant tumor. In the first stage it is hard, in the second stage it ulcerates. The seat of cancer is in the female breast, the skin, the tongue, the stomach, the womb, the lips, etc. It rarely occurs in subjects under thirty years of age. It is at first a small hard tumor, movable, but eventually it forms deep and superficial attachments. It grows in general slowly, is irregular in shape, and painful. The pain is mostly sharp, lancinating, and is much increased on pressure. In the

15*

course of time the tissue beneath the skin is absorbed, and becomes attached to it, and it presents a bluish, nodulated appearance. Ulceration usually takes place by absorption of the skin, and as sloughing proceeds, the edges become ragged and everted, having a bluish purple color, and discharges a fetid, sanious pus.

There are five varieties of cancer, though microscopically they are essentially the same.

Scirrhus is hard, firm, and transparent, and of a grayish color, occurring most frequently in the female breast, skin, etc.

Encephaloid is soft and brainlike in its appearance, and hemorrhagic in character, frequently met with in the globe of the eye, testes, nares, etc.

Colloid resembles glue or honey in the comb, and usually occurs in the internal viscera.

Melanosis, or melanotic cancer, is of a black color, either soft or hard, and occurs mostly upon serous membranes.

Epithelial cancer is usually found upon the lips.

These various forms may exist separately, or one variety may be associated with or take the place of another.

TREATMENT.—As long as this disease was regarded as purely local in character, the only treatment resorted to was extirpation either by cauterizing agents or by the knife ; but since the pathology of the disease is better understood, and its constitutional character ascertained, the treatment employed has been considerably modified. I have long ago held that cancer was a constitutional affection, so instructed my patients, and based my treatment upon that opinion.

It is well to remove the tumor by the knife or cautery, but the liability to recurrence is always great unless constitutional treatment is employed. The cauterizing agents are blood-root and chloride of zinc made into a paste, and then applied to the cancer, the skin having first been removed by a blister. This is reapplied until the whole mass is dead, when in course of time it comes away as a slough. The expressed juices of poke, laurel, blood-root, and yellow-dock answer the same purpose.

The constitutional treatment consists in toning up the general system, abstaining from fatty diet, bathing, and the employment of alterative treatment. Recently, a plant has been brought into notice by the name of *Cundurango* (*Equatoria Garciana*, see page 74) which is destined to revolutionize the treatment of cancer. I have tried it in several cases, and it answered every expectation. I regard it as a virtual specific in cancer, and shall, notwithstanding its very high price, employ it in every case, thereby hoping to make my success in the treatment of this malignant disease more certain. It is a matter of regret that spurious articles are in the market, thus bringing the genuine article, which is yet difficult to obtain, into disrepute.

SYPHILIS.

Syphilis is occasioned by a specific poison which is conveyed by con-tagion or actual contact. It first shows itself upon the genital organs in the form of a small yellowish pimple, or pimples, the presence of which is at first made manifest by itching and slight soreness. The pimples (called chancres) break, and gradually change into a red, hard-edged shallow ulcer. This ulcer is circular or oval in form, and is surrounded by a ragged border. The skin and tissue in the immediate vicinity be-come inflamed, and, unless proper remedies be immediately applied, the virus is absorbed into the system, and the consequences are of the most deplorable character. There are many kinds of chancre, viz :—inflam-matory, indurated or hard, sloughing or perishing, phagedenic or eat-ing, and gangrenous or likely to mortify. Next in order, if stringent curative measures be not adopted, is the *bubo*, which is a swelling of the glands of the groin, caused by the absorption of the poison. The bubo will usually make its appearance in about a fortnight after the sore is discovered. It advances to suppuration, and also becomes a sore, when it receives the name of "glandular chancre." Sometimes growths re-sembling certain vegetables appear, in the male, upon the organ and on the membrane lining of the foreskin. In the female, they will be found in and at the entrance of the vagina, and sometimes on the neck of the womb. These are primary symptoms, and, if quickly but radically extir-pated or cured, will not result in any very serious constitutional derange-ment; but if neglected, the virus is absorbed into the blood, and the infection reaches the entire system. When the disease becomes consti-tutional, the results are most deplorable. The syphilitic ulcer then appears at various parts of the body, more usually upon the arm and forearm, forehead, shin and chest. These ulcers are quite characteristic, so that the experienced surgeon at once knows their specific nature upon sight. The affections of the skin and mucous membrane are called *secondary*, those appearing upon the bones, etc., are *tertiary*. In these advanced stages of the disease the gravity is such as should urge each affected person to employ competent surgical or medical aid, and not longer to postpone such active treatment as is required. Neglect of so important a duty on the part of the patient will result seriously to him, as the progress of the disease is unerringly from bad to worse in every case.

TREATMENT.—In primary syphilis, the chancre should be destroyed effectually by nitrate of silver, nitric acid, or caustic potash, and heal the parts by mild dressing. If this is effectually done, with proper con-stitutional treatment, no secondary symptoms will supervene.

In secondary and tertiary syphilis the treatment is very important, and must be correct in order to eliminate the disorganizing taint.

The treatment is necessarily alterative and tonic. The following may each be specifically employed, either singly or judiciously combined :— Phytolaccin, corydalin, chimaphilin, tincture of kalmia, menispermin, ceanothus americanus, sarsaparilla, stillingia, and by some iodide of potassium, but never mercury. Mercury in any form is not a specific, and in effects most pernicious. When buboes appear, they should be discussed by a mixture of tincture of iodine, ℥ ij. ; tincture of arnica, ℨ ij. ; tincture of scrophularia, ℨ ij. This should be applied by wetting pads of linen with it and securing them by adhesive strips. If suppuration has taken place, the treatment of abscess is to be employed.

During treatment, the patient should abstain from all fat meats, spirituous liquors, and excesses of every kind.

If any person is conscious that he or she is affected with a syphilitic taint they should never marry, for the offspring will surely be miserable objects of pity, and conjugal bliss very uncertain. The taint must be thoroughly eradicated, so that not a vestige remains, before a marriage, physically pure, can occur.

If rightly treated, syphilis is not a formidable disease to cure, yet how many suffer hopelessly on, after having for years been subjected to mercurial treatment. Purely chemical herbal treatment will only remove the serious disorder from the system, as attested by the thousands of cases under my treatment, in which every trace of the disease has been obliterated from the economy.

GONORRHŒA.

This is vulgarily known as *clap*, so named from the French *clappe*, a bow-string. It received this name on account of the *chordee* occurring in the disease. This is caused by the violence of the inflammation, which abnormally expands the cavernous body of the organ and is painfully drawn downwards, so that the urethra occupies the relative position of the string to a bow-gun.

This is a disease of the mucous membrane which lines the private parts of the male and female, and is communicated as is syphilis, by contagion, or actual contact. It commences with itching and uneasiness about the private parts, and a peculiar feeling of soreness in the urethra, or urinary canal. A scalding sensation is also felt when the patient makes water. In a day or two a whitish matter makes its appearance at the orifice of the urethra, and this will soon increase greatly in quantity, and assume a greenish-yellow color. The parts will be much inflamed, and the urethra will become thickened and very sore. The consistency and quantity of the pus-like discharge vary in different persons. It usually makes its appearance in from three to five days after exposure. It may propagate itself upon other mucous membranes after inoculation.

TREATMENT.—A purgative should be taken at first, and at the same time the parts should be thoroughly packed with cold or hot water. The following are the remedies mostly employed as internal remedies : —Oil of copaiba and cubebs, matico, gelsemin, oil of erigeron, oil of turpentine, etc. These oils should be taken in medium doses, and in emulsion with acacia, etc. The internal injections are vegetable astringents, sugar of lead, sulphate of zinc, etc. The injections should not be strong, and be carefully made, otherwise orchitis may follow. Applying cold water relieves the chordee.

The treatment is not difficult, and, if properly directed, will soon relieve the patient.

GLEET.

This is one of the results of abused or neglected gonorrhœa. It is a continued discharge of a thin and clear character, after the inflammatory and painful early symptoms have disappeared. It is caused by dedebility of the parts, or by unhealthy action of the glands in the urinary passage. It is sometimes, especially in persons of a scrofulous habit, a fixture for years, and constitutes a drain upon the system, the effects of which can only be obviated by the most scrupulous care and attention. The old style of treatment involved the use of cauterizing injections, and the bougie, together with blisters applied to the perinæum. It had the effect of imperfectly remedying, or else of aggravating the complaint, and rendering it next to impossible of cure.

TREATMENT.--Same as for acute gonorrhœa, but it should be more energetic.

Those who may wish to intrust their cases to my treatment, may rest assured that they will be quickly cured, and everything held confidential. The fear of exposure does frequently much mischief, and the dread of losing caste in society, or a feeling of shame, often tempts the sufferer to withhold his case from the family physician for treatment, or he may endure his mental and physical torture in silence as long as he can, and then finally intrust his case to the ignorance of a companion, who may know some recipe, or he may employ the treatment of some incompetent, uneducated physician, found everywhere, especially in large cities, who also maltreats the case, so that finally the disease, which at first was readily curable, has become a very serious affection.

The wrong of such a course is obvious, and I advise the reader, who has or may become unfortunate in this respect, to confide his or her case to some honorable and competent physician, as soon as the disease manifests itself.

DEBILITY OR LOSS OF VITALITY.

This is a condition of the organism characterized by loss of vitality, or deterioration and diminution in the quality and tone of the vital forces. It is one of the chief predisposing causes of disease, and is of itself a condition characterized by all the elements of ill health. The principal causes of debility are improper nourishment, impure air, excessive bodily and mental exercise, want of exercise, long exposure to intense heat or cold, intemperance, depressing states of the mind, and of course a prostrative disease. When not a heritage of the organism, it is generally produced by some flagrant violation of physiological law, depleting the vital forces by the disorganization of organic functions which ensues, or by the loss of vital elements through the eliminating organs, chiefly the kidneys.

That the reader may have a correct understanding of what is meant by vitality, it may be well to give its physiological sense. Though derived from the Latin *vita*, life, it has a somewhat different signification from that which is expressed by the word life. It signifies the constituent principle or essence of life rather than the entity itself. Hence vitality is not properly life, but the element conducive to its perfection and prolongation. It is that principle that gives to the physical organization its vigor, elasticity, and tone, to the mental organs, acuteness, vivacity and sprightliness, and to the whole organism a high standard of health.

If the habits are not in violation of hygiene or physiology, and the expenditure of the vital forces not exceeding the production, the normal condition of the organism would be one of health and vigor, and almost complete immunity from disease. If the expenditure exceeds the production it engenders the condition termed debility. Improper and sinful habits of life, especially in the young, are alarmingly destructive of vitality in consequence of engendering diseases characterized by losses of vital secretions. The intemperate very frequently incur the penalty of over-indulgence in intoxicating beverages by inducing structural diseases of the internal organs, especially Bright's disease of the kidney, wherein the blood becomes devitalized by loss of its albumen through the urine. In the male economy at an age often quite immature there is induced an affection characterized by involuntary expenditure of a secretion, directly by an improper and sinful life. The element thus constantly expended, and which occurs invariably without any exercise of the voluntary powers, is beyond all question the most highly organized and more intrinsically vital than any other secretion of the organism. This affection, peculiarly masculine, is one of the most prolific causes of debility, and is conducive to greater physical misfortune than any other pathological condition induced by violation of physiological laws. The chemical nature of the secretion is highly phosphatic, and as phosphorus is a very important constituent of nerve tissue, its constant involuntary escape from the organism, whether in the urine or otherwise, preys fearfully upon the nerve tissue for phosphatic supply, and eventually, and often quite rapidly, produces atony of the nerve-centres, and a general intonicity of the nervous system, or what is more commonly known as nervous debility. Of the various systems composing the organism the nervous can least afford to lose its vitality, or to become enfeebled. It is the principal or controlling system of the organism, the others being more or less subordinate. If by any depleting causes its just complement of the vital forces becomes reduced, its individual integrity is not alone compromised or destroyed, but muscular action, circulation, digestion, assimilation, and the mental operations also become enfeebled, hence the vital standard of the nervous system is of extreme importance to the general welfare of the whole organism.

Precisely the same pathological condition results from another cause, a sedentary habit of life. It is due to such exciting causes that clergymen and other persons of sedentary habits suffer so frequently from nervous or general debility. When the muscular system is permitted to degenerate from want of proper exercise it gives to the organism a condition of laxity or intonicity which in the male induces the previously mentioned loss of a highly vitalized secretion, and in the female an uncompensated loss of nervo-electric force. Debility is the result in both cases, though the devitalization is more rapid in the male, proportionally to the physical vigor inherent to the different sexes, than in the female. This is explained by the fact that in the male economy a greater loss of the phosphates occurs. In all persons of studious habits, and where bodily exercise is insufficient, the urine is loaded with phosphates, which is indicative of the breaking down of nerve tissue. Consequently in the male there is not only the usual phosphoric loss due to nervous waste, but the super-addition of the involuntary loss of a secretion which, as has been stated, is highly phosphatic in its chemical nature, makes the depletion of the phosphorus essential to a vital condition of the organism, doubly great.

In a debilitated condition of the nervous system, or, as it is usually denominated, nervous debility, from whatever cause the loss of vitality may ensue, there is in general quite a train of symptoms, as may be supposed when this more important part of the economy has become devitalized. This form of debility may usually be recognized by a marked facial expression, a characteristic mannerism, and by a peculiar mental state. The skin of the face is pale and sallow, and usually affected with acne ; there is a dark circle around the orbits, the pupils are dilated and sluggish, the eyes become lustreless, and the face has a haggard, troubled furtive expression. These physiognomic characteristics are due to atony or want of tone in the cerebral nerve-centres, and from the same

cause the devitalized patient is listless, shy, retiring and easily confused, society loses its charms, and solitude is preferred, but has, however, no compensating or satisfying influence over the patient. There
is a want of steadiness and decision in his locomotion, his inferior extremities are deficient in power, and all the movements are suggestive
of a mind ill at ease. The mental operations are confused, speech becomes awkward and often without directness; memory is defective, and
the patient is usually absent-minded and given to reverie. Pains in the
lumbar region, and a sense of weight and aching in the loins are experienced. The appetite is capricious, and digestion feeble. The mind is
deficient in power of attention, the imagination is constantly pervaded
with vague erotic dreams, the moral sense is blunted and the perceptions
are dull and confused. Pains in the course of the principal nerves and
extreme nervous sensibility are experienced. The patient also can fix
his mind on any subject with difficulty ; his attention wanders, and he
is given to day-dreams and erotic visions.

The urine, of course, contains phosphates, the source of which,
whether nervous or secretional, is easily determined by analyzation or
microscopical examination. Urates are also found in the urine. Those
who suspect such vital loss, may with sufficient certainty for all practical purposes ascertain the fact by a simple experiment. The morning
urine should be placed in a clean half-pint bottle, and let it stand from
forty-eight to seventy-two hours. If there is then found a remarkably
peculiar or cloudy sediment or deposit at the bottom, the fact is quite
evident that some of the losses alluded to occur, and proper aid should
be sought at once.

Such, briefly, are the evidences of a devitalized nervous system. The
condition, as is palpable to every one, is fraught with danger to the
general welfare, and even to life, if the process of depletion of the vital
forces continues too long, or if, by special virulence of the exciting
cause, the devitalization is rapid in occurrence. Any loss of vital power
should be regarded with solicitude and deep concern by every one who
places a proper estimation upon vigor of the organism and its special
functions. Careful and judicious treatment must not be neglected,
as by such a course only can revitalization be speedily and adequately
effected. As soon as loss of vital force becomes apparent, so soon
should the services of a competent and experienced physician be engaged. In any stage of devitalization, rehabilitation of the organism
with vitality can again be accomplished, the only requirement being
employment of competent medical aid, and the exhibition of vitalizing
remedies. Revitalization can, however, only be effected by herbal remedies, as their organic nature alone affords the elements required for
reendowment of the system with vital force. Minerals are lifeless, and
can therefore impart no vital element.

Those desiring to consult the author with reference to debility or loss of vitality from any cause whatever, may refer to page 385, where his mode of treatment is described, and to page 390, where the necessary questions are asked.

SATYRIASIS.

This is a disease characterized by a constant and insatiable desire for coition, and so called because the satyrs of mythology were greatly addicted to excesses. The disease is accompanied by a strange power of frequent congress without exhaustion. It is a nervous disease, dependent upon a disordered state of the cerebellum.

TREATMENT.—It can be cured by a low diet, frequent shower baths, physical out-door labor, ice bags to the cerebellum, a hard bed, and hop pillows.

STRICTURE OF THE URETHRA.

This is a diminution or contracted condition of the tube, and may be either *spasmodic* or *permanent*. Spasmodic stricture depends on spasm of the muscles of the perinæum, or upon contraction of the muscular portion of the urethra. Exposure to cold and indulgence in drink favor an attack, which usually occurs after dinner. It generally occurs in persons with permanent obstruction. The urine is suddenly retained, the desire to urinate causes incessant straining, the bladder becomes distended, the countenance anxious, the pulse quick, the skin hot, and at last the urine dribbles, or the bladder may burst, and extravasation occurs into the peritonæum or perinæum. There is another variety of this affection, termed *inflammatory stricture*, caused by abuse of injections, exposure, or intemperance during acute gonorrhœa.

Permanent stricture is a contraction from permanent inflammation, plastic deposit having taken place in the tissue beneath the mucous membrane. The occasion of this inflammation may be gonorrhœa, venery, kicks or blows, riding on horseback, acrid urine, drinking, etc. It is situated most frequently in the membranous portion of the urethra, usually a few inches from the meatus. The extent and degree of contraction vary. Sometimes the stricture is very tight, but limited, as if a thread had been tied around the urethra; more frequently it is of greater extent, containing from a quarter of an inch to several inches. Several strictures may exist at once. Permanent stricture comes on gradually, occurring mostly in middle-aged men. Urination is frequent, tedious, and painful; the stream is thin, twisted, or forked; and a few drops pass after urination, which had collected behind the stricture. There is pain in the perinæum, thighs, and loins; erection is often painful; chill and fever constantly occurring as in ague; the testicles, rectum, and bowels sympathize, and the general health is greatly impaired. It is a disease that causes extreme annoyance, pain, and disorder, and should receive early and competent treatment.

TREATMENT.—The indication in spasmodic stricture is to overcome the spasm, and relieve the bladder. This is usually effected by warm hip baths, Dover's powder, laudanum enemata, and cold water upon the genitals. A favorable mental impression is made by pouring water from a can, in a small stream, from some height, into a vessel containing water, in imitation of urination. A few sniffs of ether will usually relax the spasm, but if these means fail, the urine should be drawn of by a catheter.

In permanent stricture *dilatation* by means of flexible bougies is the usual method of cure. Great caution is necessary in the use of these. Some use caustic applications, and in some cases puncturation is resorted to. In some cases opening the urethra may be necessary, as the stricture is so extensive and complete that no other means are available.

These surgical means may at times be necessary, but I have cured very many cases by purely medicinal treatment, and it is very seldom that I employ bougies, but compel absorption of the deposit by alterative treatment. In some cases, however, I frequently combine dilatation with medication. Those desiring consultation are referred to page 390.

PROSTATITIS.

This is inflammation of the prostate gland. It usually accompanies gonorrhœa, but may exist independently. The discharge is similar to that of urethral inflammation, and when the result of chronic inflammation the discharge is called prostatorrhœa. The gland is frequently enlarged. Chronic inflammation is commonly brought on by gleet, stricture, horse exercise, etc., and is most frequently met with in advanced life, and disappears upon the removal of the cause. The gland is also enlarged in old persons—a hypertrophy independent of inflammation. The bladder sympathizes, and becomes irritable ; the urine is fœtid, mucous, and its stains are often retained. It causes most intense suffering.

TREATMENT.—Leeches, rest, counter-irritation, alteratives, laxatives, and enemata constitute the usual treatment. In hypertrophy of the organ, the usual treatment should be instituted. The medicinal treatment, as in stricture, is important, and should only be intrusted to those who fully understand the anatomy of the organ, and the pathology of the disease,

ORCHITIS.

This is the *hernia humoralis* of older writers. *Swelled testicle* is a common accompaniment of mumps. It is often the result of an injury, but oftener of gonorrhœa and its treatment ; exercise, wet and cold often induce it. The gland enlarges greatly, fever attends, causing intense pain.

It is usually confined to one of the glands, and mostly the epididymis. The cord is often swollen and painful.

TREATMENT.—Low diet and the recumbent position are essential. The weight of the tumor should be supported by a suspensory bandage. After the acute symptoms have subsided, friction with astringent lotions, and compression by adhesive straps, will be useful. The hardness and swelling are likely to remain unless discussed by the alteratives.

VARICOCELE.

This is a varicose condition of the veins of the spermatic cord. The causes are such as to produce obstruction to the return of blood: constipation, corpulence, tight belts around the abdomen, and warm climate. It is usually coexistent with genital weakness. The left side is more frequently affected than the right, because the left spermatic vein is more likely to be compressed by the fæces in the sigmoid or S-shaped flexure of the rectum, and because it is longer and not so direct in its course. The swelling is pear-shaped and feels like a bunch of earth-worms.

TREATMENT.—The cause, if ascertained, should be removed, and the scrotum constantly bathed in cold water, and supported with a suspensory bandage.

The veins are sometimes obliterated by a surgical operation. It can usually be overcome by proper medical treatment, however, and the operation should only be the last resort.

I use for my patients a self-adjusting suspensory bandage, which can be so arranged that any extent of compression can be made, and which in construction is simple and very durable. It is the only perfect suspensory bandage or scrotal supporter made, and the only one from which any great benefit can be expected. It is eminently serviceable in this disease as well as in orchitis, and no one suffering from these diseases should do without them. Sent by mail, postage prepaid, on receipt of $3.

DISEASES OF THE FEMALE ORGANS OF GENERATION.

The genitalia of the female is the controlling centre of her whole economy. If the womb and its appendages are in a healthy state, the female figure preserves its artistic rotundity, her mind its sprightliness, and her humanity its benevolence and sympathy. When diseased, she becomes fretful, peevish, and inconsolable. The province of the physician, therefore, becomes one of great importance, and it is his duty that he should not only thoroughly understand the pathology of uterine diseases, but in his humanity he should combine a fine feeling of compassion, with correct ideas of the treatment required. He should prove worthy of the trust confided to him, in sympathy, considerateness, and skill.

No greater trust can fall upon him; he is not only accountable for the physical welfare of the patient, but bears a further responsibility. If his treatment is not judicious and rational, his patient becomes a victim to a gloomy depression of spirits, and to an irrepressible feeling of languor and misery, that sternly bid away all brightness of life. He will but poorly do his duty if he follows but the beaten track of a routine practice, and, after successive trials, consigns his suffering patient, by pronouncing her incurable, to a condition but little better than the grave. Uterine diseases are not incurable, but when properly treated they yield kindly to medication, as the disposition of all womb affections is to get well, needing but proper medical assistance to stimulate and encourage the forces of recuperation to overcome the assaults of disease. (See page 390)

VULVITIS.

This is characterized by redness and slight tumefaction of skin, covered with mucus, while in neglected cases the parts are found much excoriated. It generally arises from want of cleanliness, or from the acrid character of the vaginal and uterine secretions. It may, however, be produced by excessive marital indulgence or syphilitic taint. The symptoms consist of great pain and tenderness, a mucous discharge, a smarting in passing urine, and a constant pain about the loins and thighs.

TREATMENT.—This should be treated by hot packs, elm poultices, and a wash of a weak solution of sulphate of zinc, or tincture of myrrh. Quinine, macrotin and leptandrin should be given internally. The parts should be thoroughly cleansed every day.

CLITORITIS.

Inflammation of the clitoris, both acute and chronic, may exist from want of cleanliness, or be produced by indiscretions. It is accompanied with burning, itching, and smarting sensations. Enlargement is the usual result of either acute or chronic inflammation, in which case there is extension of the labia, producing irritation, and labial leucorrhœa.

TREATMENT.—When the parts are inflamed, sitz-baths, hot packs, and laxatives will usually relieve it. In case of hypertrophy, it may be painted once or twice a week with a weak tincture of iodine, and the compound syrup of stillingia given internally. When there is extensive enlargement, amputation should be resorted to.

IMPERFORATE HYMEN.

This is not likely to be discovered until the commencement of menstruation. It may then be suspected, if the female has all the symptoms which accompany the menses, without the discharge of the fluid, and if these symptoms should occur at regular periods, accompanied with a sense of weight and fulness of the vagina, especially if an enlargement is perceptible in the lower abdomen, with pain and tenderness.

The symptoms ameliorate in a few days, but return at each menstrual period. If by inspection a hemispherical tumor, of a livid or bluish color, soft and fluctuating, is discovered, the fact is most certain, that it is caused by an imperforate hymen. In most cases the membrane is thin, but it is sometimes from one-fourth to three-eighths of an inch thick.

TREATMENT.—Press the finger against it gently, and attempt to lacerate it by the finger-nail. If it will not yield, perforation should be made by a proper instrument in the hands of a surgeon.

VAGINITIS.

This consists of either acute or chronic inflammation of the vagina. It may be confined entirely to the mucous membrane, or it may extend to the cellular tissue beneath. It is attended with pain, swelling, and redness of the vaginal canal; the mucous membrane is of a vivid red color, and the folds are more developed and prominent than is natural. At the first stage there is an arrest of the secretions, but after a few days serous exudation occurs, which becomes purulent, and of a yellowish or greenish color. The disease may arise from cold, which is the most frequent cause; from injuries to the vagina by violence, imprudence in the marital association, exertion after delivery, high living, etc.

TREATMENT.—A gentle purgative should be taken, and the vagina frequently injected with warm water, the patient kept quiet, and the inflammation controlled by veratrum. Astringent injections are also useful. The chronic form should be treated as vaginal leucorrhœa.

MENSTRUATION.

Though this is not a disease but a healthy function, but as, from various causes, derangement of the function occurs, it is proper that it should be perfectly understood. Menstruation is the term applied to the phenomenon that attends the rupture of what is called the *Graafian follicles* of the ovary, and the discharge of an ova, or egg. It is a bloody discharge from the female genitals—not differing from ordinary blood, excepting that it does not coagulate, and in its peculiar odor. The blood comes from the capillaries of the womb and vagina.

Menophania, or the first appearance of the menses, is usually prece-ded by a discharge of a fluid whitish matter from the vagina, by nervous excitement, and by vague pains and heaviness in the loins and thighs; numbness of the limbs, and swelling and hardness of the breasts. The first appearance is an evidence of capacity for conception. It generally appears about the age of fourteen, but varies from nine to twenty-four years. In warm climates women begin to menstruate earlier, and cease sooner than in temperate regions ; in the cold climates the reverse of this holds as a general rule. The manifestations of approaching puberty are seen in the development of breasts, the expansion of the hips, the rounded contour of the body and limbs, appearance of the purely feminine figure, development of the voice, and the child becomes reserved, and exchanges her plays for the pursuits of womanhood.

More or less indisposition and irritability also precede each successive recurrence of the menstrual flux, such as headache, lassitude, uneasiness, pain in back, loins, etc. The periods succeed each other usually about every twenty-eight days, although it may occur every twenty-two, twenty, eighteen, fifteen, or thirty-two, thirty-five, and forty days. The most important element is the regularity of the return. In temperate climates each menstrual period ordinarily continues from three to six days, and the quantity lost from four to eight ounces. The menses continue to flow from the period of puberty till the age of forty-five or fifty. At the time of its natural cessation, the flow becomes irregular, and this irregularity is accompanied occasionally with symptoms of dropsy, glandular swellings, etc., constituting the *critical period*, *turn*, or *change of life ;* yet it does not appear that mortality is increased by it, as vital statistics show that more men die between forty and fifty than women.

It should be the duty of every mother or female in charge of a child, in whom age or actual manifestations suggest the approach of puberty, to acquaint her with the nature of her visitation, and the importance of her conduct in regard to it. She should be taught that it is perfectly natural to all females at a certain period, and that its arrival necessitates caution on her part with regard to exposure to wet or cold. The author has made the acquaintance of the history of many cases of consumption, and other diseases, which were directly induced by folly and ignorance at the first menstrual flow. The child is often kept in extreme ignorance of the liability of womanhood occurring to her at a certain age, and hence when she observes a flow of blood escaping from a part, the delicacy attached to the locality makes her reticent with regard to inquiry or exposure ;. she naturally becomes alarmed, and most likely attempts to stanch the flow, with bathing or applying cold water to the part, thus doing incalculable mischief.

This purely feminine physiological function should be well' studied and understood by all females. At least they should know that the phenomenon is a natural one, liable to disorder, and that the best interests of their general health demands care and prudence on their part to maintain regularity, etc., of the flow. Disregard of such a duty will surely entail much misery.

AMENORRHŒA.

This may occur in three forms. 1st. Where evacuation has never oc-curred, or *retention of the menses*. 2d. Where there has been no secre-tion. 3d. Suppression. There are cases where the secretion has been perfect, but the discharge prevented by occlusion of the vagina, or im-perforate hymen, etc.; again, secretion may never have occurred, owing to a congenital deficiency of the ovaries; and there are cases where the uterus and ovaries are sound, yet no flow from the vagina. The most common variety, however, is suppression after they had once been regularly established. It may cease by degrees, as in con-sumptive and scrofulous patients, or occurs as the result of cold, which induces inflammation of the uterus or ovaries. It may also be induced by excessive venery, wet feet, ice water, insufficient clothing, bathing, fear, grief, anxiety, emetics, drastic purgatives, falls, copulation during flow, etc. The symptoms are weight, pain in the head, loins, and uterine regions, hot skin, apoplexy and epilepsy in some cases, vicarious hemor-rhages, palpitation of the heart, constipation, chills, loss of appetite, etc.

TREATMENT.—Give a hot foot-bath, if the suppression be recent, and apply hot mustard poultices to the breasts. Internally give tansy, thyme or wintergreen tea, keep the patient warm, and allow but gentle exer-cise. A compound decoction of seneca, cotton root, and Indian hemp is also very beneficial. In obstinate cases, a hot sitz-bath should be given during the operation of the medicine, so as to centre the blood in the pelvis. If this does not succeed, the system should be invigorated by quinine, blue cohosh, life root, wine, etc., and then the above treatment repeated. The chronic form of the disease should be treated by sup-porting and invigorating remedies, such as bayberry, black cohosh, sitz-baths, galvanism, tonics, etc.

DYSMENORRHŒA.

Painful menstruation occurs generally in single women, and is produced by inflammation or ulceration of the mouth of the womb, neuralgia of the womb during menstruation, indiscretions, constipation, and a ner-vous irritable temperament. The symptoms are restlessness, heat, flushed face, weight and heaviness in the head, pain in the back, and pelvic regions, sometimes so severe as to cause fainting. After a time the pain becomes bearing down, accompanied by a shreddy discharge, or blood-clots. In young and plethoric subjects, but little effect is produced on the general health, but in nervous persons the health fails, and, not unfrequently, consumption ensues. Women subject to dysmenorrhœa are liable to cancer after the turn of life.

TREATMENT.—When the disease is produced by inflammation or ulceration of the mouth of the womb, hot sitz-baths, with hot vaginal injections frequently repeated, in connection with ten or fifteen drops of the tincture of crawley every two or three hours, will usually relieve it. Mild purges should also be taken. When due to neuralgia, black cohosh should be given, and the treatment of neuralgia instituted. Senecin, gossypiin, and gelsemin, are also valuable. When produced by an irritable constitution, ladies'-slipper, scullcap, etc., should be given. Out-door exercises and a nutritious diet should be prescribed.

MENORRHAGIA.

This is characterized by profuse, prolonged, or too frequent menstruation, separately or conjoined. It is accompanied by headache, hot skin, full pulse, weight in the back, hips, loins, pelvis, etc. It is caused by hot rooms, abortions, leucorrhœa, falls, marital excesses, long walks, constipation, etc. The health gives way, the patient becomes bloodless, and exhaustion ensues upon the least exercise.

TREATMENT.—This should be treated by wild cherry, gelsemin, unicorn root, beth root, and injections of a decoction of golden-seal, matico, and cinchona. If the hemorrhage is active, a strong decoction of tannin or cranesbill may be injected, and ten or fifteen grains of cayenne pepper administered. The oil of erigeron is also useful. Tonics should be given in relaxed condition of the system.

VICARIOUS MENSTRUATION.

This is a discharge from some other part than the uterus, usually occurring in the unmarried. In the married, they are usually barren. The blood may escape from any part of the skin or mucous membrane, in the form of bleeding from the nose, lungs, etc.

TREATMENT.—Ten or fifteen drops of the oil of solidago should be given four or five times a day, in connection with sitz-baths, tonics, etc. Life root is especially valuable.

CHLOROSIS.

This is a disease characterized by chronic anæmia, or bloodlessness, affecting females about the age of puberty. In some instances it is undoubtedly dependent upon a nervous affection, but in most instances it is connected with disordered menstruation and other causes. The red corpuscles of the blood are pale and small, and diminished in numbers. The countenance assumes a wax-like hue, which is so remarkably characteristic, that the disease is called by nurses "*green sickness*." The appetite is irregular, with craving for particular kinds of food, the urine is thick and full of sediment, and there is usually vertigo, headache, backache, hysterical affections, dysmenorrhœa, and leucorrhœa. The tongue is flaccid and indented at the edges, the pulse is weak and quick, and there is a feeling of general languor, with great indisposition to bodily or mental exercise.

TREATMENT.—When arising from feeble and imperfect digestion, give prickly ash, alder, golden-seal, and nux vomica, cautiously. The animal oils are also very serviceable. The great object in the treatment of this disease is to restore the general health, and not to force menstruation by agents having that power. The patient wants strength and blood, and when that is achieved, menstruation will be natural. Baths, friction, out-door exercise, and a nutritious diet should not be neglected.

CESSATION OF THE MENSES.

We have already stated that this usually occurs between the ages of forty and fifty, but in some cases it occurs much earlier, in others much later. The courses become irregular, often staying away two or three months. Nausea and vomiting, swelling of the abdomen, tenderness of the breasts, etc., are the prominent symptoms. Pregnancy may sometimes be suspected, and there are frequently uterine pains, a dragging sensation in the back and loins, accompanied by violent headache, a loaded tongue, and symptoms of indigestion. A sudden return of the menses mitigates the symptoms, which usually last longer than is natural, and also more profuse.

TREATMENT.—If the symptoms are slight, regulate the bowels and diet, bathe the surface, and occasionally wear a pack, saturated with equal parts of whiskey and water, upon the lower bowel. If more severe, take unicorn root in decoction. Ladies'-slipper, wafer-ash, and black cohosh, are also very good. The tonics should also be given in debilitated subjects. In fact the constitutional symptoms should be met with such remedies as are indicated, as soon as they manifest themselves.

LEUCORRHŒA.

This is commonly known as the *whites*. It consists of a discharge from the vagina, or inner cavity of the womb, of a catarrhal character, varying in color from a light to a yellowish-green, or reddish-brown. It is usually due to inflammation of the mouth and neck of the womb (*cervicitis*), but it is also caused by congestion and inflammation of the interior membrane of the organ (*endo-cervicitis*), in which case it is more serious, and more difficult to cure. There are few females who are not

16

occasionally subject to moderate leucorrhœa. It may be known by the
discharge, but also by the attendant pain and a sense of heaviness in the
loins, abdomen, and thighs, disordered digestive functions, palpitation of
the heart, etc. It causes great impairment of the general health when
long continued.

TREATMENT.—Wear flannels next to the skin, and pay attention to
the general health. Keep the pores open by the proper medicines. In
acute cases inject cold water, and in chronic, warm water. This will
modify the inflammation. After this, injections of a strong decoction
of golden-seal, white-oak bark, or cinchona, should be frequently used,
and witch-hazel taken internally. Dog-wood, bayberry, black and blue
cohosh, and gelsemin, are also used for the same purpose. The astringent injections are also serviceable. Rest and quiet are important in
the treatment of the disease. Patients should, however, intrust the
treatment to an intelligent physician, who should ascertain the cause,
when, if the proper treatment is given, the disease will soon be cured.

ULCERATION OF THE WOMB.

This is chiefly confined to the neck of the organ, occurring most
frequently in those who have borne children. It is caused by excesses in married life, imprudence during menstruation, as standing,
walking, lifting, etc., and very often premature efforts after abortion
or labor. There is always more or less discharge associated with ulceration, which in quality is mucous, purulent, or starchy, and in color,
milky, greenish, yellowish, or brownish,—often tenacious masses of mucus, like starch, come away. It affects the general health similarly to
leucorrhœa.

TREATMENT.—Rest should be observed, and marital excesses abandoned. The treatment for leucorrhœa should be instituted. Vaginal
injections of red-raspberry leaves and golden-seal prove very beneficial
in this disease. The constitutional treatment in this disease is more
important than any local applications, and should take precedence.

FALLING OF THE WOMB (PROLAPSUS UTERI).

This is denoted by pain in the back and loins, heat in the vagina,
painful copulation, painful and irregular menstruation, constipation
and diarrhœa in alternation, irritable bladder, etc. The mouth of the
womb can be more readily felt than is natural, feeling spongy and hot,
and very tender on pressure. It may be ulcerated, and bleed upon
the slightest touch. The patient has all the symptoms of dyspepsia,
hysteria, neuralgia, palpitation, cough, and difficulty of breathing. It is
directly caused by weakness of the broad and lateral ligaments, and
remotely by various causes. It is a disease severe in its effects, causing
much suffering and impairment of health.

TREATMENT.—The patient should observe perfect quietude. The Inflammation and ulceration of the womb treated as previously described. The womb should be gently replaced to its normal position, the bowels kept open by mild laxatives, and the vagina injected with a warm decoction of hemlock and white oak bark. Pessaries do more harm than good, but abdominal supporters to sustain the weight of the bowels should be worn in all cases. (See page 370)

UTERINE DROPSY (HYDROMETRA).

This is an accumulation of fluid in the womb, caused by inflammation and constitutional debility. During the first months the symptoms resemble those of pregnancy; but by introducing the finger, so as to touch the neck of the womb, and pressing the tumor, fluctuation of fluids is felt. The menses are usually suppressed, and general debility will appear, if the disease continues. The patient may die from exhaustion, or the walls of the womb may be ruptured from the pressure of the fluid, causing fatal peritonitis.

TREATMENT.—A tonic and hygienic treatment should be prescribed, and if you can introduce a catheter into the womb and evacuate the fluid, it should be done, but it is better to intrust this to an able physician.

ANTEVERSION AND RETROVERSION.

If the womb falls forward upon the bladder, and towards the pubes, it constitutes *anteversion*. In this case the top or fundus of the womb is turned forward to the bladder, and the mouth towards the rectum. When the womb falls over backwards, between the rectum and the vagina, it is said to be *retroverted*. In this case the fundus is turned towards the rectum, and the neck towards the bladder. If the womb is anteverted and turned upon itself, it is *anteflexed*, and when retroverted and turned upon itself it is called *retroflexion*. These displacements may occur suddenly or gradually, causing great distress. The usual symptoms are costiveness and straining at stool, frequent urination, painful menstruation, pain in the lumbar region, and down the limbs, neuralgia, hysterics, and nervous debility. It is a serious affection, and should receive early attention and proper treatment.

TREATMENT.—The organ is first to be replaced to its normal position, and then the treatment for falling of the womb instituted. Such important diseases should, however, be confided to the care and direction of a competent physician. Great relief is at all times gained by wearing abdominal supporters.

HYDATIDS.

These consist of a formation of small cysts or bladders of water in the uterus, developed from the inner membrane, and vary in size from half a pear to a partridge's egg. They are usually oval, with a thin wall, opaque, and contain a thin fluid. They are most frequently in clusters, and numerous. The symptoms simulate those of early pregnancy, such as nausea, vomiting, enlargement of the womb, fulness of the breasts, suppression of the menses, etc. In a few months, the patient feels a weight and uneasiness about the abdomen, followed by uterine pains, hemorrhage, and expulsion of the hydatids.

TREATMENT.—If the flooding is excessive, control it by injecting vinegar or astringents and administer ten or fifteen drops of the oil of erigeron every fifteen minutes. If the pain is not sufficient to expel the masses, give a warm infusion of blue cohosh or cotton root. Ergot may also be given. After the expulsion the patient should receive tonic treatment.

PREGNANCY AND ITS ACCIDENTS.

PREGNANCY.

The first sign of pregnancy is a cessation of the menstrual flow. This will generally be noticed between two and three weeks after conception, and about the same time the woman will discover her breasts to be enlarging, and notice that the rings around the nipple are darker, and cover more space than usual. She will also, to a greater or lesser degree, experience nausea in the morning, and often be afflicted by vomiting, while she will experience dull pains in the "small" of the back, a decided disinclination for exertion, and considerable nervousness. As the womb increases in size and weight (which becomes apparent between the second and third months after conception), it sinks lower into the cavity of the pelvis (or part of the trunk which bounds the abdomen below), and produces much suffering, especially when the pelvis is small or narrow. After the fourth month, the womb, finding insufficient accommodation in the pelvis, mounts higher, and seeks room in the more capacious and yielding belly. Then the distress in the back, and the sickness and vomiting are somewhat modified, or in some comparatively disappear altogether. When the condition of pregnancy is first discovered, the woman, no matter how robust, should avoid all over-exertion or excitement, and should bear in mind constantly St. Paul's motto of "moderation in all things." A state of indolence is productive of disastrous, or, at least, painful consequences. Judicious exercise, and a determination to be cheerful and contented, will do much towards suppressing the usual annoyances of pregnancy, while moping and idling will increase them, and will almost invariably bring about a hard labor. Thus the poor working woman, providing she does not labor *too* hard, or expose herself imprudently to the vicissitudes of the weather, rarely suffers so much in child-bed as the woman who lives only to be petted and admired, and who seldom breathes the air of heaven in its delicious purity. Among the many incidental afflictions of pregnacy, are costiveness and piles. These are produced by the pressure of the enlarging womb upon the lower bowel. This, becoming filled with hardened matter, in turn presses upon the womb, and endeavors to crowd it out of the way. The combined and continual pressure of the womb and bowel upon the water-pipe, causes great difficulty in making water, and their uninterrupted weight upon the ascending veins produces congestion in the lower bowel, and hence the appearance of painful and disagreeable piles. The stomach and bowels should be kept in the best possible order. To prevent or ameliorate piles, use seidlitz powders every day, and inject into the bowels half a pint of pure cold water every morning. With regard to nausea, if it continues after the first three months, eat nothing but plain, yet nourishing food, and use chamomile flower tea as a beverage.

The habit of swathing or bandaging during any period of pregnancy is decidedly injurious, unless the woman be of a very fragile form and debilitated constitution. The child quickens about the end of the fourth month, when its motions will often produce hysterics and fainting fits, and the mother (for such she then is) becomes peevish, irritable, thin, and weak. Great care must be taken to combat this peevishness and irritability by fixing the mind upon pleasant thoughts, and mixing with lively company, if it be available. It will be as well, too, for the woman to lie down a little while, two or three times a day, and not to remain in an erect position too long without taking a little rest. During the last three months, the woman will generally suffer much uneasiness "all over," and will experience trouble in the attempt to get a perfect night's rest. They should not touch opiates under these circumstances. When varicose swellings of the veins of the legs are produced, a good plan is to wear a laced stocking over the affected parts, and this should be adjusted so as not to press too tightly upon the limb. It should be arranged so that the pressure will be equal throughout its length. Sometimes delicate women have convulsive fits in the last stage of pregnancy. These are dangerous, and no time should be lost in calling in an experienced midwife to take charge of the case. However, a two-grain opium pill administered internally, an injection of warm suds, and mustard plasters applied to the feet, and between the shoulders, will not fail of giving speedy relief. Also bathe the feet in warm water. The habitual use of the warm bath will often prevent these convulsions.

Palpitation of the heart, cramps of the legs and thighs, tooth-ache, puffy swellings, suppression of urine (use parsley tea for this), lethargy and headache are always accompaniments of pregnancy. For cramps and swellings, bathe the parts with warm water and red pepper, or mustard. If the swellings are very troublesome, apply fomentations of bitter herbs. In order to prevent sore nipples (which, if neglected, merge into caked and broken breasts), bathe them daily several times with alum-water, or a decoction of white oak bark. This bathing should be commenced about six weeks before confinement. Fox-glove (digitalis) is recommended by many for palpitation of the heart; but I discountenance its use. A little compound spirits of lavender, in water, and moderate doses of Turkey rhubarb will alleviate the attacks.

All pregnant women should wear flannel drawers and keep the feet warm.

All expectant mothers may greatly render a coming labor more easy and painless, if, at about the eighth month, they thoroughly rub my "Herbal Ointment" (see page 472) externally on the abdomen once a day, and continue until labor, and at about the middle of the ninth month they should lubricate the vagina and womb with the ointment. This has the effect of making the mouth more dilatable, the soft parts more yielding, and consequently a safe and comparatively easy labor.

The time of labor to every expectant mother causes constant solicitude, and scarcely any woman approaches the period fearless of the result, but very anxious as to the suffering or safety of life. In the present condition of civilized woman, we well know that the phenomenon of childbirth is attended with pains of an agonizing character, but that the suffering is mostly owing to habits of life, dress, etc., now characterizing woman, is equally certain. It would be an anomaly in nature if a process, so natural to females as child-birth, was originally ordained to be agonizingly painful, and it is quite evident that the pain now characterizing nearly all cases of labor is an infliction imposed by nature in consequence of violation of some of her laws. We are glad to see intelligent women approaching this subject, and have seen no brighter gleam of sunshine than Mrs. Stanton's recent address at San Francisco, which no false delicacy should prevent being reproduced in every paper in the land. She said, "We must educate our daughters that motherhood is grand, and that God never cursed it. And the curse, if it be a curse, may be rolled off, as man has rolled away the curse of labor, as the curse has been rolled from the descendants of Ham." While saying that her mission among woman was to preach a new gospel, she tells the women that, if they suffer, it is not because they are cursed by God, but because they violate his laws. What an incubus it would take from woman could she be educated to know that the pains of maternity are no curse upon her kind. We know that among Indians the squaws do not suffer in child-birth. They will step aside from the ranks, even on the march, and return in a short time bearing with them the new-born child. What an absurdity, then, to suppose that only enlightened Christian women are cursed. But Mrs. Stanton says that one word of fact is worth a volume of philosophy, and gives her experience as follows: "I am the mother of seven children. My girlhood was spent mostly in the open air. I early imbibed the idea that a girl was just as good as a boy, and I carried it out. I would walk five miles before breakfast, or ride ten on horseback. After I was married I wore my clothing sensibly. The weight hung alone on my shoulders. I never compressed my body out of its natural shape. My first four children were born, and I suffered but very little. I then made up my mind that it was totally unnecessary for me to suffer at all; so I dressed lightly, walked every day, lived as much as possible in the open air, ate no condiments or spices, kept quiet, listened to music, looked at pictures, read poetry. The child was born without a particle of pain. I bathed it and dressed it and it weighed ten and one-half pounds. That same day I dined with the family. Everybody said I would die, but I never had a relapse or a moment's inconvenience from it. I know this is not being delicate and refined, but if you would be vigorous and healthy in spite of the diseases of your ancestors and your own disregard of nature's laws, try."

While we heartily endorse all that Mrs. Stanton has said in this matter, we could not advise every mother to " dine with the family " on the day of her labor. It would be an exceedingly dangerous proceeding; but if every woman would be willing to practise the same initiatory training, which is so healthful, because in accordance with physiological laws, there is probably no doubt but that she would also be able to "wash her own baby " and " dine with the family," on even as substantial a dish as pork and beans.

PUERPERAL FEVER.

Child-bed fever is a very fatal disease, and frequently follows parturition. Scrofulous women are peculiarly liable to it. The disease manifests itself in every degree of intensity. The usual symptoms are weight and soreness in the lower part of the abdomen, accompanied by lassitude and debility, capricious appetite, imperfect after-discharge, spongy condition of the gums, constipation, and scanty and high-colored urine. These symptoms continue for two or three days after delivery, when the patient will be seized with chills and rigors. These are soon followed by a hot and pungent skin, pain in the head, nausea, and sometimes vomiting. The pulse becomes hard and quick, respiration rapid, the secretions are arrested, and the pain centres in the lower part of the abdomen and becomes very severe. The bowels are bloated, and very tender, and the lochia or after-discharge is entirely suppressed. In many cases delirium is present, also agitation and a sense of impending death. The worst form is when it presents the appearance of malignant scarlet fever.

TREATMENT.—The bowels should be freely opened with a purgative, after which opium should be administered in tolerably large doses. Warm slippery-elm emulsions should be frequently injected into the vagina, with a view to bring on the lochial discharge. The fever is to be controlled by aconite or veratrum. Tonic stimulants and carminatives should be used, according as the disease shows excitement or depression. In the low form, quinine and camphor are indicated. In the gangrenous form, put charcoal and yeast poultices to the abdomen, and give a decoction of wild indigo in wine and yeast four or five times a day.

INVERSION OF THE UTERUS.

This may be partial or complete. When partial, it may be known by the absence of the fundus or top of the womb behind the pubic bones, and the presence of a large solid tumor in the vagina, accompanied by profuse hemorrhage, intense pain in the pelvis, violent straining, vomiting, fainting, cold clammy sweat, and feeble pulse. Complete inversion is recognized by the presence of a reddish livid tumor filling the vagina, and protruding beyond it. It may occur spontaneously in atony of the womb, or from irregular contractions, or it may be caused by violence in extracting the after-birth, shortness of the cord, delivery in the upright position, tumors, etc.

TREATMENT.—Watch the tumor carefully, and at the moment when there is no contraction, the fundus should be pressed with one finger, and indented like the bottom of a bottle, and make continued pressure until reposition is sure. Then control the hemorrhage, if any is present, with ice to the pelvis, or vinegar injections, and give stimulants if the patient is exhausted.

ABORTION OR MISCARRIAGE.

Abortion or miscarriage signifies the expulsion of the foetus from the uterus, before it is sufficiently developed. The causes may be either natural or violent. Among the most prevalent causes, are mercury, constitutional syphilis, either in the father or mother, small pox, sudden and violent excitement of the blood-vessels by surprise, fright, anger, etc. It may also be caused by disease of the embryo, disease of the afterbirth, or direct violence to the abdomen. If it occurs in the early stage, the patient feels languid, uneasy and despondent, and is troubled with alternate chills and flashes of heat; there is nausea, palpitation, pain in the back, and tenderness over the abdomen. The breasts become flabby, and there is more or less hemorrhage. In the more advanced stages, the pains are more severe, and frequently the hemorrhage is so violent that the life of the patient is endangered, unless the proper remedial agents are employed. If miscarriage occurs once, it is liable to recurrence, and hence pregnant women should be very careful.

TREATMENT.—Those predisposed to abortion, should carefully avoid purgatives and diuretics, should indulge in no violent exercise, and take a cold sitz-bath every morning on rising, followed by brisk friction with a crash towel. Unicorn root and bayberry should also be taken internally. The pain should be subdued by hyoscyamus, and the hemorrhage checked by the oil of erigeron, or cayenne pepper and matico may be taken. If abortion, however, defies treatment, a strong decoction of cotton root, or ergot, should be taken to promote rapid expulsion of the fœtus. After it is expelled, if hemorrhage occurs, the oil of erigeron should be given, and much care observed, until the placenta is removed. During convalescence the patient's strength should be maintained to prevent weakness of the womb.

INFLAMMATION AND ABSCESS OF THE BREASTS.

During and after pregnancy the breasts are very liable to become inflamed and sore. The patient shivers, has pain in the head, loss of appetite, is constipated, and her urine is high-colored, and pulse quick. The breasts become red, painful, and swollen, and if the inflammation is allowed to continue, an abscess is formed, which, sooner or later, opens and discharges. Cold during nursing, accumulation of milk, injuries, diseases of the womb, scrofula, etc., are the principal causes.

TREATMENT.—Subdue the inflammation by applying the following:— Take arnica flowers, ℥ j. ; lobelia leaves, ℥ ss. ; hops, ℥ ij. Make a strong decoction, and apply cloths wrung from it hot as the patient can bear, and repeat every fifteen or twenty minutes. A small dose of aconite may be given internally to control the fever. A mild purgative should also be taken, and if the patient is debilitated, the general tonics should be exhibited. If the abscess, however, will occur, it should be opened, and then poulticed with slippery-elm. For *caked breasts*, apply hot packs, and change them frequently, and between each application bathe the breasts with a liniment composed of equal parts of lime-water, sweet-oil, spirits of camphor, and oil of horsemint.

SORE NIPPLES.

This is one of the most common and troublesome difficulties connected with the breasts, after child-birth. It is very frequently caused by want of cleanliness on the part of the mother or child.

TREATMENT.—Wash with castile soap and warm water after each nursing of the child, and then sprinkle the nipple with very fine powdered hemlock bark. Or make and use the following ointment:—Take balsam of fir, ℥ j. ; white wax, ℥ ij. ; melt together, then add ten grains each of tannin and powdered bayberry. Apply this as often as necessary, previously washing the breasts. Cover the nipple with folds of linen during the intervals of nursing. My Herbal Ointment (page 472), is a speedy cure for this painful affection.

16*

RELAXATION OF THE ABDOMINAL MUSCLES.

One of the most frequent sequels of pregnancy is a permanent relaxation of the abdominal muscles, more or less in degree. The abdomen becomes pendulous, occasioning great inconvenience, suffering, and often inducing malposition of the womb, and other affections.

The only way to remedy this relaxed condition is by artificial support, which is to be kept up until the muscles have again attained their full powers of contraction. Ladies are therefore in the habit of wearing bandages, though these but inadequately supply the necessary support, owing to the difficulty of proper application, so as to secure the equalization of pressure, and the stability of position, necessary. Mechanical appliances should only be used for the purpose of support. These are called *abdominal supporters*. Decidedly the best supporter is the one

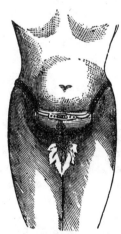

represented in the cut, an appliance so arranged as to supply the firmest support by means of elastic springs. It gives no uneasiness to the wearer; on the contrary it affords the most comfortable support, enabling the sufferer, who before could scarcely walk, to do so with the utmost facility, occasioning no pain or inconvenience. Supporters are absolutely necessary in all cases, as no medicinal treatment will overcome the relaxation, on account of the constant superimposed pressure of the bowels. These supporters should also be worn in all cases of uterine misplacements, as they afford the greatest relief, and serve as an almost indispensable adjunct to the required medicinal treatment.

Dr. O. Phelps Brown's Abdominal Supporter.

Another supporter, represented by the adjoining cut, is also a meritorious one, having many excellent qualities. It is especially well adapted to corpulent females. Equality of support under all circumstances is gained by an elastic band in the pad at front. These supporters are the result of thorough study as to the requirements of such appliances, and the author is convinced that they are the best articles for the purpose designed. Their many qualities will at once be apparent both to the professional man or to the patient.

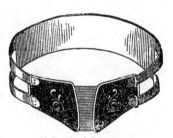

Abdominal Supporter.

Ladies, in need of supporters, may address the author for further particulars. (See page 389)

THE CONDUCT OF A CASE OF LABOR.

This should never be attempted except by a physician or competent midwife, but, as it may sometimes take place in railroad cars, in voyages, etc., the duty may fall to the lot of almost any woman or man, and hence it is important that they should know how to proceed. These hints may also be useful to perhaps many in the backwoods, where the population is scarce, and where the nearest doctor lives " a day's journey " away.

How do you Know that the Patient is in Labor?

This the mother frequently knows herself, but she may sometimes be deceived by what are *spurious pains*. If she is in labor, she will have what is called " *come and go* " pains, which at first are moderate and wide apart, but which finally become more intense and succeed each other at shorter intervals. She will describe those as *bearing down* pains, and frequently they are so severe as to cause cries and gestures, the former being of a mourning or complaining character, the other twisting and writhing. She will also have a mucous discharge from the vagina, which is called a " *show*." She will probably wish to void her urine often, and to relieve her bowels, which should be encouraged. During this stage the mouth of the womb is dilating. Now it will be well for you to pass your finger well up into the vagina, and you will most probably find that the mouth of the womb is dilated, and in extent it depends upon the time at which you may make the examination. When the pains become " thick and fast," you may again make an examination, and you will probably find a fluctuating tumor, which is the *bag of waters*. If this does not burst itself, you may rupture it with your finger, but do not allow yourself to be frightened at the forcible rush of the waters. If you have withdrawn your hand, you may again insert it, and you will most likely find the head about descending into the vagina. If it is the head or breech it will be a natural labor (which I hope it may always be, for I do not believe I could teach you how to proceed in what is called a *preternatural* labor). If the head is there, all right. You may give the soon-to-be-mother your hand, or you may tie a sheet to the bed-post and let her pull at that, or if her husband is present, or if you are he himself, let her press him around the neck whenever an expulsive pain occurs. This will greatly aid her, and you do not know how thankful a woman is in such a case, when she observes apparent assistance on your part. After a few *good* pains, the head of the child will be born, and then the worst is over, for usually one pain more will cause the birth of the whole child.

What will You do Next?

As soon as it is born, you will probably hear the child gasp and cry, which is caused by pain ensuing upon sudden expansion of its lungs.   If it does not do this, take the child, and shake it gently, give it a few slaps on the buttocks, and empty its mouth of any secretions that may be found there.   By doing this, the child may soon cry—when it is all right.   If, however, it should not be so easily resuscitated, sprinkle a little water on its face, and if it looks blue in the face, cut the cord, and let it bleed a little ; then put your mouth to that of the baby, and while holding its nose shut, blow your own breath into it and fill its lungs, and then press gently on its chest, in imitation of expiration.   Do this as long as there is any hope, and your efforts may often be crowned with success.   We will suppose, however, that the baby is a struggling, crying, healthy darling.   Then, as soon as you do no longer feel the cord pulsate, you can separate it from the mother.   To do this take a few strands of thread and tie it round the cord, not so tight as to cut through, about two inches away from the navel.   Then take a pair of scissors and cut the cord through about half an inch away from the ligature, not on the side, however, towards the navel ; you can put two ligatures on the cord, if you like, and cut between them.   Then take the baby away, but be careful how you do it, or else an accident may befall you, and hand it to the proper person to be washed and dressed. The baby is very slippery, so take it up in this way : put its neck between the thumb and forefinger of your left hand, and put the palm of the right under its buttocks ; you then have it secure, but do not be too anxious about its safety, or you might choke it.

WHAT NEXT ?

You must now pay attention to the exhausted but joyous mother, rejoiced that she has passed such an agony of pain as you can form no conception of, such that you have never felt and never can feel, unless you have been or will be a mother, and yet she will now greet you with a sweet, smiling countenance.   Her anxiety, however, is not over until she is relieved of the after-birth.   By the time that you have got through with your duty to the baby, you will probably find the after-birth expelled into the vagina, by the *after-pains*.   If such is the case, take the cord and pull gently downwards and a little upwards, but by no means pull so hard as to tear the cord, or invert the womb   If it will not come, wait, and in a short time try again, and you will most probably find it to come away readily.   If you should find her *flooding*, take a rag, saturate it with vinegar, or take a lemon, divest it of its rind, and then pass it into the womb and squeeze it.   This causes contraction of the organ, and stops the hemorrhage.   You may also apply ice to the spine for this purpose, and if you have ergot in the house, give a pretty large dose of that.   After delivery of the after-birth, take a towel, and pass it around the pelvis of the mother, and bind it pretty tightly; cover her up warmly, and allow her to sleep, and so recover strength, as you may suppose that she is very much exhausted by this time.

YOUR WORK IS NOT DONE YET.

The baby has to be washed. This is a tedious job, unless you know how to proceed. All babies are covered with more or less unctuous matter, and this should be removed, or else it is liable to get a skin disease. After you have got your rag (a soft woollen one is the best) and some pretty warm water, smear the child over with pure lard or sweet oil, and then use castile soap and water, and you will soon have it clean. Be careful, however, not to get soap into its eyes, or else you will have to treat it in a few days after for sore eyes. Now you have got it clean, but you must not put on its clothes, until you have dressed the navel, and put on its *belly-band*. To dress the navel, take a well-worn cotton rag, cut it into patches of about four inches in diameter, take three or four of these and cut a hole through the middle of them. Cut also a little bandage, half an inch wide, and wrap it round the navel string, then slip it through the patches, and lay the string pointing towards the left shoulder. Now, put on the woollen belly-band, moderately tight, and secure it with needle and thread, not with pins. You may think this caution unnecessary, but if you had seen as many torn limbs and deep scratches in infants as I have, you would not think so. After this you can put on its whole toilet, and lay it in its proper warm nest—its mother's arms.

But you may think the baby is *hungry*, and that it needs some physic; so you give it some gruel, and follow this up either with castor oil and sugar, molasses, or butter and sugar made into a paste, and force them down the little victim's throat. I say victim, because you could not easily do more harm, and yet this abomination is done every day. If the mother has milk, put it at the breast as soon as you can; if not, let it wait until she has,—it won't starve. It needs no purgative, for the *colostrum* or first of the milk is by nature designed as a laxative, and if it gets that, it will soon have the *black stools*, or discharge of *meconium*, as doctors call it. By no means give it soothing syrups nor spirits, nor put a cap on it, or wash it with spirits. If you take my advice in this matter, the baby will be the better for it, and there will not be a necessity, which is so often the case, of the early exchange of its little dresses for a tiny shroud.

In about twelve hours after delivery the mother may be cleansed, and her bed changed, and light food given to her. She should remain in bed for at least ten days, after which, if she feels strong, she may sit up, but should avoid exertion. If she has insufficient milk, follow advice given on page 328.

LOCHIA.

For some time after child-bearing, a discharge takes place from the womb which is called lochia. It is at first red; but if all goes well, in a few days the red appearance subsides and gives place to an effusion of a greenish color and a peculiar odor. When the womb is reduced to its original size, the lochia ceases. If it is checked before it should be—and in some women it ought to continue a month—or if the flow proceeds with irregularity, great distress and danger are the consequences. The immoderate flow of the lochia is not so disastrous as the suppression. The latter may be produced by cold, by chilled drink, by mental excitement, or, in fact, by any undue exertion of either mind or body. The results of the suppression of the lochia are great fever, restlessness, heat, pain in the head, back, and loins, delirium, inflammation of the womb, colic pains, costiveness, nervous excitability, muscular contractions, and, in fact, general distress. The first and only thing to be done is to restore the flow. For this purpose, if the patient can bear it, the warm bath must be used; fomentations should be applied to the abdomen; large emollient injections should be given in the rectum, and sudorific medicines (not of a mineral character), assisted by copious diluent drinks, should be administered. The acetate of ammonia will be found very useful. A profuse and general perspiration is the precursor of rapid recovery and safety. While the lochia is apparent the patient must not endeavor to get up, or to undergo any noticeable degree of exertion, or be exposed either to atmospherical changes, or imprudence in diet.

THE TREATMENT IN ACCIDENTS.

The treatment of fractures, dislocations, etc., should always be intrusted to the surgeon, but the emergency of such cases may be so great in certain instances that a few minutes' delay might prove fatal to the patient. Hence I will attempt to instruct the reader how to proceed and what to do *before the doctor comes.* In all cases where surgical help can be procured, it should be done as quickly as possible, but dangerous accidents may occur where surgical aid is impossible to procure, and, therefore, the treatment devolves upon others.

WOUNDS.

In case of wood-choppers, hunters, etc., away in the backwoods, or in any other case where this precaution is necessary, they should provide themselves always with bandages, Monsel's solution, and a roll of adhesive plaster, and then they are prepared for nearly all cases of accidents that may befall them.

The worst feature about a wound is the bleeding, unless, as in case of gun-shot wound, a vital part is injured. We will suppose, however, that unfortunately one received a wound, either from some sharp instrument, or a gun-shot wound, or some part of his body was lacerated, contused or punctured from some cause, and that the wound was bleeding freely. Before the wound is dressed the character of the bleeding is to be noticed. If the blood is dark-colored and flows regularly in a stream, it is venous blood, and you will be able to control it easily; but if it is bright-scarlet, and spurts out in jets, some artery has been wounded—always a dangerous accident. If the wound is a gun-shot one and received in the trunk, all you can do on the moment is to hermetically seal the wound. Take the adhesive plaster, and cut a piece from it large enough to cover the wound well, and then apply over the wound so as to seal it effectually against escape of blood or entrance of air; or take a rag and shape it in a pledget, and tie it on the wound firmly with a bandage or handkerchief. If internal hemorrhage occurs, you cannot do anything, and the patient will probably die.

If the wound is in the arms or legs, then you can always do something. If the bleeding is venous, you will be able to arrest it by applying cold water. Elevate the limb, and use compression. If this does not arrest it, apply some of the Monsel's Solution, which is a solution of the persulphate of iron, which quickly stanches the blood by coagulation. After the hemorrhage has ceased, apply a bandage. If the blood comes out in jets, you may know that an artery is wounded, and that no time is to be lost. No styptics will arrest hemorrhage from any important artery, but in such cases instantly apply the Spanish windlass, which is made by tying a handkerchief around the limb, and twisting it with a stick, until the hemorrhage ceases. This compression is to be maintained, until the patient can have the attention of a surgeon. Be careful, however, to apply the windlass above the wound towards the heart.

If you have to deal with any ordinary wound, cut, etc., draw the edges together with strips of adhesive plaster, and put on cold water dressings.

FRACTURES.

These accidents often happen where no surgical aid can be conveniently procured. Any one can easily detect a broken bone by the person not being able to raise the limb, by its bending where it ought not, by pain, and by *crepitation*, or crackling sound if the parts are moved. When the bone is merely separated into two parts it is called a *simple* fracture; when an open wound communicates with the fracture it is called *compound*; when the bone is broken into numerous fragments, it is termed *comminuted*, and *complicated* when attended with dislocation, laceration of large vessels, etc.

HEAD.

The bones of the head and face are liable to be broken by blows, falls, etc., and need immediate medical attendance. All you can do before the arrival of the surgeon, is to raise the head, apply cold water, avoid all noise and excitement, and arrest the bleeding by the means heretofore advised.

COLLAR BONE.

This bone is usually broken by violence upon the shoulder, arm, and hand. It is generally broken near the middle of the bone. the part is painful and swollen, and every attempt at motion produces pain; the shoulder is sunken and drawn towards the breast-bone. The patient usually is found supporting the arm with his hand, to relieve the pressure upon the sensitive network of nerves in the armpit.

TREATMENT.—Push the shoulder backwards, and press on the seat of fracture, until you get it in its place. Then make a wedge-shaped pad, and put it in the armpit and secure it there by a bandage, which surrounds the chest. Then bring the elbow to the side, and place the forearm in a sling; then take bandages, and secure the whole arm so tightly in that position that it cannot be moved. The surgeon may then be called, or, if the above advice is properly and effectually obeyed, the cure will be a good one.

BROKEN RIBS.

This is known by pain when the patient breathes, or on pressure where the injury has taken place. Crepitation is also felt when the hand is placed over the part during respiration or coughing, and if the pleura is injured, the chest swells, or emphysema appears.

TREATMENT.—If the broken ends project, apply a compress over it; if there is a depression, a compress is to be placed at each extremity. If there is a bruise, apply hot fomentations; then take a bandage six or eight inches wide, and draw it tightly around the chest over the injured part. This gives great relief, as it prevents expansion of the chest in respiration, and holds the broken ends in opposition. Keeping this bandage firmly applied is all that need be done in the way of treatment.

FRACTURE OF THE HUMERUS.

This is the bone between the elbow and shoulder. It may be detected by the ordinary methods.

TREATMENT.—Place the bones in apposition, making sure that it is right, by comparing it with the sound arm. Then take four splints, and put one in front, one behind, and one on each side of the arm. Secure these with a bandage. This dressing will do, until better attention can be given to it by a competent doctor. Place the arm in a sling.

FRACTURE OF THE BONES OF THE FOREARM.

There are two bones here, the radius and ulna. They may both be fractured, or only one of them. The fracture is easily detected.

TREATMENT.—The difficulty here is to observe the space between the bones, which is called the *interosseous* space. The fracture is readily reduced by drawing the arm forwards, and when this is done, press the muscles into the interosseous space. Now, take two splints, well padded on the inside, reaching from the elbow beyond the fingers, put one on the inside and the other on the outside of the forearm, and secure them with a bandage. The arm should be carried in a sling.

FRACTURE OF THE BONES IN THE HAND, FOOT, OR ANKLE.

These solid bones are almost always wounded by such accidents that tend to crush them, as machinery, threshing machines, heavy weights falling on them, etc.

TREATMENT.—Dress the open wound as any other, then cover the whole hand in several folds of rag, or handkerchief, dipped in cold water.

FRACTURE AT THE HIP-JOINT.

This is a very serious accident, and liable to occur in aged people. One that receives this injury cannot stand or rise from the ground. If the patient is placed upright the injured limb will be found much shorter than the other, and the foot turned outwards. What is called osseous union rarely if ever occurs in this fracture.

TREATMENT.—In old persons support the limb by pillows and restrain all motion. This is all you can do. In other cases, make two splints, one reaching from the arm-pit to about six inches longer than the foot, the other from between the legs, extending to the same length. Pad these well, especially at the upper ends. Apply them to the inner and outer side of the leg and secure them with a bandage. Now make a foot-board with two mortised holes in it, through which the splints can pass. Bore holes in the lower ends of the splints every half inch. Put on the foot-board, and attach the foot to it firmly, then pull the foot-board down so as to stretch the leg well, for this secures what is called *extension*, which is necessary in these cases. The splints resting against the arm-pit and perinæum affords what is called *counter-extension*. See in all cases that you have the leg straight.

FRACTURE OF THE THIGH-BONE.

Fracture of the shaft of this bone is easily recognized by shortening, crepitation, etc., and you should treat it just the same as advised in the fracture of this bone at the hip-joint. If this fracture should occur away from home, in the fields or elsewhere, get some stiff straw, or bits of very thin board, or if you have a "stove-pipe" hat take that, knock out the crown, take off the rim, and split it up at the sides. Bind these around the limb rather tightly with suspenders, handkerchiefs, or tear your shirt up for bandages. Then you can safely remove the patient to a place where he may receive the proper treatment.

FRACTURE OF THE CAP OF THE KNEE OR PATELLA.

This may be broken by muscular contractions or direct violence. Falling on the knee very frequently produces it. There is no crepitation felt in this fracture. The pain is not very severe, but the limb is partially bent, and the patient has no power to extend it.

TREATMENT.—Keep down the swelling with lotions, etc., and then, by means of strips of adhesive plaster, draw the fragments together and retain them firmly in that position. Prevent motion by putting a long splint on the back of the leg.

FRACTURE OF THE LEG.

There are two bones below the knee, the *tibia* and *fibula*, and a fracture, occurring in one or both of them from a fall or direct violence, is a frequent accident, the tibia being most frequently broken. The signs are evident. Crepitation, pain, want of motion, etc., declare it.

TREATMENT.—When both bones are broken, or when the fibula alone, or when the upper part of the fibula is fractured, the best and most simple apparatus is the fracture-box and pillow. Make a box considerably wider than the leg, with only one end board, and that considerably higher than the sides of the box—the box has no lid. Put a pillow, or little bags of chaff or bran in this; put the broken leg into this; see that it fits well; then secure the foot to the foot-board, so as to prevent lateral inclination.

The great object in the treatment of fractures is to keep the broken ends well together, or in apposition, and keep them there. Nature will do the healing part. In bandaging limbs, be careful that you get them smoothly on the parts, and make allowances for the swelling which occurs. If a bandage is formed too tight, it should be removed. or else mortification of the limb will ensue.

DISLOCATIONS.

The signs of limbs being out of joint are deformity, swelling, and a hollow where none should be, shortening or elongation, pain and immobility of the limb.

BROKEN NECK, OR BACK.

This is nearly always accompanied by a fracture. It may be produced by convulsions, falls, hanging, etc. The chances of life are small, on account of injury done to the spinal marrow, or the action of the diaphragm may be suspended by compression of the phrenic nerve.

TREATMENT.—Lay the person (if in the neck) on his back, plant your knees on the patient's shoulders, grasp the head firmly, pull gently, and at the same time put the head into its proper place ; but this must be properly and gently done, or else you may do great harm. If in the back, do nothing.

DISLOCATION OF THE JAW.

This is often caused by yawning, by convulsions, or by blows on the chin, when the mouth is wide open. The mouth gapes and cannot be shut, the saliva trickles, there is great pain, and the patient cannot talk.

TREATMENT.—Seat the patient on a low stool, stand in front of him, and then press your thumbs upon the last molar or grinding teeth very firmly. Be careful, however, to have your thumbs well protected with wrappings, or else you may be severely bitten. By doing this you get the articular ends of the jaw-bone from their unnatural position, and reduction is caused by the normal action of the muscles. When you hear the *snap*, you may be sure that the bone is in its proper position. After reduction, the chin should be confined by a bandage for a week or ten days.

DISLOCATION AT THE SHOULDER.

This may be displaced in three directions, viz.: inwards, downwards and backwards. By comparing the injured with the sound shoulder, you may be able to tell that it is a dislocation. Where the head of the bone ought to be, you will find a depression, and you will most likely find a tumor, near the breast, in the arm-pit, or towards the back, according to the manner of dislocation.

TREATMENT.—Lay the person on his back, and sit down beside him on the injured side, and put a round pad in the arm-pit. Then take off your boot, put your foot against the pad, grasp the patient's arm, or tie a towel to it, put it around your neck, and pull in that way. Then while you pull at the arm and push with your foot, tell the patient to turn round, or you may carry the arm across his chest. While this is done, a snap will be heard, and the bone is in its proper place.

DISLOCATIONS AT THE ELBOW.

When both radius and ulna are dislocated, the forearm is bent nearly at a right angle, and is immovable. When the ulna alone is dislocated, there is a tumor projecting posteriorly, the elbow is bent at right angles, and the forearm is turned upwards. The radius is dislocated at the elbow either forwards or backwards. When backwards the head of the bone forms a prominence behind, the arm is bent and the hand prone.

When forwards there is a distinct prominence in front, the arm is slightly bent, and the hand supine.

TREATMENT.—When both bones are dislocated, or in case the ulna is alone out of joint, make forcible extension of the forearm over your knee, placed at the elbow, to make counter-extension. Then bend the forearm while making extension, and reduction will take place. In forward dislocation of the radius make forcible extension, and while doing so, turn the hand from without inwards, called pronation. In backward dislocation make forcible extension, and turn the hand from within outward, or supination. In either case you should press the head of the bone into proper position with your thumb. Then advise rest, cold applications, and a sling.

DISLOCATIONS AT THE WRIST.

The luxation of both bones of the forearm from the bones of the hand is rare. When it occurs forward there is a great projection in front, and the hand is bent backwards ; when backwards, the projection is behind, and the hand is flexed. If the radius alone is dislocated the hand will be somewhat twisted. If the ulna is dislocated, it may be easily recognized by a projection on the back of the wrist.

TREATMENT.—The reduction of both bones is effected by making extension and pressure. If either of the bones are dislocated, the reduction is performed in the same manner. Pain, swelling, and stiffness of the joint may follow, which should be obviated by cold applications, rest, lotions, etc., and a light splint may be applied to prevent its recurrence.

DISLOCATION OF THE BONES OF THE HAND.

Displacement of the bones of the carpus or body of the hand rarely occurs. The bones of the fingers are occasionally dislocated, but more frequently the thumb is dislocated backwards.

TREATMENT.—Make extension in a curved line, by means of a narrow bandage or tape, firmly applied by a close-hitch upon the finger.

DISLOCATION OF THE RIBS.

Dislocation of the ribs from the spinal column may sometimes occur by severe falls, or blows upon the back, and from the breast bone, by violent bending of the body backwards. Great pain and difficulty of breathing follow in either case.

TREATMENT.—Tell the patient to take a deep inspiration, and slightly bend the body backwards, and while he does this, make some pressure on the projecting point. After reduction treat the same as for broken ribs.

DISLOCATION AT THE HIP.

In this case the leg is shortened and the foot is turned *inwards*. It may be dislocated in five different ways;—upwards and backwards is, however, the most common dislocation. In all cases you may know that displacement has occurred, by comparison with the articulated limb.

TREATMENT.—The accident is so serious that no attempt should be made at reduction, except by a surgeon, but if it happens when no such aid can be procured, you may proceed as in dislocation of the shoulder. If you cannot make sufficient extension in that way, you may attach pulleys to a towel fastened above the knee, and make counter-extension by means of a folded sheet in the perinæum. After full extension is accomplished, push the head into the socket, or so manipulate the leg that its movements will force reduction. After reduction, the patient should be kept at rest, and walking should not be attempted for several weeks.

DISLOCATION OF THE KNEE-CAP.

This may be dislocated in various directions. It is characterized by the leg being stretched, and a prominence formed by the patella in an abnormal situation.

TREATMENT.—Raise the patient's leg and rest it upon your shoulder. While in this position, force the bone into its place with the hand.

DISLOCATION AT THE ANKLE.

This may be forwards, backwards, inwards and outwards, and are the results of severe force. The bones' ends are usually fractured at the same time. It is a very serious accident, and when it occurs to patients whose constitutions are bad amputation may often be necessary.

TREATMENT.—Reduction is effected by bending at the knee, and while in that position, drawing the foot forwards.

In all cases of dislocations and fracture communicating with joints, the danger is anchylosis or stiffness of the joints. This is to be obviated by what is called *passive motion*, which is to be instituted in all cases, a few weeks after the accident. It is accomplished by taking hold of the limb and moving it in natural directions, as far as consistent, and repeated after suitable intervals. The patient is to be enjoined, also, when practicable, to exercise his limb at the wounded articulation. There are many other fractures and dislocations that I have not spoken of, for the reason that they are all so serious that the treatment should only be attempted by those having the proper anatomical knowledge and surgical skill.

PREVENTION OF EPIDEMIC DISEASES.

The alarming fatality consequent upon an epidemic reign of disease demands the closest scrutiny upon the part of communities, large or small, to guard against its approach or prevalence. Medical skill is unable to cope with the fearful onslaught of epidemics, and in many cases epidemic diseases are of so violent a character that the most vigorous constitutions succumb to the assault, and the profoundest medical skill and most rational medical treatment are unavailing. It is questionable if medical science will ever be able to materially decrease the rate of mortality that usually ensues upon epidemic reign; the subtle ethereal poison causing epidemics being of too violent a character to allow ascendency to be gained by material medicinal agents. Since it is questionable that mastery can be gained by medicinal or therapeutic agents, the proper remedy is suggested, not by investigating the best agents of cure, but in measures of prevention, as the author is quite certain that by proper knowledge and concerted action the spread of an epidemic can be limited, and its onset prevented. Epidemic diseases belong to the class which has been conveniently but inaccurately designated "zymotic." They are generated, according to the most modern physiological doctrine, by a specific poison, introduced into the body from without, which is capable of causing morbid changes in the blood, and of destroying life. The poisons of various epidemic diseases are distinct *inter se ;* the contagion of typhus, for instance, being altogether different from that of small-pox, and the contagion of cholera from that of diphtheria, and yet it is plain that they are all somehow related, and capable of gradual transmutation from one type into another. Some ancient types have died out—the black-death, the sweating sickness, and the plague ; but new types, undescribed by the old physicians, have arisen. We are able to note remarkable "waves of disease ;" at one time the great mortality is from typhus, at another from small-pox, at another from scarlatina. In England they have recently had a succession of epidemic. The outbreak of cholera in 1866 was followed by typhoid fever, and as the latter began to abate in violence, scarlatina appeared in the most malignant form, and attacked the metropolis. This disease had begun a year and a half ago to decline in London, but at the same time it began to spread through other parts of the kingdom, where it has since raged destructively. A little later than the scarlatina, relapsing fever, which has been rare in these countries since 1849, broke out with great severity, also attacking London first, and, when it had spent its force there, extending itself into the provincial towns. Lastly, they have been visited with an epidemic of small-pox more severe than any outbreak of that disease which has been recorded in England during the present generation. And no sooner has the small-pox begun to abate its violence than they are threatened with a return of cholera. This periodicity of disease is yet to be explained; but it is established that, given the same conditions for the reception and propagation of contagion, about the same proportion of lives will be carried away, whether the prevailing epidemic be scarlet fever or typhus, or relapsing fever or small-pox.

The blood-poisoning of the zymotic diseases, which is thus various and changing in type, is traceable, however, to the same class of causes. In some epidemics the germs of contagion are far more volatile than in others, but, in all, we know by experience that, if we can isolate the patient and submit his immediate surroundings to disinfectant agents, we check the spread of the disorder.

Pure air and pure water are irreconcilably hostile to contagious disease. The first duty, therefore, of sanitary administration is the enforcement of effective ventilation, the supply of a fixed quantity of fresh air to every person in every house. This is an innovation which will of course be resisted both by ignorance and self-interest, but no infraction of real liberty will be committed in preventing ignorant or self-interested persons from doing mischief to the community by sowing the seeds of disease broadcast. The next step in the work of prevention is to insist upon a free and well-distributed system of sewers to carry away at once from every habitation the impurities which poison the air, and which, even when they do not directly propagate contagion, insidiously weaken the constitution of those subjected to their influence and prepare them for the reception of the germs of disease. Most country villages and many small towns are almost wholly destitute of systematic drainage, and cesspools, which are the commonest substitutions, are merely traps for infection. The enforcement of drainage and the abolition of cesspools are reforms which experience has shown will never be carried out by the local authorities, and is especially an improvement which ought to be and can be carried by pressure from a strong central executive office. A third precaution is systematic disinfection, not only of everything connected with and surrounding a person suffering from contagious disease, but of all places where dirt unavoidably accumulates, and whence at any time effluvium can be perceived to proceed.

These precautions, however, though valuable in themselves, and also as tending to effect the further object to which we are now able to refer, are quite unavailing unless supplemented by securities for a pure supply of water. Cholera, as we have seen, is held to be propagated almost exclusively through polluted water, and there is scarcely a form of epidemic that is not to some extent disseminated in the same way.

We have stated that it is doubtful if sanitary reform can ever be properly enforced by local authority, and hence advocate that its requirement should be insisted upon by national statutes. The health of any country is as much a principle of political economy as its freedom, and just as worthy, if not more so, of vigilance ; and it is to be hoped that the day is not far distant when legislators in every land will see the absolute necessity to enact such laws rendering thorough disinfection and drainage obligatory upon all its citizens. Physicians have long advocated so desirable a reform, and neglected no opportunity to teach the people the virtue of and benefits to be derived from disinfection ; but the absence of any epidemic gives a false sense of security, and the advices are unheeded until the deathly blast of the epidemic is upon them, when their folly is exposed and the wisdom of precaution established.

Of the disinfectants, the following are the best :—Chloride of lime, Labarraque's solution, carbolic acid, and bromo-chloralum. Chlorine gas is probably the best, but not so practicable for universal use. Most of them are comparatively cheap, and no household should be without a sufficient quantity.

All cesspools, sinks, etc., should be thoroughly disinfected whenever they become offensive and exhale noxious vapors, and no pools of stagnant water or other filthy places should be permitted to remain undrained for any space of time. If such a desirable reform could become of universal operation, the reign of epidemics would be over and become things of the past.

TREATMENT OF CHRONIC DISEASES.

THE AUTHOR'S SPECIALTY.

Important to the Suffering Sick, Male or Female.

The aim in presenting this work to the public is to supply what is so urgently necessary in the present progressive age,—a reliable and worthy guide for self-treatment with the medicinal agents that Nature has so bounteously provided, viz., the products of the vegetable world. Aside from this work, the author is unacquainted with any other that is devoted exclusively to Herbalism. Many of the possessors of the "Herbalist" will naturally make use of it for the purpose of treating themselves or those in the household affected with disease, and if advices and directions for treatment are closely adhered to, they will be enabled to treat and cure many afflictions which otherwise would require the services of the family physician. The reader, however, must not forget that the science of medicine is not so simple and so capable of ready acquirement that a work designed as a guide for self-treatment will, in all cases, serve him or her to dispense with the services of a physician. The physician is only competent to properly combat disease and assuage human suffering after many years of profound study, patient investigation and untiring research. It would, therefore, be unreasonable for any one to suppose that an adequate knowledge of disease and its treatment can be gained in any other way than that by which the physician attains his knowledge. The design of a medical work for popular study and use is to impart to the reader a knowledge of the philosophy of the medical science in general, and to instruct him as to the proper course to pursue in emergencies. The majority of the simpler diseases constantly met with, the reader will, of course, be enabled to treat capably and successfully at all times, with the aid of a good work devoted to domestic medicine. In the graver affections, acute or chronic, the intelligent services of a physician are indispensable. In chronic diseases, a careful diagnosis is absolutely required, as the symptoms of such affections are invariably delusive, and each case is usually accompanied by a variety of sympathetic disorders; hence, it requires the educated and experienced physician to note the variations, detect the complications and identify the locality and extent of the real disorder. Patient, exhaustive, and intelligent investigation is absolutely requisite in all cases, as without such a careful diagnosis the treatment would necessarily be but experimental in kind and very possibly hurtful in effect. A work of this character is, therefore, designed to give general ideas of disease and treatment, rather than to afford the proper knowledge and skill by which the services of the educated and skillful physician can be altogether dispensed with. A simple illustration will make this quite plain to every one; the manner of making a plain and simple piece of mechanism can be so definitely and succinctly taught, that it can readily be made, but when a complex machine is to be constructed, it can only be done by the educated, skillful, and experienced mechanic. Precisely the same holds true in medicine—the treatment of simpler diseases can be fitly taught—and I trust that I have done so to the comprehension of all—and the philosophy of disease and treatment in general, can be imparted in a popular medical work; but grave, complicated, and pathologically serious affections, acute or chronic, can only be properly combatted by the physician having the requisite knowledge, skill and experience; and the patient within the grasp of the disease, or to those to whom he is near and dear, will always remain discontented as long as the watchful care and intelligent services of a physician are not provided, no matter how ably and extensively medical knowledge may be popularized. It is so now, and so it will remain as long as disease afflicts humanity.

Since I have placed myself within the sphere of authorship and in the attitude of a pronounced exponent of Herbalism, there will be thousands of invalids groaning under the remorseless grasp of disease who will seek my counsel and professional aid; and who, furthermore, may wish to be treated with the products of the Herbal world exclusively, inasmuch as all previous efforts for relief were unavailing. This has been my professional experience for many years past, and so it will probably continue as long as life exists. My professional sphere is, therefore, general, and my practice national in extent. It is due, then, to invalids everywhere (as but few, comparatively, can make it convenient to gain a personal interview) that I define my specialty, my system of practice, and my position as a physician in general.

My specialty is the treatment of *Chronic Diseases.* I very rarely give advice, unless specially and urgently solicited, with reference to acute affections, and never essay treatment unless the affections be of specific or strumous origin, as private diseases, acute phthisis, scrofula, etc. Aside from these exceptional cases, my professional attention and services are entirely absorbed in the treatment of chronic diseases, and these I can justly claim to treat with unvarying success. This assertion is certainly pardonable when the fact of my success is attested by thousands of former patients in all parts of the world. Early in my professional career it became apparent to me that only as a specialist can any physician hope for either competence or success. Aware of the folly of the attempt to become equally skilful in the treatment of both acute and chronic affections, I made chronic diseases exclusively my study, and devoted for many years all the energies at command in the endeavor to acquaint myself with all the varied and multiform manifestations, the intricate pathology or morbid aspects, the obscurity of the real seat of affection, and the many other characteristics common to chronic diseases; and I may fairly and justly claim a fair portion of the knowledge of authority relative to either the diagnosis and the indicated or required treatment. No physician, unless he be a prodigy of science, can with equal success treat both acute and chronic affections. If he is animated with the principles of professional integrity, striving to gain absolute competence, he has no time to investigate the characteristics of chronic diseases, should he even have the inclination. I aver what I know to be the truth and what many invalids have suspected,—that the physician who more commonly treats acute disorders has not the proper sympathy, the stock of patience and the inclination for pains-taking investigation absolutely required, nor has he in one case out of ten the extended acquaintance of pathology or diversified requirements of treatment, indispensable to ascertain the identity and extent of chronic disorder, or to capably and successfully treat the same. The "family physician" deals mostly with acute affections; hence it is necessary to his professional success and reputation to devote his sole attention to the study of acute disorders. It is well known that the highest perfection of mechanism demands the division of labor into special branches, and so it is with the practice of medicine—division into specialties secures greater intelligence, competence, and success of treatment. Disease thus combatted will certainly be less deplorable in its ravages and a higher standard of health would prevail in common.

It is not necessary that I should particularize each disease for which my advice may be solicited, or for the treatment of which my services may be engaged. I may be consulted with reference to every existing chronic disorder, claiming the requisite ability to give definite and conclusive advice, and provide treatment invariably successful in result, if in my estimation the affection is capable of cure. It will, however, not be out of place to particularize those affections localized in the genital part of the economy, inasmuch as their great prevalence brings me more in professional contact with them than any other class of chronic disorders. Their gravity, insidious approach, their tardy progress at times, and their want of violent manifestations tend to give to them a special interest, calling for more active and energetic medical interference because of their special enmity of the health, vigor and manhood of the race. Their very apparent mildness gives them a two-fold capacity for undermining the constitution and destroying the integrity of the general health, and in all cases this disguised feature is usually a characteristic. These affections are usually contracted by early indiscretions or violation of physiological laws, and the patient, though long aware of his indisposition, is not fully conscious of the nature or seriousness of his disease until his health is completely broken, his system wrecked, and his vitality and vigor of manhood imperilled or destroyed. Long before this he knows that all is not right; but, owing to a false delicacy, and moreover, a fallacious confidence that nature will assert its supremacy and the disease disappear, he neglects to employ competent treatment until obliged to do so by the very grave character the affection eventually assumes. I have, therefore, specially alluded to these affections, such as nervous debility, etc., inasmuch as this very negligence is attended with deplorable consequences; and the failure to early intrust their cases to the care of competent and experienced physicians for treatment causes more human suffering, more deterioration of the physical and mental capacities, than aught else by which the welfare of our race is reduced or compromised. Physiology teaches that the genital organs exert a controlling influence over the whole economy; consequently, any affection jeopardizing healthy functional action of the organs is sure to effect a general disturbance of the whole system, as well as to deteriorate the quality and capacity of manhood. Every one, then, should become reflective, look well into his own condition, and if he suspects or discovers that the integrity of the genitalia is assailed by disease, he should throw aside all diffidence and false confidence in unaided nature, and at once seek medical advice and engage effective treatment of a physician who has the requisite ability and skill to be of service to him in such a critical and serious emergency.

In the female economy, we meet with serious diseases as well, which also justify special allusion to them. By the habits of advanced civilization, she also greatly deteriorates the quality of her general health and capacity for motherhood. She suffers also, untold agony from *Uterine Diseases*. Vital statisticians assert that there scarcely exists a female in civilized life who does not suffer with uterine disorder at some period of life, and that as a rule, the adult female suffers more or less with womb disease. Why is woman, in some way or other, thus fearfully a sufferer? Is it altogether owing to injurious modes of dress, habits of life, and other agencies? Is it not possible that this prevalence of uterine disease is partially owing to irrational and inefficient treatment? If treatment was competent, this load of suffering would certainly be less grievous to bear. The pathology of uterine affections is not so exceptionally severe that all efforts to cure are unavailing; why, then, are those affections so annoying to the "family physician," and why does he pronounce them *incurable*? Simply—and I know whereof I assert—because the usual routine practice observed by such practitioners is not calculated to cure, *does* not cure, but is capable of hurtful results and of so aggravating the condition of the disease as to change a simple pathological disorder into one characterized by pain, great suffering, and extreme gravity. The long-continued suffering so generally an important feature in the history of every case of uterine disorder, is due more to harsh and inappropriate treatment than to any peculiar severity or stubbornness in the morbid elements of the affections themselves. Proper internal medication with the indicated herbal remedies, in conjunction with such local applications as may be required, will effect a cure, in a large majority of cases, of Prolapsus, Leucorrhœa, Ulcerations, the various misplacements, menstrual disorders, etc., etc.

In particularly alluding to certain affections I do not wish the reader to be impressed with the idea that the nature of my special practice is the treatment only of the affections thus particularized. On the contrary, whatever the character or condition of the chronic affection may be, I can be consulted with reference to it, and my services engaged if the sufferer so desires. The reader of this work need scarcely be told what my professional convictions are with reference to the proper remedies to be employed in the treatment of disease. It will be apparent to all that I regard as medicinal only the products of the herbal world. In herbal remedies only do I place my confidence; they alone possess safely curative properties, and these they possess by right of Nature's grand design. I have no faith whatever in minerals, regarding them as obsolete, and as much a relic of the dark ages as incantations, amulets, or talismans of health. In all parts of this work I endeavor to present the superiority of plants as medicines, and zealously advocate the exclusive employment of herbal remedies in disease, and I am sure that all candid-minded, reflective, and thinking readers will admit the correctness of my premises and the conclusions I draw from them. None but the prejudiced will deem me an enthusiast, and ascribe my advocacy of exclusively herbal medication to over-zeal and biased antipathy to minerals. How must we regard the universality of the herbal kingdom? I see in it a noble purpose of the Author of Nature; plants are living medicines, capable of exhibition in disease without any trouble, while minerals must undergo a variety of chemical manipulations before they can be administered. The natural instincts of man and beast (when not prevented by conventional schools and erroneous teachings) lead unerringly to the life-giving products of the vegetable kingdom for the alleviation of pain and cure of disease. This fact was recognized at an early age; for, over two thousand years ago, the *Herbari* of Greece, Egypt, and Rome declared that plants are the only natural provision for the cure of disease. It is very deplorable that the principles and practice of medicine have become so heterodox as to greatly ignore herbal medicines, and employing in their stead, lifeless and injurious minerals. No honest, intelligent, and progressive physician can employ minerals without offending his better knowledge or compromising his moral sense; experience soon teaches him the vast superiority of herbal agents, and the employment of minerals is only in obedience to the teachings and practice of conventional schools which enforce the closure of eyes and ears against the recognition of the grand truth of the superiority of herbal over mineral medicaments. My supreme confidence in the healing virtues of herbal medicines was gained only by observing their superiority, and not born of prejudice or antipathy; for, in the first few years devoted to the study of medicine, I was taught as others are, to regard the employment of mineral agents as right and advisable. Experience only gave me better knowledge and fuller understanding, and at the present time, should the privilege of employing the medicinal properties of plants be taken away from me, leaving me but the inert and harmful minerals, my professional knowledge would avail me nothing, and I would stand in the presence of disease with fettered hands, helpless as a child, and absolutely without power to mitigate or relieve a single pain or symptom.

The art of healing consists merely in properly ascertaining the nature and extent of the departure from healthy physiological action or morbid condition, and in the application of the medicinal qualities of plants, roots, herbs, seeds, bulbs, etc, in proper proportion, to effect the restoration of healthy physiological action or removal of the morbid elements interfering with organic functions. This I regard as the true philosophy of disease and mode of treatment, and in accordance with such views I conduct all my investigations into the pathological condition of individual cases of disease necessary for identification, and for the application of the required medicinal agencies to effect restoration to a healthy condition again. The capacity to readily recognize pathological phenomena, and aptitude in the provision of required remedies, I trust and believe I have capably attained. The eminent and gratifying success attending my treatment of chronic maladies affords unimpeachable evidence of the correctness of my philosophy and professional competence.

If my suffering readers are satisfied that my philosophy of disease and mode of treatment are correct, I cordially invite them to present their cases for my consideration. My written opinion of the nature and curableness of their affections will be promptly sent in response. (In extending this invitation, I will take occasion to remark, that it is not beneath the dignity of the profession for any physician to offer his services to afflicted humanity in an open and honest manner; such an offering is implied and fully recognized in the fact that by study and experience he has become sufficiently competent to be thus engaged.) *Consultation is, under all circumstances, free.* No patient who consults me is required to feel a sense of obligation for thus gaining gratuitous medical advice. Every invalid unable to avail himself or herself of the opportunities of personal interview who presents his or her case for my consideration, will receive promptly in return a letter giving my opinion both as to the nature of the disease and the probabilities of cure. This, of course, will absorb my time and energies, but even then, if the sufferer is not fully convinced as to the correctness of my opinions, or confident as to the honesty of my assertions, he is under no obligations to engage my professional services, whatever; for in no case do I feel disposed to treat any patient who is not fully satisfied as to my knowledge of his case, my integrity, or my ability to cure, when, in my opinion, I may feel justified in pronouncing the case a curable one. I desire the confidence and friendship of all the sufferers who may employ me, and this can only be gained and maintained by strict observance of professional honor, fair dealing, and honest, capable and effective treatment. My sympathies are with afflicted humanity, and especially do I feel great and enduring regard for the welfare of those who constantly and often heroically suffer and who enjoy but little of life's brightness in consequence of the ever present tortures of chronic disease. In behalf of all patients I call to aid my best abilities, treating no case with indifference or a culpable disregard as to the final results of the treatment.

Afflicted persons desirous of gaining my advice should give a plain statement of their affections, when contracted, the present symptoms, etc.—in fact, everything should be made known to me precisely as would occur by personal interview. The questions on the next and following pages are intended to assist invalids in properly presenting their cases. Answers to all the questions are not necessary—only those which have a particular reference to the diseased condition of the patient need be replied to. Fine nor technical writing is not required. Give all in confidence, withholding nothing that rightfully I should know. All correspondence held inviolably sacred.

In writing for advice, give legibly the post-office, town, county and state to which you wish your answer directed, and if medicines are ordered, the name of the Express Station (and that of the Express Company) to which they are to be sent. *Remittances should be made in Post Office Money Orders*, payable at Jersey City, N. J., wherever there is a Money Order Office, which is now almost universal, there being only a few exceptions. Where these exceptions do exist, REGISTER THE LETTER containing money. Either of these modes is PERFECTLY SAFE, the Postmaster always giving you a receipt for the money. No MEDICINES SENT C. O. D., unless half the money is sent in advance. The express business has reached *such perfection* within the last few years, that I can almost guarantee a DAILY DELIVERY to every hamlet in the United States.

ALL LETTERS WILL BE TREATED AS STRICTLY PRIVATE AND CONFIDENTIAL. Invalids on a visit to New York may call on me whenever convenient. Office hours, from 10 A. M. to 4 P. M.

Address DR. O. PHELPS BROWN, No. 21 Grand Street, Jersey City, N. J.

QUESTIONS TO INVALIDS.

It is not necessary that invalids should answer every question; only those having a particular reference to their cases need be responded to.

A. What is your age? Color of hair and eyes? Complexion? Weight? Are you fleshy, plump, or lean? What was your weight when in health?

B. What is the condition of your skin—soft and moist, rough or dry? Is it free from eruptions? if not, what is the character of the eruption?

C. Are your parents living? if so, at what age? If either, or both, are dead, of what did they die? Any hereditary disease in the family, present or remote? Were your parents healthy at the time of your conception? Were you fed in infancy from your mother's breast? if so, at what age was other food substituted?

D. Have you any mental trouble? if so, what is the cause? Have you had any nervous disease of any kind? Are your nerves very sensitive? Have you ever overtaxed yourself with study or mental labor? Is your memory acute and retentive, or the reverse? Have you ever suffered from intense and prolonged grief from any cause? Do you sleep well? if not, what is the cause of disturbance? What is the favorite position in sleep? Have you horrible dreams and nightmare at times? How many hours do you sleep? Do you rise refreshed, or drowsy, from your sleep? Are your emotions easily excited?

E. Have you any bodily deformity? if so, were you born with it, or was it caused by accident? Have you, or did you ever have salt-rheum, erysipelas, ulcers, abscesses, or cancer? Have you been vaccinated? if so, did it produce any unpleasant consequences? Have you ever been dosed with mercury? Have you any tumors or swellings? Are you ruptured at any part? Do you feel strong, or weak? Does walking fatigue you, and can you run far? Is exercise agreeable to you? Are your muscles hard, or soft and flabby? Are your hands and feet cold, or warm; wrist, dry or hot? Do you protect yourself with sufficient clothing?

F. What time do you go to bed, and at what hour do you arise? Are you regular in this respect? What composes your usual diet? Do you use stimulants? if so, what, and to what extent? Do you use tea or coffee? Do you use tobacco in any form? Any opium? Are you fond of condiments, pickles, and pastries, and do you eat them excessively. Are you regular with your meals?

G. Have you any headache? if so, at what part of the head? Have you catarrhal or mucous discharges from the nose or throat? if so, moderately or excessively? Have you any dizzy sensations, feelings of oppression, or rush of blood to the head? Have you ever fainted, and are you liable to do so?

H. Have you any trouble about the eyes or ears? Do the eyes water more than natural? Have you any ringing or buzzing noises in the ears? Are there any specks before your eyes, circles around bright light? Do you see and hear well? Is there any inflammation about the eyes? Do your ears secrete wax to excess? Have you any discharges from them?

I. Have you any trouble in the mouth, scurvy, canker, dryness, excessive saliva, unpleasant taste—bad breath? Have you any decayed teeth? Is the tongue coated? if so, white or yellow?

J. Have you any throat affection? Do you raise much? Have you tickling sensations, hawking, choking sensations, enlargement of tonsils? Is your voice strong? Does reading aloud fatigue the voice?

K. Are you predisposed to colds? Where do colds affect you? Do you cough much—dry or loose cough—at what time do you cough most? Is coughing usually painful, and does it yield readily to any treatment resorted to? Have you occasional or constant pain in the chest? When you take a full breath, is the pain increased? Have you any difficulty of breathing—wheezing—gasping—or sense of tightness? Do you expectorate much—and what is the character of the phlegm? Have you night sweats? Are your feet and ankles swelled?

L. How many pulsations at the wrist in a minute? Have you any soreness or pains about the heart? Have you any palpitation—sense of stoppage—disagreeable symptoms?

M. Is the appetite good, poor, variable, voracious? Does your food digest well? Does it distress you—cause any soreness—wind--belching

—nausea—sourness? Are you careful about the articles and character of diet? Are your bowels costive, loose, bloated, tender? Do you take much physic? Have you any piles?

N. Have you any pain or weakness in the lower part of back? Have you any pain or soreness about the region of the kidneys and bladder? Do you pass water often? Do you pass much, or little, at a time? Does its passage cause any smarting? Is there any sediment? if so, what is the color? If you allow your urine to stand about forty-eight hours, do you observe any peculiar sediment? What is the ordinary color of your urine—milky, high-colored, bloody?

O. Have you any pain in any part of the body? Are you troubled with rheumatism or neuralgia, occasionally? Have you any cramps? Any loss or increase of sensation at any part of the surface? Are you paralyzed at any part?

P. Are you married or single? If married, have you any children, and if so, are they healthy? Does pregnancy interfere with your general health? Are your labors severe and protracted?

Q. Have you ever injured yourself by any bad habit? If a male, do you suffer from weakness in any part? if so, where, and state full particulars? Do you suspect any secret drain upon the system? What is the most probable cause—excesses, injudicious indulgences, sedentary habits, or intemperance? Have you varicocele? Are your organs unnatural in any respect? (It is not necessary on my part to further investigate into the pathological condition of the genital organs, as every patient will see the propriety of unreservedly informing me of all the facts.)

R. If a female, do you have any womb disease, prolapsus—leucorrhœa—displacement—ulceration? Have you any bearing-down pains in the pelvic region? Have you any unnatural signs, symptoms, anxious peculiarities, or weakness about these organs? if so, state the fact. Are you regular in your courses? Do you have pain? if so, before, during, or after the flow? Is the flow scanty or profuse—and how long does it continue? Do you have any soreness, pruritus, irritation, or morbid growths about the vagina? Have you ever had any miscarriages? if so, what was the cause?

Correspondents who propose to place themselves under my treatment are required to give only a plain statement of their symptoms, when the disease first commenced, its present character, etc., etc. The above questions are merely intended to assist the patient to present his or her case. Answers to all the questions are not necessary, only those which have a particular reference to the diseased condition afflicting the patient. Any ordinary case can be sufficiently explained on one side of a letter-sheet. Fine or technical writing is not required. Write precisely as if you were conversing with me, endeavoring merely to give a plain and concise history of the case. In all cases I give advice without charge where the patient proposes to come under treatment.

All those addressing me should be particular to write their names legibly, and give the name of Post-Office, County, and State ; and when ordering medicines they will please name the Express Company and Station.

Remittances may be made by Post-office Order or registered letter, at my risk. Address Dr. O. PHELPS BROWN, 21 Grand Street, Jersey City, N. J.

17*

PART III.

THE PHILOSOPHY OF THE SEXES.

Admitting the delicacy of the subject, it is, however, eminently within the province of the medical writer to teach the scientific bearings of
the marital prerogative of the sexes, inasmuch as health, as well as civilization, is greatly dependent upon the purity of that relation. While I
condemn such literature which is elementarily and purposely suggestive,
I have but little sympathy with that prudish modesty which is outraged
by everything appertaining to the special characteristics of sex. The
author shall, in the consideration of the subject, not attempt to offend
healthy conservatism, yet, at the same time, the subject is too important to discuss it with undue reserve or by unintelligent circumlocution.
The essays are not written to gratify immoral curiosity, but to edify
those who wish to learn and be governed by the correct principles of the
philosophy appertaining to the marital union of the sexes. And as this
work is specially intended to educate the popular, and not the professional mind, it is proper and quite consonant with every moral consideration, that it should contain such general knowledge as all should know
for proper guidance in matters pertaining to the organs of reproduction.
It is quite important for all to know the anatomy of the genitalia of
both sexes. I shall, therefore, prepare this special part of this work with
the anatomy of the organs of both sexes.

ANATOMY OF THE MALE ORGANS.

These consist of the organ itself, seminal vesicles, prostate gland,
testes and scrotum.

The male organ conveys the urine from the bladder, and the seminal
sections from the seminal vesicles. Its anterior extremity is called the
glans, and its posterior extremity is the *root ;* the intervening part, the
body, which consists of two structures, the *corpus cavernosum*, or cavernous body, and the *corpus spongiosum*, or spongy body. The skin is thin
and delicate, studded with numerous sebaceous follicles. Surrounding
the glans is a loose doubling of skin called the *prepuce*, which is connected to the mouth of the urethra by a process called the *frænum*. The
thick rim or edge around the base of the glans is the crown, or *corona
glandis*, behind which the organ is narrow, and this portion is known as
the neck or *collum*. The caseous secretion found here is known as *smegma*, which is the product of the *glands* of *Tyson*, numerous about the
neck and crown.

The cavernous body forms the largest part of the organ and in shape is a double cylinder. At the root these cylinders are separate and pointed, and called the *crura* of the penis. Each of these is firmly attached to the branches of the pubes and ischium,—bones of the pelvis. The cavernous body has a thick, elastic, fibrous coating externally; internally it consists of a spongy structure made up of cells, or little caverns, which readily communicate with the arteries and veins. Those arteries that terminate in blind tufts are called *helicine*. The cylinders are partially separated from each other by a partition whose fibres resemble the teeth of a comb, whence the name *septum pectiniforme*.

The *corpus spongiosum* has the same fibrous covering as the cavernous body, and is also composed of cells, but which are larger than those of the cavernous body. Its relative position to the corpus cavernosum is about the same as a ramrod to a double-barrelled gun. Posteriorly it enlarges into what is called the *bulb*, lying between the crura of the organ. Anteriorly it forms the glans.

The urethra, or urinary canal from the bladder, perforates the spongy body. Its mouth at the glans is called *meatus urinarius*.

The *seminal vesicles* consist of two convoluted tubes placed at the posterior and inferior portion of the bladder. They are oblong in shape, about two inches in length. They act as a receptacle for the semen. When secreted by the testicles, the semen is conveyed by a tube, called the *vas deferens*, into these vesicles, where it is mixed with a little mucus, and retained until discharged.

The *prostate gland* is a dense hard structure, about the size of a horse-chestnut, surrounding the neck of the bladder, at the commencement of the urethra. It is perforated by the urethra, and also by the *ductus ejaculatorius*, which is formed by the junction of the vas deferens and the seminal duct. The semen is further liquefied by the secretion of the prostate, in its passage through the gland. It also discharges a thick and white secretion into the urethra. In front of the prostate are two glands (*Cowper's*), about the size of a pea, which also discharge a mucous secretion into the urethra.

The *scrotum* is the bag-like covering for the testicles. Its skin is loose and thin, and of a dark color. The transverse wrinkles which cold produces are due to a dense, reddish, contractile structure, intimately connected with the skin, and called the *dartos*. The scrotum has a muscular covering, next to the dartos; its internal covering is called the *tunica vaginalis*.

The *testes* or *testicles* are the glands for the secretion of semen. They are two in number, oval in shape, and flattened laterally. They are suspended by the spermatic cord. Each testicle is formed by lobules, consisting of a fine tube, very finely convoluted, which, if finely dissected and unravelled, is many feet in length. The *epididymis* is a vermiform appendage encircling the posterior edge of the testicle, as a crest upon a helmet.

The *spermatic cord* consists of an artery and vein, and nerves, together with the vas deferens.

The *erectile tissue* of the organ consists essentially of intricate networks of veins, which communicate freely with each other, presenting a cellular appearance.

These features constitute what is termed the regional anatomy of the organs—the minute anatomy being much more complex. The physiological functions of the male organs of generation are various, and inasmuch as they are associated very intimately with one of the most important of human passions, which if not properly controlled by the dictates of the moral sense, are exceedingly liable to derangement. Anything tending to cause a departure from a healthy or normal standard of action of these physiological functions, will assuredly induce a faulty condition of the organs themselves, besides impairing the integrity of the general health. Those interested in this subject may turn to page 350, and read the article on "Debility or Loss of Vitality." No one should be neglectful in this respect, but strenuously endeavor by correct habits of life to maintain the physiological functions in full purity, vigor and integrity of action.

THE SEMEN.

This is a secretion formed by the testes, which anatomically we have seen are composed of lobules formed of convoluted seminiferous tubes. The number of lobules is about 450 in each testis, and that of tubules about 840. It is apparent, then, that each testis presents a vast extent of surface for the secretion of the spermatic fluid. The testes originate in the lower part of what is called the Woolfian bodies in the embryo, while the kidneys spring from the upper part. They do not descend into the scrotum until about the ninth month, and sometimes one or both remain in the abdomen, without, however, interfering with their function.

The semen is a thick, tenacious, grayish fluid, having a peculiar odor called *spermatic,* probably dependent on the secretions mixed with it. The semen as ejected is not the same as secreted by the testes, as it receives, in its passage out, the addition of the liquefying secretions of the prostate and Cowper's glands. It is alkaline in reaction, and contains albumen and a peculiar principle called *spermatin.* It also contains *spermatazoids,* very small bodies with a tail-like process to them. They were formerly regarded as animalcules, but now known to possess no independent organic life. As viewed under the microscope they are seen floating lively around the spermatic liquor ; this is, most probably, due to ciliary vibrations. The semen also contains other minute, granular bodies, called *seminal granules.* These, in conjunction with the spermatozoids, constitute the formative agents furnished by the male in generation. They are supposed to correspond with the pollen tubes of plants. The vermicular motion of the spermatozoids evidently aids the passage of the semen, after its injection into the womb, to the ovaries of the female, and if they there meet the female elements of generation an ovule becomes impregnated, and pregnacy is the result. The semen is a very vital element, and is only secreted in proportion to the vigor of the male. It contains chlorides and phosphates, hence its waste preys upon the nervous tissue for its supply of phosphorus. The secretion takes place about the fourteenth or fifteenth year, and continues till about sixty or sixty-five, and during the whole of this time is much under the influence of the nervous system. Its presence in the seminal vesicles is required for the proper accomplishment of the virile act, and it is a well known physiological fact that full procreative quality is only gained after it has been for some time lodged in the vesicles. The involuntary expenditure of this vital fluid is therefore not only detrimental to the general health, but also seriously destructive of procreative capacity.

ANATOMY OF THE FEMALE ORGANS.

The organs of generation in the female are generally divided into the external and internal. The external consist of the *mons veneris, labia externa, clitoris, nymphæ, vestibule, meatus urinarius, hymen* in virgins, and *carunculæ myrtiformes* in matrons. The internal are the *vagina, uterus,* and the uterine appendages, the latter consisting of the *broad* and *round ligaments, ovaries,* and *Fallopian tubes.*

The mons veneris is placed at the lower part of the abdomen, and consists of dense fibro-cellular and fatty tissues, and is covered in the adult with hair. The anatomical provision of this particular covering in combination with the fatty texture is to prevent chafing and pressure upon sensitive nerves at certain periods.

The labia externa, or outer lips, are two folds of skin and mucous membrane, which commence in front of the pubic bones, and extend back to the perinæum, where they again meet. The superior junction is called the *anterior commissure,* the posterior is called the *posterior commissure,* or *fourchette.* By *vulva* some mean the whole external organs, by others the longitudinal opening between the projecting part of the external organs. The use of the external labia is to protect the organs situated between them.

The *nymphæ* or *labia interna,* or inner lips, arise from nearly the same point, at the anterior commissure, and run downwards and backwards, about an inch, to the middle of the vaginal orifice, where they disappear in the general lining of the labia externa.

The *clitoris* is seated just below the point of the junction of the labia interna. In structure it is the same as the male organ, with the exception that it has no spongy body or urethra. It is erectile and extremely sensitive. Its mucous covering is continuous with the vaginal lining. Under exciting influences it distends and enlarges. In exceptional instances and from certain causes, it becomes abnormally enlarged and elongated, and those females in whom this enlargement is observed, are the reputed hermaphrodites, especially when other congenital deficiencies are associated. This must be regarded, however, as an anotomical vagary, as in animated nature there is nothing truly epicene.

The triangular space between the sides of the labia interna and above the clitoris is known as the *vestibule*, at the lower portion of which is found the *meatus urinarius*, or orifice of the urethra. The urethra is about an inch and a half long and very dilatable.

The *hymen* is a fold of mucous membrane, generally of semilunar shape, with its concavity upwards, which is found just within the orifice of the vagina. It is generally ruptured at the first carnal intercourse. Its presence generally denotes the virgin; it is, however, not an infallible *argumentum integritatis* (one of its names), or evidence of virginal integrity. Connubial infelicity has often arisen on account of its absence in the chosen one of a man who earnestly believed its presence absolutely necessary to establish virginity. Many circumstances of an innocent character may occasion a rupture or destruction of this membrane, such as coughing, convulsive laughter, menstruation, etc. It is often, indeed, found absent in children soon after birth, whilst it may remain entire even after copulation. Cases of conception have been recorded, and yet the membrane was found intact. Hence its presence does not absolutely prove virginity, nor does its absence prove incontinence, although its presence would be what is known in law as *primâ facie* evidence of continence.

Its remains after rupture form what is known as the *carunculæ myrtiformes*, by reason of the resemblance to the leaves of the myrtle. The space between the hymen and fourchette is called the *fossa navicularis*.

The external organs in the aggregate are often called the *pudendum*.

THE INTERNAL ORGANS.

The *vagina* is that canal extending from its origin in the vulva obliquely through the cavity of the pelvis to the uterus. Its usual length is about four or five inches, and about three in circumference, though in a few females it may exceed that length, while in others it may be but a few inches long. It is shorter and more capacious in those who have borne children. It is well supplied with blood-vessels, and its mucous membrane is of a pink color, so arranged in various folds as to allow great extension. Its orifice is surrounded by a collection of mus-

cular fibres, called the *sphincter vaginæ*. It is not much under the control of the will, however, as is shown by the inability to retain injections.

The *uterus*, or womb, is placed at the upper part of the vagina, and
hangs in the centre of the pelvis, behind the bladder and before the
rectum. In shape it resembles the pear, rounder posteriorly than anteriorly, and is about two and a half to three inches long, two inches
wide, and very nearly an inch thick. Its upper part is called the *fundus*, the inferior cylindrical portion the *cervix* or *neck*, and the intervening portion the *body*. It is held in place by the broad and lateral
ligaments. Its cavity is triangular, the base being directed upwards,
and the superior angles corresponding to the points of entrance of the
Fallopian tubes; in size it is about equal to a split almond, and the interior walls are nearly always in contact. Its inferior angle communicates with the vagina through the canal of the neck, which is barrel-
shaped, and from half to three-quarters of an inch long. The contraction at the upper extremity of the canal is called the internal *mouth* or
os uteri, whilst that of the lower extremity is called the *os uteri* or *os
tincæ*, the latter name from its supposed resemblance to the mouth of a
tench. In shape the os varies, in some being transverse, in others circular or ragged, the latter especially in women who have borne children.
The uterine cavity lodges the fœtus from the commencement of conception until its birth.

The *Fallopian tubes* are cylindrical canals about four inches long,
arising from the superior angle of the uterus. Externally they are
equally thick throughout, except at their terminal extremity, where
they expand into a trumpet-shaped enlargement, called *fimbria* or
morsus diaboli, by which the ovaries are grasped. They are the ducts
for the passage of the ovules from the ovaries of the uterus. The
ovaries are the analogues of the male testes. They are situated on each
side of the uterus; three or four inches away from it. They are oval
in shape, and in removing the outer coats, the proper ovarian tissue
appears, called the *stroma*. The stroma is studded with numerous
little bodies called *Graafian vesicles*. These vary in size, the largest
being found near the surface of the ovary, and are found early in life,
but are more developed about the period of puberty. These vesicles
have two coats, the *tunic of the ovisac*, and the *ovisac*. Within the
cavity formed by these membranes is an albuminous fluid, in which is
found floating the *ovum* or *egg*, which is exceedingly small, but which
if impregnated becomes the fœtus. The human egg in all its details
resembles the egg of the chick. It contains a yolk, in the centre of
which is a little vesicle called the *germinal vesicle*, and on the walls of
the germinal vesicle is seen its *nucleus*, named the *macula germinativa*,
or germinal spot. As each Graafian vesicle rises to the surface of the
ovary it bursts, and allows the contained ovum to escape, which is seized

by the fimbriæ of the Fallopian tube, and transmitted to the womb. The scar left on the ovary after the discharge of the ovum is called the *corpus luteum* or *yellow body*.   This function in the female is named *ovulation.*

There is no correspondence between the number of yellow bodies found in the ovaries of a woman and the number of children she may have borne, as the ova are constantly discharged, irrespective of fecundation, and hence the corpus luteum is no evidence of previously existing pregnancy

SOCIAL STATUS OF THE ORGANS.

We have now described the most important anatomical features of the genital organs with the same composure and desire to instruct, as when we described the anatomy of the other organs, and I am sure that all of my correct-minded readers have read the same with equal equanimity and desire to learn.   It is altogether owing to a false and foolish modesty that everything descriptive of the anatomical differences of the sexes is declared to be indelicate or obscene.   It is only obscene when used to awaken and excite the imagination to dwell on amatory objects, and not when used for the purposes of legitimate instructions as in these pages.   Extreme reticence with regard to matters referring to the genital part of the economy is not always indicative of a pure modesty or continence, nor is it healthy conservatism, but often the promoter of disease and imbecility.   Those who are diseased at this part of their anatomy, usually became so because they were ignorant of either the anatomy or physiology of the organs.   This fact leads me to have no sympathy with any prudish illiberality, but forcibly impresses me with the great necessity existing for instruction and enlightenment relative to this part of the economy.   I will therefore break loose from the trammels of prudery, and attempt, in a measure, to properly inform my readers, in a discreet manner, of all the bearings of philosophy relative to the economy of the genitalia.   Knowledge of this kind, in obeisance to a proscriptive spirit, is now isolated within a narrow precinct of intelligence, while the demands of the highest welfare of humanity are urgent for universal dissemination.   Medical men have long been aware of the necessity of popularizing intelligence relative to this subject, but lacked the wisdom to ignore the illiberal countenance that banished it within their own limits of intelligence. If any medical knowledge is worthy of popular acceptance and guidance, it is that pertaining to the genital part of the economy ; on no other subject are unprofessional people so ignorant, and no other species of ignorance is conducive to greater misfortunes.

Discussion of this subject in the decorous language of science in a popular work, will not lead to lewdness nor encourage lechery ; on the contrary, my convictions are that such information as will be imparted will tend to give a healthy tone to modesty and encourage continence. This is my purpose, all others I ignore and condemn.

Excessive modesty is often the offspring of ignorance. The physician who is fully acquainted with the anatomy and physiology of the generative organs, finds nothing suggestive in such knowledge; it is to him as common-place as the anatomy and physiology of other parts of the economy. And should unprofessional people be possessed of proper knowledge of the anatomical features and physiological functions of the organs, any decent and necessary allusion to them would not be regarded as indelicate or offensive. Such intelligence is not subversive of the moral nature, nor provocative of impure thought; the conventional illiberality deemed proper by certain people, is far more hurtful than judicious instruction. Knowledge with refererence to the human economy is capable of great injury if permitted to be buried, and this is as true of the organs in the pelvis as of those in the thoracic region. We should all know, and not be ashamed to admit, when admission is proper and right, that Nature completed her work in case of our own persons; injudicious reservation in this respect, does a great deal of harm, as it often obliges the unfortunate to suffer in secret with serious affections, the locality of which makes them ashamed or unwilling to confide in those whose counsels may be of benefit. Few parents have the wisdom to take their children in their confidence and teach them the evils consequent on solitary indulgence, and but few mothers acquaint their daughters with the phenomenon of womanhood before its appearance. The son is unwilling to seek the counsel of his father, and the daughter does not avail herself of her mother's wisdom and experience. It is the experience of every medical man whose practice extends largely among females, that questions concerning the integrity of the organs in the pelvic cavity are unwillingly answered. What young female is willing to intrust to her medical attendant the knowledge of her disordered menstruation? She refuses to answer his questions, and probably hides her chlorotic face under the bed-clothes. The doctor only gains the truth after he is taken to another room where the mother or nurse acquaints him with the fact. This round-about way of imparting the required information, places the patient in an embarrassing attitude towards her physician, and it would be far better for her own welfare and individual independence did she herself state the fact, and freely and composedly answer the interrogations of her medical attendant. Who can admire the sickly modesty of Dr. Abernethy's patient, who enveloped her wrist in a linen handkerchief before she would permit him to ascertain the condition of her pulse. The Doctor, however, gave the proper rebuke, for he immediately put his hand in his coat-tail, and remarked that " a linen patient requires a woolen physician." Those of the author's sex are also very often uncomfortable in the physician's presence, if questioned with regard to diseases of the generative organs. This is radically wrong, for such timidity and unwillingness induces the patient to defer medical treatment until absolutely driven to it by the extreme gravity the affection assumes. Modesty is an admirable virtue, as far as social intercouse is concerned, but under circumstances requiring medical aid or counsel, the re-establishment of the organs to healthy physiological action should not be embarrassed by a diseased modesty, or timid and foolish reservation. As this work is intended to bear a relation to the reader the same as the physician does to his patient, it is hoped that the knowledge contained in these essays, will receive commendation instead of condemnation, that they will be considerately read by all who have need of such intelligence; and that errors of habit may be abandoned and the proper •observance of the laws of health respecting the generative organs be followed instead.

In conclusion, I hope there are not many of my readers who are offended with Nature for making us distinct as to sex, and who endeavor to remedy her mistakes by hushing up the fact altogether.

PRESERVATION OF THE HEALTH OF THE ORGANS.

Complete health of the organs is necessary to the full vigor of the general economy, and it should be the aim and desire of all to maintain the vigor of the genitalia. The male delights in the shapely figure of the person of the female, the full development of her bust, and the vivacity of her spirits, all indicative of a healthy genitalia; and the female takes pride in the male who presents the evidences of a vigorous manhood. This is a natural selection, and no one is indifferent to it.

The greatest requirement is *cleanliness*. Ablutions of these parts should be more frequent than of the body in general. We have seen that in the male the secretion of smegma constantly accumulates at the corona. Besides, the scrotum is so situated that perspiration is at all times attendant. Its surface is also studded with numerous sebaceous follicles, whose secretions become quickly very offensive. If these secretions are not removed, they will impede the full development of the organ as well as abridge coitive power. They should therefore be daily cleansed. Cold water is preferable, as it is more stimulating, and possesses greater tonic properties than tepid or warm water.

In the female the excessive secretions render cleanliness very important. The vaginal secretions should not be allowed to accumulate at the vulva, as they soon become offensive, and if re-absorbed impair the general health. On the pubic prominence are many sebaceous follicles, whose secretions should be frequently removed by ablutions. Besides, the urine which passes through the external parts adds constantly to the uncleanly state. It is therefore very important that the parts should be frequently washed, omitting, however, cold-water ablutions during the menstrual period.

Nothing is capable of doing greater harm than excesses of any kind, and those organs should not be indulged by any unnatural means. It is promotive of disease, destructive of manhood and healthy womanhood, and, if early engaged in, arrests the full development of the organs of either sex, and so reduces the strength of these organs that it renders them incapacitated for the purposes which were ordained to them by nature, besides wrecking the nervous system very materially. It is well known that those who have thus been imprudent, having so long been accustomed to self-gratification, do not find subsequent and legitimate excitement so intense as those who have been continent. They have so long been accustomed to the gratification induced by their own electricity that the magnetism of another body becomes more or less inert in the production of a complete orgasm. The habit is morally and physically pernicious, and its prevalence should be abated by influence of a superior education in these matters.

Undue excitement of the important passion is detrimental in the extreme. Obscene literature and pictures do more harm than merely depraving the moral tastes—they so stimulate the amative passions that the seminal vesicles, by the consequent nervous excitement, will allow the semen to ooze away, inducing hidden seminal waste or losses of semen with the urine, creating an intonicity of those organs and deprive them of natural vigor. The same effect is produced by association of the sexes, where the mutual conduct is provocative of amative excitement, though modified by forbidden indulgence. Those who have the welfare of the organs in view, are therefore counselled not to permit abnormal excitement of the passions to occur. Females should, likewise, avoid reading obscene literature, from the fact that the constant expenditure of nervous force ensuing upon the engorged condition of her organs is very hurtful. It is a well-known physiological fact, that undue excitement of any passion, such as anger, mirth, etc., is always followed by a certain weakness of the general organism, and the same holds true of the amative passion also.

The occasional desire for congress is purely a natural one, and the most chaste or pure-minded person, sufficiently fortunate to possess healthy organs, cannot rise superior to the desire. It is simply a manifestation of a function of the economy in perfect obedience to a physiological law. It is readily explained. We have seen that semen is the secretory product of a gland (the testes), afterward deposited in a vesicle; the urine is also secreted by a gland, and deposited likewise in a vesicle (the bladder). When the bladder becomes filled the afferent nerves distributed to it convey intelligence of the fact to the brain, and a desire for urination arises, which continues as long as the bladder remains charged with urine. This is a natural phenomenon of organic function. In like manner the full seminal vesicles impart the sensation to the nerves distributed to them, which is also conveyed to the brain. What is the result ? Naturally, a desire for cohabitation in order to evacuate the charged vesicles. This fact is an unalterable condition of the economy, and it follows that a desire for the evacuation of the vesicles is as much a natural manifestation of functional action as that of relief of the bladder. In the female the hyperæsthetic condition of the nerves distributed, to the clitoris awakens the same desire, which remains as long as the nervous forces, are not equalized by the expenditure of a part. It is, therefore, purely a nervous phenomenon in the female. The amative passion is not a cultivated one ; it is natural to the human being, and ineradicable by the greatest exercise of continent thought and behavior, and its gratification is unquestionably hygienic. It is, of course, as subject to rational indulgence as in diet or drink.

We have seen that desires are natural in a healthy condition of either sex, and that a rational indulgence is hygienic, but I earnestly caution every reader to guard against debauching the passion by unlicensed congress. The indulgence can only be countenanced in marriage. It is, therefore, the plain duty of every male and female to marry, and as early in life as contingencies will permit. That marriage is hygenic is proven by the fact that married people live longer than the unmarried, a fact that demonstrates the marital privilege as a healthy relation between the sexes. Nature did not design total continence, and such a condition is aversive to the physical and mental well-being of the sexes. Nature, however, provides in this as she does in everything else. The amative passions do not present themselves or become inconveniently strong in either sex until a full marriageable age is attained.

MARRIAGE.

This is, in law, the conjugal union of man with woman, and is the only state in which cohabitation is considered proper and irreprehensible. The marriage relation exists in all Christian communities, and is considered the most solemn of contracts, and, excepting in Protestant countries, it is regarded as a sacrament, In some countries its celebration falls under the cognizance of ecclesiastical courts only, but in the United States it is regarded as merely a civil contract, magistrates having, equally with clergymen, the right to solemnize it, though it is usually the practice to have it performed by a clergyman, and attended with religious ceremonies, Marriage, as a legalized custom, is of very ancient origin. It is doubtful whether even the primitive man was not governed in the intercourse of the sexes by some recognition of the union being confined to one chosen one. No greater promiscuity can cer-tainly be supposed than occurs in the lower animals, where pairing is the law. The nobler animals, as the lion, elephant, etc., never have but one mate ; and even in case of death do not re-mate. As man ad-vanced, civil codes were inaugurated, and certain protection given to the choice of the parties. The earliest civil code regulating marriage of which we have any account was that of Menes, who, Herodotus tells us, was the first of the Pharaohs or native Egyptian kings, and who lived about 3,500 years before Christ. The nature of his code is not known.

The Biblical account extends further back, but it does not appear that any laws existed regulating marriage, but each one was allowed to choose his wife and concubines, and it is supposed that common consent respected the selection. Next Moses gave laws for the government of marriage among the Israelites. The early Greeks followed the code of Cecrops, and the Romans were also governed in their marital relations by stringent laws. In fact the necessity of some law regulating the in-tercourse between the sexes must have become very apparent to all nations or communities at a very early period. It certainly antedates any legal regulations with regard to the possession of property. It is very probable that every community did by common consent afford to each male one or more females, and the presumption is that such choice or assignment, as the case may have been, was respected by common agreement as inviolable. It is doubtful if ever promiscuity was the law or privilege with any community of men, even in their primitive state. The possession of reason is antagonistic to such a belief ; and man was most probably elevated above the beast by the faculty of rea-son in this respect as in others. Promiscuous indulgence is always evi-dence of debauchery, and a departure from that natural course which is prompted by an innate sense of propriety characterizing mankind. The law is very indefinite with regard to what constitutes a legal marriage. It is an unsettled question, both in England and in this country, whether a marriage solemnized by customary formalities alone is legal, or if one characterized by the mere consent of the parties is illegal. The latter has been held as legal in some instances in both countries. Kent, in his *Commentaries*, lays down the law that contracts made so that either party recognizes it from the moment of contract, and even not followed by cohabitation, amounts to a valid marriage ; and also that a contract to be recognized at some future period, and followed by consummation, is equally valid. It is unfortunate that the law is so un-decided in this respect. The decisions arrived at, for or against, were not dependent upon any recognized law, but seem to be influenced by the character of the cases, either for favor or discountenance. As long as the law recognizes cohabitation legal only in marriage, it seems to me that if consummated under consent of the parties to bear marital relations with each other, or promise of marriage, the act should be unhesitatingly pronounced as the equivalent of a valid marriage in all instances. If cohabitation is only a marital prerogative the law should not stultify itself by recognizing it as possible to occur in any other relation. If either of the parties are married the law defines it as adultery, and, very properly, defines the punishment. It is necessary to the progress of the age that some such principle should be recognized in common law, so as not to subject the decision of the question to the individual opinion of any judge. It would at once obviate the confusion of sentiment now held in regard to it, and besides arrest the decision in test cases from mere caprice of the tribunal. It is certainly as correct a principle as any in common law, and would, in its operations as a statute law, be free from injustice, and capable of doing much good.

POLYGAMY.

This is a state in which a man has at the same time one or more wives, or a woman more than one husband. The latter custom is more properly called polyandry, and prevails in Thibet and a few other places. Polygamy has existed from time immemorial, especially among the nations of the East. In sacred history we find that it prevailed before the flood. Lamech had two wives, and the patriarchs were nearly all polygamists. The custom was tolerated by the laws of Moses, and, in fact, no positive injunction against it is found in the whole of the Old Testament. It is questionable whether more than one was recognized as the *bonâ-fide* wife, the other simply being wives by right of concubinage. But if polygamy was in its strictest sense the legal custom, it soon grew unpopular, for no trace of it is met in the records of the New Testament, where all the passages referring to marriage imply monogamy as alone lawful. The custom has been almost universal in the East, being sanctioned by all the religions existing there. The religion of Mohammed allows four wives, but the permission is rarely exercised except by the rich. The custom is accounted for on the ground of the premature old age of the female in those regions, and also on the ground of excess of the number of females, though the latter, by the authority of recent travellers, is probably not the truth. The marriage code of Fu-hi, who primarily established civilization among the Chinese, gave most probably superiority to but one wife, but raised the concubine to the dignity of a wife to a certain extent.

Among the Greeks, at least of later times, monogamy was the custom, though in the time of Homer polygamy prevailed to some extent. It was not known in the republic of Rome, but during the existence of the empire the prevalence of divorce gave rise to a state almost analogous to it. It prevailed among the barbarous nations of antiquity, excepting the Germans, who, according to Tacitus, "were content with a single wife." In some countries more than one wife was allowable if the husband could extend the dowry ; a wife without a dowry was considered only a concubine. This was the case in Judea, when it became a dependency of Rome.

In Christian countries polygamy was never tolerated, the tenets of the church forbidding it, though Charlemagne had two wives, and Sigibert and Chilperic also had a plurality. John of Leyden, an Anabaptist leader, was the husband of seventeen wives, and he held that it was his moral right to marry as many as he chose.

In England the punishment of polygamy was originally in the hands of the ecclesiastics. It was considered a capital crime by a statute of Edward I., but it did not come entirely under the control of the temporal power until a statute of James I. made it a felony, punishable with death. George III. made it punishable by imprisonment or transportation for seven years. By the laws of ancient and modern Sweden the penalty is death. The Prussian Code of 1794 subjected the criminal to confinement in a house of correction for not less than two years. In the United States the second marriage is a nullity, and the punishment varies in the different States, though usually imprisonment for a certain period, or fine, or both, is the penalty. The term bigamy is most in use, however, as the plurality seldom extends beyond two. Polygamy has had some defenders even in modern times, most of whom have grounded their defence on the absence of an express prohibition in the Scriptures. Bernard Ochinus, general of the Catholic Order of Capuchins, though afterwards a Protestant, wrote in the sixteenth century a work in which he advocated it. It was also boldly defended by the Rev. M. Madan, in a treatise called *Thelyphthoro*, but limited the privilege to men.

It is the offspring of licentiousness, and its advocates merely wish to give legal color to licentious habits. Every student of history will find that as soon as a nation became morally depraved, polygamy was practised, and that monogamy was the rule in all countries truly civilized. Monogamy is an element of civilization, and, as a true child, fosters and maintains its parent.

Polygamy has of late years been most shamefully revived, and outrageously practised in face of law, by the Mormons. They claim it as a religious duty, and defend the system by claiming that unmarried women can in the future life reach only the position of angels who occupy in the Mormon theocratic system a very subordinate rank, being simply ministering servants to those more worthy, thus proclaiming that it is a virtual necessity of the male to practise the vilest immorality in order to advance the female to the highest place in Heaven.

Mormonism is a religion founded by Joseph Smith, who was born in Sharon, Vt., December 23, 1805, and killed at Carthage, Ill., June 27, 1844. The Smith family removed from Vermont to Palmyra, N. Y., in 1815, and, according to testimony, the reputation of the family was bad, and that Joseph was the worst of the lot. They were untruthful, intemperate, and commonly suspected of vile practices, which were probably true in some cases, and false in others. These statements are not contradicted even by the Mormons. Joseph claims that in 1823 (Sept. 21), he had a vision, in which the angel Moroni appeared to him and made known that in a hill near Manchester, N. Y., he would find a record written on golden plates. giving an account of the ancient inhabitants of America, and the dealings of God with them, and with the record, two transparent stones in silver bows like spectacles, which were anciently called Urim and Thummim, on looking through which the golden plates would become intelligible. These he claimed were placed in his hand September 22, 1827, by the angel of the Lord. The language was called the reformed Egyptian, not then known on earth, and the contents of the plates formed the "Book of Mormon." The book of Mormon has been proven to have been written by Solomon Spaulding. It will thus be seen that Mormonism was the development of a stupendous fraud, and it is exceedingly singular, that a sect of such numbers as Mormonism is now, or has been, could have been formed, when everything connected with it is fraudulent and perniciously immoral. Polygamy was not introduced among the Mormons until 1843, when Smith ordered it as a doctrine of the church by virtue of a revelation. The Mormons also aim to prove its right by claiming that St. Paul's injunction that a bishop "should be the husband of one wife," implies that other men should have as many as they choose, and that if a bishop should be the husband of one wife at least, the passage does not express a prohibition of his having more if he wishes.

It is a most singular fact that a sect like the Mormons could have been established in a country peopled with such law-abiding people as of the United States, and maintain a system of marriage antagonistic to the law and religion of the land. Neither could they have done so, if they had not possessed two great virtues, temperance and industry. It is to be hoped that the legal process now instituted for its abolition will effectually remove the blot from the national escutcheon.

The " Oneida Communists " are essentially polygamic, although they have no marriage system. They do not marry, and ignore all marriage codes. Cohabitation is under no restrictions between the sexes. Marriage is also not observed among the Shakers.

Monogamy.

This is the conjugal union of a male with one female only. We have
seen that monogamy was co-equal with the dawn of civilization, and that
most probably the majority of the males had but one wife, even among
polygamic nations. Universal polygamy is practically impossible, the
scarcity of females and the poverty of the males forbidding it. The
excess of females is not so great in any country as to allow to each male
more than one wife, except the male portion is depleted by long and
disastrous wars. Monogamy has done more for the elevation of the female than any other custom of civilization. The rich could only afford
to practise polygamy, and should the poor imitate the example, it would
necessarily subject the wives to a state of serfdom. In the economy of
nature it is designed that the male should be the protector of the female,
and that by his exertions the provision of food and raiment should be
secured. In polygamous nations the female has not attained that social
state that she has reached in countries where the male is entitled to but
one female as his wife. Woman's highest sphere is not in the Harem or
the Zenani, but in that dignified state in which she is the sole connubial
companion of but one man. It is debasing to her nature, and subversive of her dignity in the rank of humanity, to make her the equal only
with others in the marital union with one male. She becomes only the
true, noble, and affectionate being when she is conscious of a superiority
to others in the connubial companionship with her accepted one. The
female of birds chirps but for her single mate, and she is pugnaciously
monogamic as well as virtuous, allowing neither male nor female at or
near her home. The spirit of independence she gains by being the
mate of but one male gains for her the victory over the intruders.

The physical and mental welfare of the female is also dependent upon
monogamic marriage. I have demontrated that temperate indulgence
is conducive to the sanitary condition of the sexes, and that absolute
abstinence is opposed to the designs of nature. It is also evident that
the male is not endowed with greater power, vigor or capacity than
the female; therefore, confinement or limitation of the congress to the
companionship of one male with one female, as in monogamic marriage,
gives the healthy balance to the marital union. The polygamic husband must either suffer from the consequences of excessive indulgence,
or his wives from poverty of uxorial gratification; probably both would
be the case. Polyandry is equally as proper as polygamy, yet it never
in the history of man obtained a permanent foothold. The female is
equally capable, if not more so, to capacitate more husbands than one
as the male more than one wife, and the physical deterioration would
not be greater. The system is more logical than polygamy, because
her dependence would be distributed between two or more husbands, in

18

which case she would be better insured against poverty, and her support would be guaranteed by greater probability.

We have now described the history and aspect of the two customs, and will conclude this subject by remarking that a man is morally and physically entitled to but one wife, and that a plurality is a great wrong to the female, and in total opposition to the ordinance of Nature. Wherever polygamy is the custom the female is held in slavish subjection. It only prospers in proportion to the ignorance of the sex. Intelligent and civilized woman will always rebel against such uxorial debasement and servitude.

MARRIAGE CUSTOMS.

It would probably be interesting to many to describe the marriage ceremonies observed by different nations, but to enter into a descriptive detail would occupy too much space. It is sufficient to say that while some wives are wooed and won, others are bought and sold ; while in some countries the husband brings the wife to his home, in others, as in Formosa, the daughter brings her husband to her father's house, and is considered one of the family, while the sons, upon marriage, leave the family forever. In civilized countries the ceremonies are either ministerial or magisterial, and are more or less religious in character, while in others less civilized the gaining of a wife depends upon a foot-race, in which the female has the start of one-third the distance of the course, as is the custom in Lapland. In Caffraria the lover must first fight himself into the affections of his lady-love, and if he defeats all his rivals she becomes his wife without further ceremony. Among the Congo tribes a wife is taken upon trial for a year, and if not suited to the standard of taste of the husband he returns her to her parents. In Persia the wife's status depends upon her fruitfulness : if she be barren she can be put aside. In the same country they have also permanent marriages, and marriages for a certain period only—the latter never allowed to exceed ninety years.

In fact the marriage ceremonies differ nearly in all countries. Tc us some may appear very absurd, and yet our customs may be just as amazing to them. It matters but little how a conjugal union is effected as long as sanctioned by law or custom, and obligates the parties, by common opinion, to observe the duties pertaining to married life.

THE BASIS OF A HAPPY MARRIAGE.

The state of conjugal union should be the happiest in the whole of the existence of either man or woman, and is such in a congenial marriage. Yet in the history of very many marriages contentment or happiness is palpably absent, and an almost insufferable misery is the heritage of both parties. It is therefore important that previous to the marital union the parties should take everything in consideration that foreshadows happiness after marriage, as well as everything calculated to despoil conjugal felicity.

The first requisite of congenial marriage is *love*. Without being cemented by this element the conjugal union is sure to be uncongenial. It is the strongest bond, the firmest cord, uniting two hearts inseparably together. Love for the opposite sex has always been a controlling influence with mankind. It is the most elevating of all the emotions, and the purest and tenderest of all sentiments. It exerts a wonderful power, and by its influence the grandest human actions have been achieved. Of what infinite worth it is to either sex to be compensated with a worthy and satisfying love, and how ennobling to the impulses and actions it is to bestow the sentiment upon one worthy to receive and willing to return.

Love is only given to that which we admire and esteem. The man who admires the shapely hand, the comely figure, the pretty foot, the handsome features, the well-formed waist, etc., will naturally love the woman possessing such attractions. The woman will love the man who favorably approaches her standard of conception as to manly excellence and beauty. Others admire moral purity, vivacity of disposition, superior talents, genius, etc., and hence naturally will love the possessors. In fact this proposition is founded upon a law of mind; love cannot be generated by forces that antagonize our ideals of esteem and admiration. The love that engenders matrimonial happiness must be reciprocal. Reciprocity of love will naturally induce matrimonial alliance. It should not be inspired by a passional nature only, nor should it be platonic entirely, but the two intimately blended together will render the love one of adaptation, and secure conjugal placidity. The love that is created in us by the Venus-like form of the female, or Apollo-like character of the male, is not that love that alone insures happiness, the moral and mental nature must also be congenial. Candidates for marriage should carefully consult themselves, and without ulterior motives ascertain if the love they have for the one to be chosen or accepted is adequate to compensate the yearning of this sentiment. If the one selected has all the characteristics that inspire love, that will be the proper one to marry. Love is the main-spring that regulates the harmony of conjugal life, and without it there is a void in the machinery, productive only of jars, convulsive movement, and a grating and inharmonious action. The soul yearns for love and to love, and unless the desire is compensated, human life is a blank, and becomes a purposeless existence. Love ever stimulates the good and suppresses the bad, if kept in a proper channel, and guided by pure affections.

Another requisite of a happy marriage is *health*. No person has a moral right to engage in wedlock who cannot bring to his partner the offering of good health. It may be apparently a cruelty to the consumptive to deny to him the gratification of his affections or passions, but it would be a greater cruelty to encourage him or her in a step the consequences of which would engender anything but happiness. Is it a pleasing thing to contemplate that you throw upon the bosom of your spouse but the body of an invalid, and one that will be the constant object of care and solicitation on the part of either husband or wife? Is it consoling to your justness that you can but offer a limited period of your life to the one of your choice, and that the inevitable consequences of your affection will at an early period leave but one at the hearthstone? Is it encouraging to know that the offspring of your union will in all probability be equally tainted as yourself, and that on those upon whom you conjointly place your hopes and pride are destined to perhaps an early grave? It is intrinsically wrong for those in whom the taint of consumption, scrofula, syphilis, insanity, etc., to marry, unless they feel convinced that by proper medical treatment they have been or can be thoroughly cured. Intermarriage of the cachectic would be far more judicious than the union of the healthy to the diseased. Vigor and debility are constitutional opposites, and cannot exist together in the physical economy, and the marital union of the physically healthy to the physically unhealthy does also produces nothing but discord in the economy of marital existence.

A very important consideration is the knowledge of what marriage really implies. It obliges the encountering of duties and circumstances which press considerations and plans of life upon the most careless minds. The change in the habit and manner of life, the divided responsibility, the inexorable demands of marital duties to be complied with, and various other matters incident to wedded association should be fully pre-considered, and the relation assumed only after thorough deliberation and satisfactory self-examination. It is the duty of the eligible of either sex to marry, but a marital alliance should be consumated intelligently, not thoughtlessly or ignorantly. "Look before you leap," is an adage that has profound significance in its application to candidates for connubial association. If an error is made in selection, scarcely an other error that may be committed by man or woman is so difficult of rectification, and none will result in greater misery, mental anguish, and destruction of all the joys of life. If, on the contrary, the selection or acceptance is wisely and discreetly made on both sides, the conjugal pair will be blest with all the earthly joys capable of attainment.

It is invariably those who thoughtlessly entered into marital companionship that make mistakes. They shrink before the realities incident to married life on their first presentation, simply because they never dreamed, much less thought, that such exigencies are inevitable to the marital sphere. They are ignorant of the duties incumbent upon either husband or wife, hence they leave them unperformed ; opportunities for advancement are not improved ; neglect becomes the basis of action with only one possible result—marital infelicity. If we trace the cause, we find that in the majority of cases, infelicity is owing to neglect in the performance of marital duty ; and this disregard is ascribable to utter ignorance previous to marriage of the duties inherent to the marital sphere ; consequently, as soon as they confront the wedded pair they are not met with a fixed determination to discharge them satisfactorily as emergencies will admit, but are shirked and postponed, and finally, when the necessity for action becomes absolute, they are inadequately performed ; a fault which is sure to engender dissatisfaction, petulance, or reproach on the part of either husband or wife.

Marriage implies the utter abandonment of the interests and advancement of self to the exclusion of the other marital companion. If circumspect, by noting marital conduct in others, a fair conception of marriage and its consequences will soon be known. Then, the individual must ask himself, or herself : Am I capable and willing to do my duty ? Could I rise superior to all the trials, vexations, and perplexities that present themselves to those in marriage ? Would I never weary of doing the best under all circumstances ? If you can satisfactorily answer these and others, you can enter fitly and nobly into the marital sphere.

Another consideration is *evenness of temper*. In the wooing days every one is a lamb, and only becomes the howling wolf after marriage. Circumstances that ruffle the temper in the presence of the intended are but like the harmless squib, but would become like the explosive torpedo in his or her absence, or in after-marriage. Quarrelling caused by matrimonial differences is the most frequent cause of infelicity, and most of them are caused by an innate irate temper of either the husband or wife. Differences that would be amicably adjusted by the exercise of a little reason and temperance in argument or judgment, are to the irascible the subject for the most vehement and angry logic, and the solution is inevitably discord. It is difficult, I acknowledge, to ascertain previously the mental disposition of persons, when they have occasion to conceal the defect in order to enhance their own interest. It is quite possible that Socrates, when he wooed the *lovely* Xanthippe, deemed her perfection, called her his "darling," his "pet," his "angel," if philosophers ever make use of such endearing expressions. Her conduct evidently deceived him as to her real nature, for the poor old philosopher was egregiously deceived and inexpressibly tortured in his married life by the historically renowned virago and termagant. "Love is blind," but its eyes should not be blindly closed against any such imperfection as naturally tends to destroy wedded bliss. Careful observation in a variety of circumstances will often disclose the real disposition, and the mask is sometimes unwittingly let fall, so that you may gain a cursory glance of the features, which if uncomely, should be enough.

The *tastes* should not be *dissimilar*. Some of them may be unimportant, but others are a fruitful source of disagreement. The social wife will never be contented with the unsocial husband, and the gay husband, though his gayety may not be commendable, will always accuse his wife if she lacks a social disposition to a great extent. The religious wife will never excuse a tendency to irreligion in her husband, and though he may be far from being immoral, she is unhappy if he does not participate in her devotions. The one devoted to children will never be happy with one having a natural repugnance for them. In this way we might multiply facts illustrative of the importance of an investigation into the similarity of taste, previous to marriage. Great love, however, overcomes almost every obstacle.

The parties should be nearly of one age, the husband should be the older. The union of the old husband to the young wife, or the reverse, is seldom a happy one. There is seldom that such a marriage occurs in which the incentive is not the wealth of either of the parties. The young graft on the old tree does not thrive well, the vitality required by the one is not afforded by the other. The magnetism of the old is not suited to the young, and there never can be a concord in their union. It is a law of nature that animals of like age should only mate together. The old male bird does not mate with the young female bird, but mating always occurs between those of the same year's brood. It is only in their domestication that they lose this law of instinct, and it is only through a vice of civilization that marriages between the old and young are contracted, in opposition to the original design of marital union. Such marriages are but seldom the result of a mutual love ; one of the party is sure to be actuated by motives other than the one of conjugal happiness, and the union is usually enforced by the opportune chance of enhancement in respect to wealth or station in society. The progeny of such a union is very seldom endowed with either physical or mental vigor, which is easily accounted for. The physiologist knows that the mental emotions of the mother, during the period of pregnancy, is very apt to affect development of the child *in utero*, either favorably or unfavorably. How, then, can a young mother be actually comfortable, how can her emotions be elevated, how can she have that solicitude which is prompted by love, if she bears but little more than respect for her elderly or old husband ? She has not that intense solicitude or hope that her child shall be all that is excellent ; she has not that incentive of love that prompts her to a revery of desire that her child shall be all that she deems noble and beautiful ; her conjugal relation is not calculated to inspire her highest and purest emotions, and the pride of her husband is not great enough for her to yearn for the day when she can present, with all the joys of maternity, an heir to her lord. It is, therefore, a union not calculated to promote domestic contentment, and there must be in the heart of either a husband or wife an aching void, and a longing for other than a senile embrace.

There are other considerations to be viewed before a union is effected. No one should neglect the moral character, the habits of frugality and industry, etc., etc. A marriage should only be consummated when both of the parties are morally certain that they are necessary to each other's existence ; that life would be a dreary waste without the oasis of the loved one ; that the intended one possesses all you admire and esteem ; and that the journey of life in his or her companionship will be one of serenity and happiness ;—the union will then, by the endeavors of both, be attended by all the joy, contentment, and happiness that it is in the power of mortals to obtain here below.

I cannot more appropriately close this subject than by quoting an abstract from a well-known author, who presents his case in full color, but it exposes the undercurrent that leads to the marriage-tie only too truthfully. He asks: "Who dared first to say that marriages are made in heaven ? We know that there are not only blunders but roguery in the marriage-office. Do not mistakes occur every day, and are not the wrong people coupled ? Had heaven anything to do with the bargain by which young Miss Blushrose was sold to old Mr. Hoarfrost ? Did heaven order young Miss Fripper to throw over poor Tom Spooner, and marry the wealthy Mr. Bung ? You may as well say that horses are sold in heaven, which, as you know, are groomed, are doctored, are chanted on the market, and warranted by dexterous horse-venders as possessing every quality of blood, pace, temper, and age. Against these Mr. Greenhorn has his remedy sometimes ; but against a mother who sells a warranted daughter what remedy is there ? You have been jockeyed by false representations into bidding for the Cecilia, and the animal is yours for life. She shys, kicks, stumbles, has an infernal temper, is a crib-biter, and she is warranted to you by her mother as the most perfect, good-tempered creature, whom the most timid could manage ! You have bought her. She is yours. Heaven bless you ! Take her home, and be miserable for the rest of your days. You have no redress. You have done the deed. Marriages were made in heaven, you know ; and in yours you were as much sold as Moses Primrose was when he bought the gross of green spectacles."

Marriages are usually contracted to gratify various desires, as love, fortune, or position. The results are most truthfully stated by an eminent divine in the following passages :—

"Who marries for love, takes a wife ; who marries for fortune, takes a mistress ; who marries for position, takes a lady. You are loved by your wife, regarded by your mistress, tolerated by your lady. You have a wife for yourself, a mistress for your house and friends, a lady for the world and society. Your wife will agree with you, your mistress will rule you, your lady will manage you. Your wife will take care of your household, your mistress of your house, your lady of your appearances. If you are sick, your wife will nurse you, your mistress will visit you, your lady will inquire after your health. You take a walk with your wife, a ride with your mistress, and go to a party with your lady. Your wife will share your grief, your mistress your money, and your lady your debts. If you die, your wife will weep, your mistress lament, and your lady wear mourning. Which will you have?"

To man there is but one choice that he can rationally make, a marriage of love. My female readers, I hope, will also decide rather to wed a husband than the master or the elegant gentleman.

A little foresight, a little prudence, and a little caution, will prevent in most cases the entrance into a marriage which, by the very nature of the alliance, is certain to be an unhappy and improper one.

MARRIED LIFE.

Two sparrows, votaries of Love,
The Mars and Venus of the grove,
Had been for years such constant mates.
You would have sworn the very Fates
Were impotent to break the bond,
That joined a pair so true and fond;
Together still they sought their food;
Together played in field and wood;
Together built the cosy nest
That served for shelter and for rest;
Together fought the feathered foes
With whom they came to words and blows;
In fine, they lived as lovers ought,
Without a single selfish thought,
Save such as might concern the twain,
Their mutual joy or mutual pain.
At last, one day, they chanced to get
Their feet entangled in a net,
(A vagrant boy had spread the snare
To catch and keep the pretty pair!)
And soon, despite their noisy rage,

They both were prisoned in a cage;
Where—much I grieve the tale to tell—
A sorry scandal now befell;
They scold, recriminate and fight,
Like arrant foes, from morn till night;
Until, at length, the wretched birds
In cruel acts and bitter words
The very furies emulate—
And all their love is turned to hate!

L'ENVOI.

Full many a couple come to strife
And hatred in connubial life,
Whose days of courtship promised fair
As those of this unhappy pair;
But, like the sparrows in my tale,
When trouble comes their tempers fail;
They blame each other for the fate
Which both should strive to mitigate,
With patience helping to endure
The ills that kindness fails to cure!

What an interesting lesson is contained in the above—a lesson that should be well conned and thoroughly learned by every married couple for practical use and guidance.

The physician, in his advices as to the conduct that should be observed by the husband and wife, is more properly confined to physiological aspects, but as the behavior in every respect is so intimately blended, it is not amiss, in a medical work, to state what the conduct should be in general. Unhappiness in wedded life is the result frequently of a couple being joined who should not on any account have been thrown into marital companionship. It is found that they are uncongenial in every respect, and hence the natural and inevitable result is dissension and a mutual regret of marriage. The pharmaceutist knows that if a chemical element is incompatible in a mixture that no amount of shaking, trituration, or commotion that he may produce will make the contrary element act affinitively ; on the contrary, the more violent his endeavors the more the incompatibility is manifested. It is precisely so in the union of the man and woman who are by nature and purposes of life incompatible. Discord is evident at the first contact, which in time increases to ebullitions and explosions of temper, and the more they attempt to reconcile their differences the greater they become ; the affections are destroyed, and each one becomes conscious that they have made the greatest mistake of their lives. Each blames their misfortune to the other when both are to blame, not so much on account of their combativeness, as that is but a law of their nature, but because neither of them had the wisdom to abstain from entering into the marital relation. It is, of course, commendable that both should be desirous of making the best of their union, and that each should display prudence in their conduct, but in the face of all their endeavors the galling fact of incompatibility is ever present, and no amount of the best efforts will make the union a happy one. If children are born to them they will in all probability be of a vicious nature, lacking in all the noble qualities, and who, born with the innate disposition, and reared and schooled in the midst of family discord, will almost inevitably "go to the bad," thus adding materially to the general misery of the parents, both of whom are ready and honest in their belief and averment that the disposition of the children is the heritage from the other. It is unfortunate that such marriages are consummated, for the diversity in all the actions and purposes of life naturally manifested by both is too great to be reconciled by the most earnest exercise of either prudence or forbearance. Such a union has always been, and will always be, an unhappy one, and the best endeavors will scarcely make it tolerable. It may be poetical to say that such a man and woman are *one*, but they are decidedly *two* on all subjects and conditions of married life.

It is not to be supposed, however, that every infelicitous episode in married life is to be ascribed to incompatibility. The turbulence in many cases is owing to decided misconduct on the part of either husband or wife. Many unions would be very happy if but a generous effort would be made to render it so ; but if either one is actuated by a spirit in opposition to mutual confidence, mutual welfare, and mutual enjoyment, it will either create a slavish submission on the part of one, or the assertion of mutual equality. In both cases the result is detri-

18*

mental to conjugal bliss. A tame submission begets disrespect, and the
assertion of the right generates the "family jar." In the social and
commercial intercourse of man and wife, mutual confidence, mutual
endeavor, and mutual benefit should be the objective point. Conceal-
ment of purpose is as wrong as deception in action, and neither should
be for a moment entertained. The wife should be the possessor of the
husband's secrets, and the husband the custodian of the wife's confi-
dences. To be actuated by secrecy either in intent or action is nothing
more than duplicity, and an attitude in entire opposition to the spirit
of wedded life ; but, while the author in every instance advocates an
open and candid intercourse between the husband and wife, he can
only hurl anathemas upon the one who betrays the confidence. To be
worthy of confidence, and to be entrusted with secrets, demands the
fidelity that will not betray the one or divulge the other. Deception on
the part of either husband or wife will, in spite of all attempts at con-
cealment, often be detected, causing justly indignation and loss of respect. It is an evidence that the one to whom everything should be
confided is deemed unworthy of trust, and it puts at an end that harmony and confidence that should exist.

Married couples should most carefully husband their affections for
each other. It is a most deplorable fact, that the love between many
too soon loses its fervor. This loss is not due to familiarity, nor is it a
natural result of daily association ; but decidedly the effect of a reprehensible disregard of a mutual endeavor to maintain it. We love only that
which is lovely ; and the person who makes himself lovely will be loved.
It is more frequently the case that the wife loses her husband's affections
than the reverse. This is not so much the result of the inferior affectionate nature of man as it is of neglect and imprudence on the part of woman.
Women, if they would rule men's hearts, must deserve and unwittingly
exact the approval and admiration of their minds. Her variability of temper is most unfortunate. It goes up like a rocket and comes down like an
aërolite ; a miracle of smiles or weeping Niobe, a driving tempest or a flash-
ing sunbeam. A never-varying, bland, lullaby-sort of temperament is
most deplorable ; sparkle, buoyancy, and even an irrepressible dash of fun,
now and then, are most healthful and appetizing ; but mere feminine diplo-
macy should forbid the not unfrequent dovetailing of winsome caresses
and childish poutings on the part of the wife, and so should the whimsical
interplay of foolish indulgence and churlish neglect on the part of the husband be abandoned. Principle, not caprice, should be the energizing and
controlling motive. The most charming views of wedded life are to be
taken from the higher mounts of vision—those of settled design and
steady purpose. There must, of course, be mutual concessions and mutual agreements to disagree. There is a way to win by commanding,
and a way to command by winning. By the wise interblending of self-

centred strength, and a prodigal wifely affection, she may achieve mar-
vels of wifely management. The husband may unconsciously lead ; but
never essay to drive. At the same time, we are frank enough to con-
fess that there are too many women who need the flaming sword of an
archangel to awe and repress them. There is no such thing as conquer-
ing them by love ; as well prate of love to a blackbird. But if kindness
fails, severity will fail all the more surely. Flies still continue to take
more kindly to molasses than to vinegar. If they but knew how a
cheerful temper, joined with innocence, will make their beauty more
attractive, knowledge more delightful, and wit more good-natured,
they surely would endeavor to cultivate and cherish it. It is an un-
questioned fact that too many wives neglect the most important elements of wifely conduct.

To her is entrusted the care and management of the home—if it is
agreeable, it is her work, if it is attractive, it is to her credit alone that
it should be ascribed. If the home is not a cheery place, it is because
she does not render it so. It is not requisite that elegance and luxury
—that only wealth can procure—should characterize it; cleanliness,
order, and, above all, her bright, sunny smiles, and cheerful company,
adorn it more than the richest household furniture. The atmosphere of
the home must not be darkened by the clouds of discontent, perplexity or
anger, but lit up by the effulgence of social conviviality, good-nature,
and buoyancy of spirit. The husband coming from his daily task must,
in return for the bright smiles of the wife and children that welcome
him home, throw aside all cares of business, and devote himself to their
enjoyment. It will put a new life in him as well as in his wife and
children. If exhausted and fatigued, or if his mental energies have
been overtaxed, he must not thrust the fact too forcibly upon his
family, but on the contrary bring freshness and buoyancy of spirit into
the family circle. He must not recuperate his energies at the expense
of the vitality of his wife and little ones. The wife should also as early
as possible dispense with household duties, and, until the retiring hour,
be ever ready to engage in that social communion, which is so healthful,
and so conducive to happiness of married life. But how frequently is
it the case that the weary husband, who would gladly engage in that
relaxation afforded by domestic conference in play, reading, etc., is
only beguiled by the din of pots and kettles, the clatter of dishes, the
music of a wash-tub, etc., in the kitchen, which often is incessant, until
the poor husband, desirous of social comforts, but weary of waiting for
them, goes to bed with nothing to lull him to sleep but the confused
noises that come from the kitchen, made by his busy and industrious,
but indiscreet spouse. We would not deprecate industry on the part of
the wife. We well know that many a wife, whose household duties and
personal attention to the children absorb most of her time, can find but

little opportunity to engage in recreation or social enjoyment, but while we admire thrift, coupled with industrious habits, we cannot but deplore the state which robs from her the best energies, instead of applying some, at least, upon the effort to render the atmosphere of the home, not one of incessant labor only, but also one that is brightened and rendered cheerful by the relaxation afforded by an occasional leisure hour, in which the man, wife, and children are brought in contact, and stimulated and refreshed by social concourse. As well might the husband file his saws, grind his axes, and chop his wood at the same time, as the wife to be continuously drawn from. his presence by the labor of the home. It is, we know, not a pleasing contrast, to compare a thrifty and industrious wife with one who is indolent and careless, but we only argue for a limit, as we know that matrimonial happiness, health, and noble qualities of children are dependent in a great measure upon enlivened social intercourse in the family. We would have no wife merit the exclamation of " *How shiftless!* " from an Aunt Priscilla, but they must not be so busy either, that her husband has in her no social companion. Such wives cannot much blame their husbands if they seek social pastime in the club, in the inn, or even in his neighbor's house, where Mrs. Sparkle makes everything so pleasant. It is the duty of the husband, whenever possible, to give his leisure hours to the companionship of his wife and children, but it is also a duty that the wife so arranges everything that they can not only be passed tolerably but agreeably. It should be the effort of both husband and wife to make the home the dearest place on earth to them, and when that is accomplished, connubial happiness is certainly achieved. It is often that the best-meant efforts are fruitless, simply because they are driven in the wrong direction, and the disappointment occurring in consequence of misapplied energy is full hard to bear ; but if the married man or woman would study the wants and desires of their consorts a little more, and make earnest effort to supply them, the apple of discord would not be eaten in so many instances.

I cannot two strongly impress the importance of fidelity. Could I have but one word of advice to give to the conjugal pair, I would say :—"*Be true to each other.*" Disloyalty in the marriage bond is the cause of infinite trouble, misery, and ruin. It is the rock upon whose ugly and jagged contour lie the wrecks of numberless matrimonial vessels. Fidelity is the rudder that guides the bark safely through the course, let adversity and all else assail her, as long as not without her rudder, she will out-ride the storms, and glide triumphantly and peacefully along in smooth water. Disloyalty pitches her at once into the breakers, where she will pitch and toss, heave and thump, and should she even escape, it is only at the expense of important appanages, and most frequently the best directed efforts will not save her from utter ruin.

It is not only the duty of physicians, but of every one who has the welfare of society at heart, to put their voices against the doctrine of "free love," which has of late been promulgated and defended by certain persons who wish to make it a matter of creed or principle of society. It is to the shame of the sex that the majority of its adherents are women, in whom virtue is supposed to have its staunchest defenders and supporters. It is not ostensibly advanced in advocacy of unrestraint in cohabitation, but if thoroughly analyzed, its objective principle amounts to the same. It is a scortatory love at best, and its tendency is to give still greater laxity to the morals of society. It is veiled under the sophistical dogma that every woman, if she desires to become a mother, should be privileged to select her own male to be the father, and that every man should be licensed to choose the woman he desires to be the mother of his progeny. This, they advocate, would insure higher development of the race, and that mankind would soon be superior in intellectual, moral, and physical qualifications. The fact is undeniable that a superior offspring would be the result, if the most eligible individuals would copulatively unite, but it could never be accomplished by licensed libertinism. It can only be gained by judicious marriage, and in no other way. If the doctrine of unrestraint they promulgate is best adapted to promote higher development of offspring, it would naturally be exemplified in the issue of those who "*loved not wisely, but too well*," or in those of the lowest grades of society or savage races, where chastity is unknown as a virtue. All the principles of free love characterize such an intercourse; but it has yet to be ascertained whether such progeny are in any respect superior; on the contrary, it is quite probable that they are in many respects inferior. This may be, however, accounted for by the mental emotions of the mother, which are naturally caused by grief, fear, shame, etc. If, even, such unfavorable mental emotions could be removed by sanction from society for such issue, the case would not be modified to a more favorable extent than is now possible by legitimization of offspring by marriage. They also prate of "affinities" and spiritual attraction; but let the candid and virtuous mind investigate the full import of these cohesions, he will find that the spirit of attraction is the cohesive power of gratification of the animal passions. The hideous form of lechery is veiled with but the thinnest gauze; and disguise it as they will, they cannot hide the fact that it is lewdness, and not virtue, which they attempt to honor. The doctrine, if philosophically reviewed, presents no advantages over marriage, but is one pregnant with defects and immoralities, and if carried into effect would unmistakably prove itself to be the death-blow to morality and civilization. The barrier to promiscuity is to be made even more impregnable, and the sacred precinct of the prerogative legitimatized by marriage is not to be over-stepped by the husband or suffered to be invaded by the wife. Lechery has never been, nor can never become a standard principle of moral philosophy, and " free love " is but its synonym.

Is it a consoling picture to those with whom moral rectitude is a cardinal principle to see disloyalty to the marriage-tie openly and shamelessly displayed? Is it ennobling to man's moral nature to cut loose the shackles put upon him by a well-organized society with regard to his conduct in amorous matters? Can it be justified by the most liberal views of right and wrong? Unalterably, no ; the man who comes to the abode of his wife, with his lips tainted by contact with others, and yet excited by an unlawful orgasm, commits the greatest offence against his wife, against nature, and against high heaven. The wife who receives the embraces of an unsuspecting husband, while at the same time she is guilty of illicit dealings with others, is worse than the lowest prostitute, and is entitled to no sympathy or condonement. It is only by the most scrupulous adherence to the loyalty that should be observed by man and wife, that marital happiness is to be gained or maintained ; infringement is the element of its decay and destruction.

Jealousy is one of the most common visitors at the hearth of a family, and is a great destroyer of its peace. Entertained to a moderate degree it is quite natural, but when it becomes a morbid feeling, it is worthy of severe denunciation. The exhibition of slight jealousy is an unerring manifestation of love, and should be accepted as such by either man or wife. We are jealous of what we love, and unconcerned only about that which we do not appreciate, therefore a certain degree of jealousy entertained by the husband or wife in respect to each other should be elevating to their pride, respectively, and not condemned as a sickly sentimentality. It is only when it becomes a ruling passion that it exerts mischief and discord. When it is so morbid that it becomes a matter of dislike and reproach for the husband to bestow but the ordinary civilities of social intercourse to the opposite sex, or for the wife to receive them, it amounts to but little more than insanity. If the wife is so jealous as to impugn all the motives of the husband, that he dare not even look askance at any other woman, that to speak with other women subject him to one of those infinitely pleasant curtain-lectures, and his personal liberty denied to him with regard to social intercourse, it is then that it becomes disruptive to marital felicity ; for the husband, if erring though he be, will surely chafe under the injustice which she will be sure to commit. On the other hand, the jealous husband is just as extravagant in his folly, and instead of guarding his wife's love, takes the best means of repelling it. Confidence, not suspicion, should be the controlling motive, and its mutual entertainment should not be disregarded until the most indubitable proofs are presented to guarantee a disbelief of the partner's honor. Then, if you have bombshells, set them off; but even then, I think, it would comport more with reason and dignity, if the error could be calmly adjudicated, and if that is impossible, a quiet and dignified separation is unquestionably the best course. Reproach, recrimination, and parade of the cause of disruption before the public are by no means a philosophic action, or part of an honorable conduct. It is so with all matrimonial differences, they should not be made public property, for they will surely become disgusting scandal before the scandal-loving people, to be found in every community, are done with them. It will receive such additions, and will be so manipulated and distorted, that, which at its fountain-head was but a peccadillo, will at its terminus be magnified into the greatest crime. What was at first but a slight immorality, is sure to become at the end the grossest violation of decency. If Mr. John Smith in a playful moment is found to kiss Mrs. Sarah Jones, the critics of society will wink and blink, they will hem and haw, look wise, toss their heads superciliously, and before they have ceased their comments, there will be no doubt in their minds but that Mr. Smith and Mrs. Jones were found in *flagrante delicto*. Finally, when the scandal has assumed its worst aspect, some order-loving Christian (!) will with considerable embellishment acquaint Mrs. Smith of her husband's *crime*, and Mr. Jones of his wife's *sins*, and then comes the sequel. The fact would scarcely produce a ruffle, at best but a gentle breeze, but the monster created by scandal produces the commotion of a tornado. Then these vampires who feed upon the peace and reputation of society are satisfied, but they at all times go round like " roaring lions seeking whom they may devour." It is to these scandal-mongers that matrimonial infelicity is often due, from the fact that a husband or a wife may be guided by their opinion rather than to rely implicitly upon each other's honor. If respect is shown to scandal connubial peace is at a discount. The only way to circumvent it, is to isolate adjustment of differences to the family circle, and not allow it to be the property of the unconcerned. The advice of disinterested and honorable people may at times be very serviceable, and not to be disregarded, but to array any or every matrimonial variance before the public for their comments is reprehensibly imprudent and foolish..

It is, however, not to be understood that selfishness should extend to social intercourse with the neighbors, for next to an affectionate family an agreeable neighborhood and good society become objects of desire, because calculated to create happiness. As far as friendship is not abused it should be freely given to the neighbors, and it should be the endeavor of every one to make the relations of a neighborhood of a most friendly and accommodating character. How consoling it is to the bride, who leaves the bosom of her own family and accompanies her husband to a locality where all are strangers, to find in her new home

neighbors who manifest a friendly spirit, and are willing to extend cordial greetings to the stranger. She is at once set at ease. The duty that
families owe to society is only second in importance to the duty that
husband and wife owe to each other, and domestic happiness is not
complete unless its social surroundings are congenial and agreeable.
An ascetic married life is abusive of the order of nature.

The conjugal pair should in reality be *helpmates*. They should (to
use a homely phrase) pull in one direction, and, if the direction is proper
and right, pull together. The combination of similar forces has a two-
fold effect, but forces opposed to each other weakens one and annuls
the other, or brings them both to a *quietus*. This simple law of physics
is peculiarly applicable to the behavior of the married pair. A harmonious progress requires a combination of purpose and exertion. If
the husband is devoted to literature or science, the wife should manifest interest in the same, but if her taste is not for either, she should
by no means show displeasure at her husband's devotion to them. It is
her duty, in case of improvidence on his part in consequence of his
studies, to ask him to improve his negligence, but never in a tone of
anger or reproach. The husband should, in like manner, never frown
upon any of his wife's delights. If she is devoted to flowers, to music,
to painting, etc., it should be he that should stimulate by approval. In
case the husband is desirous to accumulate a fortune, and exerts himself to that effect, the wife should not dispirit him, or render his efforts
abortive by extravagance. If he is not successful, or fails in business,
she should be his comforter and stimulate him to further exertion ; and
in case the manner of living will in consequence be rendered less luxurious, she should exhibit such a contentment and willingness as to rob
the misfortune of half its bitterness. The noble wife is one who does
not sink under the crucial test of her husband's misfortunes, but rises
to a higher mount of greatness and action by her cheerful resignation
to the loss, and encouragement to her husband's drooping spirits. The
husband should ever be ready with his approving smiles to cheer his
wife's labors, even if to him it appears but a trivial affair. Woman
only thrives under the approbation of man, and if that is withheld,
especially from the one whom she values most, she soon becomes purposeless and fretful. How many a good wife's heart has been wounded
by her husband's indifference with regard to matters which she in her
simplicity of heart hoped would delight her companion ? It may be
but a trifle, but so exceedingly tender is the plant of connubial love,
and so susceptible of being lacerated, that "trifles light as air" often
impede its growth and embitter its fruit. It is the "*little* foxes that
spoil the vines." A single tart remark or unkind tone of voice will
penetrate the inner recesses of the heart of the wife who loves, and
render her most wretched. *Oneness* should be particularly exhibited in

purpose and design, the respective action should be one of accord, and the faculties of each other should be mutually gratified. It is only by such a concert that love is perpetuated and wedlock made an Elysium.

If the husband or wife have vices, the conduct to be pursued is peculiarly delicate. If it is judicious, the vice may be corrected; if otherwise, the habit may become intensified. If the husband is intemperate, the wife should address his highest sentiments, and not attempt to bring about repentance and reform by angry reproach, unkind remarks, or undignified aspersions. No one has a keener sense of his depravity than the drunkard, and he is by no means dead to the finer sensibilities, hence any inhumane treatment, or reproof insulting to inherent dignity, is not calculated to achieve reformation. He is to be approached as a man, his nobility is to be addressed, and his better feelings excited. He is to be shown that he is none the less loved for his noble qualities, that aside from his folly he is still the being who possesses his wife's affections, and that only his vice and not he himself is abhorred. It is only by such a procedure that vices, or a disposition to vice, can be cured. It is the mild and gentle force that works reform, revolutions scarcely ever do.

We have now in many aspects considered the prudent course for the conjugal pair to pursue in search of wedded bliss. We have confined ourselves merely to their social relation, there yet remains for us to discuss a not less important subject, namely, that of connubial commerce. From what we have already written the inference is plain, that we advocate a dignified conduct, benignity of temper, subjection of anger, co-operation of purpose, etc., etc., and though there may be, nay, are, many other rocks upon which the matrimonial bark will impinge, the reflective mind will be guided in his behavior in every possible contingency by what we have more lengthily dwelt upon. The indices to marital happiness are reason, prudence, justice, and equality, and they who shape their course by them must attain the object. It shall now be our purpose to consider a subject that is not less important, and much less understood. In its discussion we will confine ourselves to particulars which married people mostly inquire after, and in which they need the most enlightenment.

The discussion of this delicate relation between the married pair is necessary, inasmuch as the unprofessional have access to scarcely any work of standard value and excellence from which they may gather the knowledge so indispensable, unless they are fortunate enough to have the privilege of reading the works of an extensive medical library. Even if this opportunity is afforded, the truth is not clearly presented to them, as such works are intended usually for the professional reader. I, therefore, am confident that I discharge an important duty, especially as I write particularly for the instruction of the popular mind, in presenting to my many readers the philosophy of that relation legitimatized by marriage. In consideration of the subject, I shall employ plain but decorous language, and attempt to present the facts so that they may be intelligible to all, and yet not wound any of the finer sensibilities of my readers. I have previously stated my aim to be merely to afford instruction to the masses relative to such medical subjects as have never been capably popularized, but have been, and are yet a theme on which incompetent charlatans have so ignorantly dwelt upon, and disseminated so much offensive literature. The medical profession is to blame for this. If they had not neglected to teach the popular mind the physiology of cohabitation, empirics would have found no market for their offensive and pernicious works, excepting, perhaps, among the morally depraved.

The married, which I positively know from the many opportunities afforded me in my professional career, are extremely ignorant of the philosophy and physiology appertaining to the special connubial relation, and absolutely know nothing of the hygienic limit or period. I know also that every married man and woman is extremely anxious to possess proper knowledge. As the access to works of scientific authority is extremely limited, they are led to accept the teachings of ignorant empirics, and thus unwittingly do much that is wrong and hurtful. The diffidence characterizing the marital pair to interrogate the family physician as to the proper course to pursue, also tends to keep them in ignorance. It is only when the abuse of the marital privilege becomes painfully apparent that the physician feels warranted to interpose his cautions, and counsel reform and moderation. This, however, occurs only in exceptional instances, the great majority are uninformed and unadvised, controlled only by self-interpretation of the right or wrong of their conduct, or by such information as is commonly possessed by the heads of families, which is often traditional, and usually faulty in its conclusions.

To supply, then, in a medical work for general circulation, the proper instruction as regards the important marital relation alluded to, needs no further justification, but every person actuated by a catholic spirit will, I am sure, deem the discussion eminently appropriate. The underlying purpose of wedded association is of greater importance than half who assume the relation are aware of. Marriage implies much more than a mere association of the sexes—it is rather an institution devised by society to regulate cohabitation and the propogation of species in the best manner. This is the only legitimate purpose of marriage, as aside from this relation between the sexes, every other one could be secured and maintained without matrimonial ties or obligations. Any system of rules or regulations subserving the purpose of controlling this particular marital relation so as to accord with the best known laws of physiology and hygiene, and best adapted for the requirements of propogation of the species, so that offspring will not be recklessly brought into the world, but calculated to secure to it the highest possible endowment of all the nobler human qualities, is decidedly the best marriage code. As an institution, marriage should be governed more by physiological laws than by statute regulations, and the time may yet come when wilful disregard of physiological laws applicable to the matrimonial association of the sexes will be regarded as reprehensible or criminal as the violation of the statute laws governing the institution. It is then quite important that those in marriage as well as those who contemplate matrimonial alliance, should possess adequate knowledge of the incumbent duties, contemplate the dignity and importance of wedlock, endeavor to promote the grand interests and welfare which the marital pair have at stake, avoid animalization and debasement of the connubial repast, endeavor to fitly endow their offspring, and so conduct themselves throughout the whole course of wedded association, that they may be rewarded with all the manifold blessings that should be gained by the grandest and closest association of human interests, purposes, and hearts.

It should never be forgotten by the married that our passions can be over-indulged precisely the same as our appetites. Hygiene requires that our appetites for food or drink should only be appeased to such an extent as will not create a loathing for that which was eaten or drunk, upon quitting the repast. If indulgence is carried to such an extent it amounts to intemperance and will be followed by the usual consequences of violation of hygienic law. It is precisely so with the marital repast: if the relation is assumed too frequently the temperate limit will be over-reached and hurtful consequences ensue. Excess is not only deleterious because destructive of the natural tone of the excitement, generative of nervous disorder, and other hurtful consequences ; it is extremely apt to engender indifference after a certain period on the part of either or both of the conjugal pair. By indifference I mean to express that feeling of insatiety after indulgence, that want of mutual accord, or sense of unsatisfactory awakening of the emotions, which is sure to follow excesses. The desires are present but cannot be satisfactorily appeased, precisely as an appetite for a certain article or kind of food remains unsatiated if not within reach to be partaken of. This condition, directly a sequal to immoderation, is one of the greatest incentives to adultery. I am well satisfied that this unpardonable violation of matrimonial trust and fidelity is, in the majority of instances, due to neglect of observing temperance in the early years of marriage. The results of coitive intemperance should thus be strongly impressed upon the minds of every one married or contemplating marriage, as by moderation they will surely attain a higher altitude of connubial enjoyment,

besides avoiding the violation of the highest and purest of all human
trusts which if committed, is irreparably destructive of the integrity of
matrimonial alliance.

The married pair should carefully guard against all excesses. Excess
of connubial commerce is a severe tax to the nervous system, and very
detrimental to health. The class of diseases met with by the physician,
of which the remote cause is immoderation, is scarcely second to none
in frequency. Besides, the orgasm is less profound if the banquet is
too freely partaken of. The physician is frequently asked the question
how often intercourse may be indulged in without injury. To this no
answer can be given with numerical preciseness; but both sexes possess an unerring monitor, whose voice they should promptly heed.
Whenever a sense of exhaustion is felt, after copulation, the violation
of a physiological law is made manifest. No coitive act should be completed when it requires fatiguing efforts to accomplish it. It is sure to
be followed by exhaustion, and the orgasm is neither elevating or satisfactory, and apt to generate an inharmony quite antagonistic to the de
signs of nature.

Frequency of indulgence does not only deteriorate the moral tone of
the coitive act, but it often provides the germinal agencies of serious
diseases. The remote cause of insanity and consumption is not infre-
quently intemperance in marital union. The children who are the products of the earlier periods of married life, at which time coitive intemperance is most frequently indulged, are more mentally imbecile,
and more pallid in hue and attenuated in form than those born at a later
period. This is in consequence, that, sooner or later, the parents are
forced to abstain from excess by the ensuing ruination of health, allowing nature to gather up the shattered powers and assert anew the control of the organism. In the early years of marriage excesses should
therefore, by no means transpire.

During the period of the catamenial presence, strict continence must
be observed by the conjugal pair. I should not give this caution were
I not aware that in many instances the marital prerogative is thus griev-
ously abused. Propriety and privilege in this respect are particularly at
variance, and duty demands observance of propriety.

During the period of pregnancy the husband's conduct should be characterized by kindness, forbearance, and encouragement. While the
germ of an immortal being is in her loins, that husband is no more than
a brute, who would in any way neglect her wishes, or refuse to join
with her in the solicitude for its welfare. The expectant mother must
also control every appetite or mental passion that might injure the
precious trust committed to her. The best and noblest thoughts should
occupy her mind, and the purest sentiments prevail in her heart, while
the babe is hid beneath it, so that her shortcomings and caprices may

not be communicated to the product of her conception. She should be, and her husband should assist her to be, patient under any weariness or sorrow belonging to her condition. She should strengthen her heart against the hour of her labor with the thoughts of joy she shall feel, when her child shall see the light, and the process of maternity fulfilled. It is she who bore and in agony gave birth to the link that unites the parents all the more closely together, and that strengthens the hymeneal compact. To her the husband owes devotion, allegiance, and comforting encouragement. He must make her feel that the joys of maternity are not to be centered entirely in the little helpless babe nestling in her arms, but also her heart is to be rejoiced in witnessing the paternal pride of the product of connubial union—the jewel of their conjoint love. The component parts of the family are then complete, the husband, the wife, and the child, nothing is wanting but the coupling of energy and intent, to procure the highest share of human bliss to be obtained on this side of the grave.

The author is prompted, but space will not allow, to give at length his views upon the management of children. On this point husband and wife frequently disagree, and the result of the disagreement is manifested in the child. It is more usually the case that the father is sterner and firmer than the mother, in whose heart the tender elements of humanity prevail. It is, however, not necessary to be stern in the management of children, but an unflinching firmness is at all times essential, and absolutely necessary in both parents to gain a healthy control over their children. Firmness must, however, be exhibited in the same direction, and that direction the right one.

There is a tendency, we think, at the present day to put children too forward, not so much for the sake of showing off their extraordinary merits to an admiring world, as from the better motive of early accustoming them to the conversation of grown people and the usages of society, and of inspiring them with confidence, ease, and self-possession. No doubt these results are very valuable, but the mistake which many people make is in forgetting that children are something like dogs, which require to be very well trained before they can safely be recommended to the familiarity of strangers. And it is to be remembered that the moment children cease to respect any of the grown-up people with whom they associate, not only is the whole benefit of the intercourse lost at once, but real injury is inflicted on the moral tone of the child. For this reason children should be brought as little as possible into the society of men and women who cannot command their respect; while those who can, the influence should be hedged round by all the numerous impalpable barriers which judicious parents know perfectly well how to interpose between children and the most popular and careless of their adult play-fellows. The confidence which well-bred chil-

dren at once repose in an eligible stranger, without being rude or troublesome, is charming to everybody, who has any natural taste for their
society. It is not pleasant, on the other hand, to see children who are
shy, timid, and sheepishly speechless in the presence of strangers, but a
confidence and unobtrusive ease of manners can be inspired without
thrusting them constantly into the society of elders.

Closely allied with the mistaken license allowed to children in matters
like the above, is the disposition to laugh at, and thereby to encourage,
all traits of singularity, oddness or affectation, which children may exhibit, as marks of genius which ought not to be repressed. Of all the
dangerous errors into which parents can fall, this, in our opinion, is the
worst. For nothing so soon hardens into second nature as juvenile
eccentricity; and few things are more injurious to success in life than
marked oddities of manner and gesture when they reach the point of
grotesqueness. The fond parents dote upon the eccentric child as an
original, but the author in this respect agrees perfectly with Mr. Peter
Magnus ; he does not see the necessity of originals. And what is more,
so many " originals " are only sham ones after all. That is to say, their
singularity is merely a bad habit which they can't shake off, and is only
very partially innate. When parents see their child doing anything
unlike other children, anything queer, surprising, or uncouth, however
comic or however clever it may seem, they should never laugh at or
applaud it. Children naturally self-willed, and with real natural peculiarities, can soon be broken of such tricks, if treated with absolute
indifference. But soon let the idea find its way into their brains that
such sallies, naughty though they be, are regarded as marks of genius,
and the mischief is done. It is not necessary that parents should engage
harsh reproof or exhibit anger to correct such pertness or disposition to
oddity, but if approbation is withheld, and probably displeasure shows,
the mischief will soon be corrected. Children, like their elders, delight
in approbation, and if they can only secure it by doing what is right
and proper, the inclination to do that which is wrong or displeasing, is
robbed of its greatest incentive.

To come back to the point from which we started—the management,
namely, of young children—there is one thing to be laid down : let
there be no divided rule in a house. Do not let children see that
the father means one thing and the mother another in their bringing
up. They see the difference in a moment, and when they do, farewell
to all wholesome parental influence. The starting-point of ruined manhood or womanhood, in many cases, is just this diversity of parental
control. That mother urges her child towards destruction who
offers condolence to it, after reproof or correction by the father, no
matter how harsh or cruel it may have been. Such matters must be
corrected by conference, at which the children are not present. She is

not to show any displeasure at the exercise of authority by the father in the presence of the child ; if she does, the child's self-will is gratified by a mother's alliance, and a certain importance is given to the improper conduct of the child, which, in accordance with the human liability to err, is hard to resist. The parents in this respect must be the allies, not the children with the father and mother.

Husbands and mothers may talk too freely before their children, forgetful of their rising intelligence. And, indeed, nothing is more common than to get a wink from the head of the house, implying that you are to be on your guard before Johnny or Tommy, Kitty or Lucy, who are listening open-mouthed to your witty narrative, while they themselves in the next moment will offend against their own precautions in the most barefaced manner by plunging headlong into your domestic controversy, in which, to speak metaphorically, knives are freely used on both sides. Again, parents should be extremely careful in commenting upon the conduct of their neighbors in the society of their children, or that self-same Tom will at the first opportunity acquaint neighbor Jones that, in the opinion of his father, " he is a confounded old fool ; " or the same little Kitty will tell Mrs. Robinson that her mother says she is a " lazy, good-for-nothing woman." Trouncing Tommy or Kitty for such imprudence is hardly fair, when the fault lies at the door of the parents. At best, it gives children but a poor example, and instills within them a disrespect of the neighbors, which, probably, they do not deserve, and which may in later years possibly stand in the way of individual advancement. Parents, in rearing their children, have a greater trust than is commonly supposed, and they owe a double duty—one to the child, and the other to society in general. If the child is inclined to vice, the fault lies in many cases with the parents, and the right to thrust upon society either a son or daughter who will constitute but a useless or vicious member thereof, is not properly one of the privileges of humanity. No man has the right to set at large a lot of ferocious animals, who, in the exercise of their ferocity, may do harm to his fellow-men ; neither has that parent a moral right to send adrift in the world sons and daughters, who, in the exercise of the vicious culture they have received, prove annoying and harmful to their fellow-beings. There is no deeper stratum of thought in moral economy than this, and none that receives less attention.

It is to mothers that society and mankind are indebted for its morality and uprightness. By her efforts the only real work of reformation can be achieved. The training of children is mainly intrusted to her hands ; if her duty is properly performed, the moral tone of society is to be placed to her credit ; if carelessly and imprudently attended to, she is the one that is mainly accountable for its vices. It may seem a cruelty to add to the travails of maternity and to her household duties the further responsibility of rearing the moral structure of society ; but who is to assume it, if she be not the proper person ?   The child is, to a certain age, mainly in her presence alone, and this association cannot be shirked or changed ; for it is true to a natural law that the mother is to be the closest companion of her children.   It is during this period of companionship that the foundation of the moral superstructure is to be laid, and the mother must be the artisan.   She may be aided by her husband and others ; but the chief duty to form and direct is her own, and the structure she rears, whether good or bad, is her work.

Her duty to her offspring commences at the moment of conception. While the product is yet hidden within the confines of her womb she must have its future welfare at heart, and lend her thoughts only upon that which is good and noble.   She should in her mind select the career of the child, and that such a one that is characterized by all the noble qualities, and freedom from vices.   Who can gainsay the fact, that when the babe is assuming its physical character, while yet in the mysterious depth of the gravid womb, that the mother is not enabled by the purity of her thoughts and exalted character of her emotions to give it also the endowment of its moral character ?   Who will deny that the transmission of hereditary qualities give the original bias, which subsequent to birth is hard to overcome ?   The law of transmitting talent and virtue from mother to child is based on physiological principles, as demonstrable as material matter.   I would then say to every expectant mother : Let your thoughts be good, your emotions pure, your imaginations morally exalted ; be brave, be strong, be good, and centre all and only the purest feelings upon that helpless atom of humanity reposing in your womb, so that at the hour of your labor you are fortified against its agony by the consciousness that the babe you usher into the world is endowed with qualities, which, by subsequent development and culture, will enable it, when of proper years, to take its place among the good and noble of this earth.

Subsequent to birth the mother must continue her efforts.   She must impose barriers against everything that has an unwholesome influence on the moral tone of her child.   She must not intrust the training of her precious darlings to nurses or governesses.   A mother who reposes the development of character of her children to salaried persons is prostituting the high estate of maternity, and sins against Nature and her God.   It is she who must take the hand of the child while yet in its innocence, and lead it in the path of virtue and truth ; her hand must remove all the lures and seductive temptations that beset its path, and she alone must assume the cultivation of its moral nature.

Men may build prisons, asylums, reformatories, create midnight missions, etc., but reformation by these means is uncertain, expensive, and at best very ineffectual.   It is the hardened criminal they deal with—

one in whom vice has become the second nature. No real reformation is accomplished by any such means, none will ever ensue; and as long as mothers are not alive to the importance of properly training the pliant child, vice will increase and baffle every other mode of reformation. One wiser than myself has said—"Train up a child in a way he should go, and when he is old he will not depart from it." The truth of this is self-evident, and is supported by another, whose figurative language is equally truthful—

"As the twig is bent the tree 's inclined."

It is, therefore, the mother who must nourish the truth in her arms, so that when it leaves them it will walk strongly forth alone, blessing and blest of all men.

ADVICE TO THE CHILDLESS.

The most impressive words in the whole range of language are Father and Mother. Their full significance is only realized and understood when the prattling babe stretches out its tiny arms and first lispingly pronounces the tender words. The heart must, indeed, be dead to all emotion, which at that moment does not pulsate with pride and exalted love. The first words taught to it, and the first words learned, are those tender names, and the proudest moment of the whole of parentage is when the lesson is learned by, and let fall from, the lips of the smiling babe. The soul is elevated above material things, the tenderest chords of love are vibrated. the joys of the world but this one are forgotten, and the whole heart embraces but the innocent babe that sprung from their loins. The entity of the family is incomplete without children, and the action of its machinery is unharmonious without those little wheels. The integrity is faulty in the absence of offspring; it is like the pillar of which the capital and pedestal exist, but the shaft is wanting to give it dignity. The childless family is not a pleasant one to contemplate; the husband and wife grow old, but there is no young life to inspirit them, or to give cheer to their existence. Childless longevity is at best but a dismal life—there is always an aching void—a palpable evidence of a lacking integer. Barrenness is a condition from which every woman instinctively recoils. The desire for children may or may not be entertained, yet to know that she is incapable of motherhood is to know that she is lacking in the most important element of womanhood. It is a physical condition abhorrent to every female, because she feels that she is beneath the dignity that distinctively characterizes her sex. Motherhood is the ideal state of womanhood, and the yearning for maternity is one born of nature. The woman in whose bosom such a desire makes no response is unworthy of her sex, and she deserves none of the elevated joys and honor which woman is sent here

19

to achieve, and she will reap none. It is the highest honor her sex can reach, as productiveness entitles her to the proud position of one of the prime factors in the propagation of species.

None but physicians know how great the desire for children is in those whose married life has been passed for some time without issue. To them the secret yearnings of their hearts is intrusted, and to their confidence is reposed the animated impulse that is ceaselessly throbbing in the bosom of those whose hearth-stone is desolate, and around which gathers not a child. The outside world may not know of the painful vacancy that is ever confronting them, nor the despair that has possession of their hearts; but the physician, to whose skill they so earnestly appeal to accomplish the realizatian of their hope, is ever, and probably the only *confidante*. He alone knows the elevation of spirits, the fulness of pride, and the intensity of satisfaction that is manifested if he has removed the barrier to productiveness, and that the process of maternity is in progress. But let him say that the barriers to conception are insuperable, it causes a painful despondency, and that exquisite anguish resulting from unappeased yearnings of the soul. It is, however, a providential ordination that few women are hopelessly barren, and but few men unprocreative. Circumstances may for a certain time make them practically unproductive, but such a physical condition can in almost every case be removed by consistent treatment, and by observing such measures and precautions tending to promote fruitfulness. The causes of childlessness with certain married parties are various. It may be due to deformities of the womb, Fallopian tubes, and ovaries of the female ; or testes, spermatic cord, and of the male organ. The pathological conditions are many, which occur in both sexes, that produce barrenness, while in some cases the anatomy of the parts render conception and child-bearing utterly impossible. It may be caused by stricture of the womb and Fallopian tubes, misplacement of the tubes, adhesions of the uterine walls, etc., etc., or through malformation, as occlusion of the vagina, etc. It may also be due to degeneracy of the testes of the male, epispadias, hypospadias, etc. Conception may also temporarily be prevented by uterine and ovarian diseases, or to a diseased condition of the spermatozoids of the male semen. Unproductiveness is frequently due to a devitalized condition of those animalculoids, in which state they have no fecundating properties. Sterility, dependent upon some vicious conformation of the genital organs of either sex, apparent or concealed, is called *absolute*. Infecundity, due to the conditions already enumerated, are absolute causes of sterility, and can only be removed by medical treatment, which in most cases, if of a rational and appropriate character, can effectually be accomplished. When a female does not conceive with one individual, but has or may with another, the condition is called *relative* sterility. Relative infecundity is frequently met with, and in many cases presents such features that the atociac condition cannot be overcome without calling to aid artificial means. It is often observed that a woman in her second mar· riage is sterile who in her first marriage was prolific in offspring ; again, the widower in his first marriage gave evidence of fecundating power, but in his second alliance no impregnation ensues. Absolute and relative sterility may exist at the same time, thus a female may be married to a man who is physically incapable of impregnating her, yet at the same time the conformation of her genital organs may be such as to render her absolutely sterile. It is therefore necessary in all cases of sterility to fully investigate the causes, both absolute and relative. Sterility in some females is often dependent upon a condition of the womb characterized by membranous menstruation. Conception is prevented in such cases by devitalization of the semen by the vitiated secretion and discharges from the uterine surface. In all cases of absolute sterility, medical treatment offers the only hope of obliteration of the causes. The diseases of the female genitalia which are causative of infecundity must be treated as required by their pathological character ; and it is necessary that such treatment should be admirably adapted to the conditions of the case, and most carefully instituted. Such cases should only be intrusted to physicians who by skill and experience have the requisite ability, and who are conversant with the precautions that studiously are to be observed. Improper treatment is exceedingly apt to render sterility an irremediable condition, which under rational treatment would have resulted in the removal of all the barriers to impregnation. If the cause lies in the male, whose formative material is devitalized by a diseased condition of the fabricating organs, seminiferous ducts, or seminal vesicles, medical treatment likewise is the only means of making the patient procreative. The male often renders himself powerless to procreate by imprudence or various excesses, in which case the semen is not fully organized and deficient in procreative elements. All these varied conditions of husband and wife contributing to childlessness are mainly remediable, so that under the care of an intelligent physician parentage to them is not always a forlorn hope. The prospect for issue is favorable in most cases under rational treatment, hence the gloom of the childless need not be perpetual if they but employ the counsel and aid of the competent physician. Neglect of so important a duty is very common, the conjugal pair stolidly agreeing that their childless state is owing to Divine ordinance, little dreaming that their unproductive union is in opposition to the requirements of the Deity, and that the fault of non-conception is due to incapacity and not to dispensation.

Relative sterility is not amenable to medical treatment. The most common cause of infecundity of this character is the want of adaptation or fitness of the genital organs of the conjugal pair to each other. This want of adaptation is a very frequent cause of sterilty, and should receive proper attention by the medical man to whom is intrusted the rectification of an unproductive union. Of itself, inadaptation may not be the cause of the atociac condition, but when associated with an atonic condition of the uterus, procreation rarely, if ever, ensues. It will not be necessary for me to detail the various forms of inadaptation, as the consideration of such causes of sterility more immediately concerns the medical attendant, but it is quite appropriate to make allusion to such causes, as the childless very properly desire information relative to all possible conditions hindering fructification. Self-treatment is not to be thought of; but a proper knowledge of all the physiological or anatomical causes of sterility should be possessed by all in conjugal association, especially by those who have not as yet attained the full measure of matrimonial enjoyment, by reason of an exceptional provision of fate by which their union is left without the graces and endearments of childhood.

One of the most common causes of barrenness is unquestionably what has been already alluded to, atony of the womb or appendages; in fact some pathological condition of the reproductive organs of the female is, in the large majority of cases, the sole cause. Uterine atony, or intonicity of the womb, may be of every degree of intensity—ranging from a slight feebleness to complete exhaustion—the latter condition being known as paralysis of the womb. This atonic state is owing not to any structural or organic disease of the womb itself, but is merely a secondary pathological condition, the actual seat of the disorder being in the sacral plexus, or that nervous net-work situated near the sacrum, from which the genital organs receive their nervous supply. A paralyzed condition of the womb is aptly illustrated by a paralyzed arm or leg; the loss of natural power, motion, or functions resulting from a diseased condition of some cerebral or spinal nerve-centre, and not from any morbid condition of the part affected. In all cases, therefore, where the cause of sterility has been ascertained to be uterine paralysis, the proper treatment is to restore the tonic powers of the sacral plexus. This is best accomplished by the intelligent application of the electric or galvanic current, or by the employment of the appropriate cerebro-spinal tonics and other medicinal agents. The treatment is, however, to be intrusted to careful, able, and experienced physicians.

The physiological function of the womb, favoring the transmission of the male formative material from the *os uteri* to the ovarium, is a certain suction power or intro-staltic motion. This is accomplished by short and wave-like contractions upward of the uterine muscles. In a paralyzed condition of the womb, which is usually of a chronic character, there is a complete absence of this uterine motion, and consequently the respective formative materials necessary for procreation never come in contact.

Membranous menstruation has already been stated as one of the causes of sterility. This painful affection is characterized by either partial or complete denudation of the uterine cavity of its mucous covering at each menstrual period, leaving the uterine walls in an abraded condition, entirely unfitted for the purposes of gestation. Conception may, however, take place in these cases, but at the arrival of the first period for the occurrence of the menstrual exacerbation, the placenta and membranes are dislodged with the mucous membrane.

The childless wife will note that a pathological or abnormal condition of her pelvic organs is relatively the most frequent cause of sterility, all of the affections being characterized by more or less gravity and requiring the most appropriate and energetic treatment in order to restore the organs to health, and at the same time establish functional integrity and maternal capacity. As most of these uterine affections result from a wilful disregard of the laws of health, slavish obedience to the behests of fashion, and bad habits in general, the author hopes that all females, married or unmarried, who properly appreciate the grandeur of womanhood and motherhood will not wilfully violate physiological law, but strenuously endeavor to preserve uterine health and integrity of the maternal capacity.

Congenital phymosis is a condition of the male organ depriving him of procreative power in nearly every instance. The intervention of the prepuce in this case arrests the ejaculatory force of the seminal expenditure, preventing impulsion into the womb. This deformity is easily obliterated by a surgical operation, which is very frequently performed in my office. It causes but little pain, no inconvenience, and heals rapidly. Circumcision among the Jews is a custom having for its object the removal of this frequent obstacle to multiplication, as existing in the male. Infecundity, especially in the earlier years of marriage, is often a consequence of exhaustion, induced by improper excesses. Intemperate indulgence often renders both husband and wife sterile. The semen must, in order to have procreative perfection, necessarily remain in the seminal vesicles for a certain time, where its procreative qualities are fully developed. After its escape from the vesicles, it further receives the intermixture of prostatic fluid, liquefying it to the proper consistence for easy propulsion into the uterine cavity. Marital excess is therefore preventive of full procreative quality of the semen. Excessive indulgence on the part of the wife causes a feebleness of peristaltic motion of the uterine muscles, or, as it may be otherwise termed, the suction power of the womb. Feebleness of the upward propelling forces of the womb and Fallopian tubes is caused by the excesses alluded to, and hence, if even the semen is introduced within the uterine embrace, the absence of retentive power allows its escape through the mouth of the womb. Sterility from such cause can only be overcome by the observance of moderation by the conjugal pair, and in most cases restorative medical treatment becomes also a necessity.

The most susceptible period for the occurrence of conception is immediately after the complete cessation of the menstrual flow. This susceptibility continues for eight or ten days, but is necessarily greatest at an early period after the menstrual discharge. The menstrual flow in its discharge carries away all obstructions that exist in the mouth of the womb, thus facilitating intro-propulsion of the semen, and the womb at that period has also its greatest tonic power. It is, however, not to be supposed that conception will not take place at the period just preceding the menstrual flow ; on the contrary, it may occur at any period between the cessation and onset of the catamenial discharge.

It will thus be seen that many causes, both absolute and relative, tend to sterility. In but few cases, however, is sterility a fixed fact, or an irremediable condition. The greatest triumphs achieved by the medical profession were in the study of the causes of sterility, and the best means for their removal. No physician, alive to the importance and exalted character of his calling, should neglect the study of the subject ; on the contrary, he should be conversant with all the pathological features sterility presents, and. be able to intelligently ascertain the causes. An important trust is confided to his professional care ; the intensest longing capable of the human heart depends upon his skill, either to be appeased or unrequited. Professional acumen is in no respect more essential than in this, and the medical counsellor, unworthy of the trust by reason of imperfect knowledge of the subject, does a grievous wrong by attempting treatment, or venturing decisive advice. The childless pair should at all times seek the most intelligent counsel and most competent treatment, and not allow themselves to become victims of despondency before they have made such a definite attempt.

The author has devoted much time and study upon this subject, feeling that no greater field of usefulness is presented to the physician for the exercise of his skill and professional attainments. The success attained in this sphere of professional activity has only been gained at the expense of laborious study and by the advantages conferred by extensive practice. Competence can only be gained by study and experience in every subject of intelligence—-proficiency being only the reward of intellectual labor and. opportunity'for exercise of the secured knowledge.

The author will gladly give advice to those to whom this chapter refers, being justified by previous success and long professional experience to give proper and definite ad\ice and appropriate treatment. Those desiring to avail themselves of such an opportunity are referred to page 390 for guidance as to the proper information to submit for my consideration.

IMPOTENCE OF THE MALE.

By this is generally considered the inability to engage in the virile act. It essentially signifies a loss of the virile powers. Impotency may be either *partial* or *complete*, and, like sterility, *absolute*, and *relative*. The term impotence is frequently used synonomously with sterility; but, as sterility has been considered in another place, we shall discuss the subject in this place only in the sense implying loss of capacity.

The loss of virile power is owing to a variety of causes. The process of loss in idiopathic cases is usually slow, though in some cases invirility ensues quite rapidly. When due to traumatic causes virile power is lost synchronously with the occurrence of the injury. Impotence usually follows injuries received by the spine and base of the brain, but in these cases the loss is not of itself a pathological disorder, but essentially symptomatic of the injury.

The most common cause of impotence is nervous debility, apparent or concealed and unsuspected. It is the usual sequel to that disease, if it is allowed an unchecked career, manifesting itself at first by a slight incapacity, but which gradually progresses until finally the virile power is completely lost. That impotence is the inevitable result to nervous debility is quite natural, the ceaseless waste of such a vital element of the male economy as semen can have no other finality. The general disturbance of the nervous system caused by involuntary spermatic losses is manifested first in the virile organs, as the erectile property of the organ, purely a nervous phenomenon, and consequently any function so directly under the control of nervous power as the erectile quality, is the one first to succumb to nervous disorganization. Impotence in such cases is, therefore, due to feebleness or insufficiency of the nervous stimuli necessary to provoke a copulative aspect of the male organ. This condition of invirility is also caused by immoderate indulgence, the pathological disorder produced being in all respects the same as that following seminal incontinence, though as a general thing masculine power is lost less rapidly.

Spinal and cerebral diseases are usually associated with a low condition of the virile power. This manifestation is quite in accordance with the physiological laws governing the virile functions, as it will be remembered that the nervous supply that the organs of generation receive is the pudental nerve, which arises from the sacral plexus. This nerve and branches afford the requisite stimuli necessary to promote congestion of the organ, which phenomenon constitutes an erection. The brain gives the necessary sensory stimulus, without which the nerves are not excited to action. Phrenologists place amativeness in the lower lobe of the cerebellum, but it is quite probable that its locality, though most evidently in the base of the brain, is not in that situation, as analogy will not comport with such a view. Observation teaches that the chanticleer is the most amorous of animals, yet anatomists find no lower lobe of the cerebellum in the brain of the fowl. External violence, however, upon the sacral and occipital regions usually cause virile imbecility, and hence we know that a healthy condition of the base of the brain and sacral plexus is necessary to the existence of virility. Diseases, excessive study, intemperate use of tobacco, violent and prolonged grief, etc., are therefore causes of impotency, from the fact that the cerebral disorganization which follows produces inertia of the nervous stimuli. Apoplexy is also a cause of temporary impotence, in consequence of the paralysis of the sacral plexus ensuing. It is therefore vitally important that in the consideration of any case of impotence every predisposing cause should receive attention, so that restorative efforts are based upon correct principles. No pathological condition requires such nicety of treatment as impotence, and none that will so readily be remedied if the medication is thoroughly adapted to the case. Although impotence is the usual concomitant to long-continued seminal losses, my experience teaches me that a fair proportion of impotent cases are the results of habits and practices which are perfectly legitimate, and to which no shadow of blame or disgrace can be properly attached. It is a well-established fact that too much mental application, also constant confinement within doors in a vitiated atmosphere, or habitual or sudden exposure to heats and colds, or the destroying influences of extreme grief and care, will produce all the evil effects upon the mental and physical organization that are caused by and attributed to solitary habits. Nervous debility, which is quite a common and comprehensive name for all failures of the intellectual or physical organs or faculties to perform their functions properly, is originated and nurtured, in both sexes, by a variety of causes as countless as the leaves of the forest. Consequently, people should not be backward about making their deficiencies of mind or body known to physicians in such a clear and confidential way as to secure to them the full restoration of their normal health and vigor. Any course of life which is inordinately irksome or, involves heavy tasks, is liable to cause the loss of virile power, or especially in middle age, IMPOTENCY, which is the aggravated form of the same difficulty. Thus we find that clergymen, merchants, book-keepers, literary workers, men who are overtaxed by care and labor, lawyers, judges, boys confined too closely at school, young men who seldom take out-of-door exercise, clerks, heads of public departments, and all others who are constantly wearing and tearing both mind and body without seeking the neutralizing aid of *rest*, amusement, and change of scene, are subjected to some of the numerous ills developed in disabilities and incapabilities which impose untold suffering. These ills are the inheritance of everybody physically and mentally overworked, no matter in what capacity they may labor. It is to be lamented that many of these innocent individuals, from the fear of being charged with guilt, suffer long years in silence when the truly judicious course is to engage medical aid as soon as the fact becomes known. The old-class physicians have used the most powerful minerals within their reach, and, with the earnest and honest desire to do good, have accomplished much that has been of *temporary* benefit. But the reaction from the use of these minerals has been, in all instances, of a non-curative character, the patient purchasing for temporary enjoyment many after-years of incapacity and local weakness.

There is nothing so discomforting to man as the loss of virile power. He may not be a sensual being, yet manhood is a pride to him, the possession of which is always a gratifying knowledge. Impotence implies more than mere virile imbecility, it signifies also a loss of vigor and elasticity of the whole organism, and a gloomy state and impairment of the mental faculties. It has elsewhere been observed that the well-being of the whole economy is greatly dependent upon healthy genitalia; and mental composure, vitality and acuteness of intellect, graceful and easy manners, etc., are no less independent of the virile faculties. Impotency is, therefore, always a deplorable condition, and he who permits himself to be long without the legacy of virility, commits a great injury upon his own personal welfare, and places but a poor value upon the choice powers of manhood. Man without virile power is an anomaly; he has lost his status of sex, and is practically a eunuch as long as the unmanly condition is tolerated. There is a higher motive in possession of virile power than the ability to gratify amorous passion. If that alone gave chief value to virility, its loss would be but inconsiderate, but as we have seen that vigorous manhood is consonant to vitality of the mental and physical economies, it gains a value not to be despised, but greatly cherished, even by the most continent and virtuous men. Healthy functions of the genital organs are as requisite to the integrity of the whole organism as healthy functional action of the thoracic and abdominal organs, and any derangement of the pelvic organs is capable of precisely as much, if not more, disorganization of the general health as a disordered digestive or circulatory apparatus. I will close the consideration of this subject by inviting all those who are deficient in masculine tone or capacity to call on me in person or consult me by letter. (See page 385.)

THE PHILOSOPHY OF GENERATION.

The greatness, importance, and responsibility of the marital relation are but improperly appreciated and understood by the majority of males and females who enter into that relation. There is a momentous duty to be performed, far more important than those generally supposed to be

19*

incumbent upon husband and wife. We have in other places considered the more general duties devolving upon husband and wife to be discharged ; we will in this place dwell upon a subject which of all others pertaining to the conjugal association of the sexes is the most important, and which as a duty is more universally neglected and improperly performed because the principles and laws governing generation are but imperfectly understood or not at all. The precise question relative to generation which we purpose to discuss is the transmission to children of the best possible mental, physical and moral attainments.

We have in another part of this work stated that the legitimate object of marriage is to legalize the sexual covenant, and to confine it within a healthful and moral atmosphere. This is not only the legitimate, but technically it is the only aspect of which the law takes cognizance. Such a congress is, therefore, legal between a male and female who have been bound together in wedlock. This is all right and proper ; but not by mere legalized association can the welfare of the race be best advanced or secured. The distinguishment of animal creation into two sexes was only designed by Nature for one purpose—the multiplication of species ; but it never was the purpose of Nature that the sexes should indiscriminately associate, or that the intent and design of multiplication would be fitly subserved in all cases by merely allowing any male to covenant with any female, irrespective of selection. In the lower animals this is avoided by instinct, but in man the restraint is given by the higher impulses of reason. Yet, notwithstanding this high quality in man, the purpose of Nature is often defeated or controverted by wilful disregard of the promptings of an innate intelligence or disobedience to what is known as physiological law.

The first requisite is circumspect marriage. Without the marital union of eligible parties human progress would be slow, or unpromising. A circumspect marriage tends, however, to bring into conjugal union the more highly endowed male with the more highly endowed female ; or, in other words, the *best* man would marry only the *best* woman. The man having highly developed physical, mental, and moral, faculties would only be content in marrying a woman with similarly developed faculties, and in such a union we have the basis for highly endowed offspring. In another essay are given the precautions candidates should observe prior to consummating marriage, and if the instructions therein given should be heeded, unfit marriages would be of rarer occurrence.

But in marriage, proper or improper, a duty has to be performed, neglect of which is sinning against the welfare of the whole race. The aim of all married people should be the bringing into the world of healthy children, not physically only, but mentally and morally also. The greatest achievement and proudest monument of parentage is in giving to the world such offspring as will act well their part in the great

drama of life. How is it to be done ? Can parents so regulate the gestatory process as to give their children at birth the heritage of physical
excellence, large mental capacity, and superior moral disposition ? Assuredly they can ; it requires but willingness and effort in the right direction. The mother who imparts to the being hid away in her loins
her personal features, her disposition, etc., can impart much more by
proper effort. The father, from whom the male formative material is
received, can do much for the welfare of that being evolved from that
material. For all that it is, the child is indebted to either one of the
parents; from them is received the human qualities it possesses or exhibits. Subsequent care, training, and education may do much, but the
original bias is received within the confines of the womb.

Not much need be said as to the transmission of mental superiority
to children. If the parents are intelligent and educated, the children
will also have large mental capacity. Subsequent mental training will
serve to give offspring that mental culture which in the present progressive period of the human race each individual being should possess.
Intelligence, not ignorance, now holds sway ; and no one can harmoni-
ously glide along with the current of human progress without a cultivated mind. If mothers, therefore, have tastes for the intellectual pursuits, let them not abandon them while another life is developing.

The transmission of moral qualities is more readily accomplished. To
what extent they can be transmitted is not readily definable, but it is a
well-settled fact in psychology that the moral habit readily descends
from parent to child. This fact is exemplified in the history of nearly
every family, for in nearly every case the moral tone of the children
represents that of the parents, at least as far as disposition is concerned.
Vicious association may destroy the moral tone, even if the disposition
is unfavorable ; but when the disposition is favorable to moral excellence
the inclination to vice is strongly curbed, and moral degeneration is not
so easily effected, even if the child is surrounded by all the allurements
of vice. On the mother, then, a high duty rests—she is chargeable with
the moral tone of society, not by neglecting the supervision of the moral
faculties of her born children so much as by indifference when a
human soul is undergoing intra-uterine development. Motherhood
comes to many most unwelcomely ; the trials and cares incident to it are
not favorably regarded ; but there are few women in whom the maternal instinct is so deficient that they would, with sheer malice, endeavor
to give birth to a babe so weighted with the destiny of a bad organization, as to make them through life utterly insensible to all the moral relations of life. Yet such a legacy is completely within the power of a
mother to give. If she is not elevated by purity of thought and of action, if not ennobled by intensity of maternal feeling, and if not actuated by constant solicitude for the welfare of her unborn babe, the or-

ganization of the child will be unquestionably vicious. She should remember that the child in uterine life has no blood but that of its
mother; all that courses through its veins and arteries also courses
through the blood-vessels of the mother. How important it is then for
mothers to guard against everything calculated to disturb the harmony
and regularity of the vascular current!

The child *in utero* is technically but an appendage or parasite, over
which the maternal mind and body exerts a marked influence; consequently, if mothers in the pregnant state pay heed to the moral relations
of life, curb for the time any evil disposition they may have, take pleasure
only in that which is pure and upright—in short, lead a blameless moral
life—they will most surely be blest with offspring in whom the disposition will be kind and the moral tone exalted. Let me then say to expectant mothers : enlighten and elevate the moral sentiments, exercise desirable talents, cultivate beautiful qualities; for if you do, they will certainly bloom in great brilliancy in your children and children's children. So,
too, if there exists among the subtleties of your character any dark
spot, exert all your moral strength in order to eradicate it. Surround
the growing soul with good influences; cultivate all noble impulses, all
holy aspirations; breathe into the opening flower, by the magic power
of a mother's love, such knowledge and moral legacy as will prepare it
for the world in all its antagonisms; and you will see in the final fruit
the reward for all your care, self-denial, and self-abnegation. Husbands
must learn to recognize this supreme power of their wives over the
ante-natal life (both mental and physical), and they must observe such
a line of conduct as not to frustrate any endeavor to exercise it rightly,
but should give them the best possible conditions to improve it.

How can parents have healthy children? This is a question of such
significant importance to married people that it should engage their
most earnest thought and liveliest interest, for parents can by judicious
care and careful practice endow their offspring with most excellent physical vigor. To effect this it is only necessary that they should themselves be healthy, or to render inert by proper medication the tendency
of transmission of any infirmity or disease with which they may themselves be afflicted. The most potential cause of degenerate health in
offspring is the ruinous effect of nervous debility. Any male who previous to marriage practised self-abuse, and who married while suffering from the effects of such a pernicious habit, cannot furnish for
the purposes of generation such perfection of formative material as
will insure full health in the being that evolves therefrom. The seminal
liquid is diseased, and carries with it the germs of low vitality and
poverty of physical endurance or capacity. For this reason the author
discountenances marriage in those who by youthful errors induced
the involuntary expenditure of semen, because that affection destroys

the instinct of propagation, and renders the sufferer incapable or unfit to afford such formative material as will result in healthy products of conception. I therefore adjure all these suffering from this infirmity not to marry until by proper and skilful treatment a healthy integrity of the organs is fully re-established. If those who are married suffer from the unmanly losses of semen, they should by all means make early endeavors to have their manhood restored in all its fulness. Those who are partially impotent should not neglect to secure the required treatment—such as will restore virile vigor and healthy procreating power. Medical treatment is of the greatest importance, and, assuredly, it is only those who have full manly vigor and integrity that can hope for healthy offspring. It is scarcely an allowable exercise of privilege for any male to marry if suffering from the effects of indiscretions, as it is well known to every physiologist that procreative capacity is lessened thereby, and offspring usually of feeble mind and body and low moral tone. Let all such sufferers then fully appreciate the responsibility of the married state, and only enter its portals with healthy genital organs and proper virile capacity. This advice should be heeded by all who properly estimate marital eligibility. Their first duty is to engage the services of a competent physician, who will by proper treatment restore the proper integrity of the organs, impart the required vigor, and secure the necessary conditions for healthy propagation.

Eligibility for motherhood requires full integrity of womanhood. No healthy babe can be born if its ante-natal life is passed in a diseased uterine cavity. Women suffering from inflammation or ulceration of the mucous membrane lining the uterine cavity cannot possibly give birth to a healthy child. It is then a high duty for all wives to make all possible effort to become sexually healthy, and if they have the prudence to engage the proper herbal treatment they will certainly regain the required feminine vigor and motherhood will be a blessing instead of a curse.

Proper treatment will even avert the transmission of scrofula, epilepsy, consumption, and other diseases capable of hereditation. This must be given while the child is developing within the uterine cavity. The disease in the parent may not be cured, but rational treatment, under the guidance of a skillful physician, can so modify the gestatory process as to effectually prevent the child from being born with a similar diathesis.

This subject is one of the most important within the whole range of medicine, and should engage the interest of all; it concerns not only individual welfare, but the health and the mental and moral well-being of the whole human race.

The author gladly gives advice to those who may need counsel or treatment. Parents who submit their cases for my consideration will be fully advised what course should be pursued. All communications held inviolably secret. (See page 385 for guidance as to consultation.)

DIVORCE.

This implies the separation of the married pair, by legal dissolution of the matrimonial bonds. Divorces are most commonly given by the courts for causes occurring after marriage ; but jurists, in treating upon this subject, also include those causes by which a marriage may be rendered null upon antecedent grounds; as where a marriage was accomplished by forcible or fraudulent means, or where, in consequence of near consanguinity, the act of cohabitation between the pair is by law considered incestuous. Where a physical incapacity for marriage prevails in one of the parties, divorces are usually granted by nearly all courts, provided such an incapacity existed previous to marriage.

It is not our purpose, however, to discuss the subject in its legal aspect, however interesting it might be, but to consider it rather in its popular sense. It is not within the province of the medical writer to consider the subject relative to its legal bearings, though he may with propriety give the subject the attention it claims with reference to abuse of the marital privilege. There are practically many divorces between husbands and wives, of which the law takes no cognizance, and for causes for which no court would grant a dispensation. The author is fully aware that the divorce laws are not any too stringent, and probably too facile in many commonwealths ; but, while he is by no means in favor of easy divorce laws, he is ready to admit that the strong hand of the law sometimes is not waved to the side of justice, but inflicts intolerable anguish by enforcing a matrimonial existence which in its very nature is adverse to the very spirit and essence of matrimony.

It is practically divorcing the marriage tie when mutual love no longer characterizes the union. The only bond that unites and that makes the union an inseparable one is love, and not the mere formal ceremony of espousal. The law, however, does not and cannot recognize anything but the *vinculum matrimonii* as binding, but the philosopher delves deeper, and while he does not dispute the necessity of legal ceremonies, he nevertheless knows that marriage is in its very essence not such a union as defined by law, but a linking of affections, a union of souls and hearts. Marriage is practically annulled when love is no longer the cord of union ; without mutual affection the association becomes intolerable, the higher purposes of the tie are defeated, and the sacred precinct is invaded by elements foreign to the psychical character of the marital atmosphere. Law can, however, not remedy this ; the candidates for marriage must, as before advised, exercise such precautions, that they may not deceive themselves, and only form a matrimonial alliance that augurs a congenial wedded life. Divorces cannot be

granted for uncongeniality, provided no actual infringement of the marriage bond has been committed, and cannot extend a dispensation
because married life is loveless. Abuse of its privileges would follow,
and divorce laws should therefore of necessity be stringent, so that
marriages be not recklessly contracted, and obliging intended union to
be the result of guarded and careful deliberation, as it is easier to prevent
mistakes than to rectify them. Negligence of consulting the better
knowledge brings its own reward, and, however intolerable the punishment, a separation cannot ensue by virtue of law. Humanity would
grant the dissolution of the tie, but the purity and purpose of law must
be protected. Stringency must shield it from disgrace, or the possible
chance of its becoming the agent whereby injury may be done, or flagrant
violations of matrimonial duty may be prompted by its laxity. Every
candidate should lose sight of every consideration except that of happiness in married life, and see that no one can exclaim

> "She (or he) whom the law calls yours,
> Is by her (or his) love made mine."

In nearly all courts, adultery is sufficient cause for divorce, and very
properly so. It is the most heinous violation of the duty and trust attached to a conjugal union. Everything besides pales in comparison
with adultery in the enormity of its malfeasance in the marital sphere.
It is such a flagrant abuse of duty and fidelity that the conjugal pair
owe to each other, that it has even been recognized by divine law as
sufficient cause for divorce, and as long as civilization has a foothold,
and morality considered a virtue, so long will adultery be regarded
subversive to the integrity of the conjugal union. It is a crime admitting of no extenuation, and incapable of condonement by the
morally upright or the virtuous pure. It is the brand that inflames the
worst passions in the one who has thus been injured and disgraced by
his or her conjugal associate, surely engendering hate and detestation if
the proper value is placed upon marital loyalty. The bubble that has
just burst is as easily reconstructed as to again establish confidence,
peace and happiness in that family, of which either the husband or
wife has sinned. The wound is incurable, and prolongation of the
wedded association only aggravates. Therefore, the only remedy is a
legal separation from the one who has proved so unworthy of marital
trust. It is not enough that the husband and wife should be guiltless
of adultery, but their conduct must be such as to arouse no suspicion
of neighbors or others. The conduct must be so guarded that loyalty
is not doubted, but manifested even under circumstances where the
liability to err is great, so that fidelity is established, and suspicion dis-
armed.

That wife, who, by her conduct in society, or in her social intercourse with other men, brings upon her mistrust, and who provokes public scandal by her vagaries and lax conduct, actually debauches her husband's good name, and does him as much injury as she would were she guilty of adultery. She may never have committed the act, and probably never would, but her deportment is such as to lead observers to the opinion that she would prove disloyal if circumstances favored, thereby committing a grievous wrong, and staining the honor and good name of her husband to an unwarrantable extent. The man that brings to his bride the legacy of honor and respectability is greatly injured if she by her immoral conduct begets the suspicion as to loyalty of his friends and neighbors, and she is unworthy of his love and protection if she so far forgets her duty as bring a stain upon his character by her own imprudence. She is guilty of adulterous proclivities, which should be considered sufficient cause for divorce, even if adultery cannot be proven. On the other hand, the husband, who by improper behavior in company, is so unguarded as to be suspected for his loyalty and attachment to his wife, is unworthy of her, and cannot justify his conduct by even the most liberal interpretation of the marriage contract. It would, unquestionably, be well if the law would recognize conduct that suggests an adulterous proclivity as sufficient for divorce, even if adultery *per se* could not be proven, as it would most probably have a salutary effect in counteracting the tendency to the degeneracy of modern free-loveism.

The cry of many wives of the present day, who think that their duty to society is paramount to the duty they owe to their husbands is— Would you exclude us from society? Am I to be imprisoned in the home you afford me and not be allowed to receive my friends, or to mingle again with society? No, not at all; the seclusivism of the harem is not calculated to promote the best interests of conjugal life; but it is to be insisted upon that when wives are in society their conduct should be so dignified, so hedged in with propriety, that their reputation remains unsullied, that the most suspicious need not suspect, and that the libertine is given no opportunity to make his offensive proposals, nor his heart gratified by a passive submission to his lascivious conversation, looks, and hints. Cæsar claimed not too much in his requirements of a wife—she should in all respects be above suspicion. The wife's greatest pride should be the observance of such a line of conduct as meets her husband's approval. All her actions should be characterized by purity and fidelity, and no cause should be given for unpleasant comment. Such noble wives are denominated the oppressed, the slaves of men, etc., etc., by the Women's Rights women; but they are not,—they and they only are the idols of men, at least of those whose affections are pure and worth having. The angelic quality of women, so often the theme of poets and lovers, is surely only manifested by the virtuous and in the faithful. The very existence of civilization is dependent upon virtuous women and faithful wives; men may become depraved, but as long as women remain pure, civilization, morality, and religion will be fostered and propagated. If women live the truth and act the truth, humanity will ever be blessed with the benefits of civilization.

To the sterner sex the mantle of virtue is no less becoming; and fidelity is as much of an adornment and requirement to them as of the gentler sex. The libertine is a despicable creature; and the adulterer is so lost to honor and nobility of character, that his presence in the society of the pure and good should be considered an outrage upon decency and propriety. Chastity is a superior virtue, and loyalty in wedlock a noble attribute; and whichever one of the conjugal pair proves reckless to these connubial trusts is unworthy of marital companionship and defiles a sacred institution.

BRIDAL TOURS.

"Some essays have been written on the barbarisms of civilization; many more might be. Many of the habits prevailing in what ought to be our most refined society are at variance with almost elementary ideas of decency. Others are equally marked in their injurious physical tendencies. It is not surprising that clergymen, even when not of the strictest sect, and philosophers of no particular sect at all, have declaimed against fashionable dresses and dances at late hours. But there are other customs against which no church has fulminated its anathemas, the dangers and absurdities of which no fidgety reformer has perceived or noticed. One of these conspicuously is the Bridal Tour.

"Let us illustrate by a typical case. During one of the earliest and coldest 'cold snaps' there comes off a wedding, which, from the official standing of the parties, naturally attracts some attention. We are soon told that the 'happy couple' are off on their wedding trip to—well, not exactly Alaska or Greenland, but a territory nearly as frigid, and that part of the journey is to be made in stages or sleighs. The intense excitement in appropriateness of the proceeding, the wonderful pains taken by these people to make themselves uncomfortable on what is supposed to be the most festive occasion in their lives, would move one to Homeric laughter, did not events disastrous to the health of the conjugal pair usually follow so closely on the heels of bridal tours." If the parties are not as high in the social scale and less wealthy, the mischief done is as great, if not greater, for in their tour they may lack substantial comforts which the wealthy alone can afford. To all married couples a bridal tour seems to be considered as absolutely essential to give the marital union an importance, without which it would, in their opinion, be an unromantic and but partial marriage.

Looking at the custom from an æsthetic and sentimental point of view, nothing can be more repulsive. An American marriage is theoretically a love match, and it is generally so in practice. Now two persons in love want to see as much as possible of each other, and as little as possible of other people. It is to that we find exceptions; there are individuals whose diseased vanity desires to give publicity to every act of their life. It is a misfortune that these vulgarians are not rarer in every class. An instinct of seclusion and modesty should be the general rule, but this absurd custom forces a new-married couple to put on an unnatural restraint on their legitimate affection, or to make themselves ridiculous before the public. Love, both emotional and passionate, is usually most exuberant to those recently joined in wedlock, and philosophy would suggest the exercise to be confined more to seclusion than the sporadic opportunities afforded in a wedding tour.

Now, in the common-sense, practical, man-of-the-world point of view, the fashionable practice is equally objectionable. It is notorious that nothing, except marriage itself, tries the temper more than joint travel. Therefore, at the very outset of their life-partnership, the quality on which the happiness of that union principally depends is put to the rudest strain. The happy couple expose themselves to the insolence of hackmen and hotel-clerks, the discomforts of rail and hotel, irregular hours and uncertain meals. The Irishman, in the song, married a wife to make him "unaisy." A wedding tour on one of our great thoroughfares of travel is admirably contrived to accomplish this result for both parties.

All this, however, it may be suggested, is matter of taste. We cannot expect to shape the caprices of fashion or custom by the dictates of deliberate philosophy. But what follows is not a questionable point of taste or comfort; it is a matter of downright fact, as certain as if it could be mathematically demonstrated.

The consummation of marriage is, with the exception of child-birth, the most critical period, physically, of the woman's life. After the moral and physical excitement which attends it, her system demands rest, repose, quiet, regular and good living, a supporting and restorative way of life. If these can be secured for some weeks, so much the better, but at any rate they are necessary for some days. Her emotional nature attains the highest state of excitement, in consequence of assisting in a repast which is approached only by intense agitation, no matter how much she may feel it to be a legitimate incident to marriage. This makes it doubly exhaustive, and not only her health for the rest of her mortal existence, but the health and strength of her offspring may be, and often are, materially affected by the want of proper care at this time. Instead of which, the bridal tour piles on additional excitement and fatigue, makes regularity of life impossible—in short, the act involves the reverse of all that the rules of health and physiology require. There is an underlying sense of modesty which may urge the bride on to a journey immediately after marriage. The new condition of life exacts changes which she rather would fulfil among strangers than in her own or husband's domicile. It may confuse the modest and retiring woman to assume the conjugal associations in presence of her parents, brothers, and sisters; but as this is one of the modesties not really commendable, however natural it may be, it does not afford sufficient inducement for encountering all the vicissitudes of a wedding tour.

For man too, at this time, repose and calm, though not so necessary, are highly desirable. It constantly happens, in the case of both sexes, that a slight indisposition, which passed unnoticed in the hurry of preparation, is aggravated to a serious and even fatal extent by the excitement, exposure, and neglect consequent on the wedding tour. No man, for instance, would think of postponing his marriage on account of a slight cold. If he stayed quietly at home afterward, and took care of himself, it would pass away like other slight colds ; but he goes off on a bridal tour in the depth of winter, and the malady develops into a chronic pulmonary complaint. Nor would a young woman put off her marriage because she felt a little extra lassitude and want of appetite, with an occasional headache, which, however, *may* be premonitory symptoms of typhoid fever. If you take typhoid fever in time, there is nothing specially dangerous about it ; care, patience, and slight treatment are only necessary, and it runs its course. But, if neglected at first, it is almost inevitably fatal. Many cases of brides and bridegrooms, in my profesional experience, came under my observation, dying of typhoid fever just after a wedding trip, which had caused the early symptoms to be misunderstood and neglected. And I have known things worse than death to happen—insanity, temporary or permanent, brought on by the extra fatigue and excitement of the wedding journey.

One old New York custom, and probably to some extent prevailing in other places, was infinitely more rational. The new-married couple took up their quarters at the house of the bride's father, and remained there in seclusion for a week. The only fault about this arrangement was the shortness of time, but for a week, at any rate, they had absolute repose and quiet, and enjoyed all the comforts of a home without the trouble of housekeeping. For one week, at least, the inter-communion of the conjugal pair was unhampered, and secured against the criticism and gaze of the public.

The present fashion of bridal tours is an unmeaning and unreasonable imitation of the European, especially the English practice. The original English theory of a wedding trip is, driving in a comfortable carriage, at a rate of speed just sufficient to exhilarate without fatiguing, over good roads, in weather which may be pleasant or unpleasant, but is never **dangerously** cold or dangerously hot, to some secluded country-place or seaside village, and resting there a month. The new mode of continental tours is in some respects just as absurd as ours, though the advantage of climate lessens the fatigue and physical risk to some extent. The notorious mutability of our climate is in itself reason enough why a bride should not be exposed to the accidents of travel.

It will thus be seen that the medical aspect of a bridal tour is sufficiently important, and the risk incurred sufficiently great, to cause the wedded pair, if they wish to be actuated with impulses of reason and prudence, rather than by the dictates of custom, to pause before they undergo the trials of a wedding journey. It would certainly be more conducive to their health and happiness if they were guided by a better reason in this respect, and leave wedding trips to be indulged in by those who would rather run the risk of injuring their health and general well-being than offend a fashionable practice. It is a fashionable vulgarity, and not prompted by the behests of good-breeding and social dignity.

POISONS AND THEIR ANTIDOTES.

Nothing that appertains to domestic treatment is of greater value than a knowledge of poisons, and the treatment necessary in cases of accidental or premeditated poisoning. So many substances of a poisonous nature are used in manufactures among farmers, mechanics, and also in private houses, it will be useful to have a guide to refer to in case of accident, for in almost every case of poisoning the antidote must be instantly given or else success cannot be expected. In all cases, unless the physician is within immediate call, no time is allowed to engage his services; hence the great importance of every one supplying himself with the requisite knowledge to treat any or all cases of poisoning.

Precaution with regard to poisons is very necessary. In every family, manufactory, etc., where poisons are required and used, the antidotes should also be kept for use whenever occasion calls for them. Again, when poisons are used for any purpose, it is not enough to know that they *are poisonous*, but it should also be known of what they are composed. For instance, corrosive sublimate may be used, and by accident a poisonous dose may be taken of it; but, unless known that it is a preparation of mercury, the treatment must necessarily be of a vague and uncertain character.

As a general rule, in all cases of poisoning, especially if seen immediately after the poison has been swallowed, the indication is to make the person *vomit*. To bring this about give a teaspoonful of mustard in a tumbler of water, or two or three teaspoonfuls of powdered alum in the same way. Vomiting can in all cases be promoted by tickling the throat with a feather.

ARSENIC.

ARTICLES.—Scheele's green, arsenious acid, orpiment, king's yellow, realgar, fly powder, ague drops, arsenical paste and arsenical soap, rat poison.

SYMPTOMS.—Pain and burning in the stomach, dryness of throat, cramps, purging, vomiting, hoarseness and difficulty of speech, eyes red and sparkling, suppression of urine, matter vomited greenish or yellowish.

TREATMENT.—Give large quantities of milk and raw eggs, lime-water, or flour and water. Then castor-oil; or, if tincture of iron is within reach, take from half to a full teaspoonful of it, and mix with it a little bicarbonate of soda or saleratus, and administer it to the person, and follow it with an emetic. This acts as a real antidote—the chemical combination resulting being insoluble in the fluids of the stomach.

ACIDS.

ARTICLES.—Oxalic (salts of sorrel), sulphuric (oil of vitriol), nitric (aquafortis), muriatic (spirit of salt), but not prussic acid.

SYMPTOMS.—These acids are all corrosive, and hence produce horrible burning and sour pain from the mouth downwards. The skin and mucous membrane of the lips, mouth, and throat is eaten away. The patient experiences great thirst, and purges blood, and has excruciating pain in the stomach.

TREATMENT.—Put an ounce of calcined magnesia into a pint of water, and give a wineglassful every two or three minutes. If you cannot get magnesia, use whiting, chalk, soda, or lime-water, or even knock a piece of mortar from the wall, pound it fine, and give it with milk or water. While one person is attending to this, let another cut common soap into small pieces and give a tea-spoonful with water, or a table-spoonful of soft soap. Also give plenty of warm water to drink.

Citric and *acetic* acids are also poisonous in large doses. The treatment is the same as for the above.

ANTIMONY.

ARTICLES.—Tartar emetic, butter of antimony, oxide of antimony.

SYMPTOMS.—Severe vomiting (if this does not occur it should be induced), cramps, faintness, purging, colicky pains, sense of tightness in the chest, recurrence of vomiting repeatedly.

TREATMENT.—Give plenty of strong tea. If no common tea is at hand, use an infusion of oak, elm, sloe, currant, or blackberry bark or leaves, the requirements being a vegetable astringent. If the butter of antimony has been taken, resort to the treatment advised for acids. In all cases the strength should be supported with stimulants.

BISMUTH.

ARTICLES.—Nitrate, pearl powder, face powders.

SYMPTOMS.—General inflammation of the whole alimentary canal, suppression of urine, hiccough, vomiting, cramps.

TREATMENT.—Plenty of milk, flaxseed tea, infusion of slippery elm, marsh mallow.

COPPER.

ARTICLES.—Blue copperas, blue verditer, mineral green, verdigris, food cooked in copper vessels, pickles made green by copper.

SYMPTOMS.—Coppery taste in the mouth, tongue dry and parched, very painful colic, bloody stools, convulsions.

TREATMENT.—Large quantities of milk and white of eggs, afterwards strong tea. *Vinegar should not be given.*

GOLD.

ARTICLES.—Chloride of gold, fulminating gold.

SYMPTOMS.—Similar to other irritant poisons. Pink patches about the lips and mouth.

TREATMENT.—Give sulphate of iron, which decomposes the substances.

IODINE.

ARTICLES.—Iodides of potassium, mercury, iron, or sodium.

SYMPTOMS.—Burning pain in throat, lacerating pain in stomach, heartburn, vomiting, colicky pains, very likely salivation.

TREATMENT.—Large quantities of starch and water, flour and water, grated potatoes, or anything that you know contains starch. If the iodides are taken in overdose, produce vomiting as soon as possible.

IRON.

ARTICLES.—Sulphate of iron (copperas), green vitriol, chloride of iron.

SYMPTOMS.—Colic pains, constant vomiting and purging, violent pain in throat, coldness of skin, feeble pulse.

TREATMENT—Give an emetic, afterwards magnesia or carbonate of soda and water. Also mucilaginous drinks.

LEAD.

ARTICLES.—Acetate or sugar of lead, white lead, red lead, litharge.

SYMPTOMS.—Metallic taste in mouth, pain in stomach and bowels, painful vomiting, often blood, hiccough. If taken for some time, obstinate colic, paralysis, partial or complete ; obstinate constipation, diminution of urine.

TREATMENT. — Put two ounces of epsom salts into a pint of water and give a wineglassful every ten minutes until it operates freely. If the solid forms have been taken, give dilute sulphuric acid, but very carefully.

MERCURY.

ARTICLES.—Calomel, corrosive sublimate, red precipitate, vermilion, white precipitate, turbith mineral.

SYMPTOMS.—Harsh metallic astringent taste, burning pain in the stomach, vomiting and purging frequently of bloody matter, tightness and burning in the throat, tendency to doze, stupor.

TREATMENT.—Albumen in some form must be instantly given ; either the white of eggs beaten up with water, milk or wheat flour beaten up. Iron filings can also be given. After these give linseed tea.

PHOSPHORUS.

ARTICLES.—Lucifer matches.

SYMPTOMS.—Pain in stomach and bowels, vomiting, diarrhœa, tenderness and tension of the abdomen, great excitement of the whole system.

TREATMENT.—Prompt emetic, copious draughts of warm water containing magnesia, chalk, whiting, or even flour. No oils or fat should be given.

SILVER.

ARTICLES.—Nitrate, or lunar caustic.

SYMPTOMS.—Similar to other irritant poisons, especially arsenic.

TREATMENT.—Give a large teaspoonful of common salt in a glass of water, and repeat this in ten minutes. Then a dose of castor-oil, and linseed tea, or barley water for a drink.

TIN.

ARTICLES.—Chloride, called muriate by dyers, oxide, or putty powder.

SYMPTOMS.—Vomiting, pain in stomach, purging, convulsive twitchings.

TREATMENT.—Milk must be given copiously. The milk may contain magnesia, chalk, or whiting, if handy. Also raw eggs beaten up with water and milk.

ZINC.

ARTICLES.—Sulphate, or white vitriol. Acetate, chloride (Burnett's disinfecting fluid, also used to destroy cancers).

SYMPTOMS.—Violent vomiting, astringent taste, burning pain in stomach, pale countenance, cold extremities, dull eyes.

TREATMENT.—Plenty of milk with white of eggs in it. If it is the sulphate give carbonate of soda. If excessive vomiting occurs, it can be relieved by copious draughts of warm water.

VOLATILE OILS.

ARTICLES.—Creasote, Dippel's animal oil, oil of tar, oil of tobacco, oil of turpentine, fusel oil.

SYMPTOMS.—Burning pain, vomiting, pungent taste, purging. The oils of tobacco and turpentine affect the nervous system, and will be recognized by their peculiar odor in the matter vomited.

TREATMENT.—Creasote is immediately coagulated by albumen, as milk, white of eggs. Dippel's animal oil may be counteracted by dilute sulphuric acid, and castor or linseed oil. For the others give milk, and promote vomiting, and probably some stimulant.

ALKALIES.

AMMONIA.—Spirits of hartshorn, muriate, or sal ammoniac.

POTASSA.—Caustic potash, liquor potassa, carbonate, or pearl ash, salts of tartar, nitrate, or saltpetre, or liver of sulphur.

SYMPTOMS.—Violent, caustic, acrid taste, great heat in throat, destruction of the mucous membrane of mouth and throat, cold sweats, weakness, hiccough, colic pains, bloody stools.

TREATMENT.—Vinegar, lemon juice, citric or tartaric acids. If the free alkalies are taken give castor or linseed oils, which will form soap in combination with them. For saltpetre give a mixture of acacia, marsh-mallow, flax-seed tea, and for liver of sulphur give common salt.

PRUSSIC ACID.

ARTICLES.—Oil of bitter almonds, laurel water, peach-kernels, cyanide of potassium, used by photographers.

SYMPTOMS.—If the quantity be large, death instantly ensues. In smaller quantities, nausea, giddiness, debility, weight and pain in the head.

TREATMENT.—Give spirits of hartshorn very much diluted, and apply a bottle of smelling-salts to the nose, dash cold water on the head, give stimulants, and make the patient stir about.

VEGETABLE POISONS.

OPIUM.

ARTICLES.—Laudanum, paregoric, black drop, soothing syrups, cordials, syrup of poppies, morphine, Dover's powder, etc.

SYMPTOMS.—Giddiness, stupor, gradually increasing to a deep sleep, pupil of the eyes very small, lips blue, skin cold, heavy, slow breathing.

TREATMENT.—Make the patient vomit as quickly as possible. If a full-grown person give fifteen grains of sulphate of zinc in a little water, to a young person half the quantity, to an infant a teaspoonful of syrup of ipecac. If these drugs cannot be had, use mustard and warm water, salt and water, and tickle the throat with a feather. After vomiting, give plenty of strong coffee, and place a mustard poultice round the calf of each leg, and if the patient is cold and sinking, give stimulants, and rouse him to walking or running by your assistance. Beat the soles of his feet, dash cold water on the face, and do anything to prevent him from sleeping until the effects are passed off, for if he goes to sleep, it is the sleep of death.

STRYCHNINE.

ARTICLES.—Rat poison, nux vomica, St. Ignatius' bean.

SYMPTOMS.—Lockjaw, twitching of the muscles, convulsions, the body is bent backwards, so as to rest on the feet and head only.

TREATMENT.—Empty the stomach by an emetic, then give linseed tea or barley water, and to an adult give thirty drops of laudanum, to relieve the spasms. A tea-spoonful of ether can also be given.

OTHER POISONOUS PLANTS, OR SEEDS,

Such as false mushrooms, belladonna, henbane, or anything a child may have eaten, or taken in mistake by any person. Vegetable poisons act either as an irritant, acro-narcotic, or narcotic. If it an irritant, the symptoms are an acrid, pungent taste, with more or less bitterness, excessive heat, great dryness of the mouth and throat, with sense of tightness there, violent vomiting, purging, with great pain in the stomach and bowels, breathing often quick and difficult, appearance of intoxication, eye frequently dilated, insensibility resembling death. The symptoms of narcotic poisons are described under opium.

TREATMENT.—If an irritant and vomiting does occur and continues, render it easier by large draughts of warm water, but if symptoms of insensibility have come on without vomiting, empty the stomach with any emetic that may be at hand,—sulphate of zinc, mustard; and after the operation of the emetic give a sharp purgative. After as much as is possible of the poison is got rid of, very strong coffee, or vinegar di-

20

luted with water, may be given with advantage. Camphor mixture with a little ether may be taken frequently, and if the insensibility is considerable, warmth, frictions, and blisters may be employed. For the narcotics proceed as in opium.

ANIMAL POISONS.

POISONOUS FISH.—Old wife, crawfish, land crab, gray snapper, hyne, dolphin, conger eel, mussel, barracuda, smooth bottle fish, grooper, rock fish, Spanish mackerel, king fish, bonetta, porgee, tunny, blower, etc.

SYMPTOMS.—In an hour or two, or much sooner after the fish has been eaten, a weight at the stomach comes, with slight vertigo and headache, sense of heat about the head and eyes, considerable thirst, and often an eruption of the skin resembling nettle rash.

TREATMENT.—Give a brisk emetic. After full vomiting an active purgative should be given. Vinegar and water may be drunk after the above remedies have operated, and the body may be sponged with the same. Water made very sweet with sugar, to which a little ether may be added, may also be drunk freely. If spasms occur, give laudanum.

POISONOUS SERPENTS.—Copperhead, moccasin, viper, black viper, rattlesnake, water viper.

SYMPTOMS.—A sharp pain in the wounded part, which soon extends over the limb or body; great swelling, at first hard and pale, then reddish, livid, and gangrenous in appearance, faintings, vomitings, convulsions, pulse small, breathing difficult, cold sweats, failing sight, and derangement of the intellectual faculties.

TREATMENT.—Tie a string tightly above the wound, wash it well, apply a cupping glass, or let the person bitten suck the wound well if he can. If lunar caustic or butter of antimony are at hand, rub them well in, to the very bottom of the wound, or take a very small poker, or a steel used for sharpening knives; make the point of this red hot—to a white heat, if you can—and press this for a moment into the wound. This is not such a dreadful operation as it seems to be, for one moment's application is sufficient, and, if the steel is really hot enough, gives scarcely any pain at the time. Small doses of hartshorn may also be given, and if gangrene is threatened, give wine freely. In case of rattlesnake bite, give whiskey freely. Bibron's antidote and the Tanjore Pills may also be used,—the latter carefully, as they contain arsenic.

POISONOUS INSECTS.—Spanish fly, potato fly.

SYMPTOMS.—Nauseous odor of the breath, acrid taste, burning heat in the throat, stomach, and abdomen, bloody vomiting, excruciating pain in the stomach, heat in the bladder, strangury or retention of urine, frightful convulsions.

TREATMENT.—Excite vomiting by giving sweet-oil, sugar and water, milk or linseed tea, very freely. Rub camphor dissolved in oil over the belly and thighs.

VENOMOUS INSECTS.—Tarantula, scorpion, hornet, wasp, bee, gnat, gad-fly.

SYMPTOMS.—In general, the sting of these insects occasions only a slight degree of pain and swelling, but occasionally the symptoms are more violent, and sickness and fever are produced by the intensity of the pain.

TREATMENT.—Hartshorn and oil may be rubbed on the affected part, and a piece of rag moistened with the same, or with salt and water, may be kept upon it till the pain is over. A few drops of hartshorn may also be frequently given internally, in a little water. The sting may in general be removed by making strong pressure with the barrel of a watch-key around it.

RABID ANIMALS.—See Hydrophobia, in its proper place among diseases.

RECIPES.

In the following pages will be found a variety of recipes, applicable to many diseases and afflictions for which symptomatic treatment is all that is required. They will be found to be very valuable for domestic treatment. They are not all strictly herbal, but essentially eclectic, so as to be easily prepared and the ingredients readily procured. Nothing capable of harm is, however, admitted,—the few mineral substances that are prescribed being only inserted for therapeutic effects, in consequence of their vegetable analogues being hard to procure or difficult to prepare. Availability was studied more than scientific arrangement, though the merit of each is retained. For handy recipes, therefore, the following are sufficiently diversified for a wide range of application.

In complicated cases, or in diseases requiring systematic treatment, recipes are not to be depended upon. Such cases, of course, require treatment in accordance with the demands of the pathological conditions observed in the disease, and which should in all cases be directed by a competent physician. The remedies, for which the recipes are given in this connection, are designed merely for diseases or affections not ordinarily grave in character, or which do not require more than simple medication. Those desiring to make use of them should have them prepared by a druggist, if they do not have the necessary pharmaceutical appliances to insure correct weight, quantity, mixture, division, etc. The purity and worth of the article are also to be ascertained before being administered.

GOLDEN TINCTURE.

No. 1. Balsam of tolu, two ounces; gum guaiacum, two ounces; gum hemlock, two ounces; gum myrrh, two ounces; each coarsely powdered; oil of hemlock, three ounces; oil of wintergreen, two ounces; alcohol, one gallon. Let it stand fourteen days. Shake frequently in the meantime.

Dose.—From one to two teaspoonfuls, according to severity and obstinacy of the case, in half a glass of sweetened water. This mixture has proved highly useful as an internal remedy for rheumatism, colic, pains, chills, soreness, lameness, sour stomach, languor, depressed spirits, palpitations, water brash, flatulency, and a variety of painful affections.

PULMONARY REMEDY.

No. 2. Take of the roots of spikenard, elecampane, comfrey and blood-root: of the leaves and flowers of hoarhound, and of the bark of wild cherry, each one pound. These may all be ground and tinctured, by adding alcohol, water, and sugar sufficient to make three gallons of syrup, or any portion of the above compound may be tinctured in sufficient alcohol to cover them, when the herbs may be boiled until their strength is obtained, and the tincture and watery infusion may be mixed, and a sufficient amount of refined sugar added to make a thick syrup. For coughs and colds, to be taken in teaspoonful doses as required.

LIVER CORDIAL.

No. 3. Thorough-wort, two ounces; ginger, half ounce; cloves, half ounce; extract dandelion, four ounces; water, one and a half pints. Boil to one-third, and add sugar one and one-half pounds, and brandy, one pint.

Dose.—A wineglassful once or twice a day. An excellent cordial cathartic to act upon the liver. The herbs must be gathered at the proper season or they will be worthless.

ANTI-BILIOUS PILL.

No. 4. Aloes, pulverized, five ounces; fine, dry castile soap, half a drachm; gamboge, pulverized, one ounce; colocynth, one ounce; extract of gentian, one ounce; mandrake, one ounce; cayenne pepper, two ounces; oil of peppermint, half a drachm. Mix well together, and form into three-grain pills.

Dose.—Three to five pills.

AN EXPECTORANT.

No. 5. For asthma and cough, to promote expectoration, and remove tightness of the chest, the following is a valuable compound preparation. Fluid extracts of skunk cabbage, one ounce; lobelia, one ounce; blood-root, one ounce; pleurisy-root, one ounce; ginger, one ounce; water, one pint; alcohol, three pints.

Dose.—Two to four teaspoonfuls. (See Fluid Extracts, page 475.)

FOR PRODUCING SLEEP.

No. 6. The following is a useful preparation for producing sleep, in wakeful or excited conditions, viz.: fluid extract of ladies' slipper, one ounce; fluid extract of pleurisy-root, one ounce; fluid extract of skunk cabbage, one ounce; fluid extract scull-cap, one ounce. Mix.

Dose.—Half a drachm to a drachm three times a day.

FOR SICK AND NERVOUS HEADACHE.

No. 7. For sick-and nervous headache, dependent on an acid stomach, the following is useful: fluid extract of ladies' slipper, half an ounce; fluid extract of catnip, half an ounce; fluid extract of scull-cap, half an ounce; water, one pint.

Dose.—One to three teaspoonfuls. Mix.

TONIC TINCTURE.

No. 8. Old cider, four gallons; white oak bark, ten ounces; horse-radish root, one pound; seneca snake-root, six ounces; golden seal root, four ounces; cayenne pepper, two ounces; bruise all fine, add the cider, let stand for ten days, frequently shaking up the mixture in the meantime.

Dose.—For an adult, half to two-thirds of a wine-glassful, three times a day.

SARSAPARILLA SYRUP.

No. 9. Good sarsaparilla, two pounds; guaiacum, three ounces; rose leaves, two ounces; senna, two ounces; liquorice root, two ounces; oil of sassafras, five drops; oil of aniseed, five drops; oil of wintergreen, three drops; diluted alcohol, ten pints; sugar, eight pounds.

Dose.—A tablespoonful two or three times a day.

RHEUMATIC TINCTURE.

No. 10. Peppermint water, one and one-half ounces; wine of colchicum root, half an ounce; sulphate of morphia, one grain; magnesia, one scruple.

Dose.—One teaspoonful three or four times a day.

FOR BRONCHITIS.

No. 11. Tannin, three grains; extract of belladonna, three-fourths of a grain; extract of conium, two and a half grains; infusion of senna, three ounces; fennel water, one and a half ounces; syrup of marsh-mallow, one and a half ounces. Mix.

Dose.—A tablespoonful to be taken every two hours in chronic bronchitis.

COMPOUND SPIRITS OF LAVENDER.

No. 12. Dried lavender flowers, two drachms; nutmeg, 2 drachms; mace, two drachms; cloves, two ounces; cinnamon, two ounces. Pulverize all these, and add a quart of spirits. Let it then stand for a week, and then strain off the liquid.

Dose.—One or two teaspoonfuls may be taken often in a little water, with loaf sugar. Useful in nervous affections.

NERVE TONIC.

No. 13. Extract of scull-cap, two drachms; extract of chamomile, two drachms; extract of boneset, one drachm; pulverized cayenne, one scruple; quinine, one drachm; oil of valerian, half a drachm. Beat well together, and make ninety pills.

Dose.—For an adult, one pill every two or three hours.

STOMACHIC BITTERS.

No. 14. Gentian root, two ounces; dried orange peel, one ounce; cardamon seed, half an ounce (all bruised); diluted alcohol or common whiskey, one quart. Let it stand for two weeks.

Use.—Dyspepsia, loss of appetite, general weakness, etc.

Dose.—One or two tablespoonfuls in water, three times a day.

FEVER AND AGUE.

No. 15. Take of boneset, two ounces; b.ue vervain, two ounces; scull-cap, one ounce; Virginia snake-root, half an ounce. Make an infusion, and drink freely while warm. If it produces vomiting, reduce the dose. This will be found highly beneficial. If the bowels are constipated, use one of my " Renovating Pills" every night until all constipation has been removed or remedied.

STRENGTHENING PLASTER.

No. 16. Resin, one pound; beeswax, one ounce; Burgundy pitch, one ounce; mutton tallow, one ounce. Melt them together, and add olive oil, pulverized camphor and sassafras oil, of each one-sixteenth of an ounce, and West India rum, one fluid ounce. Stir well together, pour into cold water, and form into rolls with the hands; spread with a knife on a piece of linen cloth, and apply in weakness of the joints, rheumatism, weak chest, weak back, ulcers. This is an excellent plaster for all such purposes.

ACETIC BLOOD-ROOT SYRUP.

No. 17. Blood-root in powder, one drachm; acetic acid, or vinegar, one pint; water, one pint. Add the blood-root to the vinegar and water mixed, and steep for two hours; then strain and add two pounds of white sugar, simmer until a syrup is formed.

This is a *specific* remedy for pseudo-membranous croup. It is also used in infantile pneumonia and bronchitis, but the "Acacian Balsam" should be used with it.

Dose.—For croup, from half a teaspoonful to a tablespoonful, but it should not be given in quantities sufficient to provoke vomiting, unless there is imminent danger of suffocation, and then only sufficient to eject the mucus adhering to the upper part of the bronchia and trachea.

A GOOD EMETIC.

No. 18. Pulverized lobelia, one ounce; pulverized blood-root, one ounce; pulv. ipecacuanha, six drachms; pulv. cayenne, four scruples; seneca, one scruple. Mix. An excellent emetic in all cases where one is required. My "Renovating Pills" should be used to cleanse the system of all remaining particles of lobelia.

Dose.—Half a teaspoonful in a cup of warm water, and repeat every fifteen minutes until it operates.

NERVE TONIC AND ANTISPASMODIC.

No. 19. High cranberry bark, one ounce; skunk cabbage-root, half an ounce; scull-cap, half an ounce; cardamon seeds, two drachms; pulv. cayenne, two drachms. Put these into a pint of wine. Shake it well every day for three or four days.

Dose.—A tablespoonful four times a day.

DYSENTERY SYRUP.

No. 20. Best Turkey rhubarb, two drachms; leptandrin, two drachms; white sugar, one pound; hot water, one pint. Triturate well together; add essence of peppermint, one drachm; essence of anise, one drachm; tincture of catechu, two drachms.

Dose.—For dysentery, one teaspoonful every half hour.

COUGH PREPARATION.

No. 21. Tincture of lobelia, half an ounce; tincture of blood-root, two ounces; oil of spearmint, half a drachm; molasses, five ounces.

Dose.—Take one-half of a teaspoonful as often as needed. Useful merely as a palliative.

PULMONARY SYRUP.

No. 22. Spikenard root, sixteen ounces; white root, sixteen ounces; blood-root, eight ounces; elecampane, eight ounces; colts-foot, eight ounces; boneset, eight ounces; poplar bark, four ounces; seneca snake-root, two ounces; lobelia, two ounces; slippery elm bark, eight ounces; proof spirits, three gallons. Bruise or pulverize all, and digest in the spirits for fourteen days; then strain, and add white sugar sufficient to form a syrup.

Dose.—A tablespoonful occasionally, in a mucilage of slippery elm.

Use.—This is a fair relief in all coughs and pulmonary affections.

CHRONIC DISEASES OF THE MUCOUS SURFACES.

No. 23. Hard balsam copaiba, three and a half drachms; fresh ground cubebs, three and a half drachms; carbonate of ammonia, one drachm. Make one hundred pills.

Dose.—One pill three times a day, between meals.

LINIMENT FOR CHILBLAINS.

No. 24. Sulphuric acid, one drachm; spirits of turpentine, one drachm; olive oil, three drachms. Mix the oil and turpentine first, then gradually add the sulphuric acid.
A valuable liniment for chilblains. To be rubbed on two or three times a day.

LINIMENT FOR NEURALGIA, ETC.

No. 25. Sweet oil, one ounce; water of ammonia, strong, one ounce. Mix. To be rubbed on with a piece of flannel. A temporary relief for crick in the neck, and rheumatic and neuralgic pains.

SLEEPLESSNESS.

No. 26. Camphor, one grain, formed into a pill, followed by a draught of an ounce and a half of the infusion of hops, with five drops of sulphuric ether.

CHRONIC RHEUMATISM.

No. 27. The remedies given below will be found generally useful:
First.—Warm salt bath. When the pain is very severe at night, take tincture of guaiacum, one drachm; tincture of aloes, half a drachm; spirits of turpentine, thirty drops. Mix, and take in a pint of gruel at bedtime.
Second.—Should the pains continue very severe, give the following: Aloes, half a scruple; opium, three grains; syrup of buckthorn sufficient to form a pill mass. Mix, and make three pills; one at bedtime.
Third.—Compound powder of ipecacuanha, eight grains; camphor mixture, one and a half ounces. Mix, and give a draught every night.
Fourth.—Take wine of colchicum seeds, one ounce; give from ten to twenty drops in gruel or water three times a day, with one of the following pills: sulphate of quinia, twenty-four grains; and syrup sufficient to form into twelve pills; *or:*
Fifth.—Iodide of potassium, one drachm; distilled water, two ounces.
Mix, and give a teaspoonful in a wine-glass of water—morning, noon, and night. This seldom ever fails to give relief.

REMEDY FOR BOWEL COMPLAINT.

No. 28. Rhubarb, pulverized, one ounce; saleratus, one teaspoonful; pour on a pint of boiling water. When cold, add a tablespoonful of essence of peppermint.
Dose.—From one to three tablespoonfuls two or three times a day.

WORM MIXTURE.

No. 29. Populin, one drachm; santonine, twenty grains; tincture of pink root, four ounces; neutralizing mixture, one pint. Rub the santonine in the neutralizing mixture, until thoroughly mixed, then add the other ingredients. Excellent for removing worms in children.
Dose.—From thirty to forty drops every half hour, until it acts on the bowels as a purge. If the worms are not removed, repeat every two or three days; but be cautious to get *good* pink root, as much of the plant sold for pink root by the druggists is poisonous. This is inferior, however, to my "Male Fern Vermifuge," see page 471.

PAINFUL MENSTRUATION.

No. 30. Extract of hyoscyamus, gum camphor, and Dover's powder, of each one scruple. Mix, and make into twenty pills.
Dose.—One pill twice a day for painful menstruation.

STOMACH PILL.

No. 31.—Pulverized rhubarb, and guaiacum, of each eight grains; galbanum, two grains; ipecacuanha, two grains. Mix, and make eight pills.
Dose.—Take one or two pills, night and morning. Excellent for a weak stomach, and a bilious condition.

BRONCHIAL TROCHES. (*For Temporary Relief.*)

No. 32. Extract of liquorice, one pound; sugar, one and a half pounds; cubebs, four ounces; gum arabic, four ounces; all pulverized; extract of conium, one ounce. Mix, and take a piece as big as a pea and dissolve it in the mouth, several times a day; rubbing the neck three times a day with the "Herbal Ointment."

DIARRHŒA.

No. 33.   Syrup of orange peel, one ounce; acetate of morphia, two grains; tincture of cinnamon, six drachms; tincture of cardamon, two drachms.   Mix.
Dose.—A teaspoonful.   Valuable in diarrhœa.

NEURALGIA.

No. 34.   Tincture of American hellebore, one drachm; tincture of black cohosh, two ounces.   Mix.
Dose.—One teaspoonful, from three to six times a day.

PILE OINTMENT.

No. 35.   Extract of stramonium, one ounce; extract of tobacco, one ounce; tannin, ten grains.   Make an ointment, and bathe or lubricate the parts, if you cannot at once get the "Herbal Ointment."

STOMACHIC PILL.

No. 36.   Powdered cayenne pepper, one drachm; rhubarb, two drachms.   Make into a mass with syrup, and divide into sixty pills.
Dose.—Two to three every day, an hour before dinner.

AROMATIC BITTERS.   (*Stimulant.*)

No. 37.   *First.*—ABSINTHIUM (*Wormwood*).   Infuse three drachms in twenty ounces of water.
Dose.—From a half to two tablespoonfuls.
Use.—In debilitated state of the digestive organs.
Second.—ACORUS—Calamus (*Sweet flag root*).   Infuse one ounce in twenty ounces of water.   Joined with other tonics.
Use.—In uneasiness from flatulence.

TONIC TEA.   (*Debility.*)

No. 38.   Chamomile, scull-cap, and queen of the meadow, each one pound.   Reduce them to powder, and mix well together.
Dose.—To one tablespoonful of this powder add one pint of water; make a tea, and drink during the day.   This is a good tonic in all cases of debility.

SPICED BITTERS.   (*For weak patients.*)

No. 39.   Poplar bark, ten pounds; bayberry bark, two pounds; balmony bark, two pounds; golden seal, one pound; cloves, one pound; cayenne pepper, half a pound; loaf sugar, sixteen pounds.
Let these articles all be made fine and well mixed.   Put a tablespoonful of this compound, with four ounces of sugar, into a quart of boiling water.   Take a wineglassful three times a day before eating, or a teaspoonful of these powders may be taken in a cup of hot water, half an hour before each meal.

TONIC.   (*For Chlorosis, or Green Sickness.*)

No. 40.   Sulphate of quinia, fifteen grains; diluted sulphuric acid, fifteen drops; compound tincture of cardamon, three drachms; tincture of hops, three drachms; compound infusion of roses, six ounces.   Mix.
Dose.—A teaspoonful two or three times a day.

WHOOPING COUGH MIXTURE.

No. 41.   Tincture of blood-root, one ounce; tincture of red root, two ounces; tincture of black cohosh, one ounce; tincture of lobelia, half an ounce; tincture of belladonna, twenty drops.   Mix, and shake well before using.
Dose.—For a child one year old, fifteen or twenty drops in sweetened water.   The fluid extracts (see page 475) can be used instead of the tinctures.   Dose, when fluid extracts are used, three to five drops.

TINCTURE FOR FEVER AND AGUE, ETC.

No. 42.   Peruvian bark and wild cherry bark, each two ounces; cinnamon, cloves, and nutmeg, each one drachm; wine, two quarts.   Let it stand for a few days to extract the strength.
Dose.—A wineglassful every two or three hours.
Use.—A very good remedy for intermittent fever, or fever and ague, after suitable evacuants.   It frequently removes the disease when all other means fail.

ANTI-SPASMODICS.

MISTURA CAMPHORÆ. (*Aqua Camphora, U. S.*)

No. 43. *First.*—Camphor, two drachms; alcohol, forty drops; carbonate magnesia, four drachms; distilled water, two pints.

Dose.—One to two tablespoonfuls.

Use.—In typhoid conditions, with delirium, for after pains. TINCT. CAMPHORÆ COMP. (*Paragoric Elix., Tinct. Opii Camph.*).

Second.—Pulverized opium, one drachm; benzoic acid, one drachm; oil of aniseed, one drachm; sugar, two ounces; camphor, two scruples; diluted alcohol, two pints. Macerate for fourteen days. Half a drachm contains less than one grain of opium.

Dose.—For infants, from five to twenty drops; adults, one to two tablespoonfuls.

Use.—To allay cough or nausea, to check diarrhœa, to relieve pain.

MOSCHUS. Preputial secretion of the musk animal.

Dose and *Form.*—Five to ten grains, in pill, bolus, or emulsion.

Use.—Hiccough, epilepsy, asthma, cough, palpitation.

TONIC AND CATHARTIC.

No. 44. Aloes, gentian, orange peel, juniper berries, and bruised aniseed, each one ounce; gin, one pint. Mix. Macerate for two weeks, and then strain.

Dose.—A tablespoonful once or twice a day. Good for bilious habits.

DISCUTIENT OINTMENT.

(*For scrofulous and glandular tumors.*)

No. 45. Bark of bitter-sweet root, stramonium leaves, cicuta leaves, deadly nightshade, and yellow dock root, each two ounces; lard, one pound. Bruise and simmer the roots and leaves in spirits; then add the lard, and simmer till the ingredients are crisped or thickened into an ointment.

FOR SUPPRESSION OF URINE IN CHILDREN.

No. 46. Oil of solidago, one drachm; alcohol, eight drachms.

Dose.—From five to twenty drops on sugar at a dose, to be repeated at suitable intervals. Proportionably larger doses of this are also very beneficial for flatulence, faintness, etc., in adults.

GARGLES.

No. 47. *First.*—Raspberry leaves, geranium, blackberry root, and leptandria root, each ounce. Mix, and make three pints of strong decoction. Suitable for a gargle.

Second.—Geranium, golden-seal, marsh-mallow, wild indigo root, and rosemary, each half an ounce. Mix, and make one pint of strong infusion. After straining, add two drachms of powdered borax, and one gill of honey. An excellent astringent gargle.

HONEY BALSAM.

No. 48. Balsam of tolu, balsam of fir, each two ounces; opium, two drachms. Dissolve all three in one quart of alcohol.

Dose.—A teaspoonful occasionally. Valuable for the relief of pulmonary diseases.

ANTI-DYSENTERY CORDIAL.

No. 49. Birch bark and peach pits, each two pounds; bayberry bark, half a pound; wild cherry bark, one pound; water, two gallons. Boil down to one and a half gallons, after which add a gallon of good brandy, and loaf sugar sufficient to make it palatable.

Dose.—A wineglassful three or four times a day.

FOR GRAVEL, DROPSY, ETC.

No. 50. Queen of the meadow, milk weed, juniper berries, dwarf elder, spearmint, wild carrot seed, of each two ounces. Put all in a mortar and bruise, and boil the whole in a gallon of water, till half a gallon of the liquid is left, and then strain.

Dose.—Half a pint of the decoction is to be taken several times during the day.

COUGH SYRUP.

No. 51. Acetate of morphia, four grains; tincture of blood-root, two drachms; antimonial wine, three drachms; ipecacuanha, three drachms; syrup of wild cherry, three ounces. Mix.

Dose.—A teaspoonful two or three times a day.

20*

FOR DYSMENORRHŒA.

No. 52. Viburnin, aulophyllin, each one scruple; gelsemin, five grains. Mix, and divide into ten powders. *Dose.*—One every two hours until relieved.

FOR DIARRHŒA.

No. 53. Tincture of catechu, half an ounce; spirits of camphor, tincture of myrrh, and tincture of cayenne, each two drachms. Mix.
Dose.—From half a teaspoonful to a teaspoonful in diarrhœa.

INJECTION.

No. 54. Castor oil, one gill; pulv. cayenne, ten grains; table salt, one teaspoonful; molasses, one gill; warm water, one pint. Inject.

FOR THE BLUES, OR LOW SPIRITS.

No. 55. A pleasant cordial for low spirits is the following: aniseed, four drachms; oil of angelica, one drachm; oil of cassia, forty drops; oil of caraway, thirty drops; proof spirits, two gallons. Mix well.
Dose.—Half a tablespoonful in water.

SKIN DISEASES WITH MUCH IRRITATION.

No. 56. Decoctions of bitter-sweet and mallows, of each half a pint; mix, and make a liniment. Use the " Renovating Pills " internally.

CHILBLAIN OINTMENT.

No. 57. Lard, two quarts; turpentine, one pint; camphor, quarter of a pound. Rub into the parts. This will be found a capital remedy.

ACIDITY OF THE STOMACH.

No. 58. Hard wood ashes, one quart; common soot, half a gill; water, six pints. Digest, settle, and filter.
Dose.—Take one tablespoonful three times a day in acidity of the stomach.

HEMORRHOIDS. PILES.

No. 59. Opium, one scruple; pulverized nut-galls, one drachm; ointment althæa. Mix, and anoint the parts.

SORE THROAT.

No. 60. Those subject to sore throat should make a wash of warm water, in which wood ashes have been dissolved, and apply externally every morning. The "Herbal Ointment" should be applied at night, and well rubbed in. If the disease has become permanent or chronic, the "Acacian Balsam " must be used according to directions. (See page 470.)

INJECTION FOR COSTIVENESS.

No. 61. Castor oil, two ounces; tincture of prickly ash bark, half an ounce; compound tincture of Virginia snake root, two drachms; infusion of boneset and senna, equal parts, half a pint. Mix, and inject. It is by no means, however, as good as the "Renovating Pills." See page 473.

TO PRODUCE PERSPIRATION.

No. 62. Blood-root, golden-seal, sumach berries, bayberry bark, of each two drachms; all pulverized. Mix.
Dose.—Make an infusion in a pint of hot water, and give a tablespoonful every half hour.

POULTICE FOR A FESTER.

No. 63. Boil bread in the settlings of strong beer; apply the poultice in the common manner. This has saved many an hour of suffering.

CATAPLASMS, OR POULTICES.

No. 64. May be made by moistening bread crumbs with milk. They may also be made of flaxseed, roasted onions, snake-root, hops, etc.
Poultices are useful in nearly all cases of local inflammation.

TOOTHACHE.

No. 65. Gum opium, gum camphor, spirits of turpentine, each one scruple. Rub in a mortar to a paste. Put it in the hollow tooth.

Use.—This will cure and even prevent the toothache.

A FRAGRANT BREATH.

No. 66. Take sherry wine, one gill; ground cloves and grated nutmeg, each one drachm; cinnamon and bruised caraway seeds, each a quarter of an ounce. Place all these dry substances into the wine or spirits, in a half pint bottle, and let them stand for several days, shaking the bottle every night and morning. Strain off the tincture through linen to get it bright, then add about ten drops of lavender, or five drops of the otto of roses.

A few drops on a lump of sugar dissolved in the mouth, will secure a breath of flowers.

It may be also used with advantage on the toothbrush, in lieu of tooth powder, or, mixed with water, it makes an excellent gargle.

FOOT BATH.

No. 67. A bucket of warm water; pulv. cayenne pepper, one tablespoonful; ground mustard, two tablespoonfuls. Mix.

Use.—As a foot bath in suppression of menses.

TO IMPROVE THE VOICE.

No. 68. Beeswax, two drachms; balsam of copaiba, three drachms; powdered liquorice root, four drachms. Melt the copaiba with the wax in a new earthen pipkin. When they are melted, remove them from the fire, and, while in a liquid state, mix in the powdered liquorice.

Make pills of three grains each. Two of these pills to be taken occasionally, or three or four times a day if necessary.

Use.—This is a good remedy for clearing and cleaning the voice, and is much used by professional singers.

HEADACHE. NEURALGIC PAINS.

No. 69. Take of opodeldoc, spirits of wine, sal ammoniac, equal parts, and apply like any other lotion.

STINGS.

No. 70. Bind on the place a thick plaster of common salt or saleratus moistened; it will soon extract the venom.

A STOMACHIC.

No. 71. Fresh ground cubebs.

Dose. From five to twenty grains.

Use.—As a stomachic in disorders of the digestive organs.

FOR FEVERS AND OTHER ACUTE DISEASES.

No. 72. Asclepin, one-half drachm; warm water, four ounces; compound tincture of American hellebore, thirty drops. Dissolve the asclepin in the warm water, and afterwards add the hellebore.

Dose.—From one to three teaspoonfuls once in every two hours as long as the fever is raging. If nausea occurs, omit the medicine until it subsides. Shake the mixture well before using.

OFFENSIVE BREATH.

No. 73. Solution chlorinated of soda, six drops; water, two ounces. Mix.

Use. A sure remedy for an offensive breath emanating from a deranged stomach.

ANTIDOTE FOR RATTLESNAKE POISON.

No. 74. The *Medical Journal* says the following is an infallible cure for the poison of a rattlesnake bite. Iodide of potass, four grains; corrosive sublimate, two grains; bromine, five drachms. Mix together, and keep the mixture in a glass-stoppered vial, well secured.

Dose.—Ten drops of this mixture, diluted with a tablespoonful of brandy, constitutes a dose. The quantity to be repeated, if necessary, according to the exigencies of the case.

FOR CANCER.

No. 75. Take equal parts of fresh poke-weed, yellow dock, and blood-root; evaporate the juice by the means of a sand bath to the consistency of tar. The ointment should be applied, after the cuticle has been removed by a blister, three times a day. The parts should be washed with good French brandy after each application of the ointment. Before this is used, the advice of a physician should first be secured.

FOR HIP DISEASE.

No. 76. Take of iodine, one ounce; phosphate of lime, two ounces; water, one pint. Dissolve the iodine and lime in the water, and add twenty grains of tannin. Inject with a small syringe three or four times a day.

Use.—A valuable injection in hip disease, where the head of the bone is decayed.

FOR BRUISES.

No. 77. Take pulv. slippery elm and pulv. indigo weed, each one pound; gum myrrh, half a pound; pulv. prickly ash, a quarter of a pound. Wet with good brewer's yeast and apply. A very good poultice for bruises.

FOR DIPHTHERIA.

No. 78. Saturated tincture of scrophularia, one drachm, added to half a tumbler of water.

Triturated macrotin, twenty grains, added to a tumblerful of water.

Dose.—One teaspoonful of each every hour.

GARGLE FOR THE ELONGATION OF THE UVULA.

No. 79. Fluid extract of rhus, one drachm; fluid extract of bayberry, two drachms; water, two ounces. Mix, and gargle the throat three or four times a day. Also bathe the throat upon the outside in strong salt and water. (See fluid extracts, page 475.)

FOR BILIOUS COLIC.

No. 80. Fluid extract of wild yam, two ounces; fluid extract of pleurisy root, one ounce. Mix, and take a teaspoonful as often as is required.

TO REMOVE WARTS AND CORNS.

No. 81. Apply the juice of the leaves of the great celandine or tetter-wort, and keep applying until the fungous growth is removed.

FOR THE TEETH.

No. 82. Make charcoal of bread, pulverize it until it is reduced to an impalpable powder, then apply daily, morning and evening, with a soft brush and pure cold water.

Use.—This will keep the teeth white, and cure diseases of the gums.

A GOOD MEDICATED WINE.

No. 83. Take of powdered colchicum seed, two ounces; of sherry wine, twelve fluid ounces. Put them together in a close glass bottle, and let them stand for fourteen days, giving a good shaking every day. Filter through a fine muslin cloth, and drink as required.

INJECTION FOR ASIATIC CHOLERA.

No. 84. Take of water, one fluid ounce; tincture of prickly ash berries, one fluid drachm; tincture of opium, twenty drops. Mix together. Inject in ordinary quantity until the desired effect has been produced.

BLEEDING AT THE NOSE.

No. 85. Powder of rhatany (for internal use), ten grains.

FOR OLD ULCERS.

No. 86. Take of red chickweed, which is common both in America and Europe, the leaves and flowers, and apply in the form of a poultice, frequently changing them.

DR. O. PHELPS BROWN'S

STANDARD HERBAL REMEDIES.

BELOW will be found a list of Herbal Remedies that have stood the most crucial tests for years, by which their efficacy has been incontestably proven, and their great and deserved popularity established. Their prominence of virtues and popularity have been gained in consequence of being compounded only with the view to having the greatest concentration of curative properties for the diseases they are designed to cure that the profoundest medical skill is able to suggest, and prepared exclusively from herbs selected in localities best calculated for the development of their medicinal properties. Every herbal constituent, before selection, is subjected to a careful analysis, in order to ascertain the precise quantity of medicinal properties, thus enabling me to prepare these remedies of uniform strength, and endowing them with the highest excellence of curative properties. These remedies are in every way superior, and the use of them by invalids is recommended because of their manifest superiority. In these Remedies they will find positive cures for numberless ills, and the supreme confidence with which they are recommended as unfailing specifics is justified by the universal success they have achieved in a countless number of cases where everything else had failed. In brief, they need but an adequate trial to manifest their restorative and health-giving properties.

These medicines can be procured from all respectable druggists throughout the world. They can also be had from the author by remitting price, on receipt of which he will send them by express.

THE RESTORATIVE ASSIMILANT.

PRICE—$2 *per pint bottle;* $5 *for three bottles.*

This invaluable remedy is a distilled compound, composed of blue-vervain, water pepper, chamomile, etc., and constitutes one of the triumphs of pharmaceutical science. It is an unfailing remedy for EPILEPSY or Fits, curing even the most hopeless cases. A cure has been effected in every case in which a proper trial was given to the medicine. It is none the less effectual in Dyspepsia, for which disease it is an actual specific. It speedily cures all bowel complaints, instantly checking diarrhœa, dysentery, and has given great success in cholera. It is also the best remedy ever discovered for all liver complaints, kidney diseases, diabetes, gravel, weak nerves, general debility, etc., etc., etc.

Testimonials. —COLLINS BROS., wholesale druggists, St. Louis, Mo., say : "Your Restorative Assimilant sells very rapidly. Its universal and astonishing success in curing epilepsy, dyspepsia, etc., exceeds everything we have ever known or expected from any medicine.' Joseph P. Day, Cassville, Geo., writes : "I would have sixty or seventy epileptic spasms, and once had *fifty-two* inside of four hours, all of which were so severe as to nearly kill me. I sent for some of your Restorative Assimilant, Herbal Ointment, and Renovating Pills, which quickly cured me. I have not had a fit during the past eighteen months." Mary P. Driver, Washington, Pa., says : "I will write you again, and take pleasure in informing you that your Restorative Assimilant has cured me of my very bad case of dyspepsia that I have had for *twelve years.*" John S. King, Cincinnati, Ohio, writes : "My gratitude obliges me to inform you that your Restorative Assimilant has radically cured me of diabetes, which was pronounced hopeless by *sixteen* physicians of this city, whom I had previously consulted."

THE ACACIAN BALSAM.

PRICE—$1 *per bottle ;* $5 *for six bottles.*

This is a highly concentrated compound fluid-extract of Aya-pana, Indian Hemp plant, Coca, Nicaya, Lungwort, etc., rendered highly agreeable with the addition of Paraguayan Wild Honey. This unsurpassed remedy affords speedy Relief and Permanent Cure of Consumption, Bronchitis, Asthma, Coughs, Colds, all Diseases of the Lungs, Chest, and Throat. The cures this great remedy performs exceed the most sanguine expectations, and no one should fail to give it a proper trial, if suffering from some disease of the pulmonary organs.

Testimonials. —SETH S. HANCE, wholesale druggist, Baltimore, Md., says : "I have yet to hear that your Balsam has failed to give entire satisfaction in every case that it has been tried ; and, furthermore, the most miraculous cures of consumption, bronchitis, etc., from its use, are constantly reported to me." Abram Shoemaker, Conesville, N. Y., writes : "Having for years suffered with catarrh in its worst form, for which every remedy as well as the treatment of several eminent physicians failed, I was induced by a friend to try your Acacian Balsam, and I am happy to say that I am now entirely free from the disease, and firmly believe permanently cured." Dr. John Maxwell, M.D., Lime Lake, Ontario, says : "I have used your Balsam in my practice with perfect success in all cases of consumption, asthma, bronchitis, etc." Samuel Wellman, Bethlehem, Conn., writes : "I was pronounced hopelessly consumpted by all physicians whom I consulted, and when I first commenced taking your Acacian Balsam, I myself expected to live but a few days, but I commenced to improve very rapidly, and in a few months was strong and healthy." James P. Lindstrom, Chisago Lake, Minn., writes: "I am living testimony to the great value of your Balsam. For two years past I have been unable to speak on account of bronchitis, but the Balsam quickly cured the bronchial affection, and my voice is now perfectly strong."

THE BLOOD PURIFIER.

PRICE—$1.00 *per bottle ;* $5.00 *for six bottles.*

This is a compound extract of rock rose, stillingia, etc., and is the best alterative and depurative ever discovered. It is an unfailing cure for scrofula, syphilis, skin diseases, ulcers, sores, glandular swellings, and all other affections owing their existence to depravity of the blood, and derangement of the lymphatic system. It thoroughly eradicates at once and forever every contaminating element in the system, and as a special and positive antidote to all blood-poisoning material, it is not only unequalled, but far superior to any other known remedy.

Testimonials.—JOHN D. PARK, wholesale druggist, Cincinnati, O., writes: "I have for many years sold every kind of prepared remedies, but the praises bestowed upon your Blood Purifier by all who have used it, convinces me that in point of virtue it far surpasses every remedy I have ever sold. Its sales are immense." Winslow N. Bennett, Pembroke, Me., says: "I was for many years troubled with salt rheum, which lately became so bad that I was obliged to quit work. I took your Blood Purifier, and I wish you could see me now. I have not the least symptom of the disease now, nor has it shown itself during the past year." Miss Sarah K. Chester, Lynchburg, Va., testifies that she has been cured by the Blood Purifier of a very bad case of hereditary scrofula of twenty years' standing. James Foster, Keokuk, Iowa, writes: "My syphilitic affection, which had become tertiary, has been so effectually cured by your Blood Purifier, that I am satisfied not a vestige remains in my system."

THE MALE FERN VERMIFUGE.

PRICE—50 *cents per bottle.*

This is a syrupized compound fluid extract of male fern, pinkroot, kousso, etc., and warranted to expel every species of worms from the intestinal canal almost instantly. It is just as deadly to the dreadful tape-worm as it is to the round, pin, or thread worm, and is the only vermifuge known that is so positively destructive to all worms, and yet so perfectly harmless to the human subject. It causes no disturbance of the system, is safe to use, and pleasant to take. The wholesale houses consider this vermifuge superior to any they have ever sold.

Testimonials.—Mrs. JAMES VAN VLEET, Newark, N. J., writes: "I gave my little daughter, who for years was troubled with worms, but two doses of your Male Fern Vermifuge, and she expelled in two evacu·ations, *one hundred and eighty-four worms.*" Peter Moore, Troy, N. Y., writes: "The tape-worm with which I was troubled for many years is no more, thanks to the virtue of your Male Fern Vermifuge. I took four doses of the vermifuge, and three days ago, I discharged the miserable pest, which was forty-eight feet long." Simon K. Percival, Lexington, Ky., says: "I cannot too highly extol the efficacy of your Male Fern Vermifuge. It relieved me like magic of the seat worms, which for years greatly troubled me." Mrs. Sarah A. Beard, Albany, N. Y., writes: "My younger children were all troubled with worms, and nothing that I could give would be of benefit, until I finally tried your vermifuge, which, I must say, proved efficacious—relieving each one very quickly."

THE HERBAL OINTMENT.

PRICE—50 *cents per pot. When ordered by mail, Four cents additional must be sent for each pot to prepay postage.*

This ointment is composed of the extractive virtues of bitter sweet, skunk cabbage, green ozier, lobelia, etc., making it the most elegant and efficacious ointment that the pharmaceutic art is capable of producing. It is capable of a wide range of application, and as an external remedy it can never be equalled in point of virtue. It speedily cures all inflammations, all lung and heart complaints, swellings, croup, ulcers, tumors, abscesses, wens, cuts, wounds, burns, skin diseases, in fact every disorder arising from inflammation, morbid nutrition, etc. It is used in practice by the best physicians in the world, and its praises daily to be heard from those who have tested its great and manifold virtues are almost too remarkable for credence. Its most wondrous efficacy is particularly exhibited in all lung and heart diseases, relieving all pain quickly, and curing them in a short space of time.

Testimonials.—LORD & SMITH, wholesale druggists, Chicago, Ills., write: "Send us at once fifteen gross of the Herbal Ointment. It is the only ointment now called for by our patrons, which must be accepted as positive proof of its superior excellence." Ranson C. Scott, Richford, Vt., writes: "I feel it my duty to let you know what your Herbal Ointment has done for me. It healed up in three weeks a fever sore that had been running for five years, and which of late had laid me up completely." Dr. Wm. Steele, Windsor, Ohio, says: "I cured with your ointment a wen of twenty-two years' standing. It was of enormous size—twenty-seven inches round. It commenced to disappear gradually after the first application, and at the end of six weeks not a vestige remained." Dr. S. Farley, Palmyra, Iowa, writes that he cured his wife of sore eyes with the Ointment, when he and the best oculists in State had failed. James McIntosh, Buffalo, N. Y., writes: "Your Ointment is the best Pain Killer in the world."

THE RENOVATING PILL.

PRICE—50 *cents per box. Two cents additional for each box must be sent when ordered by mail, to prepay postage. Each box contains about seventy pills.*

This excellent pill is composed of mandrake, leptandrin, Turkey rhubarb, soapwort, etc., etc. It is a purely vegetable concentration for keeping the bowels in natural order. cleansing the system of all impurities, and positively curing costiveness. These pills unload the liver of bilious matter, and by their tonic action upon the alimentary canal they aid digestion, promote assimilation of nutriment, and produce regular and healthy action of the bowels. Their action is thoroughly effective, but so easy and painless that they can be given with great benefit in even the most diseased condition of the intestines.

Testimonials.— GEO. C. GOODWIN & Co., Wholesale Druggists, Boston, Mass., write : "The Renovating Pill is certainly the best family pill we have ever sold." Mrs. H. E. Smith, Janesville, Wis., writes— "The Renovating Pills are the best I have ever used. They have cured me of chronic constipation of sixteen years' standing." T. J. Sherwood, Marysville, Cal., says : "I have for ten years past used every kind of pills, but yours are the only ones that ever helped the sluggish motion of my bowels." Mrs. Sallie Newell, Diamond Hill, R. I., says : "I have found your pills most excellent, far superior to any I have ever used." Annie A. Guestner, Salem, N. J., writes : "Your pills are superior to any which I have ever been acquainted with." Rev. E. Barber, Cazenovia, N. Y., writes : "Please send to my address, as soon as you can, two boxes of your Renovating Pills ; they are the best cathartic pills I have ever used."

THE WOODLAND BALM.

PRICE—50 *cents per pot. Four cents additional per pot must be sent when ordered by mail, to prepay postage.*

This vegetable production is so compounded as to give moisture, warmth and action, to the hair follicles. It positively reproduces hair, cures all diseases of the scalp, prevents the hair from falling out, and often restores gray hair to its original color. One application will convince the most skeptic of its wonderful hair-producing and hair-restoring power. It produces a wealth of hair on almost any head, and causes a luxuriant growth to the beard and moustache. It is the finest hairdresser in the world, rendering the hair pliant, richly glossy, and straight or curly as desirable.

Testimonials.— J. F. SMITH, New Orleans, La., writes : "I have used your Woodland Balm but three weeks, but already there is a full growth of hair, about one-fourth of an inch long, on the crown of my head, which was previously perfectly bald." Mrs. J. J. Walker, Rockland, Ind., writes: "My hair is now thirty-six inches long, while previous to using your balm it was so short that I could not arrange it at all, but was obliged to wear it short." John C. Penrose, Kensington, Pa., says: "My beard was but a tame affair before using your Woodland Balm. It exhibited itself in scattered spots of delicate growth at various parts of my face, and the moustache was *non est inventus.* The balm was used, and I have now a fierce moustache, and a beard that would do justice to a Spanish cavalier." C. K. McClintock, Watertown, N. Y., writes: "I am pleased to state that your Woodland Balm has restored my hair, which was nearly white, to its original color."

LIVER INVIGORATOR.

PRICES —$1.00 *per bottle ; six bottles*, $5.00.

This grand specific is a distilled compound, composed of mandrake, gentian, wild yam, dandelion, and other plants valuable for their curative qualities in all bilious disorders. It arrests all inflammatory processes, removes engorgement and all noxious bilious matter, promotes secretion of healthy bile, stimulates and tones the liver, and so invigorates the organ as to speedily restore healthy functional action of both secretion and elimination. It is applicable to all hepatic diseases, and unfailingly efficacious in every case. No class of diseases is more prevalent than hepatic affections, and none, perhaps, attended with more serious effects to the general organism. The Liver Invigorator is a certain curative for these complaints.

Testimonials.—ALLEN & Co., Wholesale Druggists, Cincinnati, Ohio, write:—"Nothing could exceed the popularity of your 'Liver Invigorator;'—we hear daily of its performing very remarkable cures." John K. Simmons, Laporte, Ind., writes:—"Two bottles of your 'Liver Invigorator' effectually restored my liver to healthy action, after being torpid for many years." Chas. Janeway, Springfield, Ill., writes:—"After suffering for years from chronic congestion of the liver, I am happy to report to you a thorough cure by the use of your Liver Invigorator."

––––––

When it will become known that the Herbal Kingdom is capable of affording materials from which a list of remedies like the foregoing, containing every requisite of a remedy—elegance, efficacy, and reliability, can be prepared, there will scarcely be any who will not abandon the use of pernicious mineral drugs, and resort only to the life-giving remedial agents afforded everywhere by plants.

These remedies every one can depend upon—they embody so much virtue that good results must follow. Besides the few testimonials we

have given, the author, did space allow, could readily give tens of thou·
sands of but a few years' accumulation.

These remedies can be obtained from nearly every druggist, or they
can be had from the author of this work by express.

DR. O. PHELPS BROWN,
21 *Grand st., Jersey City, N. J.*

DR. O. PHELPS BROWN'S

STANDARD FLUID EXTRACTS.

The fluid extract is the most elegant form for administering medicinal
agents, being concentrated, and containing just enough alcohol to preserve them from degeneration by age. They can, therefore, be administered in all inflammatory conditions, in which tinctures containing a
greater quantity of alcohol are not admissible.

My fluid extracts are superior to any that are manufactured. They
are prepared without the aid of heat, in perfect vacuum, and from plants
gathered at the proper seasons, in soils best adapted for medicinal perfection, and in climates to which they are indigenous, and in which they
attain their richest medicinal development. This is not the case with
other manufacturers—they prepare them from plants of indiscriminate
selection, which accounts for their frequent worthlessness. These fluid-
extracts are guaranteed for high character and reliability, and physicians
can depend upon their action with all confidence.

It is my particular desire in preparing them to offer to households
good and convenient remedies, by which they can treat all cases of sickness occurring. They will find them, by the aid of this work, very advantageous for domestic medication. To meet the wants of families,
the author sells them in standard small quantities, as it is not to be
supposed that they desire or have use for such large quantities that
physicians or druggists ordinarily purchase.

It will be seen that the list is very complete, and so systematically
arranged that no error can occur, as the virtues and doses of each are
appended. Those marked with a star * should not be used without the
advice of a physician, and even then the administering should be very
carefully and watchfully done.

These extracts are sent by express, on receipt of price, carefully

packed in strong boxes. All of them are warranted to possess the hihg-
est excellence of virtue, and to exert the full therapeutic effects desired.

Address, DR. O. PHELPS BROWN,

21 *Grand st., Jersey City, N. J.*

FLUID EXTRACTS.

FLUID EXTRACT OF	MEDICINAL PROPERTIES.	DOSE.	Price per oz.
			$ cts.
Aconite* (leaves).......	Narcotic and sedative....................	2 to 5 drops	20
Aconite* (root)	" " "	2 or 3 "	25
Agrimony.............	Tonic, alterative, and astringent....	30 to 60 "	20
American Valerian.....	Tonic, stimulant, diaphoretic, and antispas-modic..................................	30 to 60 "	25
Arnica Flowers........	Stimulant and tonic.......................	10 to 30 "	15
Avens Root..........	Tonic and astringent......................	10 to 30 "	15
Balm...	Stimulant, diaphoretic, and antispasmodic..	30 to 60 "	15
Balmony	Tonic, cathartic, and anthelmintic........	30 to 60 "	15
Barberry.............	Tonic and laxative........................	30 to 60 "	15
Bayberry	Astringent and stimulant..................	30 to 60 "	15
Belladonna*...........	Anodyne, relaxant, antispasmodic..........	2 to 5 "	30
Beth Root.............	Astringent, tonic, antiseptic..............	30 to 60 "	20
Bitter Root...........	Emetic, diaphoretic, tonic, and laxative....	10 to 20 "	25
Bittersweet...........	Narcotic, diuretic, alterative, diaphoretic, discutient..............................	20 to 40 "	20
Black Alder..........	Tonic, alterative, and astringent..........	30 to 60 "	20
Blackberry Root.......	Astringent...............................	20 to 40 "	15
Blood Root...........	Emetic, diaphoretic, stimulant, tonic......	5 to 30 "	20
Blue Flag.......... ...	Cathartic, alterative, sialagogue, diuretic...	20 to 40 "	20
Boneset..............	Tonic, aperient, diaphoretic, emetic.......	30 to 60 "	15
Boxwood	Tonic, astringent, antiperiodic, stimulant...	20 to 40 "	15
Buchu...............	Diuretic, stimulant, tonic.................	20 to 40 "	30
" Comp...........	" " "	10 to 30 "	30
Buckhorn.............	Mucilaginous, tonic, and styptic..........	30 to 60 "	15
Buckthorn...........	Cathartic................................	30 to 60 "	20
Bugle Weed..........	Sedative, tonic, astringent, narcotic	30 to 60 "	15
Butternut............	Cathartic................................	30 to 60 "	15
Button Snakeroot......	Diuretic, tonic, stimulant, emmenagogue...	30 to 60 "	20
Cannabis Indica*......	Narcotic, diuretic, diaphoretic............	2 to 5 "	75
Canella....	Aromatic, stimulant, tonic................	10 to 20 "	15
Centaury.............	Tonic and antiperiodic....................	10 to 30 "	15
Cinchona (Calisaya)....	Tonic, antiperiodic, febrifuge.............	20 to 40 "	75
Chamomile	Tonic, carminative, antispasmodic..	30 to 60 "	20
Checkerberry	Stimulant, aromatic, astringent...........	30 to 60 "	15
Cherry Bark..........	Tonic, stimulant, expectorant.............	20 to 60 "	20
" Comp......	" " "	20 to 60 "	25
Cleavers.............	Refrigerant and diuretic..................	30 to 60 "	15
Coca	Tonic and vivifier........................	30 to 60 "	3 00
Colocynth*	Drastic cathartic.........................	10 to 30 "	35
Cohosh, black.........	Tonic, antispasmodic, diuretic............	10 to 30 "	25
Cohosh, blue.........	Emmenagogue, parturient, antispasmodic...	10 to 30 "	20
Colchicum Root.......	Sedative, cathartic, diuretic, emetic.......	3 to 10 "	25
" Seeds.......	" " " "	5 to 15 "	30
Coltsfoot.....	Emollient, demulcent, tonic..............	30 to 60 "	15
Columbo.............	Bitter tonic..............................	10 to 30 "	35
Comfrey.............	Demulcent and astringent.................	30 to 60. "	20
Conium*	Narcotic.................................	5 to 10 "	25
Cotton Root*.........	Emmenagogue, parturient.................	30 to 60 "	35
Cramp Bark..........	Antispasmodic...........................	30 to 60 "	15
Cranesbill............	Astringent.................	20 to 40 "	20
Cubebs..............	Diuretic, stimulant, tonic.................	30 to 40 "	35

FLUID EXTRACT OF	MEDICINAL PROPERTIES.	DOSE.	Price per oz.
			$ cts.
Culver's Root	Cathartic, cholagogue, tonic	10 to 30 drops	25
Cundurango	Alterative, anticarcinomous	10 to 30 "	2 00
Dandelion	Cathartic, tonic, alterative, diuretic	30 to 60 "	25
Digitalis*	Sedative, diuretic, diaphoretic	2 to 5 "	20
Dragon Root	Expectorant and diaphoretic	10 to 30 "	15
Dwarf Elder	Sudorific, diuretic, alterative	30 to 60 "	15
Elecampane	Stimulant and tonic	30 to 60 "	15
Ergot*	Parturient	10 to 30 "	50
Fever few	Emmenagogue, tonic, stimulant	20 to 40 "	15
Fireweed	Emetic, cathartic, tonic	30 to 60 "	20
Frostwort	Alterative, anti-scrofulous	20 to 40 "	15
Garden Celandine	Stimulant, alterative, diuretic, diaphoretic, vulnerary	30 to 60 "	20
Gelseminum*	Febrifuge, antispasmodic	5 to 10 "	40
Gentian	Bitter tonic	20 to 40 "	30
Gillenia	Emetic, cathartic, tonic	30 to 60 "	20
Golden Seal	Tonic, calmative	20 to 40 "	30
Golden Rod	Stimulant, carminative	30 to 60 "	20
Gold Thread	Bitter tonic	20 to 40 "	20
Hardhack	Astringent	5 to 15 "	10
Helebore, black*	Antispasmodic, diuretic, emmenagogue	5 to 10 "	20
Henbane*	Narcotic	5 to 15 "	40
Hop	Tonic, hypnotic, febrifuge, antilithic	30 to 60 "	40
Hydrangea	Diuretic, anticalculus	20 to 40 "	20
Hyssop	Stimulant, aromatic, tonic	30 to 60 "	15
Ignatia Bean*	Cerebro-spinal tonic	3 to 5 "	50
Ipecac	Expectorant, emetic	5 to 30 "	1 00
Jalap*	Drastic cathartic	10 to 30 "	50
John's Wort	Astringent, sedative, and diuretic	30 to 60 "	20
Juniper Berries	Stimulant, carminative, diuretic	30 to 60 "	15
Kousso	Anthelmintic, anti-tape-worm	30 to 60 "	50
Ladies' Slipper	Tonic, stimulant, diaphoretic, antispasmodic	20 to 40 "	25
Life Everlasting	Astringent	30 to 60 "	20
Life Root	Diuretic, pectoral, diaphoretic, tonic	10 to 30 "	25
Lily Root	Astringent, demulcent, anodyne, anti-scrofulous	10 to 30 "	20
Liverwort	Mucilaginous, astringent	1 dram	20
Lobelia	Emetic, expectorant, relaxant, antispasmodic, discutient, and anodyne, externally	10 to 30 drops	25
Logwood	Tonic, astringent	20 to 40 "	15
Lovage (Privet)	Astringent	30 to 60 "	20
Lungwort	Demulcent and mucilaginous	30 to 60 "	20
Male Fern	Anthelmintic	20 to 40 "	30
Mandrake	Cathartic, cholagogue, tonic	10 to 60 "	30
Marshmallow	Demulcent and diuretic	20 to 40 "	25
Matico	Stimulant, diuretic, astringent, alterative	10 to 30 "	40
Motherwort	Emmenagogue, nervine, antispasmodic, laxative	30 to 60 "	20
Mugwort	Tonic, narcotic	20 to 40 "	20
Nux Vomica*	Cerebro-spinal tonic	3 to 10 "	35
Opium, deodorized*	Anodyne	3 to 10 "	40
Pareira Brava	Tonic, diuretic, aperient	30 to 60 "	30
Pennyroyal	Stimulant, diaphoretic, emmenagogue, and carminative	30 to 60 "	20
Pinkroot	Anthelmintic	20 to 40 "	40
Pipsissewa	Diuretic, tonic, alterative, astringent	20 to 40 "	20
Pleurisy Root	Expectorant, diaphoretic, tonic	20 to 40 "	30
Poke Root	Emetic, cathartic, alterative, narcotic	10 to 30 "	20
Poplar Bark	Tonic and febrifuge	20 to 40 "	15
Prickly Ash	Stimulant, tonic, alterative, sialagogue	10 to 30 "	20
Ptelea	Tonic, antiperiodic	10 to 30 "	20

FLUID EXTRACT OF	MEDICINAL PROPERTIES.	DOSE.	Price per oz.
			$ cts.
Quassia................	Bitter tonic.............................	20 to 40 drops	15
Queen of the Meadow..	Diuretic, stimulant, tonic................	20 to 40 "	15
Rhatany..............	A powerful astringent...................	20 to 40 "	30
Rhubarb..............	Cathartic.............................	10 to 30 "	50
Rosin Weed...........	Tonic, diaphoretic, alterative...........	20 to 60 "	30
Sage	Tonic, astringent, expectorant, diaphoretic.	30 to 60 "	20
Sarsaparilla (American)	Alterative.............................	30 to 60 "	25
" (Foreign)..	Alterative.............................	30 to 60 "	30
Sassafras.............	Alterative.........................\....	30 to 60 "	20
Savine*..............	Emmenagogue, diuretic, diaphoretic.......	10 to 20 "	20
Savory	Stimulant, carminative, emmenagogue.....	20 to 40 "	25
Scullcap.............	Antispasmodic.........................	20 to 40 "	20
Seneka........	Emetic and cathartic....................	15 to 30 "	40
Senna...............	Cathartic...............	30 to 60 "	20
Skunk Cabbage.......	Emetic, stimulant, antispasmodic, discutient, externally ....•.........	20 to 50 "	20
Snake Root...........	Tonic, diuretic, diaphoretic.............	10 to 30 "	30
Soap Wort...........	Tonic, diaphoretic, alterative...........	10 to 60 "	20
Solomon's Seal.......	Tonic, astringent.....................	20 to 40 "	20
Spearmint............	Carminative...........................	30 to 60 "	20
Spikenard............	Alterative	30 to 60 "	20
Squill...............	Emetic, expectorant....................	2 to 15 "	40
Stillingia...........	An unequalled alterative................	10 to 30 "	30
Stoneroot......	Stimulant	10 to 30 "	25
Stramonium*........	Energetic narcotic......................	3 to 10 "	20
Sumach.............	Tonic, astringent, antiseptic............	30 to 60 "	15
Sweet Gale (Myrica)..	Astringent and stimulant................	30 to 60 "	15
Tag Alder...........	Alterative, emetic, astringent...........	30 to 60 "	15
Tansy..............	Emmenagogue, diaphoretic..............	30 to 60 "	15
Thoroughwort........	Tonic, aperient, diaphoretic, expectorant...	30 to 60 "	15
Thyme	Emmenagogue, diaphoretic..............	30 to 60 "	15
Turkey Corn.........	Alterative	10 to 30 "	25
Unicorn Root.........	Tonic, diuretic, sialagogue...............	30 to 60 "	30
Uva Ursi............	Astringent and tonic....................	20 to 40 "	30
Valerian............	Sedative..............................	20 to 40 "	30
Vervain........	Tonic, antispasmodic..............•....	20 to 40 "	25
Veratrum*........ ...	Sedative. diaphoretic...................	2 "	40
Wahoo	Tonic, alterative, expectorant...........	30 to 60 "	30
Water Pepper........	Stimulant, diuretic, diaphoretic, excellent, external remedy......................	10 to 30 "	15
Wild Indigo..........	Purgative, emetic, stimulant.............	10 to 30 "	15
Wild Yam............	Antispasmodic.........................	10 to 30 "	20
Witch Hazel..........	Tonic, astringent, sedative..............	30 to 60 "	15
Wormwood	Tonic, anthelmintic....................	10 to 30 "	15
Wormseed............	Anthelmintic	10 to 30 "	20
Yarrow.............	Astringent, diuretic, alterative...........	10 to 40 "	15
Yellow Dock........	Alterative, tonic, detergent.............	30 to 60 "	30
Yellow Parilla........	Tonic, laxative, alterative..............	10 to 30 "	30

In the administration of these fluid-extracts the minimum dose should first be given, and if the desired effect is not fully responsive, the doses should be gradually increased to the maximum dose. In some cases even larger doses may be required than those given as ordinarily sufficient for inducing their therapeutic effects.

In consequence of trouble in packing, not less than TWO DOLLARS' worth of these fluid-extracts will be sent at one time, unless ordered in connection with some of my Standard Remedies. The quantity may either consist of one medicine, or of an indiscriminate selection from the whole list. They are packed in strong bottles, fully labelled, and guaranteed pure. They can only be sent by express.

All orders should be addressed to

DR. O. PHELPS BROWN,
21 *Grand st., Jersey City, N. J.*

GLOSSARY.

IT is confidently believed that all the technical terms introduced into this work are fully defined in this Glossary. Many of the medical terms are explained where they occur, and even some of those that are here defined are explained at the place where first employed, but are inserted here also, so as to make this Glossary sufficiently complete for ready reference by the most casual reader.

ACRO-NARCOTIC, Medicines that act on the brain, or spinal marrow, or both, but at the same time irritate the parts to which they are applied.

ADJUVANT, A medicine that aids the operation of the principal ingredient of a mixture or compound.

ADYNAMIC, Pertaining to adynamia, or debility of the vital powers.

AERATION, Charging with air; the transformation of venous blood and chyle into arterial blood by respiration; arterialization.

AFFERENT, Conveying inward, nerves that convey impressions towards the nervous centres.

ALBUMEN, The immediate principle of animals and vegetables; it constitutes the chief part of the white of an egg.

ALKALOID, Having the property of or pertaining to an alkali.

ALVINE, Relating to the lower belly, as alvine dejections, etc.

AMAROUS, Bitter.

ANÆSTHETIC, Relating to privation of feeling; a medicine that prevents feeling.

ANÆMIA, A bloodless condition.

ANTAPHRODISIAC, A substance capable of blunting venereal desires.

ANTIPERIODIC, A medicine which possesses the power of arresting morbid periodical movements, as Peruvian bark.

APERIENT, A medicine that gently opens the bowels.

APHONIA, A voiceless condition; loss of voice.

APHRODISIAC, A substance that excites the venereal passions.

ANTISEPTIC, Opposed to putrefaction.

APHTHOUS, Pertaining to aphthæ or thrush.

AREOLAR, Appertaining to an areola, or the space between the fibres, composing organs, or between vessels which interlace each other.

ASTHENIC, Debilitated; pertaining to asthenia, or want of strength.

ATOCIAC, Pertaining to atocia or sterility; sterile.

ATONIC, Wanting tone; weakness of every organ, and particularly of those that are contractile.

ATROPHY, Defective nutrition; a diminution in the bulk of the whole body, or of a part.

BOUGIE, An instrument used for the purpose of dilating the urethra.

CACHECTIC, Belonging or pertaining to cachexia; depraved nutrition or a bad habit of the body.

CADAVEROUS, Pertaining to or resembling the cadaver, or dead body.

CALISTHENIC, Pertaining to calisthenics, or the art of promoting, by appropriate exercises, strength of body and grace of movements.

CAPILLARY, Hair-like; small.

CARIES, Death or decay of a bone.

CARMINATIVE, A remedy that allays pain or promotes the expulsion of flatus, or wind, from the bowels.

CARDIAC, Pertaining to the heart.

CARTILAGE, A solid part of the body of a medium consistence between bone and ligament.

CASEINE, The chief constituent of milk.

CATAMENIAL, Pertaining to catamenia, or menstrual flow.

CATHARSIS, A natural or artificial purgation, or movement of the bowels.

CEREBRAL, Pertaining to the brain.

CERVICAL, Pertaining or belonging to the cervix or neck.

CHOLAGOGUE, A medicine that causes a flow of bile.

CHOLESTERINE, An inodorous, insipid substance, forming the crystalline part of a biliary calculus, and contained in neurine and various other tumors; also in the seeds of many plants, olive oil, etc.

CHRONIC, Of long duration.

CHYMIFICATION, Formation of chyme, or the pulp formed by the food and various secretions, after it has been for some time in the stomach.

CLONIC, Irregular convulsive motions; convulsion with alternate relaxation.

COLLIQUATIVE, Profuse; exhausting; a term applied to discharges which produce rapid exhaustion.

COMATOSE, Pertaining to coma, or a profound state of sleep, from which it is difficult to arouse the individual.

CORRIGENT, Corrective; a medicine that mollifies or corrects the action of a pharmaceutical preparation.

DEGLUTITION, The action of swallowing.

DELIRIUM, Straying from the rules of reason; wandering of the mind.

DEOBSTRUENT, A medicine having the power of removing obstructions.

21

DEODORIZED, Deprived of odor or smell.

DESQUAMATION, Exfoliation, or separation of the scarf-skin, in the form of scales.

DETERGENTS, Medicines that cleanse parts, as wounds, ulcers, etc.

DIAGNOSTICATE, Forming a diagnosis or character of a disease by its symptoms.

DIAPHORESIS, A greater degree of perspiration than natural, but less than sweating.

DIATHESIS, Disposition of the body; predisposition to a certain disease.

DISCUTIENT, A medicine having the power to discuss, repel, or resolve tumors.

DIURESIS, A greater discharge of urine than natural.

DRASTIC, Active; a name given to those cathartics that operate powerfully.

DUCT, The canal leading from a gland or vesicle.

DYSPNŒA, Difficulty of breathing.

ECTOZOA, Parasitic animals that infest the exterior of the body, as lice, etc.

EFFERENT, Conveying outwards; nerves that convey nervous stimulus from the brain to other parts.

EFFLUVIA, Emanations, miasms, noxious matter.

EJACULATOR, That which effects the emission of sperm.

EMBRYO, The fecundated germ in the early stages of its development in the womb.

EMULSION, A pharmaceutical preparation, in which oil is suspended in water by means of mucilage.

EMUNCTORY, Any organ whose office it is to excrete or expel matters.

ENDEMIC, Diseases which are owing to some peculiarity in a situation or locality. Thus, ague is endemic in marshy countries.

ENTOZOA, Parasitic animals that infest the interior of the body, as worms.

EPHEMERAL, Of short duration.

EPIGASTRIUM, That portion of the surface of the body lying over the stomach.

EPIDEMIC, A disease that attacks a number of persons at the same time, and referable to some condition of the atmosphere.

EPISPADIAS, A condition of the penis in which the urethra opens at the upper part of the organ.

ERUCTATION, A sonorous emission of flatus, by the mouth, from the stomach.

EXACERBATION, Increase in the symptoms of a disorder; paroxysm.

EXANTHEMATOUS, Relating to the exanthems, or eruptive diseases.

EXCRESCENCE, A tumor which forms at the surface of organs, especially the skin, mucous membranes, and ulcerated surfaces.

EXFOLIATION, The separation of dead portions from the various tissues.

EXTRAVASATION, Escape of a fluid from the vessel which contains it, as blood from the veins.

EXUDATION, The oozing of a matter from the pores of a membrane; also the matter that issues in such a manner.

FACIAL, Relating to the face.

FÆCAL, Relating to the fæces or stools.

FALX, A name given to several membranous reflections having the shape of a scythe.

FARINACEOUS, Having the appearance or nature of farina, or the powder obtained by grinding the seeds of certain plants.

FEBRIFUGE, Having the power of abating or driving away fever.

FEBRILE, Relating to or having the character of fever.

FIBRIN, An immediate animal principle entering into the composition of the chyle and the blood; it is the coagulable material of blood.

FLEXOR, Muscles whose office it is to bend certain parts.

FLUCTUATION, The undulation of a fluid which is felt by pressure, properly practised.

FŒTUS, Usually this name is applied to the product of conception after quickening, or more advanced stage of utero-gestation; more vaguely, it is used synonymously with embryo.

FOLLICLE, A small secreting cavity formed by a depression of the skin or mucous membrane.

FUNGOUS, Relating to funga, or certain growths resembling the mushroom, which have no external ulceration, as warts, etc.

GANGLION, A name generally given to a knot-like enlargement in the course of a nerve.

GANGRENE, Privation of life or partial death of an organ; mortification.

GASTRIC, Relating to the stomach.

GELATINE, An immediate animal principle of jelly-like character.

GENITALIA, The genital or sexual organs.

GLAND, Organs which separate from the blood any fluid whatever; a secreting organ; the reddish and spongy, knot-like bodies met with in the course of the lymphatics.

GLUTEN, An immediate principle of vegetables; it is soft, of a grayish white, viscid consistence, and very elastic.

GRANULATION, Granulations are the reddish, conical, flesh-like shoots which form at the surface of wounds and ulcers.

GRAVID, Pregnant.

GRUMOUS, Clotted ; grumous blood is coagulated or clotted blood.

HALLUCINATION, A morbid error in one or more senses ; a delusion.
HELICINE, Resembling in form the tendrils of a vine.
HEMORRHAGE, A flow of blood.
HEPATIC, Relating to the liver.
HYGIENIC, Relating to hygiene, or that part of medicine whose object
    is the preservation of health.
HYPERTROPHY, The state of a part in which nutrition is performed with
    greater activity. Unusual bulk of a part.
HYPNOTIC, A medicine having the power to promote or cause sleep.
HYPOSPADIAS, A malformation, in which the urethra opens at the base
    or beneath the penis.

IDIOPATHIC, A primary disease ; one not dependent on any other.
IDIOSYNCRASY, A peculiarity of constitution, in which one person is
    affected by an agent which in many others would produce no effect.
INDOLENT, This, in a medical sense, means *painless.*
INDURATION, The hardness which occasionally follows in an inflamed
    part.
INFUSORIA, The animalcules originating in decomposition of matter.
INGESTA, Substances introduced into the body by the mouth as food.
INSPISSATED, Rendered thick, as an extract.
INTEGUMENT, Anything which serves to cover or envelop.
INTEROSSEOUS, Between the bones.

JACTATION, Extreme anxiety, excessive restlessness—a symptom ob-
    served in serious diseases.

KYESTEIN, A peculiar pellicle forming on the urine of a pregnant wo-
    man, when allowed to stand for a few days.

LACHRYMAL, Belonging to the tears.
LESION, Derangement, disorder, any morbid change.
LIGAMENT, A fibrous substance, serving to unite bones and to form
    joints.
LIGATURE, A cord or thread with which an artery or tumor is tied.
LUMBAR, Pertaining to the loins.
LYMPH, A name given to the fluids contained in the lymphatic vessels.
LYMPHATICS, The vessels conveying lymph.

MACERATION, An operation which consists in infusing, usually with
    heat, a solid substance, so as to extract its virtues.
MAMMARY, Relating to the mammæ, or female breasts.

MASTICATION, The act of chewing.

MATERIA MEDICA, The knowledge of medicines; the substances used as medicines.

MATURATION, The state of an abscess which has reached maturity.

MEDULLA, The base of the brain; marrow.

MENSES, The monthly flow.

MENSTRUAL, Pertaining to the menses.

MENSTRUUM, A solvent; a substance possessing the property of dissolving others.

METASTASIS, Changing from one place to another.

MICTURITION, Urination, discharge of urine.

MUCILAGINOUS, Having the character of mucilage; resembling gum.

MUCUS, The substance found at the surface of mucous membranes.

NARCOTIC, Substances which have the property of stupefying.

NASAL, Relating to the nose.

NAUSEA, Inclination to vomit; sickness of stomach.

NECROSIS, Death of a bone.

NEPHRITIC, Relating to the kidneys.

NERVINE, A medicine which acts on the nervous system.

NEURINE, Relating to the nerves.

NODE, A hard concretion or incrustation gathering around the joints attacked with rheumatism or gout.

NOSOLOGIST, One versed in nosology, or classification of diseases.

OBSTETRICIAN, One skilled, or practising midwifery.

OPHTHALMIA, Relating or belonging to the eye.

ORGASM, The height of venereal excitement in sexual intercourse.

ORTHOPNŒA, Necessity of being in the erect posture to be able to breathe.

OSSEOUS, Relating to or having the character of bones.

PABULUM, Food, aliment.

PAPILLA, An eminence resembling a nipple.

PARACENTESIS, The act of tapping to evacuate a fluid in a cavity, as in dropsy of the abdomen.

PAROXYSM, A periodical exacerbation or fit of a disease.

PARTURIENT, Bringing forth young.

PARTURITION, Delivery, labor, child-birth.

PATHOLOGICAL, Relating to pathology.

PATHOLOGY, A branch of medicine whose object is the knowledge of disease.

PECTIN, A principle which forms the basis of vegetable jelly.

PECTORAL, Relating to the breast; a medicine that relieves or removes affections of the chest.

PELLICLE, A thin skin or membrane, a film.

PERISTALTIC, A motion consisting of alternate contraction and dilatation.

PERITONEUM, The serous membrane lining the abdominal cavity.

PHAGEDENIC, Appearing as if it was gnawed.

PHARMACEUTIC, Relating to pharmacy.

PHARMACOPŒIA, A work containing the formulæ for the preparation, etc., of medicines.

PHARMACY, The art which teaches the knowledge, choice, preservation, preparation, and combination of medicines.

PHLEGMONOUS, Relating to inflammation which is confined to the areolar texture.

PHLYZACIOUS, Relating to tumors formed by the accumulation of a serous fluid under the scarf-skin.

PHYSIOLOGY, The science which teaches the functions of organs or tissues.

PLETHORA, A superabundance of blood.

PNEUMOGASTRIC, Belonging to the lungs and stomach.

PORTAL CIRCULATION, The circulation of blood in the system of vessels in the kidneys and liver.

PTYALISM, Profuse salivation.

PUERPERAL, Relating to child-birth and its consequences.

PULMONARY, Relating or belonging to the lungs.

PURULENT, Having the character of pus.

PUS, The secretion from inflamed textures.

PUSTULE, An elevation of the skin, having an inflamed base.

PYOGENIC, Having a relation to the formation of pus.

REGIMEN, Diet; the rational and methodical use of food.

RENAL, Relating to the kidneys.

RESPIRATION, The function of breathing, by which is accomplished the mixture of venous blood with lymph and chyle.

REVELLENT, Derivative; a remedy causing an abstraction from the morbid condition of some organ or tissue.

REVULSION, The act of turning a disease from a part in which it seems to have taken its seat.

SAC, A bag-like cavity, formed by any serous membrane.

SACCULATED, Enclosed in a sac; having the character of a sac.

SALIVARY, Relating to the saliva; glands whose function it is to secrete saliva.

SANGUINEOUS, Plethoric; relating to the blood.

SCORBUTIC, Relating to, or having the character of scurvy.

SCYBALA, Hard fæcal matter, discharged in round lumps.

SEBACEOUS, Small hollow organs seated in the substance of the skin, and which secrete a matter having a peculiar odor.

SECRETION, An organic function, chiefly confined to the glands; also the matter secreted.

SEPTUM, Partition; a part separating two cavities.

SERUM, The most watery portion of the animal fluids, exhaled by serous membranes.

SINAPISM, A mustard plaster.

SINUS, Any cavity, the interior of which is more expanded than the entrance.

SORDES, The black substance collecting on the teeth in low fevers.

SPASMODIC, Having the character of a spasm.

SPLENETIC, Relating or belonging to the spleen.

SPUTA, Expectorated matter.

SQUAMOUS, Scaly; having the character of scales.

STERCORACEOUS, Fæcal.

STERTOROUS, Of a snoring character.

STRANGURY, Extreme difficulty in evacuating the urine.

STRUMOUS, Scrofulous.

STYPTIC, Astringent; a medicine which stanches the flow of blood.

SUBLUXATION, A sprain; a partial dislocation.

SUDORIFIC, A medicine which provokes sweating.

SUPPURATION, Formation or secretion of pus.

SYNCOPE; Fainting; loss of sensation and motion.

SYNOVIAL, Relating to the membranes lining the joints.

TAXIS, A pressure exerted by the hand on a hernial tumor for the purpose of reducing it.

TISSUE, The various parts which, by union, form the organs.

THORACIC, Relating or belonging to the chest.

TOPICAL, Local; remedies locally applied.

TOXICAL, Poisonous.

TUBERCLE, A tumor in the substance of an organ, as of the lung.

URINE, The secretion of the kidney.

URINARY, Relating to the urine.

UTERUS, The womb.

UTERINE, Relating or belonging to the womb.

VACCINE, Relating to the matter used for vaccination.

VASCULAR, Relating to vessels; arterial, venous or lymphatic.

VENEREAL, Relating to the pleasures of love.

VERTEBRÆ, Bones of the spinal column.

VESICLE, A small bladder or cyst.

VIROSE, Possessed of noxious properties.

VIRUS, Literally, a poison ; an unknown principle, inappreciable by the senses, which is the agent for the transmission of infectious diseases.

VISCERAL, Relating or belonging to the viscera, or entrails.

VULNERARY, Medicines considered capable of favoring the consolidating of wounds ; only a property of plants.

ZYMOTIC, Relating or appertaining to fermentation.

INDEX.